Practices in Children's Nursing

Practices in Children's Nursing

Guidelines for Hospital and Community

Edited by

Ethel Trigg MBA RN RSCN DMS FETC
Head of Continuing Healthcare, East Sussex Downs and Weald and Hastings and Rother Primary Care Trusts, Sussex, UK

Toby Aslam Mohammed MN(Specialty in Education) PGCE RGN RSCN RNT
Head of Practice Development (Acute Services Division), RPDU, Yorkhill Site, NHS Greater Glasgow and Clyde, Glasgow, UK

THIRD EDITION

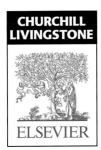

EDINBURGH LONDON NEW YORK OXFORD PHILADELPHIA ST LOUIS SYDNEY TORONTO 2010

CHURCHILL
LIVINGSTONE
ELSEVIER

First edition © Harcourt Publishers Limited 2000
Second edition © 2006, Elsevier Limited.
Third edition © 2010, Elsevier Limited.

ISBN 978-0-7020-3160-1

British Library Cataloguing in Publication Data
A catalogue record for this book is available from the British Library

Library of Congress Cataloging in Publication Data
A catalog record for this book is available from the Library of Congress

Notices
Knowledge and best practice in this field are constantly changing. As new research and experience broaden our understanding, changes in research methods, professional practices, or medical treatment may become necessary. Practitioners and researchers must always rely on their own experience and knowledge in evaluating and using any information, methods, compounds, or experiments described herein. In using such information or methods they should be mindful of their own safety and the safety of others, including parties for whom they have a professional responsibility. With respect to any drug or pharmaceutical products identified, readers are advised to check the most current information provided (i) on procedures featured or (ii) by the manufacturer of each product to be administered, to verify the recommended dose or formula, the method and duration of administration, and contraindications. It is the responsibility of practitioners, relying on their own experience and knowledge of their patients, to make diagnoses, to determine dosages and the best treatment for each individual patient, and to take all appropriate safety precautions. To the fullest extent of the law, neither the Publisher nor the authors, contributors, or editors, assume any liability for any injury and/or damage to persons or property as a matter of products liability, negligence or otherwise, or from any use or operation of any methods, products, instructions, or ideas contained in the material herein.

The Publisher

Printed in China

Contents

Alphabetical list of practices   vii
Acknowledgements   viii
Preface   ix
Clinical coordinators   x
Contributors   xi

SECTION 1: INTRODUCTORY TOPICS

1. Key concepts   3
   Dave Clarke, Jane Davies

2. Communicating with children   22
   Anne Finnegan, with a contribution by Joyce Stebbings

3. Introduction to community   32
   Dawn Moss

4. Control of infection   41
   Helen Cheney

5. Complementary therapies   57
   Julia Fearon

SECTION 2: CARE COMPASSION AND COMMUNICATION

6. Assessment   67
   Kerry Cook, Hermione Montgomery

7. Caring for the child who has died   81
   Bernadette McCormick

8. Cardiopulmonary resuscitation   94
   Fiona Clements

9. Hygiene   104
   Emma Moore, Beryl Pearson

10. Play   120
    Joyce Stebbings

11. Skin care   131
    Jacqueline Denyer, Rosemary Turnbull

SECTION 3: ORGANISATIONAL ASPECTS OF CARE

12. Bowel care   141
    Louise Ford

13. Central lines   152
    Barbara Doyle

14. Chest drainage   163
    Michaela Dixon

15. Incubator care   170
    Susan Alexander

16. Lumbar puncture   175
    Gaynor Pettitt

17. Neurological observations and coma scales   182
Alison Warren

18. Phototherapy   195
Susan Alexander

19. Cast care   200
Lynne Chadburn

20. Positioning, handling and exercises   211
Victoria Demery & Susan Rideout

21. Postoperative care   222
Jennifer McKenna

22. Preoperative care   228
Jennifer McKenna

23. Pressure area care   234
Louise Ford

24. Radiography   240
Joanne Moore

25. Removal of drains and packs   251
Jennifer McKenna

26. Seizures   257
Louise Simmons

27. Stoma care   265
Stella Snell

28. Suctioning   274
Michaela Dixon

29. Temperature control   280
Toby Aslam Mohammed

30. Tracheostomy care   284
Sue Fidment

31. Traction   299
Kathy Gracey

32. Urine testing and urinary catheterisation   308
Jacqueline Winter

33. Venepuncture and cannulation   320
Maureen Lilley

SECTION 4: INFECTION CONTROL AND PREVENTION

34. Aseptic non-touch technique   329
Stephen Rowley, Simon Clare

35. Isolation nursing   337
Rachel Sales

36. Specimen collection   344
Christina Maddox, Beryl Pearson

37. Wound care   354
Angela Deliah Rodgers

SECTION 5: NUTRITIONAL AND FLUID MANAGEMENT

38. Blood glucose estimation   369
Mark Denial

39. Feeding 1: Breast and bottle   374
Carolyn Patchell

40. Feeding 2: Enteral feeding   388
Christopher Bunford

41. Intravenous therapy   401
Nan D McIntosh

SECTION 6: MEDICINES MANAGEMENT

42. The safe management of medicines for children   417
Louise Ford, Christina Maddox, Emma Moore, Rachel Sales

43. Oxygen therapy   446
Rebecca Clarke

44. Pain management   454
Rebecca Reaney, Catherine Trower

Alphabetical list of practices

Assessment 67

Aseptic non-touch technique 329

Bowel care 141

Blood glucose estimation 369

Cast care 200

Caring for the child who has died 81

Cardiopulmonary resuscitation 94

Central lines 152

Chest drainage 163

Feeding 1: Breast and bottle 374

Feeding 2: Enteral feeding 388

Hygiene 104

Intravenous therapy 401

Isolation nursing 337

Incubator care 170

Lumbar puncture 175

Neurological observations and coma scales 182

Oxygen therapy 446

Phototherapy 195

Pain management 454

Play 120

Positioning, handling and exercises 211

Postoperative care 222

Preoperative care 228

Pressure area care 234

Radiography 240

Removal of drains and packs 251

Seizures 257

Skin care 131

Specimen collection 344

Stoma care 265

Suctioning 274

Temperature control 280

The safe management of medicines for children 417

Tracheostomy care 284

Traction 299

Urine testing and urinary catherterisation 308

Venepuncture and cannulation 320

Wound care 354

Acknowledgements

The Editors would like to acknowledge the support and contributions of the following people during the preparation of this Third Edition.

From Birmingham, all of the contributors who updated practices including: Jeanette Hawkins (Lead Cancer Nurse/ANP), Jay Kumar (Clinical Skills Educator) and Janette Vyse (Family Support Sister, PICU) for reviewing a chapter and Dr Vinod Diwaker (Consultant Paediatrician) for his input to the Lumbar puncture chapter.

From Sheffield, all nursing staff who have undertaken the practice reviews, and their peers and colleagues for their support and goodwill.

The support and contribution of Heather Dennis, Clinical Nurse Specialist (Stoma Care) and Nicole Dos Santos (Principle Paediatric Dietician), St George's Healthcare NHS Trust, London, are appreciated, along with those of Theresa Tchehrazi, Clinical Educator, Julie Smith, Project Nurse, Alison McGuire, IV Educator and Elaine Harrision, Transfusion Practitioner, who were all peer reviewers in Glasgow.

Preface

Toby and I were again delighted when the publishers invited us to update the 2nd edition shortly after it had entered the bookshops. We approached the original authors and although the majority were happy to contribute to the update, it also identified how people move around the children's nursing world and also how busy both professional and personal lives have become. You will see throughout this edition that new contributors have updated some the chapters. This does not negate the work from the original authors which still forms the foundation for this book. We would like to acknowledge and thank all of our contributors both current and past as their work has made this book a key text for undergraduate programmes and clinical/community areas alike.

This update has highlighted how busy the contributors have been and time commitments for nearly all of our authors have proved challenging and that includes both of us as editors. However, the update has been achieved and we remain proud of the contribution this book makes to the care of sick children within the hospital and the community setting.

The original five centre approach has also changed and although not all of the original centres remain involved we have still maintained an approach that involved cross centre peer review and additionally now involves three of the UK countries.

Prior to commencement of this update the book was sent out for review, with the reviewers coming from both service and the higher education sector north and south of the border and we have taken on many of the comments of the reviewers in the layout of contents and order of the book. You will see that former appendices have become core chapters to reflect the importance of these areas to current practice. In addition we have included an individual chapter on communication, which is key to all of the practices. We have structured the layout of the chapters to reflect the essential skills clusters identified by the NMC, which are being incorporated into undergraduate education. We hope that this will aid the articulation of theory and practice within the undergraduate curriculum.

There has been significant update in the concepts chapter, which underpins every practice in the book. We feel that it has been beneficial to the book to have this core chapter updated by a third country of the UK.

The community sections have been updated and additions made, as the emphasis for the sick child to remain in the community wherever possible is still key.

We again hope that you will continue to find the book useful; and well used to underpin your learning, guide good practice and safe care.

Ethel Trigg
Sussex, England 2009.
Toby Aslam Mohammed
Glasgow, Scotland 2009.

Clinical Coordinators

BIRMINGHAM
Hermione Montgomery RGN RSCN RM BSc(Hons) LTHE
Lead Nurse, Quality of Care, Birmingham
Children's Hospital NHS Trust, Birmingham, UK
Chapters 6, 16, 17, 20, 26, 39, 40 and 43

BRISTOL
Louise Ford MSc BSc(Hons) RNT(Cert Ed) RCNT RSCN RN
Senior Lecturer, School of Maternal and Child
Health, University of the West of England,
Bristol, UK
Chapters 9, 12, 14, 23, 28, 35, 36 and 42

GLASGOW
Toby Aslam Mohammed MN(Specialty in Education)
PGCE RGN RSCN RNT
Head of Practice Development (Acute Services
Division), NHS Greater Glasgow and Clyde,
Glasgow, UK
Chapters 1, 2, 5, 7, 8, 15, 18, 29, 32, 33, 37 and 41

SHEFFIELD
Vicky Vidler MA RGN RSCN
Nurse Consultant (Paediatric Haematology), Roald
Dahl Centre, Sheffield Children's NHS Trust,
Sheffield, UK
Chapters 13, 19, 21, 22, 25, 30, 31, 38 and 44

SUSSEX
Ethel Trigg MBA RN RSCN DMS FETC
Head of Continuing Healthcare, Sussex
Downs and Weald Primary Care Trust, Sussex, UK
Chapters 3, 4, 10, 11, 24, 27, 34

Contributors

Susan Alexander MN BA RGN RM ENB 405
The Royal Hospital for Sick Children, Women
and Children's Directorate, Acute Services
Division, NHS Greater Glasgow and Clyde,
Yorkhill, Glasgow, UK

Christopher Bunford RGN RSCN
Senior Specialist Nutritional Care Nurse,
Birmingham Children's Hospitals NHS Trust,
Birmingham, UK

Lynne Chadburn EN RSCN BOA OrthTechCert
Paediatric Casting Practitioner, A&E Department,
Sheffield Children's Hospital, Sheffield, UK

Helen Cheney EN(G) RN(G) ENB 148, 998 PGCE(HE).
Senior Community Infection Control Nurse,
Newhaven Rehabilitation Centre, East Sussex, UK

Simon Clare RGN BA(Hons)
Clinical Nurse Specialist, Haematology Nursing
Research & Practice Development, University
College London Hospital NHS Foundation Trust,
London, UK

Dave Clarke MA(Ed) PGDip(FAHE) BSc(Hons) RSCN RGN
ENB 100
Lecturer and Programme Manager, Children and
Young People, School of Nursing and Midwifery,
Cardiff University, Cardiff, UK

Rebecca Clarke RN(Child) BSc(Hons) ENB 415
Junior Sister, Paediatric Intensive Care Unit,
Birmingham Children's Hospitals NHS Trust,
Birmingham, UK

Fiona Clements BSc(Hons) RGN
The Royal Hospital for Sick Children, Women and
Children's Directorate, Acute Services Division,
NHS Greater Glasgow and Clyde, Yorkhill,
Glasgow, UK

Kerry Cook RGN BSc(Hons) RN (Child) ENB 160 MSc(ANP)
PGHE
Senior Lecturer, Children's and Young People's
Nursing Team, Faculty of Health and Life Sciences,
Coventry University, Coventry, UK

Jane Davies LLM BSc(Hons) DipAppSS(Open) PGCE RGN
RSCN
Lecturer and Professional Head, Children and
Young Peoples Nursing, Cardiff School of Nursing
and Midwifery Studies, Cardiff University,
Cardiff, UK

Victoria Demery RNCB BN(Hons)
Moving and Handling Facilitator, Birmingham
Children's Hospitals NHS Trust, Birmingham, UK

Mark Denial EN(G) RGN RSCN
Paediatric Diabetes Nurse Specialist, Sheffield
Children's Hospital, Sheffield, UK

Jacqueline Denyer RGN RSCN RHV
Clinical Nurse Specialist for Epidermolysis Bullosa, Department of Dermatology, Great Ormond Street Hospital for Sick Children, London, UK

Michaela Dixon RGN RSCN BSc(Hons) PGCE PGDip
Senior Lecturer, School of Health & Social Care, University of the West of England, Bristol; Clinical Development Nurse, Paediatric Intensive Care Unit, Bristol Royal Hospital for Children, Bristol, UK

Barbara Doyle MA RGN RSCN
Lead Cancer Nurse, Sheffield Children's Hospital, Sheffield, UK

Julia Fearon RGN RSCN BSc
Independent Therapist, formerly Laser Nurse Specialist, Birmingham Children's Hospitals NHS Trust, Birmingham, UK

Sue Fidment PG Dip NT BSc RSCN RGN
Lecturer/Practitioner for Paediatric Critical Care, Sheffield, Children's Hospitals NHS Trust, Sheffield, UK

Anne Finnegan MSc BSc(Hons) RSCN RGN PGCE
Senior Lecturer in Child Health, School of Health and Social Care, Teesside University, Middlesbrough, UK

Louise Ford MSc Bsc(Hons) RNT(Cert Ed) RCNT RSCN RN
Senior Lecturer in Children's Nursing, The Faculty of Health and Life Sciences, University of the West of England, Bristol, UK

Kathy Gracey
Sheffield Children's Hospital, Sheffield, UK

Sandi Hillery RGN RSCN BSc(Hons) Community Specialist
Practice in Community Health Care, Community Children's Nursing FETC ENB 923
Outreach Team Leader, Shooting Star House, Children's Hospice, Hampton, UK (Creator of *Community perspective boxes*)

Maureen Lilley MSc Bsc(Hons) AdvPractDip RGN RSCN
The Royal Hospital for Sick Children, Women and Children's Directorate, Acute Services Division, NHS Greater Glasgow and Clyde, Yorkhill, Glasgow, UK

Bernadette McCormick BSc RSCN
The Royal Hospital for Sick Children, Women and Children's Directorate, Acute Services Division, NHS Greater Glasgow and Clyde, Yorkhill, Glasgow, UK

Nan McIntosh BSc(Hons) AdvPractDip RSCN RGN
The Royal Hospital for Sick Children, Women and Children's Directorate, Acute Services Division, NHS Greater Glasgow and Clyde, Yorkhill, Glasgow, UK

Jennifer McKenna RGN RSCN
Senior Staff Nurse, Sheffield Children's Hospital, Sheffield, UK

Christina Maddox MA RNT PGCE DipHE RGN
Senior Lecturer in Children's Nursing, School of Maternal and Child Health, University of the West of England, Bristol, UK

Toby Aslam Mohammed MN(Specialty in Education) PGCE RGN RSCN RNT
Senior Nurse (Practice Development), Yorkhill Operating Division of NHS Greater Glasgow, Glasgow, UK (co-editor)

Hermione Montgomery RGN RSCN RM BSc(Hons) LTHE
Lead Nurse for Quality of Care, Birmingham Children's Hospital NHS Trust, Birmingham, UK

Joanne Moore RGN RSCN
Junior Sister Radiology/Day Services, Birmingham Children's Hospitals NHS Trust, Birmingham, UK

Emma Moore PGDip BA(Hons) RGN RSCN
Course Leader in Children's Nursing, School of Nursing and Midwifery, University of Cumbria, Lancaster, UK

Dawn Moss RGN RSCN MSc HV CCN SN
Nurse Consultant in Child Health, NHS Borders, Melrose, and Napier University, Edinburgh, UK

Carolyn Patchell BSc SRD
Head of Dietetic Services, Dietetic Department, Birmingham Children's Hospital NHS Trust, Birmingham, UK

Beryl Pearson RN RSCN RCNT CertEd(FE/HE) Med(FE/HE)
Staff Tutor Nursing, Open University, Bristol, UK

Gaynor Pettitt
Advanced Nurse Practitioner (Paediatrics),
Birmingham Children's Hospital NHS Trust,
Birmingham, UK

Rebecca Reaney RGN/RSCN ENB N53
Clinical Nurse Specialist (Paediatric Pain
Management), Sheffield Children's NHS
Foundation Trust, Sheffield, UK

Angela Deliah Rodgers BSc DipHEN(Child) RGN
The Royal Hospital for Sick Children, Women and
Children's Directorate, Acute Services Division,
NHS Greater Glasgow and Clyde, Yorkhill,
Glasgow, UK

Stephen Rowley RGN RSCN MSc BSc(Hons)
Clinical Lead and Senior Nurse Haematology,
UCLH NHS Hospital Trust, London, UK

Rachel Sales MA(Ed) BSc(Hons) RN
Senior Lecturer, School of Health and Social Care,
University of the West of England, Bristol, UK

Louise Simmons RN(Child) ENB 970
Metabolic Nurse Specialist, Birmingham
Children's Hospitals NHS Trust, Birmingham, UK

Stella Snell RGN RSCN ENB 998, 923, R92
Clinical Nurse Specialist – Paediatric Continence,
St George's Healthcare NHS Trust, London, UK

Joyce Stebbings NNEB HPS
Play Service Manager, Royal Alexandra Children's
Hospital, Brighton, UK

Ethel Trigg MBA RN RSCN DMS FETC
Head of Continuing Healthcare, East Sussex
Downs and Weald and Hastings and Rother
Primary Care Trusts, Sussex, UK (co-editor)

Catherine Trower BSc RGN RSCN
The Royal Hospital for Sick Children, Women
and Children's Directorate, Acute Services
Division, NHS Greater Glasgow and Clyde,
Yorkhill, Glasgow, UK

Rosemary Turnbull RSCN Bsc(Hons) ENB N25, 840, 998
Paediatric Dermatology Specialist Nurse, Chelsea &
Westminster Hospital, London, UK

Alison Warren RGN RSCN ENB 415,998 APLS/EPLS Instructor
Senior Sister, Project Lead-Education,
Birmingham Children's Hospitals NHS Trust,
Birmingham, UK

Jacqueline Winter RGN RSCN BSc
The Royal Hospital for Sick Children, Women and
Children's Directorate, Acute Services Division,
NHS Greater Glasgow and Clyde, Yorkhill,
Glasgow, UK

SECTION 1

Introductory topics

SECTION CONTENTS

1. Key concepts   3

2. Communicating with children   22

3. Introduction to community   32

4. Control of infection   41

5. Complementary therapies   57

Chapter 1

Key concepts

Dave Clarke, Jane Davies

CHAPTER CONTENTS

Introduction   3

Policy context   4

The preparation of children's nurses   5

Legal and professional frameworks   6

Accountability   6

Advocacy   8

Principles of consent to treatment   10

Competence in consent to treatment   11

Parental responsibilities   12

Clinical governance and risk management   12

Safeguarding children   16

Summary   18

INTRODUCTION

The well-being and healthcare of children and young people has a growing and continually shifting agenda in the UK. The experience of health and illness among this group has in part driven the key issues currently at the forefront of policy, strategy and recent inquiry. The increasing problems in relation to areas such as childhood obesity, substance misuse and the continuing high rates of teenage pregnancy require intervention from practitioners with expert knowledge and skills. Equally, the development of new and more effective technologies has meant that children and young people face different choices and outcomes, particularly in the context of long-term chronic illness.

Societal change is also influential in determining the lived experience of this group. Changes in the way that families may be configured and the shifting roles within those families can have an impact on a number of areas of life, including individual development, health and illness. Examples of this may include the growing number of single parent families (Self & Zealey 2007) and the change in working patterns, particularly among women (Lindsay 2003).

This is accompanied by changes in secondary socialisation, which also contribute to the overall experience of children and young people. Education, religion and in particular the role of the media has the potential to transform some of the activities in which they might become engaged. Social networking sites for example have become very popular and commonly form part of children and young people's everyday activity. This type of networking is clearly very different from that experienced as little as 6 years ago.

It is little surprise then, that those who work with children and young people in the healthcare setting require an increasingly wide range of skills and knowledge to achieve the optimum level of service delivery. Added to this, delivery needs to be collaborative, in an attempt to provide seamless care and at no time has this approach been more central since the recommendations following the tragic death of Victoria Climbié (DoH 2003a).

POLICY CONTEXT

The policy context continues to influence and shape the children and young peoples' agenda. The four countries of the UK, while having separate policies in some cases, the general emphasis is similar. The relevant policies are identified within this text and the further reading.

Following the publication of the NHS plan (DoH 2000), a number of task forces were established and among those was a children's task force whose remit is to secure the health and well-being of children throughout childhood until they reach adulthood. This was preceded by the *Waterhouse Report* (Waterhouse 2000) about allegations into child sexual abuse in North Wales. One of the recommendations from this report advocated the appointment of a children's commissioner. Wales was the first of the four countries to make such an appointment and the other three countries, most recently in England, who appointed Professor Sir Al Aynsley Green as its commissioner, have since adopted this concept. It is important for children's nurses to be aware that these commissioners have the power to speak and act independently from government and thus are in a powerful position to act in the interests of those who they serve.

There has been a plethora of policy, which has sometimes emerged as a result of major inquiries into the care and services received by children and young people. During the last decade there are a small number of these inquiries that have had a significant impact upon services. *Learning from Bristol* (Kennedy 2001) provided a backdrop to explore the expertise of those who were directly involved in carrying out complex surgery. One of the main recommendations from the inquiry was that, as a matter of priority and within a 12-month period, there should be

publication of a *National Service Framework for Children and Young People*, and this was duly produced in England in 2003 (DoH 2004a), followed swiftly by Wales in 2004 (WAG 2004).

The Victoria Climbié Inquiry (DoH 2003a) examined the circumstance in which Victoria Climbié died in February 2002 and made recommendations for all of the key agencies involved in safeguarding children and young people. The consequent *Every Child Matters* publication (DoH 2004b) has been used to inform the NHS service reviews being undertaken across the UK.

Every Child Matters (DoH 2004b) is about radical change for the delivery of children's services to improve the outcomes for the child. It is about making children's services more child-centred, and integrating them around the needs of children and young people by listening to children and their families. The emphasis is about early intervention and not crisis-driven action. 'Follow the child' is the key theme. In order to follow this approach, the boundaries and traditions that have emerged in nursing will need to be broken down and care and safety located as close to the child as possible. This work will change the way children's services are delivered, with emphasis that this will be managed by frontline staff who understand the changing face of children's services.

There are five themed outcomes that set the scene for delivering improved services for children:

- Be healthy
- Stay safe
- Enjoy and achieve
- Make a positive contribution
- Achieve economic well-being.

This document is clearly one that can be applied to all those who are working in the field of children and young people in whatever specialism.

A recommendation from *Every Child Matters* suggested that the Chief Nursing Officer (CNO) of England examine the role of nursing and midwifery in the health and well-being of vulnerable children and young people. The CNO's review made a number of recommendations which included increasing the number of school nurses, strengthening the public health role of nurses, the integration and co-location of practitioners, strengthening the role of nurses who work in general practice and improving leadership on child protection (DoH 2004c). These will have an impact on the role of any nurse who works with children and young people.

It is important that practitioners recognise that there are differences between the four countries. Each country has a different population in terms of healthcare need and this is reflected in policy documents developed for this age group. Recent media health commentary in Wales expressed the changing nature of healthcare services and highlighted how services are emerging which are more tailored to specific populations.

Other policy in the context of the nursing workforce, most notably *Agenda for Change* (DoH 2004d) and *Modernising Nursing Careers* (DoH 2006a) have already begun to impact upon children's nurses. The former is the most radical change in the NHS pay system since the inception of the NHS in 1948. Although anecdotal, it does appear that this new pay structure has meant there is variation in salaries awarded to similar roles around the UK. This could potentially lead to workforce retention issues, which would in turn have a direct impact upon the care of children and young people.

Modernising Nursing Careers, launched in 2006, followed an initiative undertaken by the four Chief Nursing Officers in the UK. It explains:

> This report sets the direction for modernising nursing careers. The priorities focus on the careers of registered nurses, but it is recognised that nurses do not work in isolation and nursing teams include more than registered nurses. Nursing careers also need to take account of changes in the careers of other professional groups. Importantly, this report recognises that careers take different forms: while some will choose to climb an upward ladder of increasing responsibility and higher rewards, many other nurses choose a more lateral career journey, moving within and between care groups and settings. Our actions are for all nurses no matter what the nature of their career.
>
> (DoH 2006a, p. 3)

Nurses continue to respond to these changes by enhancing and broadening their roles and looking at how roles and care can be integrated, thus providing potential improvement in the overall quality of care which children and their families receive. This can involve moving away from the traditional nursing image and undertaking tasks which previously were performed only by doctors and other professionals.

Children's nurses must continue to develop and be recognised as professional practitioners, with an ever-extending repertoire of skills. The new practitioner is one who is educated to practise from a sound, research-based knowledge. Current practitioners in children's nursing sometimes feel that they do not have the opportunity to provide much 'hands-on care'. This feeling has to be considered in the context of changes in care. One such change is the philosophy of family-centred care and partnership being central to the service provided in children's nursing (Kenny 2003). Family-centred care is a concept that has been familiar to children's nurses for a number of years. More recently, the National Service Framework's standard for hospital services states that child-centred services are those that 'treat children, young people and parents as partners in care' (DoH 2004a, p 9). Therefore, while parents and other family members are doing what were previously considered 'nursing duties', nurses have to develop a very special set of skills that enable them to care for vulnerable children and families. These skills include the responsibility for teaching families, providing support and helping families to make decisions in the best interests of their infant or child, whether sick or healthy, and may present nurses with situations in which they have to make some difficult decisions. Nurses must feel confident about the delivery of their practical skills and that they can think in a clear and rational manner about the emotional and social care they provide. Kitson (2004) emphasises the need for nurses of the future to be able to deliver integrated care across a range of settings, undertaking a range of activities on their own initiative, such as independent prescribing, referral, admission and discharge within a variety of care settings.

THE PREPARATION OF CHILDREN'S NURSES

Throughout the development of the nursing profession, children's nurses have been educated in a number of ways and in a number of environments. During the 1980s, generic preparation, followed by specialist post-registration qualification was the favoured route. This of course changed with the emergence of 'Project 2000' and the move to higher education. This type of preparation enabled students to decide on their choice of specialism at the outset of their programme. This has continued to be the trend in education preparation with students exiting at diploma or degree level, although in Wales all graduate entry was implemented in

2004. There has also, in recent years, been a return to skills-centred programmes, with an increasing emphasis on the importance of core skills. The Nursing and Midwifery Council have also published a set of essential skills clusters, which are to be mapped against existing curricular. They have agreed that simulation can be used to represent placement hours, which recognises the usefulness of simulated learning as an added tool, which can assist in skills development (NMC 2007).

Recently however, the Nursing and Midwifery Council (NMC) have consulted throughout the UK with registered nurses with a view to deciding whether the current preparation is the most effective in meeting the needs of the public. It would appear following a press release by the NMC that the current format of pre-registration in relation to branch configuration will remain.

LEGAL AND PROFESSIONAL FRAMEWORKS

The role of children's nurses continues to change and develop. Care delivery encompasses a broad spectrum of activity, which ranges from the intensive care setting, to the provision of home support to children with long-term and complex healthcare needs. A family-centred approach is still acknowledged as the most effective way of meeting the needs of children and young people, and the increasing involvement of this group in their own management as well as the organisation of services is now an emerging phenomenon.

In all areas of practice, the qualified nurse is accountable for personal decisions and actions. This fact is emphasised in *The Code* (NMC 2008). To be able to deliver care within acute and community settings is of equal importance for children's nurses, as their roles are increasingly becoming community focused. In both of these situations the responsibility to practise intelligently is with the individual nurse.

ACCOUNTABILITY

Accountability may be defined as 'the obligation of being answerable for one's own judgements and actions' (Martin 2004, p 3). This definition provides evidence of an abstract concept which nurses should explore further. Accountability is a term frequently used by and about nurses and so each nurse should be able to define this in the context of personal practice. Student nurses often ask questions such as: 'If we give a wrong drug, who is accountable?' or 'Supposing a child injures himself while he is playing with me in the playroom, am I accountable?' Students may challenge registered nurses by posing such questions; however, it is important for them to explore the issues while they are still students. Although it is impossible to explore every conceivable situation, students should be provided with guiding principles which will help in their decision-making. The *Nursing and Midwifery Council's Guide for Students* (NMC 2005) stresses that, although not professionally accountable, students must act at all times in the interests of the patients with whom they come into contact during their practice experience. Therefore, when playing with a child in the playroom, the student nurse should make every effort to ensure that the child is supervised within a safe environment appropriate to the child's age and stage of development.

Registered nurses also have unanswered questions about accountability and their extending scope of professional practice. Registered practitioners are, on the whole, clearly aware of the implications of the ever-expanding boundaries of practice and thus realise that there is no room for complacency. The Department of Health, in the response to the Report of the Public Inquiry into children's heart surgery at the Bristol Royal Infirmary 1984–1995, called for the need to improve lines of accountability at local and national levels (DoH 2002). The later inquiry into the death of Victoria Climbié re-emphasised the need for accountability across all health and social care agencies (DoH 2003a). Therefore, it would seem that accountability has now been recognised as central to practice in the health and social care professions.

The newly revised Code from the Nursing and Midwifery Council (2008) refers to accountability on a number of occasions. *The Code* states quite clearly what a registered nurse is personally accountable for and provides guidelines for the profession, although as with all guidelines, these may be open to interpretation by individuals. Nurses should avoid individual interpretations of their professional accountability, since in so doing they may jeopardise their careers, together with the reputations of their employing institutions and the profession. Added to this is a comprehensive systematic review. Pearson et al (2006) identified the importance of accountability within teamwork in nursing. Nursing has changed and will continue to change for it to be a dynamic profession. The last decade has witnessed a greater diversity of career pathways for children's nurses (Cox et al 2003) and these new pathways have meant that accountability has been firmly placed as having a central role in practice.

Some nurses and health visitors have undertaken further academic programmes in order to support the development of their roles. One such programme, which has gained professional and media interest, is nurse prescribing. Nurses who have undertaken this educational programme are now prescribing medications from the Nurses Prescribing Formulary. In some specialist roles (e.g. the advanced neonatal nurse practitioner), nurses have developed knowledge and skills to enable them to assess, plan and deliver care that previously was considered the role of a doctor. These nurses are prepared to undertake such procedures as resuscitation and intubations in critical situations where the wrong decision or action may jeopardise the life of the infant/child. The majority of nurses undertaking these specialist skills are now educated to degree level; Masters level qualifications are increasing and there are also practitioners working at doctorate level. Nurses practising at these advanced levels are making judgements and taking actions which may involve life and death situations. Recent research (Ward Platt & Brown 2004) identifies that good-quality neonatal care can be provided by neonatal nurse practitioners without the support of junior paediatricians. The emerging role of the 'nurse consultant' enables more nurses to develop in-depth expertise in a particular area and to gain recognition of their specialist knowledge. These roles are in keeping with the recommendations made by the Department of Health in *Making a Difference* (DoH 1999), where it is stated that, by developing nurses' roles, services for patients will be improved and nurses' careers enhanced.

Increasingly, there is a need to be able to recognise and deal with the mental health problems of children and young people. This is a highly specialist area where there has been an historic lack of resources. A lack of in-patient beds in this area often means that children with mental health problems are being admitted to general children's wards, where staff do not always have the required skills in the area of adolescent mental health. These children and young people can also present in a number of other areas, including emergency departments and GP's surgeries. In these environments, they may be cared for by nurses who do not always have the specialist knowledge and skills to deal with their particular problems. Often the knowledge of the children's nurse needs to be developed to effectively help this group of children and young people (Davies & Huws-Thomas 2007). The National Service Framework (NSF) (DoH 2004a) stressed that child and adolescent mental health is an integral part of all children's services. It goes on to state that where a hospital is providing a service for children, then the staff should have an understanding of how to assess and address the emotional well-being of children. The CNO's review of nursing, midwifery and health visiting states that children in acute settings would greatly benefit from nurses who have more skills in mental health and improved access to child and adolescent mental health services (CAMHS). Staff should also be able to identify any significant mental health problems. The need for a strong liaison with CAMHS, including psychiatry, psychology and family therapy, is also stressed. Section 4.27 of the NSF (DoH 2004a) calls for all hospitals treating children and young people to have policies and liaison arrangements in place to deal with child and adolescent mental health problems, ranging from overdoses and deliberate self-harm to child safeguarding and long-term life-threatening diseases. In addition, nurses working with school-age children should have appropriate competencies for working with this age group. There are, however, still real gaps in services which have been recently highlighted (Woodgate & Garralda 2006).

The increasing move towards caring for sick children in their own homes (Hughes & Callery 2004) puts more pressure on the nurse in the community. These nurses are often isolated from colleagues for long periods during their working day, making it difficult to discuss issues when uncertainty arises. They should not feel obligated to undertake practices for which they do not have appropriate skills. However, they are responsible for their own knowledge base and effective decision-making, since their level of accountability is no more or less than that of any other nurse.

Care for a sick child at home is mainly provided by the parents, but, when visiting the family, the community nurse will be expected to provide support, guidance and some care. Parents need to see evidence of a competent and confident practitioner. Such situations provide the ultimate opportunity for nurses to exercise their professional judgement. Dowding and Thompson (2003) argue that judgement and decision-making can have a significant impact upon the outcomes for patients. Where individual nurses are working within a team of professionals, then professional development and professional dialogue are more likely to happen than when a nurse is working independently, for example in the long-term continuing care environment for a child dependent on technology at home. Children with long-term conditions can be cared for by care assistants or nursery nurses/healthcare support workers who may only have had the technical training to provide the specific care needed by that child (Beale 2002) and are supervised and supported by one or two trained nurses. In these circumstances, where does the line of accountability lie? Although these carers are part of a larger team, they will be alone with the child at home. This form of care is a growing source of support to families in need of respite and, while Beale is emphatic that the most fragile children are still cared for by qualified children's nurses, there is no doubt that the use of support workers is increasing in all care settings. The qualified nurse is accountable at all times and, by delegating work to a person who is not registered with the NMC, is accountable to ensure that the person is suitably trained to undertake care at the appropriate level.

Isolation in practice should be avoided and to that end, student nurses are not generally permitted to carry their own case loads in the community. Although in the past vacant posts in the community were seldom taken as first posts for newly qualified nurses, skill mix into community teams is now more acceptable and more newly qualified staff are interested in community career pathways. Wherever newly qualified nurses seek work, they do require support and guidance from more experienced staff in order to make the transition from student to registered practitioner (NMC 2002). To aid this process, they recommend a period of supported practice of no less than 4 months. This process is termed 'preceptorship' and involves the newly qualified practitioner working alongside an experienced practitioner who provides help, support and advice. Clinical supervision is another means of support for nurses

at all levels and can be of value to lone practitioners. Clinical supervision can be undertaken on a one-to-one basis with another colleague or as part of a group meeting of the team discussing issues related to patient care that have given concern and can be used as a vehicle to explore accountability and practice issues.

Nurses working in the current environment of constant change need to develop coping skills to manage the changing environment. In circumstances where nurses are exposed to new areas of practice, whether students or registered practitioners, they must indicate any knowledge deficit and request appropriate orientation, education and support. It is the responsibility of all nurses to question when unsure and for nurses to constantly strive to add to their personal knowledge and enhancement of their professional skills. Nurses must recognise that they can learn from each other. In addition, nurses should be proactive in seeking out appropriate study days and courses to attend, demonstrating their commitment to education and sound practice.

ADVOCACY

In a professional context, the concept of advocacy remains central to children's nursing practice. Martin (2004) defines an advocate as a practitioner, usually a nurse, who will promote and safeguard the well-being and interests of their patients by ensuring they are aware of their rights and have access to information to enable them to make informed decisions.

Changes at national level required nurses to demonstrate the ability to think about patients' rights and advocacy. *The NHS Plan* (DoH 2000) required trusts to appoint advocacy services (known as PALS) so that patient concerns may be addressed at the time of concern and in a timely manner. Patients have supported this early intervention as they feel they are having their issues addressed as soon as possible. Research has identified that effective management of complaints comes from dealing with concerns at an early stage. Using complaints as a learning framework, rather than in a negative frame, can contribute to improved patient care by acknowledging possible shortfalls and, if necessary, by instituting changes to policy and practice. Also, involving patients in the complaint process wherever possible has proven to be effective.

The recent implementation of the Mental Capacity Act (HMSO 2005) has sought to strengthen the role of the advocate and requires that where vulnerable patients are involved in decision-making and have no one to advocate for them, that they are provided with an independent mental capacity advocate (IMCA) who will act in their best interests in supporting individuals to make decisions. The Act applies to those over 16 years of age.

Frequently, circumstances in the day-to-day care given to children provide nurses with ethical dilemmas and difficult decisions. *The NHS Plan* (DoH 2000) made a clear statement about the need for partnership between patients and professionals, a concept embraced some years ago in the majority of environments where children are nursed. Where nurses are working in partnership with parents and the child, trust is an essential element. Nurses are allowed into a privileged position and it is therefore important that they are aware of their own values and principles in any given situation. Charles-Edwards (2001), in reviewing advocacy and the role of the nurse, states that children are not likely to make formal requests for representation. It is therefore important that nurses have the skills to be able to offer advocacy.

Anecdotal evidence would suggest that nurses do not view it in the terms described above; rather, they interpret it within their daily activities of caring for children, speaking out and acting on behalf of the child. Examples of good practice from nurses' reflections on their role as advocate are provided below:

> *A student nurse recalled how she had prevented a doctor from inserting an intravenous cannula into Jack's arm because he had not had a topical anaesthetic cream applied for the prescribed time.*

> *In a similar situation, Stephanie was hysterical at the thought of yet another blood test. Initially, her parents and the nurse could do nothing to calm her. The doctor was anxious to get the blood samples and requested that she should be held tightly to gain cooperation. The nurse, sensing the tensions, asked the doctor to wait while she got the 'bubble tubes'. These brightly coloured objects provided a perfect distraction and the test went ahead without further problems.*

Nurses frequently feel uncomfortable about restraining children for procedures when alternative methods may be as effective (RCN 2003). This has been re-emphasised more recently as the body of legislation and guidance about restraint has grown and the overriding message is that restraint should only take place if the child is likely to cause self-harm. The scenarios above provide evidence of nurses acting in the child's best interests based on knowledge and best practice decision-making.

These scenarios also highlight the probable imbalance of power between healthcare professionals and patients, particularly between doctors and children. They indicate the vulnerability of sick children and their need for support when confronted by paternalistic medical professionals (Charles-Edwards 2003). While it would be unjust to label all doctors as paternalistic, there has been a tradition within medicine that the doctor knows best and therefore patients and nurses will do as they are told. In fairness to medical colleagues, nurses can also sometimes be too eager to exert power over children and parents in their care. Making judgemental statements about parenting skills, displaying negative attitudes and failing to provide opportunities for parents to participate in their child's care are just some examples of how nurses might demonstrate that they think they know best.

Charles-Edwards (2003) suggest that children will say 'yes' because it is seen as what they should do. Although this refers to the involvement of children in a research study, it could be translated into a variety of other situations including treatments. Such behaviour may enable the busy nurse, working within a restricted timescale, to complete the dressing, administer the intravenous drugs or apply the skin care. Children may comply with this type of behaviour, but it does not reflect the spirit of advocacy and raises questions about whose best interests are being served. There are times when nurses may think that they are acting in a child's best interests. For example, in another case, a staff nurse returned from the operating theatre to the children's ward with a child before her operation had taken place, because the anaesthetist was not ready to receive her into the anaesthetic room. The staff nurse had decided that it was in the child's best interests to wait in the less stressful ward environment rather than in the busy corridor by the operating theatre; there is no evidence to suggest that the nurse had consulted with the child. Furthermore, the child may have been told that, by the time she returned to the ward, her operation would be over. Also the nurse may have caused the child's parents to be unnecessarily alarmed by the action of returning their child to the ward. In this scenario, the nurse may have created more tension. It would seem that, if the nurse had not consulted with the child or explained what was happening, the nurse had confused the role of advocate with that of exerting power.

In almost every case, when a child is sick, parents and immediate family are faced with uncertainty and ambiguity about the treatment and outcomes of the illness. Shields et al (2006) argue that when children are ill, the roles of parents and staff are important and that these need to be flexible and can change. It would seem that there is a strong argument for not asking parents to relinquish their parenting role, but rather enabling them to adapt. Strategies for this adaptation need to be employed by nursing staff. Such strategies provide ideal opportunities for nurses to act in the child's best interests. This may be done through negotiating what care parents wish to participate in and that which they prefer to hand over to nurses. The idea of nurses being told by parents what they may do for their child could be difficult for some nurses to accept, particularly if they have to embrace the concepts of family-centred care and partnership. If nurses view advocacy as a dimension of the nursing role, then it would seem essential that partnership would need to be incorporated into the nursing strategy.

Changes in ideology concerning public/patient involvement over the last several years have meant that nurses need to demonstrate the ability to think about patients' rights and advocacy. Within the concept of family-centred care, the child is seen as part of the family; therefore, when advocating for the child, there is an argument that the advocacy role also includes the family, particularly where the child is younger or lacks competence. This raises questions of how nurses view their advocacy role, particularly when confronted with situations where there may be conflicts of interest.

Another dimension of the nurse's advocacy role may be seen in working with parents to gain their child's cooperation in a treatment regime, for example teaching the child newly diagnosed as having diabetes about diet and administration of insulin. Similarly, an older child with cystic fibrosis may find the frequent drugs and physiotherapy tedious. Negotiation with the child and parents can enable a more positive approach, with everyone acting in the child's best interests.

When nurses act as advocates for children, they should ensure that recent national policy documents, for example the NSF (DoH 2004a) and *Every Child Matters* (DoH 2004b), are implemented in the care settings in which they work and that care and outcomes are audited, measured and evaluated against these policy frameworks.

PRINCIPLES OF CONSENT TO TREATMENT

Consent for the medical treatment of children and young people has always been a central debate for children's nurses and indeed other healthcare professionals. Legislation across all four countries of the UK, as well as international treaties, have identified the rights of children to be involved in the decision-making process. The Children Act England and Wales (1989), United Nations (1989), Children (Scotland) Act (1995) can be applied to the right to be involved in decisions about healthcare. It is however important to note that legal frameworks within the four countries have some differences and it is therefore paramount the children's nurses familiarise themselves with those frameworks which would be pertinent to their own geographical area.

The consent of children under the age of 16 years has been the subject of much debate since the late 1980s. The case involving Victoria Gillick (Gillick *v* West Norfolk and Wisbech Area Health Authority [1986] A.C. 112) heralded changes in English law that were to be reflected across the UK. The case focused on the teenage child's right to consent to medical treatment (in this case contraceptive treatment) without the parents' knowledge. The House of Lords in the case ruled that a parent's degree of control over such areas varied with the child's understanding and intelligence and that where a child was competent they should be able to consent to treatment without their parents consent or knowledge. This precedent has 'stood the test of time' as it was in part recently challenged in a case brought to the High Court by Sue Axon (R. on the application of Axon *v* Secretary of State for Health (2006) EWHC 3721), where Ms Axon argued that when seeking medical treatment young people should not have a right to confidentiality. She lost however, and this was seen by a number of commentators, including The Royal College of Nursing, as a justified victory for young people. This and other cases argued not just the concept of agreement to a particular treatment, but that the agreement should stem from a process of 'being informed', through receiving sufficient information to make an appropriate choice.

Consent is defined as:

The voluntary and continuing permission of a patient
to receive a particular medical treatment based on
an adequate knowledge of the purpose, nature and
likely effects and risks of that treatment,
including the likelihood of it success and
any alternatives to it. Permission given under
any undue pressure is not a true "consent".

(Harper 1999)

It must be made clear however, that there are a number of definitions which attempt to encompass the purpose of consent. The Department of Health (2001a) document *Good Practice Implementation Guide* which outlines consent to examination and treatment for example, has a different definition which puts the emphasis on agreement rather than permission. Commonly in practice today the concept of informed consent is the preferable route adopted by practitioners and there is a range of guidance which explains what this means. More recently, the GMC published guidance on talking to young people up to the age of 18. This comprehensive guide includes important issues such as confidentiality, capacity to consent and listening to the views of young people (GMC 2007).

Consent has a dual purpose: one is clinical and the other legal. The clinical purpose of consent is concerned with enlisting the patient's confidence and in establishing a therapeutic relationship with the patient. This can potentially lead to a more efficient recovery.

In order for consent to be legally valid it must satisfy three criteria (Beauchamp & Childress 2001): (1) The person providing the consent must be competent and have the capacity to understand the proposed treatment and its implications. (2) The person must receive sufficient information to make an informed decision. (3) Consent must be voluntary and there must be no coercion or deceit when gaining consent.

COMPETENCE IN CONSENT TO TREATMENT

Confirming whether or not a child is competent is pivotal to obtaining or involving them in the consent process and can potentially be a controversial aspect of obtaining consent. There are a number of issues, which are relevant when determining competence, these include: the child's level of cognition, the ability to reason and the need to respect autonomy in relation to the refusal of medical treatment the issues are complex. Under Scottish law the young person over the age of 16 years has the same right to consent or refuse as adults do (Marshall 1998). The situation is slightly different within England and Wales. The DoH (2001b) identifies that between the ages of 16 and 18 years, parents may sometimes become involved. When a young person consents positively to treatment there is no problem. However, if the young person refuses, then parents may intervene to allow the treatment to take place. In rare cases practitioners faced with the refusal of treatment may seek advice from the courts. The DoH (2001b) suggests that situations seldom reach this stage, although in extreme cases a court may be asked to decide. The case of a 15½-year-old girl who refused a heart transplant demonstrates the complexity of the issues in relation to refusal of medical treatment (Re M (medical treatment: consent) [1999] 2 FLR 1097).

Acquiring skills in reasoning therefore is an important step towards participation in the decision-making process. There can be an assumption that decision-making in young people is not as good as that of their adult counterparts, due to their lack of experience in making choices, but this is not necessarily the case. The Mental Capacity Act (HMSO 2005), Section 2(3a) states that 'a lack of capacity cannot be established merely by reference to a person's age or appearance'. However, the Act has limited application to children under 16 years of age. It is still primarily The Children Act (1989) which serves the purpose of protecting those under 16 by governing decisions about the care and welfare of the child. In contrast, decision-making with reference to those over 16 is covered. Section 2 of the Act covers personal welfare matters, which include medical treatment and this is particularly significant for healthcare professionals, particularly in the field of mental health.

Some children can have developed a level of competence which can be the result of skilled care that has encouraged them to participate in decision-making about what happens to them. Moules and Ramsay (2008) clearly identify that children have views and that these views can provide a rich source of information on how they feel in a given situation and want to participate in decision-making. Nonetheless, in the early years of a child's life, the child's parents normally make decisions about health and welfare.

PARENTAL RESPONSIBILITIES

Parents, as adults, are often considered to be the most appropriate people from whom to gain consent when considering children. The individual Children Acts clearly identify the responsibilities of parents regarding the issue of consent. Parental responsibility is regarded as something of utmost importance and should not to be taken lightly. Interestingly, however, this is an area that may not be fully understood by professionals working within healthcare (Russell-Johnson 2004).

The British Medical Association (BMA) clearly outlines the basic principles of parental responsibility:

> Parental responsibility refers to the rights, duties, powers and responsibilities that most parents have in respect of their children.
>
> Parental responsibility includes the right of parents to consent to treatment on behalf of their children, provided the treatment is in the interests of the child.
>
> Those with parental responsibility have a statutory right to apply for access to their children's health records, although if the child is capable of giving consent, he or she must consent to the access.
>
> Competent children can decide many aspects of their care for themselves.
>
> Where doctors believe that parental decisions are not in the best interests of the child, it may be necessary to seek a view from the courts, whilst meanwhile only providing emergency treatment that is essential to preserve life or prevent serious deterioration.
>
> (BMA 2006)

The BMA further point out the recent changes in the law in relation to those cases where parents are unmarried:

> The law in relation to parental responsibility has recently been revised. In relation to children born after 1 December 2003 (England and Wales), 15 April 2002 (Northern Ireland) or 4 May 2006 (Scotland), both of a child's parents have parental responsibility if they are registered on the child's birth certificate. This applies irrespective of whether the parents are married or not. A child's biological parents are the child's legal parents (although legal parenthood does not necessarily confer parental responsibility), unless the child has been adopted or was born as the result of some methods of assisted reproduction. Where the child has been formally adopted, the adoptive parents are the child's legal parents and automatically acquire parental responsibility. Where the child has been born as a result of assisted reproduction, there are rules under the Human Fertilisation and Embryology Act 1990 that determine the child's legal parentage.

In light of the above, it is therefore essential for the children's nurse to be fully aware of the adults who are legally responsible for giving consent for a child's treatment.

CLINICAL GOVERNANCE AND RISK MANAGEMENT

Clinical governance has been a feature of the UK health service for more than 10 years, and is now embedded as the framework for ensuring safe and high quality care. The NHS reforms launched clinical governance in the 1990s, as part of the modernisation agenda (DoH 1997; Department of Health Social Services and Public Safety 2001c; Scottish Executive 1997; Welsh Office 1998). Each of the four UK countries adopted the principles of clinical governance.

Healthcare organisations now have a duty to the communities they serve for maintaining the quality and safety of care. Whatever structures, systems and processes an organisation puts in place, it must be able to show evidence that standards are upheld. Within each of the four countries strategies for addressing the health needs and standards of the local populations have been developed and these are the focus of clinical governance arrangements and monitoring. Within England, Standards for Better Health (DoH 2006b); Wales, Healthcare Standards for Wales – Making the Connections Designed for Life (WAG 2005); Scotland, Clinical Governance and Risk Management: Achieving Safe, Effective, Patient-Focused Care and Services (NHS QIS 2005) and Northern Ireland, The Quality Standards for Health and Social Care (DHSSPS 2005). Specifically in relation to children and young people each country has developed a National Service Framework – setting standards for the care of children, young people and their families.

The Royal College of Nursing identify five themes, which feature in the clinical governance arrangements in the UK, these are: Patient Focus (quality care, respect, honest, dignity); Staff Focus (education, training, appraisal); Quality Improvement (standards and monitoring, risk management); Leadership (planning and change); Information Focus (the patients' experience, processes and outcomes) (RCN 2002). The NSFs (England and Wales) for children and young people recognise the importance of high quality clinical care, facilitated through clinical governance arrangements. For example in the English NSF, the standard relating to quality and safety of care provided, states that 'children and young people should receive high quality, evidence-based hospital care developed through clinical governance and delivered by staff who have the right set of skills' (DoH 2004a, p 21).

While clinical governance is an inherent part of service planning and delivery where children and young people are concerned, there are some aspects that will require trusts to make separate responses. The NSF (DoH 2004a) highlights the need for clinical governance systems to recognise that children and young people are potentially vulnerable and need to be provided for as a discrete group. In particular it states that:

- The care of children is given a specific focus within clinical governance arrangements
- A board level children's lead is appointed within the trust
- Clinical governance is approached on a multidisciplinary and a multiagency basis
- An action plan for additional clinical governance arrangements should be part of the process
- An annual report on children's services in the hospital should be presented to the board
- Health and safety policies should make explicit reference to children and young people
- A risk register of actual and potential risks in the care of children and young people should be developed.

While the above list is not intended to be exhaustive, it does highlight some of the key issues. The arrangements for monitoring standards in the NHS differ in each country since devolution; within England, the Healthcare Commission are responsible; within Scotland, the NHS Quality Improvement Scotland; in Wales, the Healthcare Inspectorate Wales; and in Northern Ireland, the Regulation and Improvement Authority.

There would appear to be three categories of risk, which might be identified as follows: (1) The risks for the child and parents. (2) The risks for the nurse. (3) The risks arising from research, which include both the patient and nurse.

Risk management is an integral aspect of delivering high quality care to children and families. Lewis and Noyes (2008, p 25) state that risk is the possibility of incurring misfortune or loss and that it can arise from the:

- Clinical care provided
- Clinical protocols and procedure in place
- Equipment used
- People employed by or visiting the organisation
- Communication/record systems in place
- Management systems of the organisation
- Environment.

As registered nurses, *The Code*: Standards of conduct, performance and ethics for nurses and midwives (NMC 2008) identifies the management of risk as a key role of the nurse, stating: that we must act without delay if we believe someone is at risk; that we must inform someone in authority if we are not able to comply with *The Code* and that nurses must report concerns in writing if problems in the environment of care are putting people at risk.

However, the need for the reporting and monitoring of significant events in the delivery of care to children is also highlighted and where these occur, they should be used as learning opportunities for staff at all levels. Trusts must ensure that the policies are in place to enable staff to deal with critical incidents. Guy et al (2003) identify that drug errors in the care of children are higher than in the general population. Therefore, when a drug error has occurred, staff need to know how it should be investigated and what support to give to children and their families. Staff should be able to access policies that describe individual staff roles and lines of accountability for errors. Usually errors have to be recorded on an incident form and these individual forms are part of the organisational process of monitoring risk from drug errors. At a local level, the ward manager should use the incident in a non-threatening way to create a learning experience for staff (DoH 2003a). Risk assessment and management are not only an issue for the acute hospital environment, but for all environments where clinical care is delivered to children and young people. Lewis and Noyes (2008) identify a number of environments where clinical risk management strategies apply, including the home of a child with chronic illness or disability and the school environment, especially in relation to children with complex needs. It is vital that with ever-shifting care patterns moving towards the community, that we still ensure that the safety of children, young people and their families is our highest priority.

The National Patient Safety Agency (NPSA 2004) identifies strong leadership as an important part of the process of increasing safety and reducing risk. The role of the NPSA is to improve patient care through monitoring and analysing critical patient incidents in the UK. The NPSA subsequently provides incident data, directives, alerts and guidance in areas of risk. Most recently in relation to children, the NPSA issued a national patient safety alert around the use of nasogastric tubes and testing for correct placement (NPSA 2007). The NPSA in 2004 published the second version of 'seven steps to patient safety', outlining the issues NHS organisations and individual practitioners need to consider in order to address risks within clinical care. The seven steps (NPSA 2004, p 7) are:

1. Build a safety culture – create a culture that is open and fair
2. Lead and support your staff – establish a clear and strong focus on patient safety throughout your organisation.
3. Integrate your risk management activity – develop systems and processes to manage your risks and identify and assess things that could go wrong.
4. Promote reporting – ensure your staff can easily report incidents locally and nationally.
5. Involve and communicate with patients and the public – develop ways to communicate openly with and listen to patients.
6. Learn and share safety lessons – encourage staff to use root cause analysis to learn how and why incidents happen.
7. Implement solutions to prevent harm – embed lessons through changes to practice, processes or systems.

It has been reported that of all patients admitted to hospitals in the UK, approximately 10% will experience an adverse outcome (NPSA 2004). In discussing issues of adverse outcomes, Smallman (2003) states that these figures largely apply to hospital settings, but similar issues occur in the primary care arena and other settings. Wherever the situation occurs, the reason for the complaint should be explored, issues identified and acted upon to try to prevent recurrence. Possible outcomes of this investigation can be a change of policy, practice and delivery of care. Complaints need to be dealt with promptly within the timeframes set down by the Department of Health and using the policies developed locally. Nurses need to advocate for children and families by enabling them to have a voice/opinion and by including them in decisions about their care.

Within England, the Healthcare Commission has recently published information about second stage complaints that they have dealt with specifically related to children (Healthcare Commission 2008). Within the last year, they received 500 complaints, 10% of which related to vulnerable children or safeguarding children; 39% of complaints related to primary care; 32% to the acute sector; 16% specifically about communication and 10% about diagnosis. The Healthcare Commission's previous report about the services for children in hospital (Healthcare Commission 2007) highlighted that many children had a poorer hospital experience than they should because of a lack training of staff in communication (only 24% of nurses and 7–9% of surgeons and anaesthetists had received any formal training in communication). This was coupled with highly variable access to staff who specialise in play. Communication, play and distraction are fundamental concepts within children's nursing and especially in relation to the implementation of clinical skills and clearly issues that need emphasising in relation to quality of care, complaints and risk management.

Sometimes, complaints arise from poor communication and records that lack clarity. The potential for this in children's nursing is possibly greater, owing to the tripartite relationship between child, parents and the nurse. Where a system such as individualised nursing or named nursing does not exist and everyone contributes, channels of communication may become blurred and there may be no evidence of which nurse did what procedure for which child. The implementation of a clinical supervision programme, which facilitates improvements in communication with children and parents, and the inclusion of more detail in records could go some way towards effective risk management.

Family-centred care is a concept central to philosophies in the majority of areas where children are nursed. Nurses should be aware of the risks involved when they do not define clearly what they mean by family-centred care. They should be able to provide documented evidence of negotiation, which has taken place to establish exactly who will undertake which elements of care for the child. There is too much evidence, which suggests that parents may feel unsupported and neglected in the care of their sick child (Lee 2004). The NSF (DoH 2004a) highlights the various types of support which parents need and includes effective personal and material support. Much of what is stated in this section of the NSF reiterates what has been said by others in the past, but now it is being set in standards that healthcare workers are required to show evidence of meeting.

Aspects of family-centred care provide many additional examples of risks for children, parents and nurses. Feeding, or the provision of food for children to feed themselves, is usually considered to be a normal 'parenting skill'. However, when that food is to be administered via a nasogastric tube or gastrostomy, questions may arise over who should give the feeds. If the parents wish to give the feeds, then nurses must ensure a low risk/high benefit situation by teaching the parents this 'new skill' and monitoring their ability until all parties feel equally confident that the parents can carry out the practice. The risk is in handing over to parents what has previously been conceived as nursing care; the benefit is that parents and child can share the closeness of a mealtime together. Principles from this scenario can be transferred to many other practices which may involve parents, student nurses or nurses previously unfamiliar with a particular practice.

Risks for nurses may originate from many sources. Some risks arise from complaints by parents as a result of nurses failing in their duty of care. Examples of such failure might include inadequate securing of a nasogastric tube, resulting in the infant removing the tube and necessitating the passage of another, causing the child further distress. In caring for a child who is receiving fluids via a peripheral venous line, the nurse may fail to notice a swelling on the child's arm. When the electronic pump continues to alarm, a second nurse discovers the child's arm is oedematous and hard, indicating the severity of the extravasation.

A lack of written instructions may also give rise to failure in duty of care. For example, at the changeover of shifts, one nurse tells another that Joe is having 20 ml of milk 2-hourly and that his bottles are ready in the refrigerator. Once the day staff have left, the nurse checks the care plan only to realise that her colleague has not completed this for her shift.

As the nurse completing the shift has not provided details of the care given, the new nurse has only the verbal report to rely on. This may lead to inappropriate care, with both nurses implicated for failing in their duty of care. Accurate, well-written care plans in all areas of practice need to provide clinical evidence for determining the delivery of care and minimising risk. The treatment needs of children are very different and special attention must be given to babies and small children when giving them medicines and in the interpretation of results from services such as pathology (DoH 2004a). The findings of a small study by Guy et al (2003) identified that nurses, together with pharmacists, have a key role to play in identifying and preventing errors of prescribing being translated into errors of medication administration in paediatric settings. Clinical risk management is not only a concern within the acute hospital environment; within primary care there are specific considerations for children's nurses. For example the risks of lone working where there is potential for parents and carers to be verbally abusive.

In conclusion, clinical governance is the underpinning organisational tool within the modern NHS to assess and increase the quality of clinical care, risk management is integral to clinical governance and the provision of quality care and is about the prevention or minimisation of risks within the process of providing care. Benefits of a risk management programme are improvements in the quality of patient care, reductions in damage and injury to patients, increases in patient activity and a better environment for staff. Strategies identified to achieve this include improved communication and record-keeping which involve the child and family as active participants. The child and family should be encouraged to voice their opinions of the care received through systematic channels. Finally, clinical supervision (as discussed in the section on accountability) may enable a more open and honest approach to the delivery of care, both in hospital and in the community. Utilising these strategies may enable a positive and proactive approach to risk management in the future.

SAFEGUARDING CHILDREN

Children and young people have a right to be protected and be safe from harm from others; this is a message to all of us: politicians, communities, parents, families, neighbours; as well as police, health, social work and education authorities; and people who work directly with children and young people (Scottish Executive 2004). As healthcare professionals, children's nurses are in direct contact with children on a daily basis whether in hospital or in the community, and therefore it is essential that they are aware of their own responsibilities in safeguarding children and young people. However, it must be recognised that local authorities, through their Social Services Departments, under statute, are the body responsible for protecting children (Hall 2003, Scottish Executive 2003).

Child abuse can take many forms and necessitates accurate and timely communication between all members of the multi-professional team if protection is to be provided (Chudleigh 2005). Child abuse can be categorised into four main themes: physical abuse, neglect, emotional abuse and sexual abuse.

Most recently, the Victoria Climbié Inquiry made by Lord Laming (DoH 2003a) has once again identified the issues we face in the protection of vulnerable children and young people and the extent of child abuse in the UK. The recommendations of this report have been implemented throughout the UK and the report has influenced a number of policies and recent legislation including: the amended Children Act 2004 and in England and Wales *Every Child Matters*: change for children programme (DfES 2004). In Scotland, The Protection of Children (Scotland) Act (2003) and in Northern Ireland, a revision of the Guidance for The Children (Northern Ireland) Order 1995, reinforcing the importance of communication and interagency working (DHSSPS 2003, Chudleigh 2005).

Although all aspects of this chapter have some relevance to child protection, for example listening to the voice of the child and advocating on behalf of the child, perhaps health professionals can be most effective in their recognition of the child at risk. Lack of communication and documentation have been identified as key factors that influence child protection cases (DoH 2003a, Hall 2003, Scottish Executive 2003) and indeed were viewed as

being major contributing factors to the death of Victoria. The Climbié Report made 108 recommendations, all aimed at improving services for children. However, the words of Smith (2003), outlining the Royal College of Nursing (RCN) guidance following the publication of this report, carry the strongest message that 'child protection is every nurse's responsibility'. The National Society for the Prevention of Cruelty to Children goes one step further and says it is everyone's business (NSPCC 2003). Therefore everyone who has any interaction with children in a professional capacity should be cognisant of the major recommendations of the Laming report. The 108 recommendations may, according to the RCN (Smith 2003), be summarised under the headings shown in Box 1.1.

When working with children in any care setting, all nurses should be aware of the need to be vigilant for the child who may be the victim of abuse. This can manifest itself in many ways, with some behaviours being more obvious indicators than others; for example, the frozen watchfulness of the toddler who has been subject to physical harm, and the over-friendliness of another who has been neglected and possibly harmed as well, since evidence of more than one type of abuse may be seen in a single child. Older children may be looking for a confidante and do on occasions ask nurses to keep their secret, perhaps in terms of, 'If I tell you something, do you promise not to tell anyone else?' This may be because the child has been groomed by an abuser that the sexual behaviours they are engaging in are secret and the child should not tell anyone else. Therefore the child has displayed a lot of courage to get to the point of asking the nurse to keep this secret. When a child does ask for a confidence to be kept, then the nurse must do so, providing that the child is competent (see section on informed consent), however *The Code* (NMC 2008) states that: 'You must disclose information if you believe someone may be at risk of harm, in line with the law of the country in which you are practising'. Therefore if the nurse has reasonable cause to suspect that the child is suffering or likely to suffer significant harm, then they can justify disclosure. Best practice would involve negotiation with the child in gaining their permission to disclose.

Every nurse should be familiar with the procedure for what to do when concerned that a child may be at risk or has been abused in some way. The Laming report highlighted that there were

---

BOX 1.1 Major recommendations of the Laming report

Changes in services to support children

- A children and families' board to coordinate ministerial initiatives
- A national agency for children and families which will be responsible for policy on a national basis for children, young people and families
- Local committees for children and families developing collaboration and sound working relationships
- Local authority management boards which will ensure service delivery
- Lines of accountability to run through these organisations which will be inspected and reviewed by government inspectors.

Improvements to the exchange of information

- Government should review the free exchange of information
- Staff should be accountable for using information in a clear and unambiguous manner.

National children's database

- This would enable a detailed picture of the past history of individual children to be built. This is an important aspect since some parents have deliberately avoided services by moving to different geographical locations.

Service funding

- Local authorities should engage with the community and represent their needs
- Local authorities should be funded to provide 24-hour specialist services for children and families
- The use of agency and locum staff is not appropriate.

Training and supervision

- This is identified as being essential and should:
  a. Use the report to promote better practice
  b. Train staff to protect and care for children and support their families
  c. Provide child protection training for all staff
  d. Implement an effective system of supervision in action for all services.

Practice guidance and documentation

- Documentation of guidance must be simplified and uniform (Common Assessment Framework)
- Nursing care plans must contain issues of suspected harm
- Health professionals should all contribute to the same set of records for each child.

---

many documents available relating to child protection procedures and therefore professionals might become confused or indeed be using out-of-date material. To this end, 'What to do if you're worried a child is being abused' (DoH 2003b) was released in May 2003. This comprehensive document provides a standardised approach and should eliminate the need for individual bodies to produce their own and provides staff at all levels working with children with a practical guide to help do their job. Figure 1.1 is the flow chart for reporting concerns about a child's welfare; you should also refer to your local procedures. More recently, the Royal College of Paediatrics and Child Health (2006) developed a document that set out the required knowledge, skills and competencies required for the children's workforce, in relation to safeguarding children. These have been endorsed by the Royal College of Nursing and the Royal College of Midwifes. The most recent statutory guidance for

England and Wales is the 'Working Together to Safeguard Children: A guide to inter-agency working to safeguard and promote the welfare of children' (HMSO 2006) document, which all agencies, organisations and individuals working with children should be cognisant of.

There has also been a growing recognition that some children and young people are more vulnerable than others and may require safeguarding. McDougall (2008) includes looked-after children, disabled children, children in custody and those close to domestic violence within this group. While we should not focus upon these groups of children specifically, we should be aware of their specific situations and the impact it may have upon them. For further information, Box 1.2 lists the 'Government safeguarding children' websites for the countries of the UK. It is a key priority for nurses to be aware of local procedures and to be regularly trained and updated in safeguarding children policies and procedures.

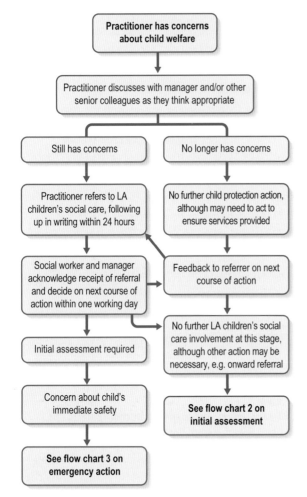

Figure 1.1 Flow chart 1: Referral. *(From Department of Health 2003b, with permission.)*

BOX 1.2   National governments' safeguarding children information

England and Wales

www.everychildmatters.gov.uk/childrens-trusts/integrated-frontline-delivery/safeguarding/

Northern Ireland

www.dhsspsni.gov.uk/publications/2003/safeguard/safeguard.asp

Scotland

www.scotland.gov.uk/about/ED/CnF/00017834/childprotection.aspx

---

SUMMARY

This chapter has explored a number of key concepts that are pertinent in the field of child and young people's nursing. The overarching statute, guidance, policy and strategy underpin the direction and delivery of care to children and families and as such, are central to the practice of all children's nurses. The latest guidance in relation to safeguarding children and young people is probably among the most significant following the tragic death of Victoria Climbié in 2000.

The preparation of the children's nurse continues to form a central part of professional, public and political debate. The key priority is that nurses are prepared in a way that effectively meets the changing needs of children and families and in so doing, can optimise their physical, social, emotional, intellectual and spiritual well-being.

The legal and professional frameworks that apply to practice are both complex and challenging and this chapter has only provided a basic explanation of legal frameworks coupled with some brief discussion of important professional principles such as advocacy. It is important that children's nurses familiarise themselves further with statutory and professional frameworks and in so doing provide protection for children, young people and families as well as themselves.

The clinical governance framework continues to be a feature of healthcare practice in the NHS today and it is important that all nurses recognise the role that governance plays in everyday practice. The public sector is increasingly audited and measured for quality and outcomes and those measures are becoming increasingly transparent and therefore open to public scrutiny.

The safeguarding of children and young people has gathered some momentum in recent years and the latest guidance and policy aims to protect the well-being of children using a collaborative multi-professional approach to practice. Again it is imperative that there is a continuous drive to raise awareness in the area of practice and that all those working with children and young people are trained and regularly updated. It is also vital that nurses undertaking undergraduate preparation are educated from the outset of their studies in an area where there have in the past been unfortunate errors leading to tragic consequences in some cases.

It remains an exciting and challenging time for children's nurses. There are however still good opportunities for change, which can enhance care delivery; continual developing academic opportunities, which give the practitioner the chance to develop advanced, expert knowledge and skills and continued optimism from those who are committed to this worthwhile area of practice.

References

Beale, H., 2002. Respite care for technology dependent children and their families. Paediatr. Nurs. 14 (7), 18–19.

Beauchamp, T., Childress, J., 2001. Principles of biomedical ethics, fifth ed. Open University Press, Oxford.

BMA British Medical Association, 2006. Parental responsibility: guidance from the British Medical Association. Ethics department. BMA, London.

Charles-Edwards, I., 2001. Children's nursing and advocacy: are we in a muddle? Paediatr. Nurs. 13 (2), 12–15.

Charles-Edwards, I., 2003. Power and control over children and young people. Paediatr. Nurs. 15 (6), 37–43.

Children (Scotland) Act, 1995. HMSO, Edinburgh.

Children's Act (England and Wales), 1989. HMSO, London.

Children's Act (England and Wales), 2004. HMSO, London.

Chudleigh, J., 2005. Safeguarding children. Paediatr. Nurs. 17 (1), 37–42.

Cox, S.J., Robinson, S., Murrells, T., 2003. Planning a career as a children's nurse: the availability of career guidance during the nurse diploma course. J. Child Healthcare 7 (4), 258–275.

Davies, J., Huws-Thomas, M., 2007. Care and management of adolescents with mental health problems and disorders. Nurs. Stand. 21 (51), 49–56.

Department for Education and Skills, 2004. Every child matters: change for children. The Stationery Office, London.

Department of Health, 1997. The new NHS: modern and dependable. The Stationery Office, London.

Department of Health, 1999. Making a difference: strengthening the nursing, midwifery and health visiting contribution to health and healthcare. The Stationery Office, London.

Department of Health, 2000. The NHS plan: a plan for investment, a plan for reform. The Stationery Office, London.

Department of Health, 2001a. Good practice implementation guide. DoH, London.

Department of Health, 2001b. Consent – what you have a right to expect. A guide for children and young people. The Stationery Office, London.

Department of Health, 2001c. Social services and public safety. DoH, London.

Department of Health, 2002. Learning from Bristol: The Department of Health's response to the report of the public inquiry into children's heart surgery at the Bristol Royal Infirmary 1984–1995. The Stationery Office, London.

Department of Health, 2003a. The Victoria Climbié inquiry: report of an inquiry by Lord Laming. The Stationery Office, London.

Department of Health, 2003b. What To do if you're worried a child is being abused. The Stationery Office, London.

Department of Health, 2004a. National service framework for children, young people and maternity services. The Stationery Office, London.

Department of Health, 2004b. Every child matters. DoH, London.

Department of Health, 2004c. The Chief Nursing Officer's review of the nursing, midwifery and health visiting contribution to vulnerable children and young people. DoH, London.

Department of Health, 2004d. Agenda for change final agreement. The Stationery Office, London.

Department of Health, 2006a. Modernising nursing careers. The Stationery Office, London.

Department of Health, 2006b. Standards for better health. DoH, London.

Department of Health, Social Services and Public Safety, 2003. Co-operating to safeguard children. DHSSPS, Belfast.

Department of Health, Social Services and Public Safety, 2005. The quality standards for health and social care. DHSSPS, Belfast.

Dowding, D., Thompson, C., 2003. Measuring the quality of judgement and decision-making in nursing. J. Adv. Nurs. 44 (1), 49–57.

Gillick *v* West Norfolk and Wisbech Area Health Authority [1986] A.C. 112.

GMC, 2007. 0–18 Guidance for all doctors. GMC, London.

Guy, J., Persaud, J., Davies, E., Harvey, D., 2003. Drug errors: what role do nurses and pharmacists have in minimising risk? J. Child Health 7 (4), 277–290.

Hall, D., 2003. Protecting children, supporting professionals. Arch. Dis. Child. 88 (7), 557–559.

Harper, R., 1999. Medical treatment and the law: the protection of adults and minors in the family division. Family Law, Bristol.

Healthcare Commission, 2007. Improving services for children in hospital. Healthcare Commission, London.

Commission, 2008. Spotlight on complaints. A report on second-stage complaints about the NHS in England. Healthcare Commission, London.

HMSO, 2006. Working together to safeguard children: A guide to inter-agency working to safeguard and promote the welfare of children. HMSO, London.

Hughes, J.M., Callery, P., 2004. Parents' experiences of caring for their child following day case surgery: a diary study. J. Child Health 8 (1), 47–58.

Human Fertilisation and Embryology Act, 1990. HMSO, London.

Kennedy, I., 2001. Learning from Bristol. The report of the public inquiry into children's heart surgery at the Bristol Royal Infirmary 1984–1995. The Stationery Office, Norwich.

Kenny, G., 2003. Skills or skilled? Children's nursing in the context of the current debate around skills. J. Child Healthcare 7 (2), 113–122.

Kitson, A., 2004. Future vision. Royal College of Nursing. RCN Magazine, Autumn.

Lee, P., 2004. Family involvement: are we asking too much? Paediatr. Nurs. 16 (10), 37–41.

Lewis, M., Noyes, J., 2008. Risk management and clinical governance for complex home-based healthcare. Paediatr. Nurs. 19 (6), 23–28.

Lindsay, C., 2003. A century of labour market change: 1900 to 2000. Labour Market Trends 111 (3), 133–144.

Marshall, K., 1998. New law on children and medical consent [advice leaflet]. University of Glasgow/Yorkhill NHS Trust, Glasgow.

Martin, E.A., 2004. Oxford dictionary of nursing. Oxford University Press, Oxford.

McDougall, T., 2008. Safeguarding vulnerable children. Paediatr. Nurs. 20 (3), 14–17.

Mental Capacity Act (England and Wales), 2005. HMSO, London.

Moules, T., Ramsay, J., 2008. The textbook of children and young peoples nursing, second ed. Wiley Blackwell, London.

National Patient Safety Agency, 2004. Seven steps to patient safety – your guide to safer patient care. NPSA, London.

National Patient Safety Agency, 2007. Advice to the NHS on reducing harm caused by the misplacement of nasogastric feeding tubes. NPSA, London.

National Society for the Prevention of Cruelty to Children, 2003. Child protection awareness in health. NSPCC EduCare, Leamington Spa.

NHS Quality Improvement Scotland, 2005. Clinical governance and risk management; achieving safe, effective, patient-focused care and services. NHS QIS, Edinburgh.

Nursing and Midwifery Council, 2007. Annex 2 to NMC Circular 07/2007: Essential skills clusters (ESCs) for pre-registration nursing programmes. NMC, London.

Nursing and Midwifery Council, 2008. The Code: Standards of conduct, performance and ethics for nurses and midwives. NMC, London.

Nursing and Midwifery Council, 2002. Supporting nurses and midwives through lifelong learning. NMC, London.

Nursing and Midwifery Council, 2005. Guide for students of nursing and midwifery. NMC, London.

Pearson, A., Porritt, K., Doran, D., et al., 2006. A comprehensive systematic review of evidence on the structure, process, characteristics and composition of a nursing team that fosters a health work environment. International Journal of Evidence Based Healthcare 4 (2), 118–157.

R. (on the application of Axon v Secretary of State for Health 2006 EWHC 3721.

Re M (medical treatment: consent) [1999] 2 FLR 1097.

RCN, 2002. Clinical governance: An RCN resource guide. RCN, London.

RCN, 2003. Restraining, holding still and containing children. Guidance for good practice. RCN, London.

Royal College of Paediatrics and Child Health, 2006. Safeguarding children: roles and competencies for healthcare staff. RCPCH, London.

Russell-Johnson, H., 2004. Parental responsibility: preparing for the change in the law. Paediatr. Nurs. 16 (1), 28–29.

Scottish Executive, 1997. Designed to care: renewing the National Health Service in Scotland. Scottish Executive Health Department, Edinburgh.

Scottish Executive, 2003. Protecting children – a shared responsibility. Scottish Executive, Edinburgh.

Scottish Executive, 2004. Protecting children and young people: framework for standards. Scottish Executive, Edinburgh.

The Scottish Government, (2003). Protection of Children (Scotland) Act. The Stationary Office. Edinburgh.

Self, A., Zealey, L. (Eds.), 2007. Social trends. Office for national statistics. Palgrave Macmillan, Basingstoke.

Shields, L., Hunter, J., Pratt, J., 2006. Family centred care: a review of qualitative studies. J. Clin. Nurs. 15 (10), 1317–1323.

Smallman, S., 2003. Keeping children safe in the healthcare system. Paediatr. Nurs. 15 (8), 20–22.

Smith, F., 2003. Safeguarding the young. Paediatr. Nurs. 15 (10), 24–25.

United Nations, 1989. Convention on the rights of the child. UN, Geneva.

Ward Platt, M.P., Brown, K., 2004. Evaluation of advanced neonatal practitioners: confidential enquiry into the management of sentinel cases. Archives of Diseases in Childhood Fetal and Neonatal edition. Online. Available: www.archdischild.com.

Waterhouse, 2000. Lost in care: Report of the Tribunal of Inquiry into the abuse of children in care in the former county council areas of Gwynedd and Clwyd since 1974

HC 201 ('the Waterhouse Report'). This inquiry was set up under the Tribunals of Inquiry (Evidence) Act 1921 on 17 June 1996.

Welsh Assembly Government, 2004. National Service Framework (NSF) for children, young people and maternity services in Wales. Welsh Assembly Government, Cardiff.

Welsh Assembly Government, 2005. Healthcare standards for Wales. Making the connections designed for life. Welsh Assembly Government, Cardiff.

Welsh Office, 1998. NHS Wales. Putting patients first. National Assembly for Wales, Cardiff.

Woodgate, M., Garralda, M.E., 2006. Paediatric liaison work by child & adolescent mental health services. Child Adolesc. Mental Health 11 (1), 19–24.

Further reading

Alderson, P., 2008. Young children's rights: exploring beliefs, principles and practice, second ed. Jessica Kingsley, London.

Archard, D., 2004. Children, rights and childhood, second ed. Routledge, London.

Baston, J., 2008. Healthcare decisions: A review of children's involvement. Paediatr. Nurs. 20 (3), 24–26.

Department of Health, Social Services and Public Safety, 2006. The quality standards for health and social care. DHSSPS, Belfast.

Elliston, S., 2007. The best interests of the child in healthcare. Routledge Cavendish, London.

Greig, A.D., Taylor, J., MacKay, T., 2007. Doing research with children, second ed. Sage, London.

Health Promotion Agency for Northern Ireland, 2005. Investing for health update 2005. HPA, Belfast.

Powell, C., 2007. Safeguarding children and young people: a guide for nurses and midwives. Open University Press, Oxford.

Scottish Executive, 2005. Building a health service fit for the future. Scottish Executive Health Department, Edinburgh.

Scottish Executive, 2005. Delivering for health. Scottish Executive Health Department, Edinburgh.

Scottish Executive, 2007. Better health, better care: a discussion document. Scottish Executive Health Department, Edinburgh.

Smith, F., 2003. 'Getting the right start': the Children's National Service Framework. Paediatr. Nurs. 15 (4), 20–21.

Welsh Assembly Government, 2005. Designed for life: creating world class health and social care services for Wales in the 21st century. Welsh Assembly Government, Cardiff.

Useful website

http://www.scotland.gov.uk/gettingitright
http://www.advancedpractice.scot.nhs.uk

Chapter 2

Communicating with children

Anne Finnegan, with a contribution by Joyce Stebbings

CHAPTER CONTENTS

Introduction   22

The key aspects of communication   23
  Verbal communication   23
  Non-verbal communication   24

The child's ability to communicate   25
  Stage 1: The sensory motor child
  (birth to 2 years)   26
  Stage 2: The pre-operational
  child (2–7 years)   27
  Stage 3: The concrete operational
  child (7–11 years)   27
  Stage 4: The formal operational
  child (11–18 years)   27

Creative communication   28

Factors that adversely affect communication   29

Written communication   29

What happens when communication
breaks down?   29
  Communication with children with
  additional needs   30

INTRODUCTION

Communication is the giving or exchange of information, ideas, or feelings. It is a two-way process where one person sends a message to another who receives it. Since the skills of communication are acquired from early infancy onward, the practitioner may feel that they are competent in this area without studying the subject further. However, poor communication is the basis of many formal complaints about healthcare Healthcare Commission for Audit and Inspection (2007) (online) and working with the child often provides particular challenges related to the child's ability to understand information and to verbalise their concerns. The practitioner is required to ensure that the language and communication needs of the children in their care are met in a way that the child can understand (NMC 2008). This requirement is a central feature of the 'Essential Care Clusters' (NMC 2007). Consequently, this chapter will focus upon the interpersonal skills needed for working effectively with children.

Effective interpersonal skills not only ensure that the practitioners meet their professional responsibilities; they ensure many benefits for the child. In any setting, a skilled communicator gives the child a role model which facilitates their socialisation, their ability to communicate with others and to work cooperatively in groups (Bellman & Peile 2006). Skilled communication should enable the practitioner to recognise at an early stage when the child is unwell, has a developmental delay or is developing a disability, and facilitate interventions to minimise severity and complications (Hall & Elliman 2007).

Where the child becomes unwell, the practitioner can help them to understand their illness, enabling them to cope with any resulting treatment (Scott et al 2007), adhere to a therapeutic regime (Wales & Crisp 2007) and where appropriate, assist early discharge and care delivery in the home setting (Department of Health 2003a, Scott et al 2007). In some instances, the practitioner can facilitate discussion about issues which affect the health of the young person or causes worry but cannot be discussed with parents or carers for some reason (Department of Health 2003b, Duderstadt 2006).

THE KEY ASPECTS OF COMMUNICATION

Interpersonal communication has verbal and non-verbal components. The practitioner needs to think carefully about both aspects in order to provide effective and sensitive communication.

VERBAL COMMUNICATION

Verbal communication is the use of words, spoken or signed, to convey information.

Practitioners are much more likely to give information to parents than to children (Pantell et al 1982) but they need to bear in mind that the child is their patient. The child's best interest must come first (Children's Act 1989), so it is important that the practitioner establishes a comfortable working relationship with the child. Most children would find it distressing and anxiety provoking to be ignored by someone who may then subject them to embarrassing or physical intrusive care. Such distress may cause the child to resist care delivery and/or leave them with anxieties, phobias and behavioural problems (Platt Report 1959). It may reduce the child's ability or desire to cooperate with healthcare providers in the future.

The effective practitioner needs to:

Begin the interaction in a warm, comfortable environment which will let the child relax quickly into their surroundings. Giving age appropriate toys and games often help this process but avoid using electronic games, radio or television, as the child can become absorbed in such activities and will be difficult to engage. Where the practitioner is unknown to the child, she or he should introduce themselves and establish the child's preferred name. The practitioner should always explain what is going to be talked about and/or will happen. Jamieson

(2006) suggests that young children often have a greater understanding of what is said to them than is realised because language comprehension usually exceeds the ability to verbalise thoughts. However, children who are anxious, unwell or have a short concentration span can be difficult to engage in meaningful interaction. So, where the child's communication abilities are unknown, it is better to use simple words and short sentences until it is certain the child can manage more complex information.

Initially, it can be helpful to focus on the parent, leaving the child to become relaxed and orientated. The watching child will usually find this interaction reassuring and a signal that they can safely join in when invited to do so (Hockenberry & Wilson 2007).

Once the practitioner begins to talk to the child, it is usually helpful to move from the least private or intrusive issue to more sensitive topics or intimate care giving (Duderstadt 2006). The practitioner needs to sound calm, confident and unhurried.

Gather information using a number of techniques including measurement, and observation, but the spoken component should give the child the chance to give their opinion and make their expectations clear (Carter 2007).

The use of questions is a common method of showing interest, seeking consent for care delivery and extending or collecting information (Box 2.1). There are many types of questions but the practitioner working with children may find that there are three types which are most useful:

- *Open questions* are broad queries which indicate to the child that there is no 'wrong answer'. They encourage description and are not threatening (Hockenberry & Wilson 2007). They give the child the opportunity to decide how much information to tell someone, in their own way and in their own time (Thomas & Monaghan 2007). They can often provide the practitioner with a comprehensive understanding of the child's abilities, needs and worries.
- *Tag questions* make a suggestion and allow the person answering to give their opinion (Schuster 2000).
- *Closed questions* are focused enquiries which do not allow or encourage discussion. Often the only response required is 'yes' or 'no'. They are often used where there is limited choice, where factual information is required, or when the situation is urgent.

Gain a focus which can be established using directional phrases. These comments highlight something the child has said and tells them more information would be beneficial (Schuster 2000), e.g. 'You said that you don't like using the school toilets, why is that?' or 'Can you tell me more about your school. What are the toilets like?'.

Try to ensure a common understanding about the purpose of any interaction. Children and practitioners have been shown to have differing conclusions about the role of communication and a satisfactory resolution to discussion. Practitioners often consider emotional support and therapeutic intervention to be the most important element of their role while the child places importance on practical support and expects the professional to ensure that their wishes are met (Macleod 2006). Ignoring these differing expectations can adversely affect the child/practitioner relationship.

Use supportive comments and compliments to which children often respond and give constructive feedback. Information given in this way lets them know when they are doing well (Csoti 2001). This technique lets them feel a sense of approval and validation for appropriate actions, e.g. 'It's really good to see you choosing the healthy food option on the menu.' It is often more effective than being critical (Green 2000).

Emphasise important points, as children often lack the experience to know what is most relevant and appropriate. When something is important, they should be told (Green 2001). Use expressions such as 'this is really important'; 'you must always remember to . . .'.

Tangible rewards reinforce positive feedback, rewarding effort and commitment. Bravery certificates, badges and fridge magnets might be offered (Green 2000).

Use silence, Use silence sparingly because it can give the child time to organise their thoughts, describe their feelings and/or formulate questions (Hockenberry & Wilson 2007). The practitioner needs to sit quietly letting the child take the lead. However, the silence should not be allowed to become oppressive or threatening (Stanton 2004). The practitioner needs to recognise when the child's silence is a sign that they do not want to talk at all. Children may find it hard to explain their discomfort or feel it is impolite to voice their preference. Generally, children are expected to respond to adult priorities. Signs that the silence is counterproductive may include the child fidgeting, changing the topic or introducing a distraction. They may look bored. Older children might look at their watch or at a clock (Hockenberry & Wilson 2007).

BOX 2.1   Different types of question

Open questions

- What are your favourite foods?
- How has your medicine made you feel?
- Can you describe your pain to me?
- Can you tell me about your friends at school?

Closed questions

- Do you eat a lot of chocolate?
- Has your medicine made you feel better?
- Do you have pain?
- Are you being bullied at school?

Tag questions

- I like chocolate, do you?
- Calpol makes a headache better, doesn't it?
- School is a good place to make friends, isn't it?

Finish the interaction clearly to tell the child the discussion is complete. But ensure that the child's questions have been answered; repeat anything that they are unsure about, recap any decisions made and actions to be taken (Thomas & Monaghan 2007).

Ensure consistency of information and record what the child has been told or has talked about. This allows other team members to ensure their information/advice is consistent (Glaspar et al 2007).

NON-VERBAL COMMUNICATION

This is a form of communication without words although it does include vocal expression such as tone, pitch and pace of speech (Stanton 2004). Facial expression, hand gestures, body position and movement contribute to this aspect of communication (Hogg & Vaughen 2008). Bruce (2004) suggests that these non-verbal actions convey about 80% of any message.

Children learn non-verbal techniques more quickly than speech (Bruce 2006). Small children may use non-verbal signals to demonstrate many of their needs and to interpret the intentions and behaviours of others. This discussion introduces some of the main features of non-verbal techniques but further reading will be needed for expert practice, particularly when working with children from ethnic minority backgrounds. Some non-verbal signals vary in their meaning between cultures (Csoti 2001).

The practitioner needs to consider these aspects of their communication technique carefully to ensure that the non-verbal message conveyed is consistent with their speech and with what is happening to the child (Hockenberry & Wilson 2007).

Facial expression enables most individuals to monitor the feelings and moods of others. It probably conveys to the child the most non-verbal information (Schuster 2000). Therefore, it is important that the practitioner looks calm, approachable and relaxed. They should try to ensure that expressions of shock, worry and discomfort are not evident even in difficult or challenging situations.

Gaze – generally we look at the person talking to us, look away when we start to speak and then look back again when we are about to stop talking (Wainwright 2003). This signals to the other person that we are ready to listen to them. This pattern regulates social interaction, signifying interest and friendliness. Even young babies will show this pattern of eye contact (Bruce 2006). However, children may avoid eye contact if they are shy or uncomfortable. The practitioner should try to delay conversation until the child has relaxed.

Active listening demonstrates that the practitioner is interested in what the child is saying. It requires concentration on the verbal and non-verbal messages the child is giving (Carter 2007). The practitioner may demonstrate they are listening by maintaining eye contact and nodding. They may use brief prompts, e.g. 'mmm' and 'uh-huh' (Hogg & Vaughen 2008) or reflective comment (Thomas & Monaghan 2007). This involves repeating a few words of the child's, e.g. 'my tummy hurts and I want some medicine' becomes 'some medicine?'

Proximity is the distance between two people. Generally, children will expect strangers to keep some distance from them with physical closeness anticipated only from family and friends (Wainwright 2003). Where nursing care requires closeness, it is often helpful to encourage a parent or carer to participate. Explain to the child what will happen and how long it will take.

Touch is often associated with the delivery of therapeutic care. Small babies/toddlers are used to adults handling them in order to support the activities of daily living such as feeding, hygiene and movement. Consequently, babies and toddlers often find touch comforting and rewarding. Patting, stroking and holding the infant can quickly alleviate distress, reduce anxiety and demonstrate support. However, the older child, particularly the adolescent may find touch provokes more anxiety than it relieves (Hogg & Vaughen 2008). They may appreciate the offer of a back rub or a hand to squeeze when distressed or uncomfortable but should always have the opportunity to refuse such gestures. Usually these should be limited to the hand, arm or shoulder. Intimate care should be negotiated wherever possible.

Orientation is the physical distance and position of the body to an object or person. Whenever possible the child and practitioner should be on the same level, facing one another with the practitioner adopting an open posture. Towering over a child in bed or because of a difference in height may give the impression that the practitioner wants to dominate the child (Wainwright 2003). Using a barrier such as a desk makes a situation more formal. The child may feel less relaxed and uneasy.

Appearance – individuals make judgements about people based on their hairstyle, make-up, clothes and jewellery. Children will do the same and will recognise the demonstration of respect through a professional and groomed appearance (Schuster 2000).

THE CHILD'S ABILITY TO COMMUNICATE

The preceding discussion indicates that the practitioner needs to consider many aspects of technique to ensure effective and sensitive communication with the child. The child is often unable to give the same level of consideration to their messages. This can be due to anxiety, illness or lack of desire to participate. But it can be related to the simple fact that children are still learning about communication. They have an incomplete knowledge of non-verbal techniques, the meaning of words and can lack expressive vocabulary.

Jean Piaget (1896–1980) spent many years researching how, why and when children learn. He developed a four-stage theory to explain how children develop their understanding of the world. Many researchers use his theory to research different aspects of childhood. The theory is open to debate (Cohen 2002), but does give the practitioner an effective framework for thinking about how children might communicate at different ages (Table 2.1).

Table 2.1 Using developmental knowledge to deliver nursing care	
AGE GROUP	STRATEGIES
The sensory motor child (birth to 2 years)	Handle gently but firmly
	Avoid loud noises and sudden movements
	Encourage the main carer(s) to participate in skills delivery wherever possible
	Where the main carer(s) cannot or does not want to actively participate in skills delivery, encourage them to hold the child or remain within sight of the child
	Minimise the number of strangers involved in the care
	Try to provide some time for social interaction before touching and handling the child
	Explain what is going to happen in short, direct sentences, just before it occurs
	Use therapeutic touch to give support, e.g. patting or stroking
	When talking to the child, leave pauses – this lets the child respond with facial expression, sounds and body movements
	Try to match tone of voice to their non-verbal expression
	Distract using sights, sounds and games which interest them, e.g. use a mobile; sing a short song
The pre-operational child (2–7 years)	Use books and equipment to teach children about what is going to happen to them
	Focus on the child's sensory experience and describe what they will see, hear and feel
	Encourage cooperation through playing games or copying others, e.g. play statues when you need to get the child to remain still
	Keep unfamiliar equipment out of sight until it is needed
	Avoid ambiguous terminology, e.g. putting to sleep
	Encourage them to make small choices, e.g. where to sit
	Ensure care delivery by their main carer whenever possible
	Accept regressive behaviours. Do not use judgemental or disparaging terms if these occur
The concrete operational child (7–11 years)	Prepare for admission, procedures and changes in condition using books and sample equipment
	Allow time for questions, give honest answers
	Facilitate expression of fears
	Build on previous experience
	Check understanding by encouraging the child to repeat the information given
	Help the child develop problem-solving skills
	Give them as much control as possible
	Teach them to deliver their own care whenever possible
The formal operational child	Treat as autonomous individuals
	Provide privacy, and explain policy about confidentiality
	Do not pry or be judgemental of their behaviour and expect mood swings
	Avoid giving advice unless it is really necessary or has been requested
	Keep to neutral topics until the adolescent shows that they are ready to talk

STAGE 1: THE SENSORY MOTOR CHILD (BIRTH TO 2 YEARS)

It can be easy for the practitioner to assume that the child's limited abilities at this age means that effective communication with them is not necessary. However, Piaget (1952) suggests even new-born babies are active learners. From birth, babies use the five senses and movement to develop an understanding of the world. A major accomplishment during this stage is an understanding of object permanence (Hockenberry & Wilson 2007). This is the ability to recognise that an object continues to exist even when the child cannot see it. The baby who has reached this stage often demonstrates distress when their parent leaves them. The child's communication skills emerge gradually during the sensory motor period.

Listening, gazing and the ability to imitate facial expression are evident during the first few days of life (Bruce 2006). By 3 months of age, the child demonstrates vocalisation, listening and turn-taking when someone talks to them (Bruce 2004). They will begin to respond to their name around 5 months of age and say their first words around 10–12 months of age (Bellman & Peile 2006). The ability to remember distressing events emerges during the first few weeks of life and the baby may become upset when similar circumstances are recognized, e.g. having a vaccination (Levy 1960).

By their first birthday, most children will probably have had several vaccinations, a number of minor ailments, and will have met a number of health practitioners including GPs, health visitors and nurses. But they will lack the vocabulary to discuss their views of these encounters and make requests about future nursing care. Therefore the practitioner needs to be acutely aware of the non-verbal cues the child will use, particularly where these indicate distress, anxiety or pain.

Babies and toddlers will often cry when in difficulty, seeking the comfort and protection of their main carers when frightened. The child may cling to their carer and avoid making eye contact (Bowlby 1969). A reluctance to spend time alone with the practitioner may be evident and the child may avoid unaccompanied visits with them, even to a neutral area such as a playroom (Green 2001). The baby or toddler may actively resist being touched and the delivery of nursing care.

STAGE 2: THE PRE-OPERATIONAL CHILD (2–7 YEARS)

These children continue to use movement and their senses to experience the world, but are more mobile and coordinated. Their vocabulary is growing. Experimentation with language and their immediate environment may be evident. However, these children are not logical or objective because of an inability to understand principles and diversity. They are egocentric in the true meaning of the word being unable to see the world from any point of view but their own (Moules & Ramsay 2008).

A range of interpersonal skills using many non-verbal techniques to express understanding, satisfaction/dissatisfaction and other emotions should be evident. Some children may be able to name parts of the body (Engel 2002) but are unlikely to know many medical or physiological terms. They may have little understanding of the interior of the body but can become acutely distressed by visible injuries (Bibace & Walsh 1980). They may recognise physical and sensory disability in others (Diamond et al 2007), but are unlikely to understand their own vulnerability during illness or following an accident.

This child may view illness and hospitalisation as a punishment (Perry 1994). Distress may be communicated through regressive behaviours such as the need for a pacifier, bedwetting or thumb sucking (Moules & Ramsay 2008). When distressed, these children may employ some of the techniques

of the younger child, but as she or he becomes more self aware, will recognise an expectation to do what an adult asks them, to be brave and to cope (Young et al 2003). Therefore communication of distress may become more subtle. The child may seek to distract others by asking questions, changing the topic or starting a game. The occasional white lie may be used, e.g. saying that they have no pain in order to avoid an unpleasant medicine.

STAGE 3: THE CONCRETE OPERATIONAL CHILD (7–11 YEARS)

These school-age children are often naturally curious, interested in their surroundings and capable of logical thought. Divergent viewpoints and options may be recognised. Problem-solving skills, an understanding of rules and an ability to follow them are features of this stage of development (Moules & Ramsay 2008). However, understanding hypothetical situations is often beyond them (Cohen 2002).

These schoolchildren should have an improving vocabulary with an ability to ask questions and express feelings and worries. They can state when something is difficult to understand.

She or he will have some knowledge about illness and healthcare delivery, recognising that illness usually has a cause, e.g. germs and can sometimes be avoided (Bibace & Walsh 1980). The value of health promoting behaviours is understood, e.g. brushing teeth, eating healthily. Sometimes events can be anticipated due to previous experience. However, the practitioner should not assume that the cooperative child is not worried or anxious.

The effects of illness and healthcare delivery may cause worry, e.g. body mutilation. Anticipation of pain may be evident during some nursing procedures. Feelings of embarrassment may emerge at times (Engel 2002) and worries about death can affect some children (Green 2000). Phobias can develop, e.g. needles, anaesthetic mask.

These issues can be expressed to the practitioner who takes the time to speak to the child and listen to their views. Schoolchildren can often seek answers to their queries or may prompt their parents to seek information for them.

STAGE 4: THE FORMAL OPERATIONAL CHILD (11–18 YEARS)

These young people will normally have the ability to think logically, deal with hypothetical situations and abstract concepts, although it is possible that some adolescents will never reach this cognitive level (Hockenberry & Wilson 2007).

Adolescents will often have a sophisticated knowledge of health and care delivery with a good understanding of the internal workings of the body and the psychological influences on health (Bibace & Walsh 1980). However, they are undergoing the major physical changes of puberty. This makes coping with illness difficult for them (Scott 2007). The adolescent may have an acute awareness of their body image and may develop a sense of dissatisfaction related to aspects of their appearance (Ogden 2000). Worry about death, handicap and disfigurement, losing control and losing face are not uncommon.

Adolescents are ready to be autonomous and make their own decisions (Moules & Ramsay 2008). Their cultural practices may be distinctive from that of their parents/family. However, they may be unwilling to communicate accurate information about lifestyle factors with a parent present. The opportunity to talk to teenagers privately should always be provided (Greydanus et al 2008). Where others question their choices, withdrawal and a lack of cooperation may be the response. Therefore, the practitioner should avoid conveying disapproval or condemnation.

Adherence to health advice may be resisted if it seems to make them different from their peer group. The adolescent may reject guidance about sexual activity, substance use and lifestyle choices where this advice conflicts with the social norms of their friends (Patton & Viner 2007). In some circumstances, rejection of health advice can extend to non-compliance with prescribed therapeutic care where the young person needs active treatment. Non-compliance is a particular issue for adolescents needing long-term therapy for enduring illnesses because treatment makes them different from their peer group. Drug regimes may be rejected, dietary advice forgotten and exercise routines avoided. The practitioner needs to be aware of this possibility and mindful that where compliance is self-reported, it is consistently exaggerated (Burkhart et al 2001). The practitioner working with the adolescent needs to be an active listener and a skilled negotiator to ensure that the young person continues their treatment as it is needed.

CREATIVE COMMUNICATION

Good communication techniques do enable the practitioner to work effectively with the child in many instances. But children can find concentrating for long periods difficult. A formal interview or examination can seem frightening and might be uncomfortable. These factors will diminish the quality and quantity of information a child will give during an assessment or remember during health promoting activities. Therefore, the practitioner should give consideration to using a more creative format such as a demonstration, story or game (Table 2.2). These techniques may improve the child's feeling of satisfaction with healthcare delivery and build their sense of trust in the practitioner. Also, remember there is nothing wrong in making healthcare fun whenever possible.

Table 2.2 Using play to communicate	
TYPE OF GAME	**POSSIBLE APPLICATIONS**
Being a nurse or doctor	Use a toy medical kit or piece of equipment with a puppet or doll. This may encourage familiarity with strange equipment and reduce anxiety. May prepare a child to deliver their own care, e.g. giving their own medication by injection
Story telling	Start a story about a child with a similar problem or in a similar situation to the patient and let the child develop it. This can help reveal their fears, anxieties and expectations
Be an artist	Ask the child to draw a picture about an aspect of their problem or nursing care. Talk to them about what the pictures shows
Be a writer	Ask the child to write a story about their problem or nursing care. Talk to them about the information in the story, e.g. how did you feel when …
Make a list	Best and worst aspects, e.g. three best things and three worst things about school, diet, hospital, etc.
Be a detective or a planner	Start with a care problem, list and discuss the options to resolve the issue. Use a mind or road map
Be a copycat	Encourage the child to copy your actions

FACTORS THAT ADVERSELY AFFECT COMMUNICATION

Just as the practitioner can employ effective communication skills, it is possible for her or him to be ineffective due to poor technique.

A lapse of concentration during interaction may lead any practitioner to make insensitive comments or demonstrate inappropriate behaviours through their non-verbal actions. There are a number of pitfalls which need to be avoided:

Not telling the truth – it can be tempting to avoid telling a child that something will hurt, take a long time, or restrict their activity. This impulse can arise because it may seem to make nursing care quicker and easier. But it can be counterproductive and unethical. Avoiding the truth can make the child unwilling to trust the practitioner in the future or to cooperate. Also, truth telling is the basis of informed consent and decision-making (NMC 2008).

Giving empty, or inappropriate reassurance that 'it will be alright' when it is unclear or untrue that this is the case. This has the same effect as not telling the truth.

Talking about 'you' i.e. direct or confrontational questioning using phrases such as 'why didn't you . . .,' can make the child feel threatened (Ireland et al 2006). The child may feel accused of something bad or inappropriate. Therefore, during discussion try to use the first person 'I' or the third person 'some'. For example, instead of saying 'You are making your condition worse by . . .,' try something like, 'Some children avoid . . . because they . . . Do you feel that?'

Not listening to the child's reply, ignoring queries, using closed questions deny the child the opportunity to clarify information, and make decisions from an informed basis.

Making stereotypical assumptions about the child based on ethnic origin, social class or gender – information, advice and nursing care should be based on an individual assessment of the child. It should not make assumptions about the child's abilities or needs based on the practitioner's views about the child's social or cultural grouping.

Showing impatience – there are many non-verbal behaviours which tell the child that they need to hurry up or be quiet. These include tapping feet or fingers, fiddling with rings or pens, nodding quickly and with vigour, frowning.

Showing lack of confidence – includes nail biting, biting of lips and wringing hands. They diminish the child's confidence in the practitioner.

Talking in an over loud voice can make the child feel bullied or indicate that you are angry with them (Csoti 2001).

Promise to keep a secret – the practitioner has an overriding responsibility to safeguard the child and must ensure that the child understands that sometimes information cannot be confidential. Information must be passed on to others if there is a risk of harm to the child (NMC 2008).

WRITTEN COMMUNICATION

Where the practitioner wants the child to remember information it is common practice to provide some form of leaflet or written directions to aid memory. However, there are limitations with this format because the child may have little or no reading ability.

Where a written format is going to be used, the use of pictures or cartoons linking to keywords should be considered (Bruce 2006). Information should be simple, direct and easy to understand. Include universal signs such as ticks, crosses, question marks, smiling and frowning faces. Alternatively, the practitioner should consider the use of technology. Information may be given using tapes, CDs and podcasts (*Every Child Matters* 2003).

WHAT HAPPENS WHEN COMMUNICATION BREAKS DOWN?

Even in situations where the practitioner employs excellent techniques, it is possible that the child will remain uncooperative and unwilling to interact. Unless the situation is urgent, it is probably best to change the topic or leave the child alone for a time. Try again later.

This enables the practitioner to discuss with the carer a strategy for moving nursing care forward. It allows time to seek advice from colleagues about gaining the child's cooperation or consent bearing in mind the Children Act (1989) and best practice related to holding and restraint (RCN 1999). Where the situation remains difficult or unclear, it may be necessary to seek advice from specialist practitioners, legal experts, or professional associations.

COMMUNICATION WITH CHILDREN WITH ADDITIONAL NEEDS

Communication is essential for us as individuals. We need it to share our ideas, likes, dislikes and how we are feeling. But what if you are not able to express in words what you want to say. Imagine everyone is ignoring you when you speak, do not understand what you say, do things to you or for you without telling you first. For some children with additional needs in hospital this is the case, 'taking for granted the easy flow of the spoken word we fail to listen to those whose speech is impaired or restricted, or who use other methods to communicate' (Morris 2001).

In February 2007, the Healthcare Commission published its findings of children's hospital services. One of the points highlighted was that of communication. It stated that, 'many children had a poorer experience of hospital than they should because of a lack of training of staff in communication (only 24% of nurses and 7–9% of surgeons and anaesthetists were formally trained).' It went on to say that Hospital Trusts 'need to recognise the benefits of communication and give it a much higher priority' (Healthcare Commission 2007).

The Department of Health in 2004 published its National Service Framework for Paediatric Services. It sets out its core standards for hospital trusts that treat children. All trusts have 10 years from its publication to bring its services in line. They will be checked periodically to make sure they are making headway to reach these targets.

This document is based on good practice. It highlights the training and skills staff need to be able to carry out their job effectively. It also raises the issue of disabled children and young people and the importance for staff to be able to communicate and understand their needs. It makes the point that, 'disabled children have the same right to high quality services as any other child, though evidence suggests many are excluded from mainstream services'. Best practice needs to be shared to change this.

References

Bellman, M., Peile, E. (Eds.), 2006. The normal child. Churchill Livingstone, Elsevier, Edinburgh.

Bibace, R., Walsh, M.E., 1980. Development of children's concepts of illness. Pediatrics 66 (6), 912–917.

Bowlby, J., 1969. Attachment and loss, vol. 1. Hogarth Press, London.

Bruce, T., 2004. Developing learning in early childhood 0–8 years. Paul Chapman Publishing, London.

Bruce, T. (Ed.), 2006. Early childhood. A guide for students. Sage, London.

Burkhart, P.V., Dunbar-Jacob, J.M., Rohay, J.M., 2001. Accuracy of children's self reported adherence to treatment. J. Nurs. Scholarsh. 33 (1), 27–32.

Carter, B., 2007. Pain narratives and narrative practitioners: a way of working 'in-relation' with children experiencing pain. J. Nurs. Manag. 12 (3), 210–216.

Children's Act 1989. (England and Wales). HMSO, London.

Cohen, D., 2002. How the child's mind develops. Routledge, Hove.

Csoti, M., 2001. Social awareness skills for children. Jessica Kingsley, London.

Department of Health, 2003a. Getting the right start: National Service Framework for Children. Standard for Hospital Services. HMSO, London.

Department of Health, 2003b. The Victoria Climbié inquiry: a report of an inquiry by Lord Laming. HMSO, London.

Department of Health, 2004. Getting the right start: National Service Framework for children, young people and maternity services. DoH, London, pp. 32.

Diamond, K.E., 2007. Preschoolers' ideas about disability. Infant and Young Child 18 (1), 37–46.

Duderstadt, K.G., 2006. Pediatric physical examination. An illustrated handbook. Mosby Elsevier, St Louis.

Engel, J., 2002. Pediatric assessment. Pocket guide series, fourth ed. Mosby, St Louis.

Every Child Matters, 2003. Online. Available at: www.everychildmatters.gov.uk.

Glaspar, A., McEwing, G., Richardson, J., 2007. Oxford handbook of children's & young people's nursing. Oxford University Press, Oxford.

Green, C., 2000. Beyond Toddlerdom. Keeping five to twelve year olds on the rails. Vermillion, London.

Green, C., 2001. New toddler training. A parents' guide to the first four years. Vermillion, London.

Greydanus, D.E., Feinberg, A.N., Patel, D.R., et al., 2008. The pediatric diagnostic examination. McGraw-Hill Medical, London.

Hall, D., Elliman, D., 2007. Health for all children, fourth ed. revised. Oxford University Press, Oxford.

Healthcare Commission for Audit and Inspection, 2007. Improving services for children in hospital. Healthcare Commission, London, pp. 4, 33. Online. Available at: www.healthcarecommission. org.uk.

Hockenberry, M.J., Wilson, D., 2007. Wong's nursing care of infants and children. Mosby Elsevier, St Louis.

Hogg, M.A., Vaughen, G.M., 2008. Social psychology, fifth ed. Pearson Education, Essex.

Ireland, J.D., Power, D.J., Woods, D.L., et al, 2006. Paediatric primary healthcare, fourth ed. Oxford University Press, Oxford.

Jamieson, J., 2006. Speech and communication. In: Bellman, M., Peile, E. (Eds.), The normal child. Elsevier, Edinburgh.

Levy, 1960. The infant's earliest memory of inoculation. J. Genet. Psychol. 96 (3), 46–50.

Macleod, A., 2006. Respect or empowerment? Alternative understandings of listening in childcare social work. Adoption Fostering 30 (4), 43–52.

Morris, J., 2001. Quoted. In: Gordon, R., Marchant, R. (Eds.), Two way street – communicating with disabled children and young people. NSPCC, Joseph Rowntree Foundation, Triangle, pp. 4.

Moules, T., Ramsay, J., 2008. The textbook of children's and young people's nursing, second ed. Blackwell, Oxford.

NMC, 2007. Essential care clusters (ESCs) for pre-registration nursing programmes. Annexe 2 to NMC Circular 07/2007. NMC, London.

NMC, 2008. The Code. Standards of conduct, performance and ethics for nurses and midwives. NMC, London.

Ogden, J., 2000. Health psychology. A textbook, second ed. Open University Press, Buckingham.

Pantell, R.H., Stewart, T.J., Dias, J.K., et al., 1982. Physician communication with children and their parents. Pediatrics 70 (3), 396–402.

Patton, G.C., Viner, R., 2007. Pubertal transitions in health. Lancet 369, 1130–1139.

Perry, 1994. Communication with toddlers in hospital. Paediatr. Nurs. 6 (5), 14–17.

Piaget, J., 1952. Play, dreams and imitation in childhood. Routledge and Kegan Paul, London.

Platt Report, 1959. The welfare of children in hospital. HMSO, London.

RCN, 1999. Restraining, holding still and containing children and young people. Guidance for nursing staff. Royal College of Nursing, London.

Schuster, P., 2000. Communication. The key to the therapeutic relationship. FA Davis, Philadelphia.

Scott, J.T., Harmsen, M., Proctor, M.J., et al., 2007. Interventions for improving communication with children and adolescents about their cancer. The Cochrane Collaboration 4.

Stanton, N., 2004. Mastering communication, fourth ed. Palgrave Macmillan, Basingstoke.

Thomas, J., Monaghan, T., 2007. Oxford handbook of clinical examination and practical skills. Oxford University Press, Oxford.

Wainwright, G.R., 2003. Teach yourself body language, third ed. Book Print, Abingdon.

Wales, S., Crisp, J., 2007. The views of nurses on adherence in school-aged children with chronic illness. Neonatal, Paediatric and Child Health Nursing 10 (2), 5–10.

Young, B., Dixon-Woods, M., Windridge, K.C., et al., 2003. Managing communication with young people who have a potentially life threatening chronic illness: qualitative study of patients and parents. Br. Med. J. 326, 305.

Chapter 3

Introduction to community

Dawn Moss

CHAPTER CONTENTS

Introduction   32

Multidisciplinary team working   33

Community children's nursing   33

Transition from hospital to home   34

Working in partnership with children,
young people and their families   35

Coordination of care and continuing care   35

Challenges of working in the community   36

Support for nurses working
in the community   37

Evaluation of the workload   38

The future for nursing children
in the community   38

INTRODUCTION

Paediatric care today has been transformed with fewer admissions to hospital and a shorter hospital stay. The emphasis is on primary health and the delivery of healthcare in the community rather than secondary care based in the hospital (Middleton 2000). Medical advances have seen an increase in the numbers of babies born prematurely and surviving with increasing levels of needs. Nurses in the community have been identified as fundamental to increasing effectiveness and improving patient satisfaction (Scottish Executive 2005). Nurses in the community also help parents of children with chronic illness by enabling, facilitating and empowering them to cope at home (Carter 2000, Olsen & Maslin-Prothero 2001) and by raising the quality of care for a range of conditions, for example eczema, incontinence problems and behavioural difficulties, which often have a low profile (Drew et al 2003).

Children with disability and technology-dependent children who need ongoing medical and nursing care are the two most common areas that require the involvement of children's services (Teare 2008). There is evidence that highlights that the outcomes are better for the child and family when they are supported to manage their child's illness at home (Wang & Burnard 2004). Benefits to the child and family include reduced levels of anxiety, positive improvements in the child's physical and mental health, financial benefits and increased educational achievement. Children's nursing in the community has a key role to play in providing the support and care needed to achieve these positive outcomes alongside the multi-agency input of social work, education and the voluntary services.

MULTIDISCIPLINARY TEAM WORKING

A joint approach to delivering care and the importance of team working is central to *Every Child Matters* (DfES 2003), The Children Act (2004) and the National Service Frameworks in England and Wales (DoH 2004a; Welsh Assembly Government 2005). The Children's Plan (Department for Children, Schools and Families 2007) brings together these existing policies and aims to ensure that services are designed around the needs of the child and their family, rather than around organisations or professionals. Doyle (2008) highlights the risks of poor communication and failure of professionals working together, which can lead to duplication of care, poor management, failure to provide care, clinical risk and the family losing confidence in the services provided. A further aim of 'The Children's Plan' is to remove existing professional barriers to improve access to services for children and families to enable effective multidisciplinary team working. 'For Scotland's Children' (Scottish Executive 2001a) states that better integrated children's services will ensure services are more responsive, and identifies the need to bring services together to meet the needs of individual children, young people and their families. The 'National Service Framework for Children, Young People and Maternity Services' (DoH 2004a) states that everyone who works with children, not just in healthcare settings, but also in schools and the wider community, will be expected to have an understanding of children's needs.

The children's nurse working in the community has a key role to play in working as part of the multidisciplinary team and meeting the holistic needs of children and their families. Examples of other professionals involved in a child's multidisciplinary team might include physiotherapist, speech and language therapist, occupational therapist, GP, health visitor, school nurse, paediatrician, social worker, teacher and all have a key role in working together to fulfill the needs of the child and family.

COMMUNITY CHILDREN'S NURSING

Community children's nurses (CCN) are registered children's nurses with additional education in caring for children at home and their wider community (Pontin & Lewis 2008). CCN services have developed and the majority of areas throughout the UK now have a service. The Royal College of Nursing (2000) states that CCN services have been developed in response to local need and circumstances instead of being based on the most effective model of provision. Models of service delivery vary and include:

- Hospital/ambulatory care outreach
- Hospital at home
- CCN team based in acute services
- CCN team working within general practice
- Community-based nurse led clinics
- Children's palliative care teams
- Multidisciplinary/multi-agency working (includes taking on a key worker role for children with complex healthcare needs, and management of complex packages of care). May also include voluntary organisations contributing to the overall package of care.

CCNs provide a wide range of care options related to the child's individual needs. They will have a caseload for which they provide a specialist or generalist service, including the following:

- Children with life-threatening or terminal conditions (e.g. cancer, degenerative conditions, organ failure)
- Children with complex healthcare needs (e.g. technology-dependent)
- Training, education, support and management of non-parent carers
- Children in schools
- Children with acute illnesses/conditions (e.g. bronchiolitis, postoperative care)
- Children with chronic conditions (e.g. constipation, epilepsy, cystic fibrosis).

CCNs have a key role in being proactive in preventing crisis through support and early intervention and providing a holistic approach that sees each child as part of a family. The concept of the nurse offering support to the child and family is widely recognised but there is a need to define what support means. Kirk and Glendinning's (2004) study with parents caring for their technology-dependent children defined support as three dimensional: (1) Emotional support (includes 'being there', easy to contact, knowing the child, listening/counselling, promoting parents' self-confidence). (2) Instrumental or practical help (includes practical support, advocacy, 'hands-on' care, organising services and equipment). (3) Information (includes advice and information giving, teaching, giving feedback and sign-posting to other care agencies).

CCNs facilitate family-led packages of care and empower the parents in care partnerships (Gould 2000). The level of care and support varies to ensure that each family is confident in the care they are able to provide.

CCNs need to have the interpersonal skills to work in partnership with the family to identify their strengths and weakness, as well as capacity, willingness and ability to get involved in their child's care. Getting to know the family in the community requires a different dynamic than nurses working in a hospital setting as the relationship develops over a longer period of time and continues on a short-term (days or weeks) or long-term (months or even years) basis. Pontin and Lewis (2008) highlight the skills that CCNs have in 'knowing' the family through gathering knowledge about the child, their condition, the family and resources available within the local community. A holistic view considers the child's views, their home circumstances and quality of life as part of the decision-making process. Knowing what to ask to find out about the child and family is one aspect of 'knowing' but there is then the need to interpret the information, understanding its relevance and then knowing what to do next.

TRANSITION FROM HOSPITAL TO HOME

Implementing a successful transition of care from hospital to home needs careful planning. The aim of this planning is to ensure that the child's care is continuous and the parents receive the support and education that enables them to provide safe care without undue stress. For children with complex healthcare needs, discharge planning needs to start some weeks before the child leaves hospital. Ideally the CCN will visit the family in hospital to enable them to develop a relationship and to start to discuss the practical issues of going home. The CCN can familiarise herself with the care that the child is currently receiving and can identify the resources that will be required in the home. This can be described

as 'hospital in-reach', where the CCN takes an active role in the discharge planning process (Royal College of Nursing 2000). While the child is still in hospital, education programmes can be initiated for the child and parents, who should be encouraged to discuss any concerns that they may have so they are able to give informed consent to the care that they are being asked to undertake. Communication between the hospital and the primary healthcare team is essential and involvement in the assessment and care planning will be a key role. The CCN is often ideally placed to act as a liaison and is able to involve the primary healthcare team at an early stage in the planning process.

When children are discharged home from hospital, any continuing hands-on care is most often provided by their parents (Thurgate & Warner 2005). Glendinning and Kirk (2000) reports on a study that aimed to look at the dynamics involved in the transfer of responsibility from professionals to parents. The findings highlighted that parents felt obliged to care for their child and this was influenced by the strong desire for their child to go home. Often there is no alternative to parents taking on the role as carer and parents in the study highlighted the lack of community services. The implications of this evidence highlight that it is essential to work in partnership with parents in planning for the child's transition from hospital to home. Parents as carers need to feel confident and competent in the care they are providing and training needs to be tailored to their needs. The nurse has a responsibility to document any training and procedures and check competency of the carers to ensure standards are being achieved. This will include regular reviews of competences and supplying training updates as necessary. This should also demonstrate that the instruction has been understood and that the parents and carers are capable of undertaking the procedure confidently and competently, being aware of all the problems that might occur and what action to take. Families should always be given the option of handing back control if they feel that they can no longer cope.

Providing care at home for children with complex healthcare needs is demanding and often exhausting for parents and families (Wang & Burnard 2004). Respite support, now known as short breaks, can offer a break for the family and may involve a range of services including respite at home, in a respite facility or children's hospice and through social services. A further example of respite support is shared care with other families taking on the caring role.

WORKING IN PARTNERSHIP WITH CHILDREN, YOUNG PEOPLE AND THEIR FAMILIES

Recognition of the need to listen to children's views about health and other services has grown over the last 10 years. Key policy documents include Article 12.1 of the UN Convention on the Rights of the Child' (1989), where it is stated that children have the right to express their views freely in matters affecting them. The Children (Scotland) Act 1995 advocates the need for professionals to listen to and take account of children's views and *Delivering a Healthy Future* (Scottish Executive 2007) and *Every Child Matters* (DfES 2003) advocates that children should be viewed as partners in decisions involving their care and treatment.

Evidence suggests that good communication between health professionals and children results in increased understanding of illness and treatment and lower levels of stress for children (Coyne 2006). Findings from Stalker et al (2003) highlighted that young people expect the following from healthcare professionals:

- Being treated as individuals
- To be asked about their care and treatment, to be listened to and to have their wished acted upon
- To have choices
- To be given information
- To know the staff involved in their care.

Kirk and Glendinning's (2002) study explored the experiences of families caring at home for a technology-dependent child and examined their needs for practical and other kinds of support. The findings highlighted that parents often have more knowledge about caring for their child than professionals. The implications for children's nurses working in the community is the need for an understanding of parents' expertise and that as professionals their role is most often focused on supporting parental care-giving rather than providing hands-on care. A family-centred approach encourages the family to become active partners with health professionals in the management, decision-making, and treatment and care of their child (Brett 2004; Thurgate 2006; Maguire & Price 2007). The CCN recognises that it is not only the sick child needing care but that a holistic approach sees each child as part of a family. The CCN works together with families as partners in planning holistic packages of care that best meets the needs of the child and family. The Royal College of Nursing (2000) states that CCNs should use networks within the community to facilitate family-centred appropriate care by teaching, supporting, advising, counselling and liaising.

COORDINATION OF CARE AND CONTINUING CARE

If there is a lack of coordination between different agencies and professionals, no holistic view of the child is obtained. Sloper (2002) states that parents report a 'constant battle' to find out what services are available and know what the roles of different professionals are. Parents can feel frustrated at trying to get professionals to understand their needs and meet their expectations. Effective care coordination prevents fragmented care and duplication of services. Townsley et al (2004) explored the impact of multi-agency working on disabled children with complex needs and concluded that well coordinated multi-agency working enables families to be supported in managing their child's care at home.

Care coordination UK (CCNUK) is an umbrella organisation promoting and supporting care coordination and key working for disabled children and their families in England, Northern Ireland, Scotland and Wales. CCNUK is an independent registered charity based at the Social Policy Research Unit at the University of York. Their purpose is to work in partnership with disabled children, their families and professionals, to ensure that all families across the UK have access to high quality care coordination. Research has shown the importance to families of key workers who help them to access services, share information and support families (Greco & Sloper 2003, Townsley et al 2004). The Royal College of Nursing (2000) identifies that the CCN fulfils the key worker role that families ask for; that is, someone who visits regularly, is approachable and easy to access and someone who listens. As a key worker, the CCN offers the family a single point of contact for any concerns, is an advocate and the source of practical, personal and emotional support and advice. The key worker role is not necessarily always undertaken by a nurse but will be the person most appropriate, such as professionals from social work, education or the voluntary services.

The 'Common Assessment Framework' (DoH 2005) aims to provide a standardised approach to gather and understand information about the needs and strengths of the child and family. As a framework for multi-agency assessment it can be used as the main tool to support inter-agency referral and multi-agency working. The framework provides assessment elements and domains to enable a holistic view to be taken of the child as part of the family. The children's nurse working in the community can utilise the framework as a tool for the child and family assessment to identify need and the resources needed to appropriately support the family. The framework includes the following elements and domains:

Development of the child

- General health, physical development and speech, language and communications development
- Emotional and social development
- Behavioural development
- Identity, including self-esteem, self-image and social presentation
- Family and social relationships
- Self-care skills and independence
- Learning, understanding, reasoning and problem-solving, participation in learning, education and employment, progress and achievement in learning, aspirations.

Parents and carers

- Basic care, ensuring safety and protection
- Emotional warmth and stability
- Guidance, boundaries and stimulation.

Family and environmental

- Family history, functioning and well-being
- Wider family
- Housing, employment and financial considerations
- Social and community elements and resources, including education.

Every Child Matters (DfES 2003) advocates support for parents and carers and the National Service Framework for Children Young People and Maternity Services (DoH 2004a) further enhances the home care concept for children with complex health needs. In 1998 the Department of Health provided funding for community children's nursing teams in Princess Diana's memory (DoH 1998). More recently in 2003, the New Opportunities Fund has provided £48 million of lottery money to expand home-based paediatric palliative care teams in selected Primary Care Trusts across the country.

In order for children with complex health needs or life-limiting conditions and their families to have their needs met, it is essential for 'continuing care' to be planned effectively. Continuing care can be defined as an individualised package of seamless care planned by health, social care and education, in partnership with children and their families. Historically, continuing care for children has always fallen under the auspices of community children's nursing teams (CCN). In recent years, CCN teams have begun to develop more robust services to ensure children with complex health needs and disabilities are having their needs met. Continuing care teams have evolved to provide home-based respite care for children with complex health needs.

There are many continuing care models for children across the country. Carers are trained, assessed, supervised and supported by community children's nurses. The most valued services identified by parents are community children's nursing services which are able to offer 24-hour contact in case of emergency; particularly in providing accessible information and advice to turn to in case of uncertainty or anxiety and practical help in obtaining services and care coordination (Kirk & Glendinning 2004). Coordinated services should ensure a referral network that can provide a seamless service between hospital and community. One of the key roles of the CCN and continuing care nurse is liaising with other professionals involved with each family from a variety of multidisciplinary teams within the hospital and throughout the community, including social care and education.

CHALLENGES OF WORKING IN THE COMMUNITY

A major role for nurses working in the community is the assessment and management of risk. In hospital, support and advice can be accessed almost immediately, whereas in the community, the nurse often has to make independent decisions about a child's care. This might be making the decision to change treatment and seek medical advice or an assessment of a child's well-being, which results in a referral for support from other agencies. Nurses working in the community are often lone-working. A survey undertaken by Smith (2007) of community nurses, identified that approximately 85% of respondents spent more than 25% of their time working alone and 66% stated that their employers did not know their whereabouts. Chapter 1 identified the issue of lone-working and highlighted the need for support through clinical supervision but there are practical issues that also need to be considered when working in the community.

Managers have the responsibility of minimising the risks experienced by lone-workers. Risk assessments need to be in place for activities such as home visits and systems established for signing in and out, to ensure the whereabouts of the practitioner is known at all times. Nurses also have a responsibility to ensure that their whereabouts are known to their colleagues (e.g. reporting to the switchboard when they have arrived at their location and when they have left to go home).

Guidance for lone-workers includes the following:

- Ensure adequate referral information is available before visiting families at home
- Withdraw immediately from situations where you feel vulnerable or threatened
- Be aware of equipment that may attract unwelcome interest such as drugs, medical equipment and mobile phones
- Undertake joint visits where areas are known to have high levels of violence and aggression
- Devise a plan of action for incidents of being trapped, attacked or injured, or car breakdown
- Carry safety equipment such as a personal panic alarm
- Park the car in well lit areas.

A further challenge of working in the community for nurses is the practicalities around risk management. Staff in the community work in a range of different environments, which often present difficult situations and their challenge is to use measures to safeguard themselves and the child and family. NICE (2003) clinical guidelines on infection control provide guidance for staff providing care within the community. The guidance includes avoiding infection through effective handwashing, using gloves and aprons, using sharps safely and educating patients and their carers about infection control. Risk assessment also needs to be made for clinical waste disposal, deciding which requires a collection service and what can be disposed of in household waste. The issue of transporting specimens also needs consideration to ensure that secure transport boxes and guidance on what to do if there is a spillage.

Primary Care Trusts may sub-contract outcare packages to nursing agencies if there is no in-house provision, and the role of the CCN as the case manager would be to ensure that the agreed care plans and packages are being achieved. The agency has a key responsibility for the supply of the agreed carer resources and the training of the agency staff but there is a need for monitoring to ensure they deliver efficiently, effectively, qualitatively, safely and competently and to report any concerns. There are a number of children with long-term ventilation needs or complex needs that are being cared for at home, supported by packages of care which can have 24-hour trained nursing care supporting the child and family in the home setting (Barnardos et al 2005).

SUPPORT FOR NURSES WORKING IN THE COMMUNITY

It has been emphasised that children and young people have a right to be protected and be safe from harm. Nurses caring for children in the community have a key role in the assessment, referral and support to the child and family. Where there are concerns about child protection, good practice includes providing help to parents and children as and when they need it, at the right time and appropriately addressing the source of risk to the child (DoH 2003, Scottish Executive 2002). Goveas (2005) reassures health professionals that if they suspect a child has been abused and go on to make a referral to social work, they are not accountable if they get it wrong, and the important thing is to communicate any concerns that they might have. Children's nurses working in the community must have the skills to work creatively and flexibly and have the right support in place to enable them to reflect on their practice.

While in hospital, the contact with the child and family may be over a short period of time, however, nurses working in the community may be involved with children and families on their caseload for many months or even years. At times, the nurse can feel 'stuck' with a family within the confines of the available resources. Clinical supervision can enable nurses to reflect on their own perceptions of how effective they consider their contribution to a family to be. The process of structured reflection is one way of enabling the nurse to come to a deeper understanding of their practice (Perry 2000). Self-challenging attitudes and practice is not always an easy or comfortable thing to do but reflection as a process of clinical supervision is a means for the nurse to become more effective and meet the needs of the child and family. Hawkins and Shohet (2000) state that knowing oneself makes you more likely to be of real help.

Reflecting in supervision can help to prevent the cycle of feeling overwhelmed, which if not addressed can lead to less effective practice, causing in turn feelings of guilt and inadequacy (Hawkins & Shohet 2000). Freshwater and Stickley (2004) argue that the clinical supervision process needs to go further than merely monitoring practice and should help staff to manage their own emotional needs. Supervision is an important part of practitioners taking care of themselves and staying open to new learning, as well as part of their ongoing development and self-awareness (Hawkins & Shohet 2000). McNeilly and Price (2007) present a model of reflection for caring for children requiring palliative care but could be used for caring for any child. Reflection is structured around three phases of discussion:

Phase 1: Describing the incident and the contributing factors, including the practitioners experience of the child and family.

Phase 2: Reflecting about the communication involved and communication with the child and family.

Phase 3: Making sense of the situation and the outcomes on a personal level and for the child and family.

EVALUATION OF THE WORKLOAD

A challenge for all nurses is identifying their workload and the resources needed to provide the service they provide. Pontin and Lewis (2008) highlight the issue of caseload management to identify workload and to identify the needs of children and families and the resources for support. Facey (2000) presents a system of dependency scoring to enable CCNs to calculate the dependency scores of the patients on their caseload to ensure appropriate use of resources. The Royal College of Nursing (2000) advises evaluation of the nurse's workload by monitoring the following:

- The child's care needs
- The quality of care delivered
- The skill mix within the team
- The time allocated to deliver the care.

The Royal College of Nursing (2000) also advises that each CCN team develops a system for monitoring the pressure of work on each nurse including the numbers of:

- Highly dependent families
- Child protection problems
- Children with life-threatening or life-limiting conditions
- Development work (non-clinical work)
- Time worked over contracted hours
- Caseload turnover.

It needs to be recognised that workload is not dependent on the child's diagnosis or condition but on the support networks in place for the family and their capacity and capability to care for their child at home. For example, a child with cerebral palsy needing home enteral feeding with a supportive family network and package of care may need less nursing input that a child with a postoperative wound where the child is complaining of pain and where there is a high level of parental anxiety. Pontin and Lewis (2008) identify that a key factor of a CCN caseload is supporting families to maintain 'usual family life' and achieving the balance of intervention with promoting independence.

A CCN workload tool has been developed that identifies the input and categories of care to enable collection of data and monitoring of caseloads.

THE FUTURE FOR NURSING CHILDREN IN THE COMMUNITY

Previous recommendations have stated that children should have access to 24-hour, 7-day CCN services (House of Commons Health Committee 1997) but while CCN services have developed, it is evident that this level of service is yet to be achieved in many areas of the UK. CCNs have the key nursing skills of providing information, advice and education, counselling, emotional support and service coordination (Kirk & Glendinning 2004). The CCN is just one of the professionals providing services to children in the community. The emphasis should be about focusing the model of team working with the child in the centre. The Department of Health (2007) recommended the development of Children's Community Teams that are multi-agency and multi-professional, easily accessible and responsive to enable them to support the care of children and young people with health needs and needs continuing support at home. The role of the community teams includes providing approachable support to children and their families and responding to local need. As part of the Community Children's Nurses (CCN) role,

the key aims are to prevent hospital admission, facilitate early discharge and caring for children with complex needs.

In England the 'Chief Nursing Officer's Review of the Nursing, Midwifery and Health Visiting Contribution to Vulnerable Children and Young People' (DoH 2004b) states that integration is needed across a number of boundaries; most importantly, health, social care and education. There is also a need to overcome the current fragmentation between hospital and primary care, and between nurses, midwives and health visitors. A key theme from this review is the need to 'follow the child', which means providing services as close to home as possible including schools and the wider community. This means that the demand for children's nursing in the community will increase as the child's continuing care needs are provided at home.

References

Barnardos, Noyes, J., Lewis, M., 2005. Care pathway for the discharge and support of children requiring long-term ventilation. Department of Health, London.

Brett, J., 2004. The journey to accepting support: how parents of profoundly disabled children experience support in their lives. Paediatr. Nurs. 16 (8), 14–18.

Carter, B., 2000. Ways of working: CCNs and chronic illness. J. Child Healthcare 4 (2), 66–72.

Children Act, 2004. HMSO, London.

Children (Scotland) Act, 1995. The Stationery Office, Edinburgh.

Coyne, I., 2006a. Consultation with children in hospital: children, parents' and nurses' perspectives. J. Clin. Nurs. 15, 61–71.

Department for Education and Skills, 2003. Every child matters. Department of Education and Skills, London.

Department for Children, Schools and Families, 2007. The Children's Plan. Department for Children. Schools and Families, London.

Department of Health, 1998. Proposals to commemorate the life and work of Diana, Princess

of Wales. Online. Available: www.hm-treasury.gov.uk/ press_105_98.htm (Accessed 28 September 2009).

Department of Health, 2003. The Victoria Climbié Inquiry: Report of an enquiry by Lord Laming. The Stationery Office, London.

Department of Health, 2004a. National Service Framework for Children, Young People and Maternity Services: Primary Care Version. DoH, London.

Department of Health, 2004b. National Service Framework for Children, Young People and Maternity Services: Supporting Local Delivery. DoH, London.

Department of Health, 2004c. The Chief Nursing Officer's Review of the Nursing, Midwifery and Health Visiting Contribution to Vulnerable Children and Young People. DoH, London.

Department of Health, 2005. Common Assessment Framework for Children and Young People: guide for service managers and practitioners. DoH, London.

Department of Health, 2007. National Service Framework for Children,

Young People and Maternity Services: Children and Young People Who Are Ill, Standard 6. Department for Education and Skills, London.

Doyle, J., 2008. Barriers and facilitators of multidisciplinary team working: a review. Paediatr. Nurs. 20 (2), 26–29.

Drew, J., Nathan, D., Hall, D., 2003. Role of a paediatric nurse in primary care 2: research findings. Br. J. Nurs. 12 (1), 34–43.

Facey, S., 2000. Chapter 19. In: Muir, J., Sidey, A. (Eds.), Textbook of community children's nursing. Baillière Tindall, Edinburgh.

Freshwater, D., Stickley, T., 2004. The heart of the art: emotional intelligence in nurse education. Nurs. Inq. 11 (2), 91–98.

Glendinning, C., Kirk, S., 2000. High-tech care: high-skilled parents. Paediatr. Nurs. 12 (6), 25–27.

Gould, C., 2000. Chapter 34. In: Muir, J., Sidey, A. (Eds.), Textbook of community children's nursing. Baillière Tindall, Edinburgh.

Goveas, A., 2005. The fallout from false diagnoses. Children Now 4–10: 12 May.

Greco, V., Sloper, P., 2003. Care co-ordination and key worker schemes for disabled children: results of a UK-wide survey. Child Care Health Dev. 30, 13–20.

Hawkins, P., Shohet, P., 2000. Supervision in the helping professions, second ed. Open University Press, Berkshire.

House of Commons Health Committee, 1997. Health Services for children and young people in the community – home and school, 3rd Report. The Stationery Office, London.

Kirk, S., Glendinning, C., 2002. Supporting 'expert' parents – professional support and families caring for a child with complex healthcare needs in the community. Int. J. Nurs. Stud. 39, 625–635.

Kirk, S., Glendinning, C., 2004. Developing services to support parents caring for a technology-dependent child at home. Child Care Health Dev. 30 (3), 209–218.

Maguire, A., Price, J., 2007. Reflecting on practice in children's palliative care. Paediatr. Nurs. 19 (3), 30–37.

McNeilly, P., Price, J., 2007. A reflective model for paediatric palliative care. Paediatr. Nurs. 19 (3), 33–34.

Middleton, C., 2000. Chapter 1. In: Muir, J., Sidey, A. (Eds.), Textbook of community children's nursing. Baillière Tindall, London.

NICE National Institute for Health and Clinical Excellence, 2003. Infection control, prevention of healthcare-associated infection in primary and community Care. NICE, London.

Olsen, R., Maslin-Prothero, P., 2001. Dilemmas in the provision of own-home respite support for parents of young children with complex healthcare needs: evidence from an evaluation. J. Adv. Nurs. 34 (5), 603–610.

Perry, M.A., 2000. Reflections on intuition and expertise. J. Clin. Nurs. 9, 137–145.

Pontin, D., Lewis, M., 2008. Managing the caseload: a qualitative action research study exploring how community children's nurses deliver services to children living with life-limiting, life-threatening, and chronic conditions. J. Spec. Paediatr. Nurs. 13 (1), 26–35.

Royal College of Nursing, 2000. Children's Community Nursing: Promoting effective teamworking for children and their families. Royal College of Nursing, London.

Scottish Executive, 2001a. For Scotland's children. Scottish Executive, Edinburgh.

Scottish Executive, 2002. It's everyone's job to make sure I'm alright. Report of the Child Protection Audit and Review. Scottish Executive, Edinburgh.

Scottish Executive, 2005. Delivering for health. Scottish Executive, Edinburgh.

Scottish Executive, 2007. Delivering a healthy future: an action framework for children and young people's health in Scotland. Scottish Executive, Edinburgh.

Sloper, T., 2002. Meeting the needs of disabled children. Quality Protects Research Briefings 6.

Department of Health, Research in Practice.

Smith, M., 2007. Royal College of Nursing lone working survey. Sheffield Hallam University, Sheffield.

Stalker, K., Carpenter, J., Phillips, R., et al., 2003. Care and treatment. Joseph Rowntree Foundation, East Sussex.

Teare, J., 2008. Caring for children with complex needs in the community. Blackwell, Oxford.

Thurgate, C., Warner, H., 2005. Living with disability: Part 1. Paediatr. Nurs. 17 (10), 37–43.

Thurgate, C., 2006. Living with disability: Part 3. Paediatr. Nurs. 18 (5), 40–44.

Townsley, R., Abbott, D., Watson, D., 2004. Making a difference? Exploring the impact of multi-agency working on disabled children with complex healthcare needs, their families and the professionals who support them. The Policy Press, Bristol.

UN Convention on the Rights of the Child, 1989. UN General Assembly Document A/RES/44.25.

Wang, K., Burnard, A., 2004. Technology-dependent children and their families: a review. J. Adv. Nurs. 45 (1), 36–46.

Welsh Assembly Government, 2005. National service framework for children, young people and maternity services in Wales. Welsh Assembly Government, Cardiff.

Chapter 4

Control of infection

Helen Cheney

CHAPTER CONTENTS

Introduction   41

The chain of infection   43
  The microorganism   43
  The source of infection   43
  Mode of transmission   44
  The host   44

Precautions to be taken   44
  Hand hygiene   46
  Protective clothing   48
  Factors to note   49
  Waste disposal   49
  Eating utensils such as dishes, cups, glasses, baby bottles   51
  Factors to note   51
  The use of disinfectants in the environment and with equipment   51
  Factors to note   52
  Equipment   52
  Factors to note   52

Occupational health   53

Surveillance of infection and auditing practice   53

INTRODUCTION

The prevention and control of healthcare-associated infection (HCAI) is the responsibility of all those involved in the care of patients. Healthcare-associated infections can impact on the quality of care delivered to patients, resulting in significant harm, unnecessary patient suffering, pain, anxiety, disability and possible death. HCAIs are avoidable and costly to both the health services and the patients (Health Protection Scotland 2007). Consequently, all healthcare workers are responsible for ensuring good healthcare practice that is focussed towards the avoidance and reduction of HCAIs.

Infection control is an important part of risk management and there is a legal obligation to take appropriate precautions (Public Health (Infectious Disease) Regulations (HMSO 1988, NHS QIS 2001, 2008). A control's assurance standard (DoH 2003a) on infection control, first produced in 1999, provides a checklist of measures for acute hospitals to ensure that the environment is managed so as to minimise the risk of infection to patients, staff and visitors. The Department of Health (DoH) has produced a number of documents: *Getting Ahead of the Curve* (2002) outlines the changing patterns in communicable diseases and antimicrobial resistance and emphasises the need for their control. The increasing emergence of serious infections with *methicillin-resistant Staphylococcus aureus* (MRSA) in the paediatric population is cause for concern (Khairulddin et al 2004). The report *Winning Ways: working together to reduce healthcare-associated infections in England* (DoH 2003b) aims to bring infection control into the mainstream of

---

BOX 4.1   Winning ways – working together to reduce healthcare-associated infection

- Action one: active surveillance and investigation
- Action two: reducing the infection risk from use of catheters, tubes, cannulae, instruments and other devices
- Action three: reducing reservoirs of infection
- Action four: high standards of hygiene in clinical areas
- Action five: prudent use of antibiotics
- Action six: management and organisation
- Action seven: research and development.

---

healthcare by setting out a strategy (Box 4.1). With the advent of new and emerging infectious diseases, it is important that there are written management procedures with formal risk assessment and audit trails where there may be hazards from infection towards patients, visitors or staff in the workplace. This includes all healthcare institutions within the hospital and community settings.

The most recent documents are: *Saving Lives: A delivery programme to reduce healthcare-associated infections including MRSA* (DoH 2007) and *Essential Steps to Safe Clean Care: Reducing healthcare-associated infection* (DoH 2006b). The hospital environment is a possible source of infection. The NHS Healthcare Cleaning Manual (NHS Estates 2004b) supports the 'Matron's Charter' (NHS Estates 2004a) and empowers senior nurses – modern matrons – to ensure the environment is safe to nurse patients. Cleanliness in hospital is not just about keeping the environment clean, as cleaning will not completely eradicate the microorganisms from immanent surfaces. Transmission of microorganisms from the hospital/healthcare environment may occur through direct contact with contaminated equipment and surfaces, or indirectly through touching hands. This reinforces the importance of hand hygiene before and after every direct patient contact.

The Healthcare Act 2006: Code of Practice for the Prevention and Control of Healthcare-associated Infections (DoH 2006c). The Code of Practice came into effect in October 2006. The purpose of *The Code* is to assist NHS organisations in planning and implementing strategies on how they can prevent and control HCAIs. *The Code* sets out criteria to ensure that patients are cared for in a clean environment where the risk of HCAIs is kept as low as possible. The Code has become part of the annual health check of the Healthcare Commission and failure to comply may result in an 'Improvement Notice' being issued to the NHS organisation. This is now being monitored by the newly formed (April 2009) Quality Care Commission.

The Department of Health commissioned the first national guidelines to promote evidence-based practice in infection control (EPIC) for hospitals (Pratt et al 2001) and the community (Pellowe et al 2003, Thames Valley University 2003). The guidelines develop good principles of best practice in infection control and are integrated into local infection prevention and control protocols. The evidence base for these recommendations has recently been updated and new guidelines published, known as EPIC2 (Pratt et al 2007). These guidelines include key audit criteria to monitor implantation for preventing infections and recommendations for preventing infections associated with medical devices, e.g. central venous access devices and urinary catheters (Loveday & Pellowe 2007).

The Health Protection Agency (HPA)/Health Protection Scotland (HPS) provides an integrated approach to protecting the health of the public against infectious diseases and chemical and radiological hazards by working with the NHS and local authorities. Their website provides up-to-date epidemiological data and guidelines on infectious diseases, including healthcare-associated infection (www.hpa.org.uk and www.hps.scotland.nhs.uk). Newly emerging or newly identified diseases such as severe acute respiratory syndrome (SARS), Influenza A H1N1 (commonly referred to as Swine Flu) and Pandemic Flu is an example of how rapidly the world's communicable disease network (through the World Health Organization) can communicate essential information.

Healthcare-associated infections are estimated to cost 5000 patients their lives and the NHS £1billion a year (National Audit Office 2004). About 9% of hospital in-patients acquire an infection while in hospital and between 50% and 70% of surgical wound infections occur after discharge. Between 15% and 30% of hospital-acquired infections could be prevented by better application of knowledge and implementation of realistic infection control policies (DoH 2002a). The incidence of nosocomial infection in children is higher and proportional to their age, with the highest incidence in neonates and infants under 1 year of age. It is interesting to note that some ethnographic studies (Macqueen 1995) have indicated that nurses wash their hands more frequently before aseptic procedures than after 'dirty' tasks, and that they perceive babies as being 'less dirty' than older children.

Medical and nursing cultural influences may play a part in non-compliance with evidence-based infection control practice. Across the NHS, it is recognised that the true champions of infection control are ward-based staff. The modern matrons of NHS England and Wales are charged to ensure good infection control practice is maintained. Within NHS Scotland the 'Leading Better Care' (2008) initiative clearly identifies this as a key responsibility of the Senior Charge Nurse. The introduction of care bundles associated with infection control, as seen in the Scottish Patient Safety Programme (see http://www.patientsafetyalliance.scot.nhs.uk/programme/), further strengthen the need for high standards of infection control measures. Ongoing education, training and support for all staff must therefore be an integral part of an infection control programme (Boyce & Pittet 2002).

THE CHAIN OF INFECTION

The chain of infection consists of the microorganism, a source, a susceptible host, a portal of entry and a means of transmission.

THE MICROORGANISM

Most nosocomial infections are caused by bacteria and viruses but problems with fungi are increasingly being identified, especially in immunosuppressed patients.

The most important characteristics of the organism are:

- Pathogenicity – ability to produce disease
- Infectivity – ability to spread from person to person
- Invasiveness – ability to spread within the host
- Virulence – the severity of the illness
- Properties of adherence to synthetic materials such as implanted devices, e.g. *Staphylococcus epidermidis* adheres well to some synthetic material.

When the body's natural defences are invaded, either by a pathogenic microorganism for which the body is not immune or through invasive technology (e.g. insertion of medical devices or surgery), the risk of infection increases. When foreign material is inserted into the body, the material interacts with the host's natural defence mechanism and the risk of infection increases. The surface of the foreign body (e.g. a plastic catheter) is covered with host-derived proteins such as albumin, fibrinogen, fibronectin, collagen, laminin, vitronectin and immunoglobulins. Some of these components (e.g. albumin) may serve to retard microbial adherence, while others such as fibronectin may serve as receptors for bacteria. This complex of host and bacterial constituents is known as a biofilm (Bisno 1995). It is important that nurses are aware of different catheter materials in order that the most appropriate for the procedure may be selected to reduce the risk of infection. Considerations of availability, cost, site and length of time of insertion, and chemicals with which the material may come in contact, such as drugs or intravenous solutions, must be taken into account.

The antigenic make-up of an organism may also change through the use of antibiotics and disinfectants. Outbreaks of multiply antibiotic-resistant Gram-negative bacteria such as *Klebsiella*, *Escherichia coli* and *Pseudomonas* and Gram-positive bacteria such as methicillin-resistant *Staphylococcus aureus* (MRSA) are becoming more common in both the hospital and the community setting (Kelly & Chivers 1996, O'Brien 1997). Reports on MRSA bacteraemia in the UK indicate the problem is increasing among children less than 15 years of age (Khairulddin et al 2004).

THE SOURCE OF INFECTION

Microorganisms are carried on inanimate or animate objects from a reservoir to a source. The reservoir is the place where the organism maintains its presence, metabolises and replicates. The source is the place from which the infectious agent passes to the host either by direct or indirect contact through a vehicle as the means of transmission.

The infection may be endogenous, arising from the child's own flora, or exogenous, arising from the environment. Exogenous sources may be other children, parents, staff or visitors, animals (Cotton et al 2000), equipment or a dirty environment (Dancer 1999). The source may include:

- Those with acute disease
- Those who are not infectious

- Persons who are colonised with an infectious agent but who do not have the disease (asymptomatic carriers)
- Those who are chronic carriers of an infectious agent.

Environmental transmission of the organism may be increased through air movement and dust. The following have all been cited as environmental sources of hospital-acquired infections:

- Lack of adherence by healthcare workers to basic infection control guidelines
- Overcrowding of patient wards (Harbarth et al 1999)
- A badly maintained environment, e.g. torn chairs or mattresses, soiled curtains, cracked tiles
- Inadequate decontamination and maintenance of equipment
- Inadequate disposal of clinical and household waste
- Lack of pest control, e.g. the sighting of cockroaches, mice or rats
- Inadequate food hygiene practice
- Improper air flow
- Lack of isolation facilities.

MODE OF TRANSMISSION

Transmission may occur by one or more of six different routes.

Contact

- Direct contact as in person-to-person spread when nursing or turning a child or between two children physically playing together (e.g. scabies or antimicrobial-resistant microorganisms)
- Indirect contact such as inadequate decontamination of equipment or the environment (e.g. contaminated needles or Norovirus causing acute diarrhoea and vomiting).

Droplet

Droplets are generated by the source person during sneezing, coughing or talking and during procedures such as suctioning or bronchoscopy. Transmission occurs when small particles (>5 μm) of residue-containing organisms are propelled a short distance through the air and deposited on the host's conjunctivae, nasal mucosa or mouth. Droplets do not remain suspended in the air and therefore this should not be confused with airborne transmission. Examples of droplet infection are pertussis (whooping cough) and influenza.

Air-borne

Dissemination via this route is of either airborne droplet nuclei (small particle residue of evaporated droplets ≤5 μm in size that remain suspended in the air for long periods of time) or dust particles containing the infective organism. Organisms can be widely dispersed by air currents and inhaled by susceptible hosts either in the same room or over a further distance, therefore special air-handling and ventilation may be required to prevent airborne transmission. Varicella (chickenpox), measles virus and *Mycobacterium tuberculosis* are examples of organisms transmitted by the air-borne route.

Food-borne

This applies to organisms transmitted by contaminated items such as food, water, medications, devices and equipment (e.g. salmonella or cholera).

Vector-borne

Organisms may be carried by vectors such as flies, cockroaches, mice, rats and other vermin.

Blood-borne

This is where infection is transmitted through blood or blood products (e.g. HIV, hepatitis C).

THE HOST

Host factors that influence the development of infections are the site of deposition of the organism and the host's defence mechanism (Table 4.1).

PRECAUTIONS TO BE TAKEN

The application of source isolation or protective precautions (barrier nursing) was revised by the Communicable Disease Center in Atlanta, USA, in 1996 and the terms 'standard' precautions and 'transmission-based' precautions are now felt to be more appropriate (Garner 1996). However, within the UK, 'universal' precautions, 'source

Table 4.1   Common risk factors for infection

RISK FACTORS	REASONS
Gestational age: <32 weeks	The stratum corneum is very scant and permeable to bacteria. The skin is an effective barrier by 37 weeks' gestation
	The skin of babies born full term has a pH of 6.4 which reduces to 4.9 over a few days as the body develops its protective acid mantle, a natural antibacterial protection. This can take up to 3 weeks in pre-term infants
	Humoral defence mechanism-complement activation is only 20–40% of adult values (full-term newborn is 50–80% of adult value)
	Maternal IgG begins passing transplacentally at approximately 15 weeks' gestation but does not reach the optimum until about 33 weeks. The fetus begins to synthesise IgM at about 30 weeks' gestation
Low birth weight	Risk of infection is increased in babies weighing <1000 g and reduced in babies >2500 g
Method of nutrition	Infection occurs less in breastfed babies because of protection from maternal antibody transference
	Infection occurs more in bottle-fed babies because of lack of hygiene in equipment, preparation and storage
Umbilical cord stump	Associated with infection, especially after placement of umbilical vein catheters or delayed separation of cord
Congenital abnormalities	Such as abnormal immune function (severe combined immune deficiency, DiGeorge syndrome, Down syndrome), congenital infection (rubella, cytomegalovirus, hepatitis) or congenital cardiac or renal disease
Acquired disease processes	Other infections or chronic disease processes
Invasive devices	External devices such as intravascular, urinary, endotracheal tubes, nasogastric, gastrostomy, drainage systems. Internal devices such as ventricular atrial/peritoneal shunts, heart valves and artificial patches
Surgery	Type and length of surgery
Chemotherapy	Antibiotic therapy has been associated with *Clostridium difficile* and necrotising enterocolitis. Certain drugs such as steroids alter immunity
Length of stay in hospital	Increases the risk of colonisation/invasion with pathogenic organisms
Increased handling by hospital staff	Hands of staff have been associated with cross-infection of pathogenic organisms in hospitalised patients
Equipment	Equipment includes suction apparatus, respiratory equipment, humidifiers, feeding utensils, thermometers, pedal bins, incubators, scalp electrodes, stethoscopes, laryngoscopes, surgical instruments, communal ointments

and protective isolation' continue to be terms in widespread use. This encompasses the need to control healthcare-associated infections, which include the increasing emergence of multiple antibiotic-resistant organisms, common outbreaks of viral diarrhoeal illnesses, infections with implanted devices and the recognition of blood-borne viruses. Although local practices may vary, the principles of infection control remain the same.

Standard precautions

These precautions are designed to reduce the risk of transmission of microorganisms from both recognised and unrecognised sources of infection (Pratt et al 2007). These guidelines can be appropriately used and adapted to be practised in both hospital and the community when care may involve coming into contact with:

- Blood
- All body fluids, secretions and excretions regardless of whether they contain blood
- Non-intact skin
- Mucous membrane.

The key principles include:

- Hand hygiene before and after every episode of direct patient contact
- Regular maintenance and appropriate cleaning, disinfection or sterilisation of equipment
- Position of the patient within the ward/clinical area
- Wearing protective clothing to avoid contamination of the skin or mucosal surfaces – gloves, aprons, face protection as appropriate. The decision to wear gloves should be on the risk associated with the care being given and not worn unnecessarily
- Safe handling and disposal of sharp instruments and needles – use of needle stick prevention device to reduce incidence of sharps injuries
- Safe disposal of clinical waste

- Safe disposal of foul and infected linen
- Safe handling and transportation of specimens
- Maintaining a clean environment.

Transmission-based precautions

These precautions are designed for: (1) children known or suspected to be infected or colonised with pathogens for which additional precautions are required to interrupt transmission; this may include one or more of air-borne, droplet or contact transmission and (2) children who are immunosuppressed and require an environment with a filtered clean air system to prevent the risk of acquiring air-borne fungal infections such as *Aspergillus* (MMWR 2000).

Children who have or are suspected of having highly transmissible or epidemiological important pathogens for which additional precautions are required should preferably be isolated in a single cubicle. A risk assessment should be made to include the causative organism, the route of transmission, the need for a special environment such as a negative-pressure room or clean, filtered air and resources available. The child may need to be:

- Nursed in an individual cubicle, preferably with hand hygiene and en suite toilet facilities
- Cohorted (placed with other children) in a separate area on the ward with others who are infected/colonised with the same pathogen
- Nursed in a room with negative pressure with at least 10 exchanges of air per hour. There is usually an air-lock and the door must be kept closed (NHS Estates 2005)
- Nursed in a room with high-efficiency filtered positive air pressure. There is usually an air-lock and the door must be kept closed. This is usually reserved for severely immunosuppressed children such as those undergoing transplantation
- Nursed at home away from susceptible people if the risk factor of infection to others is felt to be high, such as small babies or those with significant immunosuppression.

HAND HYGIENE

Hand hygiene is the primary intervention for preventing and controlling healthcare-associated infections (Loveday & Pellowe 2007). The purpose of hand hygiene is to remove dirt, organic material and transient microorganisms (Gould 1991).

During daily clinical practice healthcare workers hand touch a variety of surfaces and substances, including patients intact or non-intact skin, body fluids, mucous membranes, waste and inanimate objects. In this way microorganisms can spread throughout a healthcare environment within hours (Sax et al 2007). The transmission of microorganisms can occur from one infant to another via healthcare workers. Exogenous infection to an infant is a clinical risk. Pathogens have been introduced to susceptible sites for example the lungs during mechanical ventilation, intravascular cannulation and surgical site wounds.

Epidemiological studies (Pratt et al 2001) concluded that contaminated hands are responsible for transient hand carriage especially of Gram-negative organisms which has been reported in 20–30% of hospital staff and may persist for several weeks. Sneddon's (1990) study demonstrated that Gram-negative organisms were isolated from 44% of nurses' hands before washing and from 12% after washing; 40% of hands sampled after dirty activity and 25% after clean activity were contaminated. Only 52% of the hand washes were considered good. Pittet et al (1999) reported that hand hygiene decreased with higher workload and higher-risk patients. Increasing hand hygiene frequency and effective procedure among hospital staff has been associated with a decrease in hospital-acquired infection (Pittet et al 2000).

Using the Framework of the Swiss National Hand Hygiene Development Tool and Audits, The World Health Organization's (2005) first global patient safety challenge 'Clean Care is Safer Care' developed a concept for identifying when hand hygiene should be done as well as training and performance assessment criteria. This has resulted in the concept 'Five Moments for Hand Hygiene' (National Patient Safety Agency 2008, Sax et al 2007).

In 2007, Scotland's National Hand Hygiene Campaign, 'Wash Your Hands of Them' was commenced, thus raising the importance of hand hygiene within the healthcare sector (Health Protection Scotland 2009). This has progressed to a zero-tolerance of non-compliance with hand hygiene, which was introduced in January 2009. The materials developed for this work are based on the WHO's five key moments.

Cuts and abrasions of any exposed areas of skin must be covered with a dressing that is semipermeable and an effective bacterial and viral barrier. Healthcare workers with exfoliating skin lesions must report to an occupational health department. Alcohol gel hand rubs are acceptable in hand hygiene, however, it is important to note that alcohol preparations are not effective against *Clostridium difficile* and will not remove dirt or organic matter from hands.

Requirements

- A hand basin with running warm water
- An appropriate liquid soap, surgical scrub and/or alcohol hand-rub. Alcohols effectively reduce bacterial counts on hands provided they are not visibly contaminated with proteinaceous material (body fluids, dirt, grease, etc.). Personalised alcohol hand-rubs can be attached to the individual to encourage hand decontamination during high-risk tasks or busy periods
- Disposable towels. A clean, laundered non-disposable towel can be used in the home setting
- Where the above is not possible, an alcohol rub will suffice where hands are not heavily contaminated.

Hand washing method

The correct method of hand washing is shown in Figure 4.1. Table 4.2 lists types of hand hygiene practice – the method used will depend on the type of practice to be undertaken.

Risk factors for infection

- Skin lesions, e.g. eczema, paronychia, cuts and abrasions
- Nail polish, artificial nails or long nails including nail art

1. Wet hands, apply soap and use the following procedure

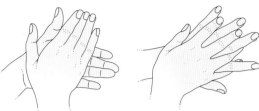

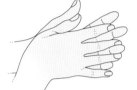

2. Rub palm to palm

3. Rub back of both hands

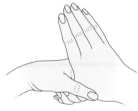

4. Rub palm to palm with fingers interlaced

5. Rub backs of fingers (interlocked)

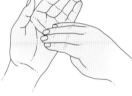

6. Rub all parts of both hands

7. Rub both palms with finger tips

7. Rinse hands under running water and dry thoroughly on a clean towel

Figure 4.1 Methods of hand washing.

- Not washing hands after removal of gloves
- Jewellery, e.g. rings, watches, bracelets. These may harbour pathogenic organisms
- Non-compliance: hand hygiene occurs in approximately half of the instances in which it is indicated

Table 4.2   Methods of hand hygiene practice

DESCRIPTION	PURPOSE	METHOD
Social hand wash	To remove soil and transient microorganisms	Liquid soap or detergent for at least 10–15 s
Hand antisepsis	To remove or destroy transient microorganisms	Antimicrobial soap or detergent or alcohol-based hand-rub for at least 10–15 s
Surgical hand-scrub	To remove or destroy transient microorganisms and reduce resident flora	Antimicrobial soap or detergent preparation with brush (sterile) to achieve friction for at least 120 s or alcohol-based preparation for at least 20 s

- Communal hand lotion
- Cloth hand towels in an institutional setting
- Large reusable containers and 'topping up' antiseptics and liquid soap
- Communal bar soap
- Alcohol hand-rub is not as effective in the presence of physical dirt
- Moisturising agents and surfactants may interfere with the residual activity of chlorhexidine
- Lack of sufficient hand hygiene facilities
- Waste pedal bins with broken lids which have to be opened with the hand.

PROTECTIVE CLOTHING

The primary use of personal protective equipment (PPE) is to offer protection to the healthcare workers and reduce the likelihood for transmission of microorganisms. Personal protective equipment must be made available for all healthcare workers. The decision to use PPE should be based upon a risk assessment of the task to be performed (Fig. 4.2) in order that the correct protective clothing may be worn. The assessment may differ between parents and healthcare workers who are more exposed to a variety of pathogens during their duties. However, risk factors in association with blood-borne viruses such as HIV, hepatitis B or C, for example, may be the same. The increasing recognition of latex allergy in both patients and healthcare workers must be taken into consideration (Markey 1994, Johnson 1997). Manufacturers

are being asked to minimise or abolish the use of latex in medical equipment and consumables.

Any blood or body secretions/excretions may contain microbial pathogens and must be handled as potentially infectious. In young children, especially in the nappy-wearing age, the bowel flora is commonly distributed over the skin and in the upper respiratory tract.

Gloves are the most commonly used PPE, these should not be worn unnecessarily as prolonged and inappropriate use may cause allergic skin reaction and sensitivities.

Disposable gloves

- Gloves provide added protection when the risk of microbial contamination is increased such as during nappy changing or when handling contaminated material as in specimen collection
- Non-sterile gloves must be worn for direct contact with blood or body fluids, non-intact skin and mucous membrane
- Wear gloves for all care if intact skin is a source of contamination, such as when the child is colonised with multiple antibiotic-resistant organisms. Certain pathogens such as *Klebsiella* have increased adherence properties to the skin and may be found on the hands after social hand hygiene (Casewell & Phillips 1977)
- Gloves should be disposable and discarded between patients or contaminated body sites
- Hands have become contaminated even when wearing gloves and therefore a soap and water hand wash or alcohol hand-rub is recommended after removal of gloves
- Wear gloves when handling disinfectants or cleaning.

Risks factors for infection

- Quality of gloves: leakage has been reported in 4–63% of vinyl gloves and 3–52% of latex gloves (Korniewicz et al 1989)
- Petroleum-based or oil emollients may affect the integrity of latex
- Dermatitis due to allergy to latex or glove powder
- Not removing stoned rings, watches and jewellery before hand hygiene.

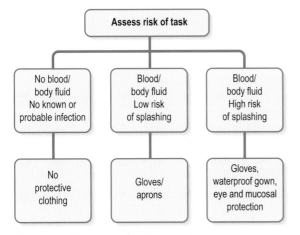

Figure 4.2 Risk assessment for protective clothing.

Plastic aprons

Cotton gowns offer minimal microbial protection (Donowitz 1986) and therefore should be replaced with single-use disposable plastic aprons. Hands must be washed after removal of the apron. Aprons should be changed between clean and dirty tasks and should be worn for:

- All patient care
- Aseptic technique
- Serving meals and feeding patients
- Performing dirty tasks
- Bed-making.

Facial protection

Masks, eye protection and face shields should be worn to protect mucous membranes of the eyes, nose and mouth during procedures and patient care activities which are likely to generate splashes, sprays or aerosols of blood, body fluids and secretions or excretions.

Masks may also be worn to protect the healthcare workers from droplet or air-borne infectious diseases. There are different size filters in masks and the appropriate one must be chosen for the correct protection. There are filter face pieces (FFP) class 1 (low efficiency), 2 (medium efficiency) and 3 (high efficiency). For example, a FFP 3 filtered mask should be worn when dealing with patients with diseases such as SARS, Swine Flu and in a Pandemic Flu situation. The Health and Safety Executive (2003) describes fit testing of respiratory protective equipment face pieces. Fit testing focuses on ensuring adequate suction to ensure that the healthcare workers when wearing the mask will not be exposed to droplet or air-borne infection when caring for infected children.

Surgical masks are worn in theatre to protect the patient against large particle droplets from the surgical team immediately over the operation site (Belkin 1997). More research is required as to the risk of infection to the patient from members of the circulating theatre team, especially during prolonged surgery where the risk may be higher.

FACTORS TO NOTE

- Compliance with wearing the protective device correctly
- Type of filter in mask

- Procedures which generate aerosols, e.g. bronchoscopy or suctioning
- Risk of splattering of blood or other body fluids
- Open pulmonary tuberculosis and multiply antibiotic-resistant tuberculosis (MRTB)
- Risk to and from the child and healthcare worker (HCW).

Protective gowns and headwear

These should not only be made of appropriate material to minimise 'strike through' or leakage of blood and body fluids, but also be comfortable to the wearer. Hair should be covered by the hood/hat. They should be available where the risk of contamination with blood and body fluids is increased such as in the operating theatre, intensive care or accident and emergency units.

Foot protection

Contamination of the feet with blood/body fluids will be minimised if boots/theatre shoes are worn in high-risk areas such as the operating theatre, intensive care or accident and emergency units. Theatre footwear should not be worn outside the theatre complex. Overshoes have not been shown to reduce infection and may indeed increase the risk by contaminating hands on application or removal.

WASTE DISPOSAL

Health Technical Memorandum (HTM) 07–01 *Safe Management of Healthcare Waste* (DoH 2006a) replaces the Health Services Advisory Committee's (1999) guidance document *Safe Disposal of Clinical Waste*. This document has been produced to provide a framework for best practice in waste management to help healthcare organisations and other producers of waste to meet legislative requirements. The advice in this document and any recommended courses of action are not mandatory, but healthcare organisations and others choosing not to follow them are advised that it is essential that alternative steps be taken to comply with all relevant legislation.

Key changes from *Safe Disposal of Clinical Waste* (1999) in the new HTM include:

- The definition and classification of infectious waste
- The definition and classification of medicinal waste

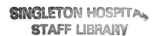

Table 4.3 Colour-coding of waste management	
COLOUR	DESCRIPTION
Yellow stream	Infectious waste which requires disposal by incineration
Orange stream	Infectious waste which may be treated to render it safe prior to disposal, or alternatively can be incinerated
Purple stream	Cytotoxic and cytostatic waste which must be incinerated in a permitted or licensed facility
Yellow/Black stream	Offensive/hygiene waste which may be land filled in a permitted or licensed site
Black stream	Domestic waste which does not contain infectious materials, sharps or medicinal products and may be land filled in a permitted or licensed site. Recyclable components should be removed through segregation. Clear or opaque receptacles can also be used for domestic waste

From: DoH (2006a).

- Changes in transport legislation
- A revised colour-code (Table 4.3)
- And packaging system
- The use of European waste catalogue (EWC) codes
- The classification of microbiological cultures for carriage and disposal.

All potentially infectious waste and autoclaved laboratory clinical waste must be placed into orange clinical sacks. The sack must be secured and the source area identified, i.e. the responsible local health authority (check local policy for hospitals and the community), before it is removed from the premises to a licensed treatment facility. Domestic waste including general refuse, i.e. confectionery and flower products must be placed in a black or clear waste bag, secured and sourced before removal to landfill.

Sharps

Sharps must not be passed directly from hand-to-hand and handling should be kept to a minimum. Needles must not be recapped, bent, broken or disassembled before use. All used sharps, needles, blades and other sharp instruments must be discarded into a sharps container conforming to UN3291 and BS7320 standards at the point of user/care contact. The sharps containers must not be filled above the mark which identifies the container is full. Discard needles and syringe as one unit into the sharps container. Do not re-sheath contaminated needles as this increases the risk of injury (Jagger et al 1990). Consider the use of needlestick prevention devices as they provide a safe system of work for healthcare workers (Loveday & Pellowe 2007). All sharps containers should be secured and placed out of reach of children at a height which enables healthcare workers safe disposal.

Risk factors for infection

- Re-sheathing needles
- Breaking the hub of the needle to take blood from neonates
- Leaving sharps lying around and not disposing of them immediately into a sharps bin
- Overfilling sharps bins or clinical waste bags
- Handing sharp instruments to another person instead of laying them down safely so that they can be picked up, especially in the operating theatre where the risk of injury may be increased
- Leaving contaminated waste unbagged or available to the public, which may encourage pests and indiscriminate searching for hypodermic needles.

Disposal of infected linen

Local policies for the handling of laundry must be followed (DoH 1995). Foul and infected linen should be segregated and placed in a red water-soluble bag contained in an outer bag and labelled 'danger of infection' as per hospital/local policy.

Soiled linen may also be contaminated with pathogenic microorganisms and should be placed directly into appropriate laundry containers. Baby clothes, blankets, etc. should be laundered centrally in an institution. If performed at a local level, a separate room with adequately maintained washing and drying facilities must be available.

Risk factors for infection

- Washing baby clothes in the kitchen or dirty utility room in an institution
- Not maintaining adequate washing temperatures for disinfection (70–71°C for at least 3 min or 65°C for 10 min)

- Inadequate maintenance of washing/drying machines
- Transporting dirty linen on the same trolley as that used for transporting and serving food
- Storing clean linen in unhygienic conditions.

EATING UTENSILS SUCH AS DISHES, CUPS, GLASSES, BABY BOTTLES

Eating utensils carry a risk of transmitting infection.

FACTORS TO NOTE

- All feeding utensils should be washed in a well-maintained dishwasher. They should be placed in the dishwasher immediately after use and not left lying around
- Where dishwashers are not available, feeding utensils should be thoroughly washed in hot water and detergent, rinsed in hot water and dried
- Baby feeding bottles and equipment should be washed in a well-maintained dishwasher or a commercial steam steriliser. It is not necessary to sterilise them in an autoclave in hospital
- Feeding utensils for severely immunosuppressed children, such as those undergoing transplantation, should be washed in a dishwasher, thoroughly dried and stored separately. Sterilisation by autoclave is not considered necessary
- Where a heat process is not available, baby bottles and feeding equipment should be thoroughly cleaned before immersion in a chemical sterilant such as hypochlorite or dichloroisocyanurate for the recommended time and stored in a clean container afterwards
- Equipment for expressing breast milk should be sterile and single use, and breast pumps should be decontaminated and maintained regularly
- It is not considered necessary to use disposable utensils if the above facilities are available.

Risk factors for infection

Food poisoning microorganisms and *Candida* can be associated with poor hygiene and the inadequate decontamination of teats and dummies.

THE USE OF DISINFECTANTS IN THE ENVIRONMENT AND WITH EQUIPMENT

The NHS Healthcare Cleaning Manual (DoH 2004b), supports the 'Standards of Cleanliness in the NHS' (NHS Estates 2003) and is intended to support existing trust policies and procedures associated with cleaning, health and safety and infection control.

Cleaning must always be undertaken before disinfection or sterilisation. The following definitions (Ayliffe et al 1993, Wilson 2002) are used to standardise different methods of decontamination.

Sterilisation

A process used to render an object free from all living organisms.

Disinfection

A process used to reduce the number of microorganisms but not usually of bacterial spores. The process does not necessarily kill or remove all microorganisms but reduces the number to a level which is not harmful to health.

Cleaning

A process that removes contaminants including dust, soil, large numbers of microorganisms and the organic matter (e.g. faeces, blood) that protects the organisms. Cleaning is always necessary before sterilisation or the use of disinfectants.

The risks to patients from the environment and equipment may be classified as follows:

- High risk: items in close contact with a break in the skin or mucous membrane or introduced into a normally sterile body area should be *sterile*
- Intermediate risk: items in contact with mucous membrane or other items contaminated with particularly virulent or readily transmissible organisms, or items to be used on highly susceptible patients should be *disinfected*
- Low risk: items in contact with normal and intact skin should be *cleaned* and dried.

Advice on the use of disinfectants should be followed (Rutala 1996, Ayliffe et al 1993) and local policies adhered to. The use of disinfectants in the paediatric setting should be kept to a minimum to ensure safety. Care must be taken to keep them locked away out of reach of children.

Hot water and detergent with thorough drying is considered adequate for most environmental cleaning. The environment must be kept clean and a high standard of housekeeping maintained. However, studies have shown that viruses (e.g. Noroviruses, including Rotavirus) causing diarrhoea can remain viable on inanimate surfaces for several days (Satter et al 1994). Touching contaminated surfaces can transfer infectious viruses to the hands and aid spread. Chlorine-based agents are an effective disinfectant against these viruses.

FACTORS TO NOTE

- Equipment must be cleaned with hot water and detergent before sterilisation or disinfection. Always follow manufacturers' instructions regarding decontamination. Chemicals may react adversely on some materials, for example alcohol will produce opaqueness on Perspex material or hypochlorites may rust metals. Always refer to the manufacturers cleaning guidance.
- Always use moist heat sterilisation and heat disinfection where possible. Some materials are heat labile and chemical sterilisation or disinfection may need to be used, such as with endoscopic equipment. Outbreaks of infection with contaminated endoscopes are not uncommon and appropriate guidelines must be followed. Equipment may require to be sent to a local decontamination unit or centre.
- A risk assessment to the child and healthcare worker must be made with any chemical used in accordance with the Control of Substances Hazardous to Health (COSHH) Regulations.
- The use of phenolic disinfectants has been associated with neonatal hyperbilirubinaemia (Wysowski et al 1978).
- Care must be taken with hypochlorite disinfectants on urine spillages as they can create toxic fumes.
- Hypochlorite disinfectant is used for:
  - 1.0% (10 000 ppm available chlorine) – disinfection of heavy spillages of blood
  - 0.1% (1000 ppm available chlorine) – general cleaning when disinfection is required
  - 0.0125% (125 ppm available chlorine) – disinfecting babies' bottles, teats, dummies.

- Walls should be cleaned if visibly dirty.
- After cleaning a room which has housed a child with an infection, it is unnecessary to leave it to air for a set period of time.

Risk factors for infection

- Not cleaning equipment before using chemical disinfection. Many disinfectants are inactivated in the presence of organic matter such as blood, dirt or grease
- 'Topping up' bottles of disinfectant or antiseptics
- Not making up fresh solutions or using the correct dilution
- Hypochlorite solutions are unstable and must be renewed every 24 h
- Mixing incompatible chemicals
- A poorly maintained environment encourages infestation and inhibits adequate cleaning.

EQUIPMENT

It is preferable that all equipment is cleaned and maintained in a central unit where documentation and quality control can be monitored. Manufacturing guidelines must be followed according to the type of equipment and level of decontamination required, e.g. sterilisation, disinfection or cleaning (Fuller 1992). The Medicines and Healthcare products Regulatory Agency (MHRA) is the government agency which is responsible for ensuring that medicines and medical devices work, and are acceptably safe.

FACTORS TO NOTE

- Equipment must be decontaminated before service or repair (see MHRA Decontamination and Sterilisation Microbiology Advisory Committee)
- Single-use items must not be reused unless the health authority have in place an adequate quality assurance programme and accept liability (see MHRA)
- Equipment such as wooden spatulas which have been used as splints for intravenous cannulation sites, a purpose for which they were not designed, consequently cause serious fungal infection (Holzel et al 1998).

Risk factors for infection

- Torn mattresses, pillow covers and chairs causing difficulty in cleaning
- Poorly maintained equipment such as suction apparatus, breast pumps or blood gas machines
- Inadequately cleaned equipment such as urine- or stool-testing equipment, thermometers, laryngoscopes, incubators and respiratory ventilators/humidifiers.

OCCUPATIONAL HEALTH

All healthcare workers should have access to an occupational health department and should report:

- For a pre-employment health review and to be advised on immunisations and relevant immunity status such as after vaccination against hepatitis B. A small percentage of people do not produce antibodies to some immunisations and therefore remain susceptible to the disease (Salisbury & Begg 1996, www.dh. gov.uk). If they are doing exposure-prone procedures (EPP) then they must provide evidence that they are not carrying the hepatitis B or C virus (DoH 2002b)
- If they have not had varicella (chickenpox), a varicella vaccine is available to HCWs
- If on immunosuppressive therapy or pregnant, when appropriate advice to reduce the risk of infection can be given (Advisory Committee on Dangerous Pathogens 1997)
- If they have suffered from an infectious disease and have been at work or wish to return to work
- If they feel that they are likely to be or are infected with a blood-borne virus such as human immunodeficiency virus, hepatitis B or C and are performing exposure-prone procedures during their work (NHSME 1993) and Addendum (DoH 1996, RCN 1997)
- For all accidents, including those involving:
  - Sharps injuries or contamination of mucosal surfaces of the eyes, nose or mouth with blood or body fluids
  - Blood or body fluids on non-intact skin (guidance on HIV post-exposure prophylaxis (DoH 2004a) must be followed)
- When allergic reactions occur such as with latex or chemicals.

Risk factors for infection

- Not adhering to hand hygiene procedures
- Not wearing recommended protective clothing
- Working with exfoliating skin lesions or uncovered broken skin
- Working with children who have certain infectious diseases such as chickenpox and not being immune
- Not being protected from infectious diseases where immunisation is available
- Travelling abroad and not taking healthcare advice
- Not reporting when you have an infectious disease or an infected skin lesion.

SURVEILLANCE OF INFECTION AND AUDITING PRACTICE

Surveillance of infection and ongoing audit of hospital-acquired infection should be seen as a collaborative multidisciplinary activity undertaking between the infection control team, clinical staff and managers (DoH 2003b).

Documentation of increased risk factors, such as insertion and removal of devices including intravascular and urinary catheters, respiratory intubation or any invasive procedure, must be maintained (DoH 2003b). Surveillance methods vary and should be discussed with the local infection control team.

The role of the nurse as a health educator can be of particular importance to the child and family when explaining about infectious diseases. Nurses must feel confident in their knowledge and be able to individualise care safely and explain basic hygiene precautions. Children and their families should have a right to expect that their health will be protected as well as promoted when receiving healthcare services.

The Scottish Surveillance of Healthcare-associated Infection Programme (SSHAIP) also outlines associated epidemiological data (see www.show. scot.nhs.uk/scieh).

The Health Protection Agency has a steering group on healthcare-associated infections (see www.hpa.org.uk).

References

Ayliffe, G.A.J., Coates, D., Hoffman, P.N., 1993. Chemical disinfection in hospitals, second ed. Public Health Laboratory Service, London.

Belkin, N.L., 1997. The evolution of the surgical mask: filtering efficiency versus effectiveness. Infect. Control Hosp. Epidemiol. 18, 49–57.

Bisno, A.L., 1995. Molecular aspects of bacterial colonisation. Infect. Control Hosp. Epidemiol. 16, 648–657.

Boyce, J.M., Pittet, D., 2002. Guidelines for hand hygiene in health-care settings: recommendations of the Healthcare Infection Control Practitioners Advisory Committee and the HICPAC/SHEA/APIC/IDSA Hygiene Task-force. MMWR Morb. Mortal. Wkly. Rep. 51 (RR16), 1–44.

Casewell, M., Phillips, I., 1977. Hands as a route of transmission for Klebsiella species. Br. Med. J. 2 (6098), 1315–1317.

Cotton, M.F., Wasserman, E., Pieper, C. H., et al., 2000. Invasive disease due to extended spectrum beta-lactamase-producing Klebsiella pneumoniae in a neonatal unit: the possible role of cockroaches. J. Hosp. Infect. 44, 13–17.

Department of Health HSG (95)18, 1995. Hospital laundry arrangements for used and infected linen. DoH, London.

Department of Health, 1996. Addendum to HSG (93)40: Protecting healthcare workers and patients from hepatitis B. DoH, Wetherby.

Department of Health, 2002a. Getting ahead of the curve: a strategy for combating infectious diseases. A report by the Chief Medical Officer. DoH, London.

Department of Health, 2002b. Hepatitis C infected healthcare workers. DoH, London.

Department of Health, 2003a. Controls assurance standard. Infection control. Online. Available: www.dh.gov.uk; search for Controls Assurance.

Department of Health, 2003b. Winning ways: working together to reduce healthcare-associated infection in England. A report by the Chief Medical Officer. DoH, London.

Department of Health, 2004a. HIV post-exposure prophylaxis: guidance from the UK Chief Medical Officer's Expert Advisory Group on AIDS. DoH, London.

Department of Health, 2004b. The NHS healthcare cleaning manual. Online. Available: www.dh.gov/publications.

Department of Health, 2006a. Health Technical Memorandum 07–01: Safe management of healthcare waste. Online. Available: www.tsoshop.co.uk.

Department of Health, 2006b. Sterilisation, disinfection and cleaning of medical equipment: Guidance on decontamination from the Microbiology Advisory Committee to Department of Health. Online. Available: www.mhra.gov.uk/Publications/Safetyguidance/Otherdevicesafetyguidance.

Department of Health, 2006c. The Healthcare Act. Code of Practice for Prevention and Control of Healthcare-associated Infections. Online. Available: www.dh.gov/publications.

Department of Health, 2007. Saving lives: Reducing infection, delivering clean safe care, revised edition. Online. Available: www.clean-safe-care.nhs.uk.

Donowitz, L.G., 1986. Failure of the overgown to prevent nosocomial infection in a paediatric intensive care unit. Pediatrics 77, 35–38.

Fuller, A., 1992. Sterilising instruments. Journal of Infection Control Nursing, Nursing Times 88 (50), 64–65.

Garner, J.S., 1996. Guidelines for isolation precautions in hospitals. Am. J. Infect. Control 24, 24–52.

Gould, D., 1991. Nurses' hands as vectors of hospital-acquired infection: a review. J. Adv. Nurs. 16, 1216–1225.

Harbarth, S., Sudre, P., Dharan, S., et al., 1999. Outbreak of Enterobacter cloacae related to understaffing, overcrowding and poor hygiene practices. Infect. Control Hosp. Epidemiol. 20 (9), 598–603.

Health and Safety Executive, 2003. OC 282/28. HSE, London.

Health Protection Scotland, 2009. Wash your hands of them. Online. Available: http://www.washyourhandsofthem.com (Accessed 26 June 2009).

Health Protection Scotland, 2007. NHS Scotland National HAI Prevalence Survey, vols. 1 and 2. Final report. HPS, Edinburgh.

Health Service Advisory Committee, 1999. Safe disposal of clinical waste. DoH, London.

HMSO, 1988. Public Health (Infectious Disease) Regulations (SI 1988:1546). HMSO, London.

Holzel, H.H., MacQueen, S., MacDonald, A., et al., 1998. Rhizopus microsporus: a major threat or minor inconvenience? J. Hosp. Infect. 38, 113–118.

Jagger, J., Hunt, E.H., Pearson, R.D., 1990. Sharp object injuries in the hospital: causes and strategies for prevention. Am. J Infect. Control. 18, 227–231.

Johnson, G., 1997. Time to take the gloves off. Occup. Health (Auckl) 49, 25–28.

Kelly, J., Chivers, G., 1996. Built-in resistance. Journal of Infection Control Nursing, Nursing Times 92 (2), 50–54.

Khairulddin, N., Bishop, L., Lamagni, T.L., et al., 2004. Emergence of methicillin resistant Staphylococcus aureus (MRSA) bacteraemia among children in England and Wales, 1990–2001. Arch. Dis. Child 89, 378–379.

Korniewicz, D.M., Laughton, B.E., Butz, E., Larson, E., 1989. Integrity of vinyl and latex procedure gloves. Nurs. Res 38 (3), 144–146.

Leading better care, 2008. Report of the senior charge nurse review and clinical quality indicators project. The Scottish Executive, Edinburgh.

Loveday, H.P., Pellowe, C.M., 2007. epic2: Updating Department of Health guidelines for preventing healthcare-associated infections. Infant 3 (2), 15–20.

Macqueen, S., 1995. Anthropology and germ theory. J. Hosp. Infect. 30 (Suppl.), 116–126.

Markey, J., 1994. Latex allergy: implications for healthcare personnel and infusion therapy patients. J. Intraven. Nurs. 17 (1), 35–39.

MMWR, 2000. Guidelines for Preventing Opportunistic Infections among Hematopoietic Stem Cells. Transplant recipients: recommendations of CDC, The Infectious Disease Society of America and The American Society of Bone and Marrow Transplantation 2000/49 (RRIO), 1–128. Online. Available: www.cdc.gov/mmwr.

National Audit Office, 2004. The management and control of healthcare-associated infections in acute NHS Trusts in England. The Stationery Office, London.

National Health Service Management Executive (NHSME), 1993. Protecting healthcare workers and patients from hepatitis B. HSG (93)40. DoH, London.

NHS Estates, 2003. Standards of cleanliness in the NHS: a framework in which to measure performance outcomes. NHS Estates, Leeds.

NHS Estates, 2004a. A matron's charter: an action plan for cleaner hospitals. Online. Available: www.nhsestates.gov.uk.

NHS Estates, 2004b. The NHS Healthcare Cleaning Manual. Online. Available: www.nhsestates.gov.uk.

NHS Estates, 2005. HBN supplement 1: Isolation facilities in acute settings. Online. Available: www.nhsestates.gov.uk.

NHS QIS, 2001. Standards for healthcare-associated infection (HAI). Infection Control. NHS Quality Improvement Scotland, Edinburgh.

NHS QIS, 2008. Standards. Healthcare-associated infection (HAI), March. NHS QIS, Edinburgh.

National Patient Safety Agency, 2008. My five moments of hand hygiene/clean your hands campaign. Online. Available: www.npsa.nhs.uk/cleanyourhands.

O'Brien, T.F., 1997. The global epidemic nature of antimicrobial resistance and the need to monitor and manage it locally. Clin. Infect. Dis. 24 (Suppl. 1), S2–S8.

Pellowe, C.M., Pratt, R.J., Harper, P., et al., 2003. Infection control: prevention of healthcare-associated infection in primary and community care. J. Hosp. Infect. 55 (Suppl. 2), S1–127. Online. Available: www.richardwellsresearch.com.

Pittet, D., Mourouga, P., Pernege, T.V., 1999. Compliance with hand washing in a teaching hospital. The members of the Infection Control Programme. Ann. Intern. Med. 130, 126–130.

Pittet, D., Hugonnet, S., Harbarth, S., et al., 2000. Effectiveness of a hospital-wide programme to improve compliance with hand hygiene. Lancet 356, 1307–1312.

Pratt, R.J., Pellowe, C., Loveday, H.P., et al., 2001. The epic project: developing national evidence-based guidelines for preventing healthcare-associated infections. Phase 1: guidelines for preventing hospital-acquired infections. J. Hosp. Infect. 47 (Suppl.), S1–S82. Online. Available: www.richardwellsresearch.com.

Pratt, R.J., Pellowe, C., Wilson, J.A., et al., 2007. epic2: National evidence-based guidelines for preventing healthcare-associated infections in NHS hospitals in England. J. Hosp. Infect. 65 (Suppl. 1), S1–S64.

The Public Health Disease Regulations 1988, Statutory Instrument No: 1546 available online www.tsoshop.co.uk, ISBN01108754.

Royal College of Nursing, 1997. Hepatitis guidelines. RCN, London.

Rutala, W.A., 1996. APIC guidelines for selection and use of disinfectants. Am. J. Infect. Control 24, 313–342.

Salisbury, D.M., Begg, N., 1996. Immunisation against infectious diseases. HMSO, London. Online. Available: www.dh.gov.uk.

Satter, S.Y., Jacobson, H., Rahman, H., et al., 1994. Interruption of rotavirus spread through chemical disinfection. Infect. Control Hosp. Epidemiol. 15, 751–756.

Sax, H., Allegran, B., Uckay, A., et al., 2007. My five moments for hand hygiene: a user-centred design approach to understand, train, monitor and report hand hygiene. J. Infect. Control 67, 9–21.

Sneddon, J.G., 1990. A preventable course of infection: carriage of Gram-negative bacilli on hands. Prof. Nurse 6 (2), 98–104.

Thames Valley University, 2003. Infection control: prevention of healthcare-associated infection in primary and community care. Clinical guidelines 2. National

Institute for Clinical Excellence, London.

Wilson, J., 2002. Infection control in clinical practice. Baillière Tindall, London.

World Health Organization, 2005. Clean care is safer care. WHO, Geneva.

Wysowski, D.M., Flynt Jr., J.W., Goldfield, M., et al., 1978. Epidemic neonatal hyperbilirubinaemia and the use of phenolic disinfection. Paediatrics 16 (2), 165–170.

Further reading

Advisory Committee on Dangerous Pathogens, 1997. Infection risks to new and expectant mothers in the workplace. HSE, London.

Advisory Committee on Dangerous Pathogens, 2003. Transmissible spongiform encephalopathy agents: safe working and the prevention of infection. Online. Available: www.advisorybodies. doh.gov.uk/acdp/publications. htm.

Association for Professionals in Infection Control and Epidemiology (APIC), 1995. APIC guideline for hand-washing and antisepsis in healthcare settings. Am. J. Infect. Control 23, 251–269.

Auditor General, 2000. A clean bill of health? A review of domestic services in Scottish hospitals. TSO, Edinburgh.

Boucher, I., 1998. Third report of group of experts. Cryptosporidium in water supply. TSO, London.

British Medical Association (BMA), 1990. A code of practice for the safe use and disposal of sharps. BMA, London.

Dancer, S.J., 1999. Mopping up hospital hygiene. J. Hosp. Infect. 43, 85–100.

Department of Health, 2000. The management and control of hospital infection. The UK Antimicrobial Strategy and Action Plan. HSC 2000/002. DoH, London.

Department of Health, 2002. Hepatitis C: Strategy for England. DoH, London.

Department of Health, 2002. Guidelines for renal dialysis transplantation units: prevention and control of blood-borne virus infections. DoH, London.

Department of Health, 2005. Saving lives: a delivery programme to reduce healthcare-associated infection including MRSA. Online. Available: www.dh.gov.uk.

Drews, M.B., Ludwig, A.C., Leititis, J.U., Daschner, F.D., 1995. Low birthweight and nosocomial infection of neonates in a neonatal intensive care unit. J. Hosp. Infect. 30, 65–72.

Emmerson, A.M., Enstone, J.E., Griffin, M., et al., 1996. The second national prevalence survey of infection in hospitals – overview of the results. J. Hosp. Infect. 32, 157–190.

Glenister, H.M., Taylor, L.J., Bartlett, C.L.R., et al., 1993. An evaluation of surveillance methods for detecting infections in hospital inpatients. J. Hosp. Infect. 23, 229–242.

Haley, R.W., Culver, D.H., White, J.W., 1985. The efficacy of infection surveillance and control programs in preventing nosocomial infections in university hospitals (SENIC study). Am. J. Epidemiol. 121, 182–205.

Hunter, P.R., 1991. Application of hazard analysis critical control point (HACCP) to the handling of expressed breast milk on a neonatal unit. J. Hosp. Infect. 17, 139–146.

Macqueen, S., 1996. Think globally, act locally: germ invasion and risk analysis. Journal of Neonatal Nursing 2 (1), 20–25.

Medical Devices Agency (MDA), 2000. Single-use medical devices: implications and consequences of reuse. MDA DB2000 (04). MDA, London.

Medical Devices Agency (MDA), 2001. Safe use and disposal of sharps. MDA SN 2001 (19). MDA, London.

Millward, S., Barnett, J., Thomlinson, D.A., 1993. A clinical infection control audit programme: evaluation of an audit tool used by infection control nurses to monitor standards and assess effective staff training. J. Hosp. Infect. 24, 219–232.

NHS Executive, 2000. The management and control of hospital infection. HSC 2000/002. NHSE, London.

NHS Quality Improvement Scotland (QIS), 2002. Healthcare-associated infection (HAI): cleaning service standards. NHS Quality Improvement Scotland, Edinburgh.

Pasquarella, C., Pitzurra, O., Savino, A., 2000. The index of microbial air contamination. J. Hosp. Infect. 46, 241–256.

Scottish Office Department of Health, 1999. Hospital acquired infection. A framework for a national system of surveillance in Scotland. TSO, Edinburgh.

Teare, E.L., Peacock, A., 1996. The development of an infection control link-nurse programme in a district general hospital. J. Hosp. Infect. 34, 267–278.

Chapter 5

Complementary therapies

Julia Fearon

CHAPTER CONTENTS

Introduction   57

Defining complementary therapy   57

Prevalence of complementary therapies
in children's care   57

Potential benefits and possible disadvantages
of therapies   58

Minimising the risks and disadvantages   59

Models of complementary therapy
provision   59
   Who should provide therapies?   59
   Consent   59

A brief explanation of the therapies   60
   Aromatherapy   60
   Therapeutic massage   61
   Reflexology/reflex zone therapy   61
   Visualisation and guided imagery   61
   Hypnotherapy   62
   Homeopathy   62

The 'clinical' environment   62

Conclusion   62

INTRODUCTION

This appendix will define and give a broad overview of the most commonly used, useful and researched therapies in children's care. The potential benefits and aims of complementary therapy integration will be discussed, as well as possible disadvantages. Questions concerning models of delivery and consent will also be considered.

DEFINING COMPLEMENTARY THERAPY

In the 1990s, the term complementary and alternative medicine (CAM) was widely used. As complementary therapy integration into orthodox medicine becomes more widespread, there is a move to re-badge the field as 'complementary and integrated medicine' (CIM) (Rankin-Box 2005). Within the context of nursing care, the term 'complementary therapies' (CTs) is preferred, implying that the most appropriate form of integration is for therapies to be an adjunct, not alternative, to conventional care. One of the most widely used definitions of complementary medicine is that from the House of Lords (2000):

> ... a diverse group of health-related therapies and disciplines which are not considered to be part of mainstream medical care.

PREVALENCE OF COMPLEMENTARY THERAPIES IN CHILDREN'S CARE

Complementary medicine continues to increase in popularity among the UK general population (Ernst & White 2000, Hollinghurst et al 2008, Ritchie

BOX 5.1   Reported complementary therapies
utilised by children

- Acupuncture (Corydon Hammond 2003, Robinson et al 2008)
- Aromatherapy (Crawford et al 2006, Scrace 2003, Robinson et al 2008)
- Guided imagery/visualisation (Kashikar-Zuck 2006, Jones & Weisenfluh 2003)
- Herbal remedies/nutritional/vitamin supplements (Crawford et al 2006, Robinson et al 2008, Simpson & Roman 2001)
- Homeopathy (Robinson et al 2008, Simpson & Roman 2001)
- Hypnotherapy (Liossi et al 2006, Richardson et al 2006)
- Massage including infant/baby massage (Barlow et al 2007, Hart et al 2003, Zealey 2005)
- Reflexology (Bishop et al 2003)

2007) and orthodox healthcare is now seeing greater integration of complementary therapies (Prince of Wales's Foundation for Integrated Health 2003). Unsurprisingly, the literature relating specifically to children is scarce and primarily from overseas, but it would appear that children and families are also using complementary medicine (Box 5.1). Therapies are commonly used for chronic illnesses, where orthodox medicine has only limited success in offering sustained relief or has unpleasant side-effects such as those for musculoskeletal disorders, skin, oncological and respiratory disease (Lueng & Verhoef 2008, Loman 2003, Robinson et al 2008, Sencer & Kelly 2007, Shaw et al 2008, Simpson & Roman 2001). It is apparent also that children and families value complementary medicine for the psychological support it can provide (Barlow et al 2007, Buckle 2003, Fearon 2003).

The debate around the quantity and quality of complementary research is ongoing. Complementary therapies present particular difficulties for traditional research methods. For most complementary therapy, there is no standardised treatment protocol. Every patient is treated individually every time with potentially different prescriptions, therefore the orthodox 'gold standard' of the double blind randomised control trial is simply not possible. Despite being hampered by lack of funding and fierce competition with orthodox medicine for existing funding, considerable time and effort is being invested into developing rigorous quality research methods appropriate for the field.

POTENTIAL BENEFITS AND POSSIBLE DISADVANTAGES OF THERAPIES

Box 5.2 outlines the potential benefits of complementary therapies for children. Although there are many perceived benefits of therapies for children, there are also some possible disadvantages. For example, many families do not disclose the use of therapies to conventional healthcare professionals – over 50% of parents 'don't tell' (Robinson et al 2008). This may be cause for concern about adverse reactions from their healthcare professionals to their choice of complementary treatment or simply that it does not occur to them to mention it and their conventional healthcare team never ask about therapy use. Parents may also self-medicate their children with over the counter (OTC) remedies rather than consult a trained therapist. Robinson et al (2008) found that over 80% of the London study population bought OTC remedies. Such treatments can bring the risk of toxicity, adverse reactions and interactions with conventional drugs. Occasionally, unscrupulous complementary practitioners have taken advantage of vulnerable families. Ramsay et al (2003) tested 24 samples of a herbal cream supplied to families by a Chinese herbalist. Of these, 22 illegally contained potent corticosteroids. Some alternative (as opposed to complementary) practitioners may advocate that parents cease conventional medication in favour of alternative approaches and there is a risk that parents may 'force' unpalatable complementary medications/diets onto their children. Cost is also a potential disadvantage of a complementary approach, as many such treatments are not widely available on the NHS.

BOX 5.2   Complementary therapies for children: potential benefits

- May offer additional or more effective symptom management for acute, chronic and terminal conditions
- Helps reduce anxiety and fear
- Encourages fun and distraction
- May help reduce the need for conventional treatments with unwanted side-effects
- Child and family empowerment → helps with better compliance with conventional treatments
- The empowered child can better realise their own healing potential.

MINIMISING THE RISKS AND DISADVANTAGES

It is possible to take steps to reduce the risks. For example:

- Establish if complementary treatment is something your patients are considering or actually doing
- Encourage open and honest discussion about therapies with children and families
- Have a basic understanding of what the therapy options are
- Signpost families to sources of reliable information.

A programme of voluntary self-regulation among those complementary therapies not yet regulated by statute is progressing well, part-funded by the department of health and led by The Prince's Foundation for Integrated Health (www.fih.org. uk). This should reduce some of the issues around identifying a properly qualified and competent therapist.

MODELS OF COMPLEMENTARY THERAPY PROVISION

WHO SHOULD PROVIDE THERAPIES?

There are several options for provision of complementary therapies into children's care. For example 50% of GP practices and 43% of primary care trusts offer some kind of access to complementary therapies – although this may not include provision for children. However, over 90% of people who use therapies do so outside the NHS (Thomson 2005). In primary care, models of provision and providers may include: enhanced service via GP – funded by charity, PCT grants, patients' contributions; or provision may be by complementary practitioners, the GPs themselves, practice nurse or other orthodox healthcare professional such as health visitor, nursery nurse or healthcare assistant.

Within secondary care, provision may be by healthcare staff qualified in a specific therapy and providing an actual therapy service. Alternatively, they may provide the therapy as part of their healthcare role if qualified to do so and it is within their job description. Some secondary services may contract in therapy services from a qualified therapy practitioner.

In any of these scenarios, when incorporating complementary therapies, it must be done carefully and within a robust policy framework if integration is to be successful (Fearon 2006). It is important to consider carefully if administration of a complementary therapy is appropriate to the nursing role or better delivered by a complementary therapy practitioner. For example it is highly unlikely a nurse would find time to be able to provide a full aromatherapy assessment and treatment within the scope of a normal nursing role, even if qualified to do so. Working together with a complementary practitioner would probably be a better option. However, there are many complementary therapy techniques, which can be legitimately incorporated into nursing care, e.g. a simple head massage during a hair wash, a brief foot massage to relax a child in preparation for sleep (Richardson 2001).

If nurses do incorporate therapies into care, they must be rigorous in their understanding of each chosen therapy in order to ensure safe integration of therapies and not fragment existing care (Avis 2003). Choosing the right training and education is vital in order for the nurse to be able to perform it and be accountable for their competence and proficiency in providing that therapy. Nurses should be rigorous and analytical of the quality of their work and also the literature they may use to argue the benefits of their chosen therapies. They should ensure that a mechanism for supervision and support by specialists in the field of complementary medicine is established (Tavares 2003).

Suggested aims of introducing therapies into care might be to:

- Improve the quality of a child's experience, communication and continuity of care
- Enhance quality of life with symptom management for acute, chronic and terminal conditions
- Reduce anxiety and fear
- Enhance relationships between child and nurse, child and parent(s), nurse and family
- Encourage fun and distraction and improve motivation
- To empower and enable children to work towards realising their potential.

CONSENT

The issue of informed consent is especially pertinent since the publication of the Report of the

Public Inquiry into Children's Heart Surgery at Bristol Royal Infirmary (2001). Informed consent for a child to receive a complementary therapy must be obtained in the same way as for any other healthcare intervention. Proof of informed consent is important not just for the child and family's sake but also serves to protect the practitioner in the event of any complaint arising following treatment.

A BRIEF EXPLANATION OF THE THERAPIES

AROMATHERAPY

The use of concentrated, aromatic plant extracts (essential oils) for their therapeutic effects, essential oils can be extracted from a variety of sources, e.g. flowers, herbs, trees, fruit and roots. The oils are used to treat the whole person in a variety of ways including massage, inhalation, compresses, creams, lotions, baths. Essential oils are highly concentrated aromatic material and must be diluted in a carrier oil or cream/lotion before being administered to the skin.

Essential oils affect an individual on a psychological, physiological and cellular level. When applied via massage, the scent of the oil activates the olfactory sense which triggers the limbic area of the brain – that which is concerned with memory and emotion (Ernst et al 2006). The oil is also absorbed into the bloodstream via the skin when the individual chemical constituents of the oils exert an effect. The therapeutic properties of essential oils relate to the pharmacology of these chemical constituents (Battaglia 2003). There are possible harmful effects associated with some constituents and the use of some oils that contain them may therefore be contraindicated in certain conditions, such as pregnancy or epilepsy.

Buckle (2003) identified positive benefits of aromatherapy for children.

- Reduce anxiety
- Relieve constipation (Shireffs 2001)
- Help relieve chronic pain
- Provide a supportive and qualitative role to play in the field of children's palliative care
- Promote parent/child bonding
- Encourage tactile development
- Improve sleep patterns
- Promote endorphin production and improve pain relief
- Empower parents by giving them control over one area of their child's care.

There is also evidence that some essential oils have antibacterial action (Battaglia 2003, Edwards-Jones et al 2004).

Some essential oils are toxic under certain conditions, while others may cause skin sensitivities. Thus, it is important that whoever uses the oils or prescribes the oils for use by another nurse or parent has a sound knowledge base and is accountable for their use. They are not the panacea for all ills and should be used with caution by appropriately qualified practitioners, whether nurse or therapist. It is important that the recipient likes the smell, because, by virtue of its links with the limbic system, it may evoke memories or emotional reactions or put in place memories for the future – either positive or negative. This is an important consideration in such areas as haematology/oncology where smells may be negatively associated with, for example, chemotherapy and may cause problems for the child and carers if they come into contact with the same smell at a later stage.

Essential oil dilutions need to be very much higher for children and even more so in newborn and pre-term infants who have fewer layers of epidermis than an older child or adult (Tisserand & Balacs 1995). Price and Price-Parr (1996) suggest 1 drop of essential oil per 12 kg of body weight to a maximum of 15 drops per 50 mL of base carrier, and a maximum of 8 drops for use in the bath, vaporiser, compress, etc. for a child weighing over 50 kg. The choice of oils is more limited in the younger age group because of the possibility of adverse reactions to some of the constituents of particular oils. This also has implications for the mode of administration. In-depth knowledge of oil derivation, constituents and actions is essential. Likewise, it is necessary to have a good knowledge of anatomy and physiology in order to understand the implications of application, e.g. the structure and development of infant skin, excretory capabilities of the immature kidney, the dynamics of dysfunctional systems and musculoskeletal splinting of an injured or unstable area.

Carrier oils are also of considerable importance, not least because of their varied therapeutic qualities and also their varying dermal uptake (Battaglia 2003). Many carrier oils are nut derived. If there is a risk of nut allergy, then use of a non-nut deriva-tive such as sunflower oil (*Helianthus annus*) is preferable.

THERAPEUTIC MASSAGE

Holey and Cook (2003) describe therapeutic mas-sage as 'the manipulation of the soft tissue of the body by a trained therapist as a component of a holistic intervention'. Massage can improve health and well-being, especially through a reduction in pain and anxiety (Holey and Cook 2003). One of the oldest therapies known to man, massage offers communication through caring touch that is very different from the 'clinical' or functional touch associated with much of nursing. Early bonding between baby and parent is vital for the infant's healthy emotional and psychological development both in early years and as the child matures into adulthood (Moyse 2005). Touch is an essential ele-ment in healthy bonding and is also influential in the development of a baby's physical well-being (Moyse 2005).

Research has demonstrated many physical and psychological benefits of massage for babies and children (Barlow et al 2007, 2008, Cullen-Powell et al 2005, Lorenz et al 2005). It has been shown to improve the outcome for neonates in terms of weight gain, length of stay in hospital and subsequent development and a reduction in corti-sol levels (Diego et al 2005, Gitau et al 2002, Vickers et al 2004). However, nerve pathways and pain modulation in the neonate need to be considered. Pre-term infants may be hypersensitive to the wrong sort of touch and handling and it may be inappropriate for some neonates to receive massage as such. Gentle touch – hand on back of head and lower back alone may be more appropriate (Rollins 2001). Similarly, nurses should be aware that chil-dren affected by autism may have heightened (or reduced) sensory responses in any of the five main senses, including touch (Cullen-Powell et al 2005). They should consider if it is more or less appropriate to instigate massage for these children.

Permission from a child or infant may be acquired through non-verbal means and it is important to identify this. Babies should always be approached with respect and openness and if a baby demonstrates, by means of facial expres-sions or other body language, that the contact is too close, that must be respected. It may be appro-priate to make contact via another part of the body.

Careful assessment of need is required, together with awareness of body language. A child who has a disordered perception of touch, as in abuse, is someone on whom massage must be used with extreme caution, if at all.

REFLEXOLOGY/REFLEX ZONE THERAPY

Gentle pressure is applied to specific areas or zones of the hands and feet which are believed to correspond with different parts of the body (Ernst et al 2006). It is suggested that stimulating these zones through specific touch can promote health and well-being (Griffiths 2001). It is reported to have been used successful in inducing a state of relaxation in an anxious person, in lowering blood pressure (Griffiths 2001), in relieving chronic constipation and encopresis (Bishop 2003) and in other functional disorders such as headache (Ernst et al 2006).

VISUALISATION AND GUIDED IMAGERY

Visualisation and guided imagery can be used as coping strategies for reducing anxiety and stress (Ball et al 2003, Kashikar-Zuck 2006, Payne 2004) and as a means of handling a difficult situation more easily (Ryman 2001), such as prior to vene-puncture. It is a form of relaxed, focused concen-tration and is a natural and powerful coping mechanism. It can be easily learned and used as an adjunct to the care of toddlers and pre-school children, as well as older children, who are experi-encing anxiety and pain (Tsao & Zeltzer 2005).

Important steps that should be taken in prepara-tion for the visualisation, involve the practitioner being very relaxed, 'centred' and focused on the children and their needs; parents should be informed of goals and permission for the visualisa-tion obtained; the practitioner should have an open and honest relationship with the child about the visualisation, listen to any expressed concerns and then help the child to refocus their anxiety on the goals and images.

However, this is not a treatment to be used with those who are experiencing emotional instability. It can be harmful to those who are suffering from mental health disorders, e.g. freely dissociating or acutely psychotic (Payne 2004). It is a useful method of teaching children and parents relaxation techniques and to enable the child to cooperate with treatment, e.g. immunisations, venepuncture, bone marrow aspirations, biopsies or radiotherapy

(Duff 2003). It can improve self-esteem by enabling children to see themselves as having coped positively with a difficult situation.

HYPNOTHERAPY

This is the conscious use of an altered level of consciousness or state of deep relaxation through suggestion to enhance the sense of health and well-being (Rankin-Box 2001). Children have shown to be generally more susceptible to hypnosis than adults (Tsao & Zeltzer 2005). It can be a valuable tool for pain management, reducing anxiety and phobias, and has many potential benefits in child care (Ernst et al 2006, Richardson et al 2006). It is often used in conjunction with or as an extension of guided imagery and visualisation.

HOMEOPATHY

Homeopathic preparations are made by diluting substances from natural sources many, many times in a water and alcohol base. Each successive solution is shaken very vigorously, a process known as succussion (Atherton 2001). Orthodox scientists state that the resulting liquid is nothing more than water, but homeopaths believe the energetic imprint or 'memory' of the original source remains in the substance. The homeopath works on the assumption that you treat like with like. The preparations when administered will produce effects that correspond to manifestations of the disorder (Ernst et al 2006). Remedy prescription will focus on the whole person, their physiology and psychology as well as symptoms, aiming to address underlying causes of illness rather than just symptom relief. Usually given orally or topically, homeopathy is thought to be extremely safe, which is probably why it is one of the more commonly used complementary therapies in children for a number of chronic conditions such as asthma and eczema (Robinson et al 2008, Shaw et al 2008). Nurses should be aware that, in around 20% of cases treated with homeopathy, a transient worsening of symptoms will be seen (Altunç et al 2007).

THE 'CLINICAL' ENVIRONMENT

The nature of the environment where therapies are offered is important. For example, consideration should be given to ambient noise, light, temperature, freedom from outside distraction where possible, privacy, lighting, warmth and so on.

Therapies can be successfully offered in a variety of settings:

- At home – by parents, therapy practitioners, duly qualified children's community nurses, play specialists, physiotherapists, occupational therapists, etc.
- In hospital wards
- In hospital departments, such as A&E, or outpatient clinics
- General practice surgeries
- Hospices
- Schools and nurseries.

CONCLUSION

The appropriate integration of complementary therapies into mainstream healthcare settings has the potential to offer many physical and psychological benefits to children and their families. It can teach children coping strategies to stand them in good stead for the future (Ball et al 2003, Barlow et al 2008, Kemper & Shannon 2007). Involving parents/carers in delivering therapies to their children can help them to feel empowered, involved in doing something positive for their child and help foster positive coping mechanisms (Buckle 2003, Fearon 2003). To apply them effectively requires sound education and skills acquisition through accredited organisations, together with access to supervision by experienced practitioners.

References

Altunç, U., Pittler, M.H., Ernst, E., 2007. Homeopathy for childhood and adolescence ailments: systematic review of randomized clinical trials. Mayo Clin. Proc. 82 (1), 69–75.

Atherton, K., 2001. Homeopathy. In: Rankin-Box, D. (Ed.), The nurses' handbook of complementary therapies. second ed. Churchill Livingstone, Edinburgh.

Avis, A., 2003. Complementary therapies in nursing, midwifery and health visiting practice: RCN guidance on integrating complementary therapies into clinical care. Royal College of Nursing, London.

Ball, T.M., Shapiro, D.E., Monheim, C.J., et al., 2003. A pilot study of the use of guided imagery for the treatment of recurrent abdominal pain in children. Clin. Pediatr. (Phila) 42 (6), 527–532.

Barlow, J.H., Cullen-Powell, L.A., Williams, H., 2007. The training and support programme for parents of children with ataxia: a pilot study. Psychol. Health Med. 12 (1), 64–69.

Barlow, J.H., Powell, L.A., Gilchrist, M., et al., 2008. The effectiveness of the Training and Support Program for parents of children with disabilities: a randomized controlled trial. J. Psychosom. Res. 64 (1), 55–62.

Battaglia, S., 2003. The complete guide to aromatherapy, second ed. The International Centre of Holistic Aromatherapy, Australia.

Bishop, E., 2003. Reflexology in the management of encopresis and chronic constipation. Paediatr. Nurs. 15 (3), 20–21.

Buckle, S., 2003. Aromatherapy and massage: the evidence. Paediatr. Nurs. 15 (6), 24–27.

Corydon Hammond, D., 2003. A phase 1 study on the feasibility and acceptability of an acupuncture/hypnosis intervention for chronic pediatric pain. Am. J. Clin. Hypn. 46 (1), 81.

Crawford, N.W., Cincotta, D.R., Lim, A., et al., 2006. A cross-sectional survey of complementary and alternative medicine use by children and adolescents attending the University Hospital of Wales. BMC Complement. Altern. Med. 6, 16.

Cullen-Powell, L.A., Barlow, J.H., Cushway, D., 2005. Exploring a massage intervention for parents and their children with autism: the implications for bonding and attachment. J. Child Health Care 9 (4), 245–255.

Diego, M.A., Field, T., Hernandez-Reif, M., 2005. Vagal activity, gastric motility, and weight gain in massaged preterm neonates. J. Pediatr. 147, 50–55.

Duff, A., 2003. Incorporating psychological approaches into routine paediatric venepuncture. Arch. Dis. Child. 88 (10), 931–937.

Edwards-Jones, V., Buck, R., Shawcross, S.G., et al., 2004. The effect of essential oils on methicillin-resistant Staphylococcus aureus using a dressing model. Burns 30 (8), 772–777.

Ernst, E., Pittler, M., Wider, B., 2006. The desktop guide to complementary and alternative medicine: an evidence based approach, second ed. Mosby Elsevier, London.

Ernst, E., White, A., 2000. The BBC survey of complementary medicine use in the UK. Complement. Ther. Med. 8 (1), 32–36.

Fearon, J., 2003. Complementary therapies: knowledge and attitudes of health professionals. Paediatr. Nurs. 15 (6), 31–35.

Fearon, J., 2006. Developing a complementary therapy policy. Br. J. Nurs. 15 (4), 228–232.

Gitau, R., Modi, N., Gianakoulopoulos, X., et al., 2002. Acute effects of maternal skin-to-skin contact and massage on saliva cortisol in preterm babies. Journal of Reproductive and Infant Psychology 20 (2), 83–88.

Griffiths, P., 2001. Reflexology. In: Rankin-Box, D. (Ed.), The nurses' handbook of complementary therapies. second ed. Churchill Livingstone, Edinburgh, pp. 133–140.

Holey, E., Cook, E., 2003. Evidence based therapeutic massage: a practical guide for therapists, second ed. Churchill Livingstone, Edinburgh.

Hollinghurst, S., Shaw, A., Thompson, E.A., 2008. Capturing the value of complementary and alternative medicine: including patient preferences in economic evaluation. Complement Ther. Med. 16 (1), 47–51.

House of Lords, 2000. Complementary and alternative medicine, Select Committee on Science and Technology, 6th Report TSO, London.

Jones, B., Weisenfluh, S., 2003. Pediatric palliative and end-of-life care: Developmental and spiritual issues of dying children. Smith College Studies in Social Work 73 (3), 423–443.

Kashikar-Zuck, S., 2006. Treatment of children with chronic unexplained pain. Lancet 367 (9508), 380–382.

Kemper, K., Shannon, S., 2007. Complementary and alternative medicine therapies to promote healthy moods. Pediatr. Clin. North Am. 54 (6), 901–926.

Liossi, C., White, P., Hatira, P., 2006. Randomized clinical trial of local anesthetic versus a combination of local anesthetic with self-hypnosis in the management of pediatric procedure-related pain. Health Psychol. 25 (3), 307–315.

Lorenz, L., Moyse, K., Surguy, H., 2005. The benefits of baby massage. Paediatr. Nurs. 17 (2), 15–18.

Lueng, B., Verhoef, M., 2008. Survey of parents on the use of naturopathic medicine in children. Complement Ther. Clin. Pract. 14 (2), 98–104.

Loman, D.G., 2003. The use of complementary and alternative health care practices among children. J. Pediatr. Health Care 17 (2), 58–63.

Moyse, K., 2005. Baby massage and baby play: promoting touch and stimulation in early childhood. Paediatr. Nurs. 17 (5), 30–32.

Payne, R., 2004. Relaxation techniques, third ed. Churchill Livingstone, Edinburgh.

Price, S., Price-Parr, P., 1996. Aromatherapy for babies and children. Thorsons, London.

Prince of Wales's Foundation for Integrated Health: 2003. Setting the agenda for the future. Prince of Wales Foundation for Integrated Health, London.

Ramsay, H.M., Goddard, W., Gill, S., et al., 2003. Herbal creams used for atopic eczema in Birmingham, UK illegally contain potent corticosteroids. Arch. Dis. Child. 88 (12), 1056–1057.

Rankin-Box, D. (Ed.), 2001. The nurses' handbook of complementary therapies, second ed. Churchill Livingstone, Edinburgh.

Rankin-Box, D., 2005. Editorial: Welcome to complementary therapies in clinical practice. Complement Ther. Clin. Pract. 11 (1), 4.

Report of the Public Inquiry into Children's Heart Surgery at the Bristol Royal Infirmary 1984–1995 Learning from Bristol (the Kennedy Report), 2001. Cmnd 5207(1). TSO, London.

Richardson, J., 2001. Integrating complementary therapies into health care education: a cautious approach. J. Clin. Nurs. 10 (6), 793–798.

Richardson, J., Smith, J.E., McCall, G., et al., 2006. Hypnosis for procedure-related pain and distress in pediatric cancer patients: a systematic review of effectiveness and methodology related to hypnosis interventions.

J. Pain Symptom Manage. 31 (1), 70–84.

Ritchie, M.R., 2007. Use of herbal supplements and nutritional supplements in the UK: what do we know about their pattern of usage? Proc. Nutr. Soc. 66 (4), 479–482.

Robinson, N., et al., 2008. Complementary medicine use in multi-ethnic paediatric outpatients. Complement Ther. Clin. Pract. 14 (1), 17–24.

Rollins, J.A., 2001. Study finds that touch helps premature babies. Pediatr. Nurs. 27 (4), 423.

Ryman, L., 2001. Relaxation and visualisation. In: Rankin-Box D (ed.), The nurses' handbook of complementary therapies, second ed. Churchill Livingstone, Edinburgh, pp. 141–149.

Scrace, J., 2003. Complementary therapies in palliative care: a literature review. Paediatr. Nurs. 15 (3), 36–39.

Sencer, S.F., Kelly, K.M., 2007. Complementary and alternative therapies in pediatric oncology. Pediatr. Clin. North Am. 54 (6), 1043–1060.

Shaw, A., Noble, A., Salisbury, C., et al., 2008. Predictors of complementary therapy use among asthma patients: results of a primary care survey. Health Soc. Care Community 16 (2), 155–164.

Shireffs, C., 2001. Aromatherapy and massage for joint pain and constipation in a patient with Guillain-Barré. Complement Ther. Nurs. Midwifery 7 (2), 78–83.

Simpson, N., Roman, K., 2001. Complementary medicine use in children: extent and reasons. A population-based study. Br. J. Gen. Pract. 51 (472), 914–916.

Tavares, M., 2003. National guidelines for the use of complementary therapies in supportive and palliative care. The Prince of Wales's Foundation for Integrated Health, London.

Thomson, A., 2005. A healthy partnership: integrating complementary healthcare into primary care. The Prince of Wales's Foundation for Integrated Health (now the Prince's Foundation for Integrated Health), London.

Tisserand, R., Balacs, T., 1995. Essential oil safety – a guide for health care professionals. Churchill Livingstone, Edinburgh.

Tsao, J.C.I., Zeltzer, L.K., 2005. Complementary and alternative medicine approaches for pediatric pain: a review of the state-of-the-science. Evidence Based Complementary and Alternative Medicine 2 (2), 149–159.

Vickers, A., Ohlsson, A., Lacy, J.B., et al., 2004. Massage for promoting growth and development of preterm and/or low birth-weight infants. Cochrane Database Syst. Rev. (Issue 2).

Zealey, C., 2005. The benefits of infant massage: a critical review. Community Pract. 78, 98–102.

Further reading and research sources

CAM Specialist Library National Library for Health. Online. Available: http://www.library.nhs.uk/cam/.

CAM on PubMed. Online. Available: http://nccam.nih.gov/camonpubmed/.

Proquest Database at Athens. Online. Available: www.athens.ac.uk.

Password available through your NHS organization, or for members of the Royal College of Nursing, through the RCN website e-library at www.rcn.org.uk.

The Prince's Foundation for Integrated Health. Online. Available: www.fih.org.uk.

Founded 1993 to promote integrated healthcare. Lots of useful information about complementary therapies, finding a therapist, the voluntary-self-regulation programme for therapy organisations, plus information about finding therapy training courses.

SECTION 2

Care compassion and communication

SECTION CONTENTS

6. Assessment   67

7. Caring for the child who has died   81

8. Cardiopulmonary resuscitation   94

9. Hygiene   104

10. Play   120

11. Skin care   131

Chapter 6

Assessment

Kerry Cook, Hermione Montgomery

CHAPTER CONTENTS

Introduction 67
    Learning outcomes 68
    Rationale 68

Model of assessment 68

Approaching the examination 68
    Subjective information (history) 69
    Objective information (physical
    examination/observation) 69
    Age-specific approaches 70

Examining the systems (obtaining
the objective information) 71
    Respiratory examination 71
    Inspection 71
    Palpation and percussion 71
    Auscultation 72
    Pulse oximetry and oxygen saturation 72
    Cardiovascular examination 73
    Neurological examination 74
    Examination of the skin 75
    Abdominal examination 76
    Genitourinary examination 76

Growth and nutrition information 76

Pulling it all together 77
    Assessment (provisional diagnosis) 77
    Plan (treatment options) 77
    Complications 78
    Dos and don'ts 78

Paediatrics is a specialty bound by age and not by system.

(Gill & O'Brien 2007)

INTRODUCTION

Assessment forms a key part of the scheduled and unscheduled healthcare journey for the infant, child or young person and their family. It can provide practitioners with important clinical, physical, social, cultural, psychological and emotional information; it can help to promote the child's understanding of their body *and* it can educate and provide health promotion (Vessey 1995), as well as assisting in detecting potential health risks and problems. These could be: developmental, psychological, nutritional and/or intellectual (Byrnes 1996).

With the growing recognition of advanced nursing roles, detailed health assessments are increasingly being undertaken by advanced nurse practitioners and nurse consultants who have expert clinical examination skills (Hamric & Spross 2004, Barnes 2003). However, despite this role development, the physical assessment skills of inspection, palpation, percussion and auscultation are not commonly utilised by nurses in general (Rushforth et al 1998). Assessment skills are necessary not only for the children and young people's nurse working in the acute setting, but also for all practitioners that come into contact with children, for example, in GP practices, walk-in clinics, NHS Direct, NHS 24, health visitors, school nurses, paramedics, emergency care practitioners and others. This chapter aims to assist these practitioners in developing an appropriate approach to the holistic assessment of the child. The term 'child' here refers to infants, children and young people. All practitioners should follow principles of good practice, particularly when the examination is of an intimate nature as outlined by the RCN (2001) guidance regarding the protection of nurses working with children and young people.

There are a variety of assessment tools currently available, such as the Paediatric Early Warning System (PEWS) (Haines et al 2005, Duncan 2007); Child and Adolescent Mental Health (CAMH) assessment tools (Honeyman 2007) and the Structured ABC approach (ALSG 2005). This chapter discusses a variety of tools used to assess the child's holistic well-being, including the subjective, objective, assessment plan (SOAP) model (Weed 1964, 1968, 1969, Epstein et al 1997, Bond & Uzelac 2004, Uzelac et al 2004).

LEARNING OUTCOMES

By the end of this section you should be able to:

- Assess the child's holistic well-being by using a systematic assessment tool
- Interpret, document and communicate the findings and take appropriate action
- Recognise when vital signs do not fall within the expected limits for the child's age, condition and developmental level
- Evaluate the child's holistic well-being during an episode of care.

RATIONALE

To obtain information via observation, history taking and physical examination, this will form a baseline for immediate action and ongoing assessment and evaluation, to assist in developing your plan of action. Assessments are undertaken at various times such as presentation to a primary healthcare setting, paramedic visits at home, on admission to hospital, and on an acute or ongoing needs basis and from shift to shift.

MODEL OF ASSESSMENT

Assessment of the child can reveal a plethora of information, which will be used towards formulating a provisional diagnosis and a plan of action. However, without a structured approach, crucial information may be missed. Using a model will ensure that the assessment and subsequent documentation is structured and incorporates all key elements, including observation, history taking and the examination. The model utilised will depend upon the setting and the severity of the child's condition. Paediatric early warning tools (PEWS) (Haines et al 2005, Duncan 2007) are being widely used in tertiary settings to identify children at risk of deterioration. These may also have a place in some primary care settings as well as the Airway, Breathing, Circulation approach (ALSG 2005).

Nurses throughout the UK are expanding their skills and responsibilities in line with current changes in healthcare. The Darzi Report (DoH 2007) highlighted the need for all staff working in areas where children are likely to be seen, to be competent in the initial assessment of ill and injured children. Proficient assessment skills are synonymous with the increase in autonomy and advanced practice that the development of the suggested 'polyclinics' will bring (DoH 2007). Practitioners need to be knowledgeable of the anatomical and pathophysiological differences in children and must be able to recognise serious illness/injury; safeguarding issues and mental health issues, particularly in adolescents; as well as being competent at basic life support and pain management (DoH 2007). Development of these skills is also a fundamental part of pre-registration education. In the meantime, this chapter will provide a guideline for students wishing to enhance their assessment skills by developing a systematic approach to holistic assessment.

The SOAP model – the Subjective Objective Assessment Plan – originally described by Lawrence L. Weed in the 1960s (Weed 1964, 1968, 1969) has been universally adopted in the medical field since its inception. It was chosen as the main structure for this chapter, as it provides a conceptual framework that can easily be adapted by other practitioners. Application of the model is taught as a fundamental part of 'assessing the ill/injured child' modules and is successfully used by other professional groups (nurses, physiotherapists and paramedics) in clinical practice.

APPROACHING THE EXAMINATION

No matter why you are undertaking an examination, the first action you take before formal evaluation is to visually appraise the well-being of the child. This will provide immediate information regarding the severity of the condition, the demeanour of the child, interactions with parents and general characteristics such as developmental milestones; for example, you would expect a 4–6 month old to smile and coo and to grasp a rattle; a 7–9 month old to transfer objects from one hand to another; at 10–12 months to pull up to stand; and at 13–18 months to walk alone with heels flat on the floor (Bee & Boyd 2007, p 103). Your plan of action may be determined by the information gained during this brief episode, which should be communicated to the appropriate professionals and agencies and must be documented in the child's records (DoH 2003a). If at this point, urgent resuscitation/emergency action needs to be taken, the airway, breathing, circulation (ABC) approach should be used (ALSG 2005); if urgent attention is not required, the assessment should continue in a more holistic way.

Before starting the formal examination, ensure that the environment is private and comfortable for the child and their parents. Providing a variety of toys and games will help the child to feel more at ease and to cooperate during the physical examination. Maintaining a non-judgemental approach is essential, recognising and respecting the individuality of the family, including culture and the religious beliefs of various ethnic groups (Engel 2006). Confidentiality and consent need to be taken into consideration at all ages but particularly for the young person, as they may wish to give information and undergo physical examination without their parents being present. You should refer to your local consent policy (DoH 2001).

SUBJECTIVE INFORMATION (HISTORY)

Subjective information refers to that obtained from the child and their parents. The child and their parents have the most intimate knowledge of the problem and are therefore the best source of data. Here you are attempting to build a profile of the child and their problems using information regarding the presenting complaint, previous hospital admissions, their prenatal, birth and neonatal history, allergies, current medications (including any over-the-counter preparations), immunisations, personal habits, nutrition, hygiene, elimination, developmental history (Bee & Boyd 2007), family, cultural and social history (Gleadle 2007), significant life events, psychosocial history, education,

physical activity and home circumstances (Engel 2006). This is a vital part of the process, however when assessing children it is sometimes difficult to get a comprehensive history due to their age or if the parent/carer is too stressed by the seriousness of the situation to articulate the relevant information; in these situations, the majority of the information may only be gathered through the objective assessment. Questioning needs to be sensitive so as not to cause undue alarm or embarrassment for the child or parents. It also needs to be delivered at the child's and parents' level of understanding, avoiding the use of medical jargon (Byrnes 1996).

It is important here to also consider assessment of the child or young person's mental health, as 10% of children are known to have a mental health problem (Office of National Statistics 2005), with 40% having a mental illness during their childhood (Health Advisory Service 1995). However, these figures are based on those children that are known to have mental health problems and therefore many are unnoticed. Additionally, the importance of assessing CAMH has been emphasised within recent governmental policies such as the Children's National Service Framework, standard 9 (DoH 2004), since a child's mental health is equally as important as their physical health for their holistic well-being (National Mental Health Association 2003). Assessment of the child should therefore routinely include a review of physical health, mental health, intelligence, school performance, family situation and behaviour in all settings (Honeyman 2007, p 40). There are a variety of tools available to assess children's mental health, such as the Paediatric Symptom Checklist (Jellinek et al 1988, which can be downloaded from www.brightfutures.org/mentalhealth/pdf/professionals/); while it will not be considered in depth in this chapter, further reading of this subject is advised (see Honeyman 2007).

OBJECTIVE INFORMATION (PHYSICAL EXAMINATION/OBSERVATION)

Objective information refers to that obtained by the practitioner through observation, physical examination and any investigative tests. The younger the child, the more important it is to observe their well-being and any physical signs from a distance; sleeping children should be observed before waking them up to examine them (Epstein et al 1997).

You can evaluate a wealth of information before touching and without abruptly handling or examining with an instrument. Examination should be approached using your eyes and hands before your ears, using the standard format of inspection, palpation, percussion and auscultation (Archer & Burch 1998). Some aspects of respiratory function and the musculoskeletal and neurological systems can be assessed while the child plays, or mobilises, around the room. For example, children with respiratory distress may exhibit the tripod position to make breathing easier; this is exhibited as an extension of the arms forward and downwards while the back is arched (Thomas 1996). The child's breathing can be observed – is it rapid, laboured, noisy or shallow? If the child is coughing, wheezing or stridulous, this may indicate respiratory distress (Thomas 1996). For the musculoskeletal system, one could observe the shape and contour of the body and assess the gait, looking for knock-knee, clubfoot, scoliosis and bowleg (Engel 2006). Asking the child to stick out their tongue and close their eyes would provide information about the cranial nerves (Engel 2006).

AGE-SPECIFIC APPROACHES

Infants are usually easier to examine and care must be taken to prevent hypothermia when exposed (ALSG 2005). The examination is best approached in a top-to-toe fashion, starting with the head and encompassing the entire body down to the feet in a systematic fashion while linking the systems together, auscultating the heart, lungs and abdomen while the infant is quiet. Palpation and percussion of areas should be conducted together. Reflexes can also be elicited as the body is being examined, but generalised primitive reflexes should be determined last. Traumatic procedures should be performed at the end of the examination, for example checking the mouth for intact palate. Many sick infants will exhibit distress and deterioration in their condition when handled to measure vital signs. In these infants, taking recordings using equipment such as blood pressure monitors can cause more harm than good; visually observing for changes will be a much more accurate indication of well-being. For example, the nurse should visually observe for changes in the respiratory rate such as increasing effort, efficacy and efficiency of breathing; grunting, wheeziness and stridor; changes in skin and mucosal colour; and changes

Table 6.1	Normal respiratory rates
AGE OF CHILD	RESPIRATORY RATE IN BREATHS/MIN
Newborn	30–60
6 months	30–45
1–2 years	25–35
3–6 years	20–30
>7 years	20–25

Reproduced by kind permission from Hull and Johnston 1993.

in movement and responsiveness before measuring rate (Table 6.1).

The older infant/toddler will prefer to be sitting on the parent's lap during examination. The advantage of this position is that the parent can also gently hold the child still if necessary (RCN 2003), since this age group strongly objects to being held in one position even when non-invasive examination is taking place, for example placing a temperature probe under the arm. It may be worthwhile gaining the assistance of a play specialist or another person to provide distraction with toys while the child is being examined. Infants from 6 months upwards may demonstrate stranger and separation anxieties (Bee & Boyd 2007), which could impede assessment. These anxieties peak at 9 and 13 months, respectively and by the age of 2 years, have usually significantly reduced. This may be overcome by having someone with the child that is familiar to them, such as one or both parents or another familiar caregiver. These children prefer minimal physical contact initially and so equipment should be introduced slowly. Areas of the body could be inspected through play, such as tickling toes, or asking toddlers to point to different parts of their body; this will also assist in gaining cooperation. Parts of the physical examination where cooperation is required can then be conducted, such as auscultating the apex beat, although it may be best to perform these when the child is quiet. Again, traumatic procedures should be left until the end of the examination (Vessey 1995). Unless the examination is being undertaken rapidly because of the severity of the child's condition, time should be taken to ensure that the child and parents feel sufficiently relaxed in order to gather a thorough history before proceeding onto the examination.

Pre-schoolers are more obliging and like to follow simple instructions. By this age, they will know most external body parts and possibly three to five internal body parts. They will prefer to be standing or sitting close to their parents, but are likely to want to undress themselves. The examination can be approached in a top-to-toe direction if they are cooperative, or as above, if not. These children like stories about the task and to examine the equipment before it is used. You should offer the child choices to assist in gaining their cooperation.

The school-age child is more knowledgeable about internal body parts and understands simple scientific explanations. They are likely to be cooperative in most positions, although prefer sitting. The older child may prefer their parents not to be present. The examination should follow the top-to-toe pattern, leaving examination of genitalia (if necessary) until last. The school-age child likes to be given an explanation of the rationale for examination and the equipment used (Vessey 1995, Hockenberry 2005).

The adolescent will generally prefer privacy; however, you should offer the option of having their parents present. They will have a basic knowledge of anatomy and physiology and hence will like to be told findings of the examination throughout. Although the top-to-toe pattern can be used, it is best to expose only the area being examined, thus allowing privacy to be maintained (Vessey 1995, Hockenberry 2005).

EXAMINING THE SYSTEMS (OBTAINING THE OBJECTIVE INFORMATION)

The examination may be undertaken using a system-based approach, as suggested below. This is by no means an exhaustive explanation of factors to consider but offers some suggestions as to the approach that could be taken, for example you may need to assess the special senses and lymphatic system, other models of assessment may also be incorporated for more specific data such as pain assessment, risk assessment, tissue viability tools and the Glasgow Coma Scale.

RESPIRATORY EXAMINATION

Respiratory disorders in infancy can be acute, life-threatening or chronic. In the acute, life-threatening situation, e.g. epiglottitis, early assessment of airway and breathing is vital if the child is to be treated effectively (ALSG 2005).

The most common reason for infants and toddlers to attend the GP surgery is an acute respiratory tract infection, normally upper, i.e. ear, nose, mouth and throat (Gill & O'Brien 2007). You may wish to refer to the NICE Asthma Guidelines (NICE 2000, 2002, 2007a). It is much better to stand back and observe rather than to immediately place your hands and stethoscope onto the child. The good observer will often be able to distinguish between an upper and lower respiratory tract infection by carefully looking and listening. Observation is also the most useful, since auscultation is frequently drowned by environmental noise.

INSPECTION

You should observe the pattern, work and rate of breathing. The respiratory rate should be counted over a full minute to ensure accuracy. In infants and children under the age of 6–7 years, the abdominal movements should be counted, as they are primarily abdominal and diaphragmatic breathers (Wong 1997) (see Tables 6.1–6.5 for normal age-related vital signs). The nurse should observe for respiratory distress, for example nasal flaring, grunting, wheezing, dyspnoea, recession, use of accessory and intercostal muscles, chest shape and movement. What is the child's colour? Is there finger clubbing? Are there traumatic petechiae around the eyelids, face and neck following a severe bout of coughing? Remember that infants are nose breathers; therefore any form of nasal obstruction will also cause problems with feeding.

PALPATION AND PERCUSSION

A more experienced practitioner, who has undertaken a nurse practitioner programme, a paediatric physical examination course or an advanced programme of education (e.g. Advanced Nursing Practice) may perform this aspect of the examination. Alternatively, these advanced assessments could be covered by in-house competency-based training.

Palpation allows the practitioner to gather information through touch about the size, shape, texture, movement of the chest wall or thorax (Candy et al 2001), location of pain or tenderness and tactile fremitus (thorax vibration palpated when the child is speaking). As the lungs are protected by the rib cage, direct palpation is not possible, however this indirect palpation of the thorax provides information about chest movement during the respiratory cycle, which is a marker of respiratory efficiency (ALSG 2005, Aylott 2007a).

Percussion allows the practitioner to assess the resonance of the thoracic cavity (reverberation/sound/noise) created by tapping the chest wall with the fingers (see, for correct method, Yernault & Bohadana 1995). Areas of the lung with excess or diminished air or fluid content can be identified as the resonance alters to either a hyper resonant (e.g. indicating pneumothorax) or a dull sound (e.g. indicating haemothorax) (ALSG 2005).

AUSCULTATION

Auscultation allows the practitioner to assess respiratory effort by identifying the presence of normal, abnormal or additional (adventitious) breath sounds, the nature of the sound, location, duration and phase (inspiratory or expiratory) (ALSG 2005, Aylott 2007b). A stethoscope with a paediatric diaphragm and bell should be used. The bell is much more useful for infants, toddlers and children because it is smaller, warmer and less surface noise penetrates, making it easier for the operator to hear the breath sounds (Gill & O'Brien 2007). Early identification of respiratory deterioration, through consecutive auscultative evaluation assists in the prevention of serious decompensation and collapse, which is linked with poor outcome (ALSG 2005, Aylott 2007b) and therefore this is an essential skill for practitioners to learn and utilise within their role of assessing ill and injured children and young people.

PULSE OXIMETRY AND OXYGEN SATURATION

The child or infant who presents with any kind of respiratory distress should have a baseline recording of oxygen saturation (SpO_2) taken with a pulse oximeter (see also Ch. 43). In the healthy child, the percentage saturation of oxygen should be 95–98% (Sims 1996). In the child with cardiac or chronic respiratory problems, their normal oxygen saturation levels may be lower. The nurse should discuss the acceptable range of oxygen saturation levels with the paediatrician, paediatric cardiologist or senior nurse/advanced nurse practitioner. Parents may also provide valuable information about their child's normal levels. Pulse oximetry is a non-invasive, painless and reliable technique for measurement of the SaO_2 (Hanna 1995). When used properly, it

will detect hypoxaemia before clinical signs become evident (Hanna 1995).

A sensor (or probe) is placed around a fleshy part of the body, e.g. a fingertip in the older child, around the nail bed of the toe in the infant or around the ball of the foot in a neonate under 3 kg in weight. Exactly which sensor to use depends on where on the body it is sited and the child's weight. The sensor packaging will clarify the weight range of child for which it is to be used.

The sensor emits red and infrared light and has a photo-detector, which detects the amount of light that is absorbed by the tissues. The different colours of oxygenated and deoxygenated blood absorb different amounts of infrared light. This information is then converted into an average value, which is displayed as percentage saturation. Pulse oximeter measurements have been shown to correlate closely to arterial blood gas values (Coull 1992).

Limitations

There are limitations to the use of an oximeter. For example, if the child's peripheral perfusion is poor (the blood supply to the extremities may be reduced under some circumstances, e.g. when the child is shocked), the readings may be inaccurate. The sensor cannot read accurately if there is excessive motion. The sensor cannot detect the difference between haemoglobin molecules saturated with oxygen and those saturated with other gases such as carbon monoxide (Carroll 1993). It is therefore not safe for use in cases of carbon monoxide poisoning. Accuracy of pulse oximetry can also be affected by the presence of direct, bright light on the sensor.

If the machine records an abnormal saturation, first look at the child. Do the physical signs fit with what the machine is telling you? Remember though, that the main reason why the pulse oximeter is used is because it can detect changes before clinical signs become evident. However, if the child's condition indicates that no changes have occurred, next check that the machine is recording properly and that the sensor is placed and secured appropriately.

If a pulse oximeter is used for prolonged periods, there is a risk of pressure sores (Coull 1992, Carroll 1993), and Sims (1996) suggests that there is a risk of burning the skin if a faulty sensor is applied. Sensors must be used in accordance with the manufacturers' instructions and the site of the sensor should be changed at least 8-hourly when continuous monitoring is in progress and more frequently in neonates or the very sick child.

CARDIOVASCULAR EXAMINATION

Inspection

Inspection would include observing for dysmorphic features, growth, skin colour (e.g. cyanosis, mottling, anaemia or polycythaemia), oedema, clubbing of the upper and lower extremities, respiratory difficulty, and chest and spine abnormalities (Engel 2006, Archer & Burch 1998, Gill & O'Brien 2007). The nurse should then move onto palpating the pulse, assessing the capillary refill time and taking the blood pressure.

Palpation – pulse

Palpate the arterial pulse over the radial, brachial and femoral arteries, preferably using your fingers rather than thumbs, as the practitioner's own pulse may interfere with the reading. The pulse should be counted for at least 1 min, particularly in infants and young children as there may be irregularities in rhythm (Hockenberry 2005). In the neonatal period, it is important to palpate and compare the brachial or axillary pulse, the femoral arterial pulse and the dorsalis pedis in the foot in the context of possible coarctation of the aorta (Archer & Burch 1998).

The brachial pulse is best felt in children under 2 years of age as an infant's neck is generally short and fat and therefore the carotid artery may be difficult to palpate (ALSG 2005). When palpating the pulse, information should be obtained regarding rate, rhythm, volume and character. Pulses can be graded according to the criteria in Table 6.2.

Table 6.2	Grading of pulses
GRADE	DESCRIPTION
0	Not palpable
+1	Difficult to palpate, thready, weak, easily obliterated with pressure
+2	Difficult to palpate, may be obliterated with pressure
+3	Easy to palpate, not easily obliterated with pressure
+4	Strong, bounding, not obliterated with pressure

After Wong (1997).

Table 6.3	Normal heart rates	
	HEART RATE IN PULSE BEATS/MIN	
AGE OF CHILD	*When child awake*	*When child asleep*
Newborn	100–180	80–160
<3 months	100–220	80–180
3 months to 2 years	80–150	70–120
3–10 years	70–110	60–100
10 years to adult	55–90	50–90

From Wong (1995), with permission.

Auscultation

Auscultation of the heart sounds is more commonly used to assess the heart rate of the infant and younger child, using a stethoscope, over the 4th intercostal space inside the nipple under 5 years of age. The apex can be auscultated over the 5th intercostal space at or inside the nipple in the over 5 year olds (Archer & Burch 1998). It may also be necessary to prioritise the order of examination, performing auscultation of the heart sounds before the baby cries. The nurse should primarily listen for the first and second heart sounds (*lub dub*). If any additional sounds are heard, the nurse should discuss the findings with relevant colleagues. Table 6.3 provides data on normal heart rates.

Recording blood pressure

It can be very difficult to gain an accurate blood pressure (BP) reading in an infant using a conventional sphygmomanometer. It is extremely hard to reliably auscultate the child's pulse beat in the cubital fossa (de Swiet et al 1989). The child is also unlikely to cooperate and hold completely still. For this reason, an electronic machine that measures blood pressure (e.g. Dinamap by Critikon, Nellcor by Hewlett Packard) by oscillometry is recommended for use in infants and younger children. However, it is important to remember the limitations of such equipment (Brennan 2008). Movement in the patient adversely affects the accuracy of an electronic blood pressure machine. It is therefore imperative that the manufacturer's instructions are followed. Unless very sick or well sedated, few children (particularly the younger ones) will hold still for the duration of the procedure. In addition, accurate recordings will only be obtained if the correct size of cuff is used. Manual blood pressure needs to be performed for renal patients and on other children when the reading is abnormally high on repeated measurements (RCN 2007, Brennan 2008).

Selection of cuff

The cuff should not be chosen dependent upon the manufacturer's age range printed on the cuff, e.g. infant cuff/adult cuff (Hockenberry 2005, Brennan 2008); it is the cuff size that is important. There are discrepancies in the research about cuff size (Iyriboz et al 1994, Clausen et al 1999, Bur et al 2000, 2003, Clark et al 2002); however, the main school of thought is that the width of the cuff should be two-thirds of the distance from the elbow to the shoulder, the inflatable part (bladder) of the cuff should reach almost all of the way around the arm, while the length of the cuff should be sufficient to cover the whole circumference of the arm (Archer & Burch 1998, Wong 2003, Hockenberry 2005) (Fig. 6.1). The nurse should document the size of cuff used to ensure that the same cuff is used on future occasions. If the cuff is too small, a false high pressure would be given and vice-versa. False readings will also be gained if the infant or child is crying or very restless.

Once you have recorded the BP, consider whether it is higher or lower than expected. Remember a low BP is a late sign of shock. A raised BP could be because the child is in pain or experiencing rising intracranial pressure. The latter would be of particular concern if the child simultaneously demonstrated a falling pulse rate. As with temperature, a single abnormal recording must be re-checked. See Table 6.4 for normal blood pressure values.

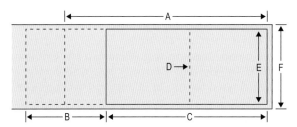

Figure 6.1 Blood pressure cuff dimensions. Dimensions of bladder and cuff in relation to arm circumference. (A) Ideal arm circumference; (B) range of acceptable arm circumferences; (C) bladder length; (D) midline of bladder; (E) bladder width; (F) cuff width *(from Perloff et al 1993, with permission. © 1993 American Heart Association).*

Table 6.4   Normal blood pressure values

AGE OF CHILD	SYSTOLIC BLOOD PRESSURE (mmHg)	DIASTOLIC BLOOD PRESSURE (mmHg)
Neonate	60–85	20–60
Infant (6 months)	75–105	40–70
Toddler (2 years)	75–110	45–80
School age (7 years)	75–115	45–80
Adolescent (15 years)	100–145	60–95

After Hull and Johnston 1993. *Note:* Blood pressure values are expressed as a range, because there are variations according to sex and the child's position on the centile chart for growth.

NEUROLOGICAL EXAMINATION

Full neurological examination (see also Ch. 17) will be undertaken by the medical clinician, including assessment of the cranial nerves, reflexes, behaviour, movement, gait and coordination (Engel 2006, Epstein et al 1997). However, the nurse needs to undertake some aspects of the examination as part of the general assessment of the infant, child or young person. Once again this can be performed initially just by observing (inspection). The AVPU scales are used: are they alert (A), how are they behaving, are they responding to their mother/father in an appropriate way? Is their cry normal or verbal (V) response normal and are they moving their limbs normally? On examination, if asleep do they wake up; if not, do they react to more robust stimulus/pain (P)? If the child's level of consciousness (U) is causing concern, or if there is a history of a head injury, or a fall, a full neurological assessment using the Glasgow Coma Scale must be carried out immediately (ALSG 2005).

Palpation – head

When examining an infant's head (lying flat on the back or sitting upright), is the anterior fontanelle depressed? This is a sign that a feed may be due or of hypovolaemia if the infant is vomiting or has diarrhoea. If this fontanelle is bulging and the infant is not coughing or crying and appears irritable, this could indicate raised intracranial pressure due to infection, injury or a number of other reasons, which need to be recorded and reported. When handling the infant, do they exhibit abnormal signs of distress, are they floppy or stiff and are they difficult to placate? This could indicate that they are acutely unwell (Gill & O'Brien 2007).

Examination of the special senses

As young children have immature immune systems, illnesses of the ear, nose and throat are common and therefore examination of the special senses should be included in a holistic assessment to identify or exclude these aetiologies (e.g. acute otitis media). Specific basic instruments are required to perform a satisfactory examination of the special senses such as an auroscope, ophthalmoscope and a Thudicum speculum (Epstein et al 1997). Assessment of cranial nerve function, such as asking a toddler to find a mint hidden in a handkerchief to assess smell (first cranial nerve, Epstein et al 1997) will also provide useful information about the function of the eyes, ears, nose, mouth and throat. More information about the aetiologies and assessment of these can be found in Barnes (2004) and NICE (2008b).

EXAMINATION OF THE SKIN

Inspection

Observation of the skin (see also Ch. 9) will yield pertinent information and is a valuable part of the assessment procedure. Inspect the colour and pigmentation of the skin, preferably in natural daylight and especially when observing for jaundice. Blue discolouration may be a result of cold or anxiety; however, it could be an indication of central cyanosis, in which case the child's nails, lips, mouth and trunk will be involved and oxygen needs to be administered. Pallor of the nails, mouth, face and conjunctivae may indicate fever, anaemia and, with clamminess, may be associated with shock. Dry mucous membranes and lack of skin turgor, accompanied with a capillary refill of more than 2 s (following cutaneous pressure of a digit or preferably the sternum for 5 s), may be a sign of dehydration (Mackay-Jones et al 2001). Observe for bruises; those of the soft tissue (e.g. on the forearm and buttocks) may be a sign of child abuse.

Palpation – skin

Examine the skin's texture and palpate for lesions, pressure ulcers and rashes; document shape, size, colour and consistency (Engel 2006). Oedematous areas should be gently pressed with the thumb to determine their nature; oedema of the lower extremities and sacrum may result from cardiac or renal disease. Petechiae that are flat, round purple/red pin-like marks, blotches or bruises, which do not blanch when gently touched, may indicate meningococcal disease and the child will require immediate treatment.

Using the back of the hand, feel the temperature of the skin for hypo- and hyperthermia. The nurse also needs to consider the racial variations in skin colour and the effect that this will have on the interpretation of signs such as cyanosis and bruises.

Taking and recording a temperature

In spite of various studies to determine the optimal site and temperature device to be used, there is no one correct way and it will differ according to the age of the child and other factors (see also Ch. 29). Rectal temperature recordings are not recommended for general use (McQueen 2001) because the thermometer needs to be inserted to a depth of at least 5 cm to obtain core temperature, which could cause injury to the fragile mucosa of the anus as well as rectal perforation (Hockenberry 2005). They are also not recommended for ethical reasons, as this can relate to rectal intrusion when continuous monitoring is in progress. When rectal temperatures are required, a dedicated rectal electronic probe should be used (McQueen 2001).

Tympanic recording of temperature is fast, easy to use and acceptable to children (Pickersgill et al 2003, Rush & Wetherall 2003); however, it should not be used in newborn infants and young children (NICE 2007b), as the earpiece is too large for the ear canal, which could result in inaccurate readings. Usage is not recommended when precision is required such as in situations of hypothermia (McQueen 2001). Rush and Wetherall's (2003) review of the literature suggests that two recordings be performed using the same ear once the child has been in an even temperature for 20 min. Tempadot is now generally accepted as a reliable way of recording temperature, especially for those children over 4 weeks (NICE 2007b) of age and can be used under the axilla, although Rush and Wetherall (2003) suggest using it sublingually where possible (see NICE guidelines for the <5 year olds; NICE 2007b). The strip should be held sublingually for 1 min and via the axilla for 3 min (Aylott 2008); after removing the strip, wait 10–15 s before reading the colour changes (Wong 1997, Aylott 2008). These strips must be stored in a cool environment. The nurse should refer to the

Table 6.5   Normal temperature

AGE OF CHILD	CORE TEMPERATURE IN DEGREES CENTIGRADE (°C)
<6 months	37.5
7 months to 1 year	37.5–37.7
2–5 years	37.2–37.0
>6 years	36.6–36.8
After Wong (1995).	

manufacturer's guidelines for more details. Where possible, the child or young person should be given a choice of whether tympanic or Tempadot recording is used (DoH 2003a, Pickersgill et al 2003). See Table 6.5 for normal temperature values.

ABDOMINAL EXAMINATION

Inspection

Much of the nurse's general examination of the abdomen can be undertaken by observation. Most toddlers and young children will have an abdomen that protrudes when standing and is often associated with exaggerated lordosis (exaggeration of the lumbar curvature). Since respiration in the younger child involves the use of the abdominal muscles, movement of the abdomen with inspiration and expiration is normal. The rectus muscle may be noted as being slightly separated (divarication) but this is normal. Small umbilical hernias are frequently noted; one might see distended veins and sometimes loops of bowel in malnourished infants. Abdominal distension is often gaseous, but can be distinguished with simple percussion.

Palpation – abdomen

This can be performed with the infant/child standing or lying down, it is important that they are relaxed and not crying (Gill & O'Brien 2007). The advanced practitioner would be trained to palpate the liver and spleen.

GENITOURINARY EXAMINATION

Examination of the genitalia is unnecessary in older children unless the presenting condition indicates the need. In infants and younger children, examination of the genitalia may be conducted through observation, for example when changing the nappy. One is looking for normality or deviation from this, such as hypospadias, undescended testes, intersex organs, size of clitoris/labia majora and male and female circumcision. If the child urinates while this is being done, then the nurse could observe for direction of flow as this may indicate whether the urethral orifice is at the normal position. A rectal examination should be performed only by doctors if the condition warrants it; this procedure should not be performed routinely. If there are concerns that the child may have a urinary tract infection, follow the NICE (2007c) guidelines on UTI in children.

Examination of the genitalia of the infant and young child can be conducted on the mother's lap (Johnson 2008). Good communication is essential prior to any external or internal examination and in the case of female examinations, a chaperone should always be present and if acceptable by the young person, this could be the mother.

As it is beyond the scope of this chapter to discuss child sexual abuse in detail, we therefore recommend that the nurse communicates any concerns regarding sexual abuse to the medical staff (Gill & O'Brien 2007).

GROWTH AND NUTRITION INFORMATION

Growth is a key indicator of normal health and development. The World Health Organization identifies growth assessment as the best single measure for defining the nutritional status and health of children, as well as being an indicator for populations as a whole for quality of life (Holden & MacDonald 2000, p 161). It is therefore essential that the nurse should take a detailed history of the eating practices of the child, determining whether the child has a special diet, any known food allergies, typical dietary intake of the child and family, recent weight loss or gain, cultural, ethnic or religious influences (Engel 2006), exercise taken and any concerns that the parents may have such as food refusal, obesity and feeding problems (Holden & MacDonald 2000). Nurses are in an ideal position to educate children and their families about nutrition, particularly since obesity is currently on the increase generally, due to lifestyle and food availability.

All children being admitted to hospital or attending any health care setting should have their weight and height measured and plotted on a centile chart (Hall 2000; DoH 2009). The measurements should be recorded on the appropriate centile chart (RCPCH 2002) and over 2009 the new WHO centile charts have been introduced across the UK (DoH 2009). Head circumference should also be measured in infants. It is imperative that all staff involved in measuring infants and children are suitably trained or supervised (DoH 2009).

When weighing children under 2 years of age, the child should be naked. Electronic scales should be calibrated following the manufacturer's instructions (NICE 2008a); the weight should then be measured to the nearest 10 g. When weighing children over 2 years, the child should be in vest and pants and weighed on sitting or standing electronic scales. When measuring height, children who are unable to stand unaided should be measured supine (under 2 years); those that can stand upright unaided (over 2 years) can have a standing height measured. Measurements should be taken to the nearest millimetre to ensure accuracy (Patel et al 2003). Further information can be gained from the Child Growth Foundation and McEwing (2007). The weight and height should be recorded along with the date and the practitioner's signature on the centile chart, medical/nursing notes and in the child's parent-held record.

There are a number of additional methods of measuring that provide a non-invasive means of assessing nutrition (e.g. the degree of obesity). Body mass index (BMI) is an alternative method of assessing nutritional status, particularly since weight and height are affected by a number of factors. This is calculated by dividing the weight (in kg) by the square of the height (in meters) (w/h^2). The BMI varies during childhood and therefore there can be some problems associated with using it (Holden & MacDonald 2000). Skin fold thickness gives an indication of subcutaneous fat and therefore an idea of nutritional status. The skin is pinched between two fingers and then the thickness of the skin fold is measured using specialised callipers (Holden & MacDonald 2000). In order to determine whether the infant, child or young person may be suffering from malnutrition, a nationally recognised nutritional screening tool should be used such as STAMP (Screening Tool for the Assessment of Malnutrition in Paediatrics) (Abbott Nutrition & Central Manchester and Manchester Children's University Hospitals NHS Trust 2008). However, more recently the PYMS (Paediatric Yorkhill Malnutrition Score) Tool has been developed and has been identified as

being a valid, reliable tool with good diagnostic accuracy to identify children at risk of malnutrition without misclassifying those at low risk (see http://www.nres.npsa.nhs.uk/researchsummaries/?entryid29=19037&p=3).

PULLING IT ALL TOGETHER

Pulling together a smooth assessment can be quite demanding, as there is no single right way to perform a physical examination. The ultimate aim is to create a method that works for you. The examination should cover all aspects so that you have a realistic chance of identifying any problem that may in fact be present. Try to link together areas that are connected spatially, even if they are detached physiologically. This allows you to be economical and efficient and also reduces the number of times the patient has to get up and down. Being effortlessly replicable ensures that you perform the examination in the same way all of the time (Goldberg 2002).

ASSESSMENT (PROVISIONAL DIAGNOSIS)

The assessment stage refers to the overall impression gained by the practitioner from the subjective and objective information obtained, i.e. the provisional diagnosis. The overall impression will indicate whether immediate action should be taken or whether the needs of the child are ongoing. The practitioner should accurately document and communicate the findings of the examination to the relevant members of the multidisciplinary team (Vessey 1995, Hockenberry 2005, DoH 2003b).

PLAN (TREATMENT OPTIONS)

In the case of a child requiring immediate treatment, your plan of action may have been determined by the information gained during the brief episode of visually appraising the child pre-assessment. Alternatively, the plan of action may be decided upon once the examination has been undertaken, a provisional diagnosis or impression has been formed and this information has been communicated to the relevant multidisciplinary team members, incorporating, for example, investigations, treatments and monitoring. Again the plan should be documented clearly and updated as necessary (Vessey 1995, Hockenberry 2005).

COMPLICATIONS

There are few risks associated with assessment or taking observations. The biggest problem arises when the individual performing the task does not recognise the importance of the results obtained, misinterprets the results and takes an inappropriate action in consequence, or does not act on them at all (DoH 2003b). The nurse must: (1) Have an idea of whether or not the information obtained is normal or abnormal. (2) Be able to assess if the result obtained was due to malfunction or misuse of equipment (if used). (3) Know how to act on the results – what must be done and who must be informed. Failure in any of these three areas could adversely affect the child.

COMMUNITY PERSPECTIVE

While assessment of the child is integral in the role of the CCN, consideration must be given to the necessity of formal monitoring of vital signs, remembering that the aim of care is to make the home as unclinical an environment as possible while maintaining the safety of the child. When the child's condition requires this monitoring, the parents should be given a full explanation.

DOS AND DON'TS

- Do ensure that you have been properly trained in the use of electrical equipment such as pulse oximeters and blood pressure machines.
- Do note and inform medical staff of any bruising or anything unusual.
- Do remember to *record* and *report* your information.
- Do ensure that assessments are undertaken in a safe environment.
- Do ensure that consent has been obtained.

References

Abbott Nutrition and Central Manchester and Manchester Children's University Hospitals NHS Trust, 2008. STAMP. Online. Available: www.stampscreeningtool.org.

ALSG Advanced Life Support Group, 2005. Advanced Paediatric Life Support: the practical approach, third ed. BMJ publishing, London.

Archer, N., Burch, M., 1998. Paediatric cardiology. An introduction. Chapman and Hall Medical, London.

Aylott, M., 2007a. Observing the sick child: Part 2b Respiratory palpation. Paediatr. Nurs. 19 (1), 38–45.

Aylott, M., 2007b. Observing the sick child: Part 2c Respiratory auscultation. Paediatr. Nurs. 19 (3), 38–45.

Aylott, M., 2008. Assessment of temperature, pulse and respiration. In: Kelsey, J., McEwing, G. (Eds.), Clinical skills in child health practice. Churchill Livingstone Elsevier, Edinburgh.

Barnes, K. (Ed.), 2003. Paediatrics: a clinical guide for nurse practitioners. Butterworth-Heinemann, London.

Barnes, K., 2004. Paediatrics: A clinical guide for nurse practitioners. Butterworth Heinemann, London, p. 88.

Bee, H., Boyd, D., 2007. The developing child, eleventh ed. Pearson Education, New York.

Bond, M., Uzelac, P.S., 2004. SOAP for emergency medicine. Blackwell Publishing, Oxford.

Brennan, E.P., 2008. Assessment of blood pressure. In: Kelsey, J., McEwing, G. (Eds.), Clinical skills in child health practice. Churchill Livingstone Elsevier, Edinburgh, p. 88.

Bur, A., Hirschl, M.M., Herkner, H., et al., 2000. Accuracy of oscillometric blood pressure measurement according to the relation between cuff size and upper arm circumference in critically ill patients. Crit. Care Med. 28 (2), 371–376.

Bur, A., Herkner, H., Vlcek, M., et al., 2003. Factors influencing the accuracy of oscillometric blood pressure measurement in critically ill patients. Crit. Care Med. 31 (3), 793–799.

Byrnes, K., 1996. Conducting the pediatric health history: a guide. Pediatr. Nurs. 22 (2), 135–137.

Candy, D., Davies, G., Ross, E., 2001. Clinical paediatrics and child health. WB Saunders, Edinburgh.

Carroll, P., 1993. Clinical application of pulse oximetry. Pediatr. Nurs. 19 (2), 150–151.

Clark, J.A., Lieh-Lai, M.W., Sarnaik, A., et al., 2002. Discrepancies between direct and indirect blood pressure measurements using various recommendations for arm cuff selection. Pediatrics 110 (5), 920–923.

Clausen, L.R., Olsen, C.A., Olsen, J.A., et al., 1999. Influence of cuff size on blood pressure among schoolchildren. Blood Press. 8 (3), 172–176.

Coull, A., 1992. Making sense of pulse oximetry. Nurs. Times 88 (32), 42–43.

de Swiet, M., Dillon, M.J., Littler, W., et al., 1989. Measurement of blood pressure in children – recommendations of a working party of the British Hypertension Society. Br. Med. J. 299, 497.

Department of Health, 2001. Seeking consent: working with children. DoH, London.

Department of Health, 2003a. Getting the right start: National Service Framework standard for hospital services. DoH, London.

Department of Health, 2003b. The Victoria Cxlimbie inquiry. Report by Lord Laming. TSO, London.

Department of Health, 2004. The National Service Framework for children, young people and maternity services – standard for hospital services. DoH, London.

Department of Health, 2007. The Darzi Report. DoH, London.

DoH, 2009. UK-World Health Organisation 0 - 4 Growth Charts. DoH, London.

Duncan, H., 2007. The paediatric early warning score. Br. J. Intensive Care, Winter 133–139.

Engel, J., 2006. Pocket guide to pediatric assessment, fifth ed. Mosby, St Louis.

Epstein, O., Perkin, G.D., de Bono, D.P., et al., 1997. Pocket guide to clinical examination, second ed. Mosby, London.

Gill, D., O'Brien, N., 2007. Paediatric clinical examination, fifth ed. Churchill Livingstone, Edinburgh.

Gleadle, J., 2007. History and examination, second ed. Blackwell, Oxford.

Goldberg, C., 2002. A practical guide to clinical medicine: pulling it all together. University of California, San Diego.

Hall, D.M., 2000. Growth monitoring. Arch. Dis. Child. 82, 10–15.

Haines, C., Perrott, M., Weir, P., 2005. Promoting care for acutely ill children – development and evaluation of a paediatric early warning tool. Intensive Crit. Care Nurs. 22, 73–81.

Hamric, A.B., Spross, J.A., Hanson, C., 2004. Advanced practice nursing. An integrative approach. Saunders, Philadelphia.

Hanna, D., 1995. Guidelines for pulse oximetry use in pediatrics. J. Pediatr. Nurs. 10 (2), 124–126.

Health Advisory Service, 1995. The commissioning role and management of child and adolescent mental health services: together we stand. The NHS Advisory Thematic Review. HMSO, London.

Hockenberry, M., 2005. Wong's essentials of pediatric nursing, seventh ed. Elsevier, Edinburgh.

Holden, C., MacDonald, A., 2000. Nutrition and child health. Baillière Tindall and RCN, London.

Honeyman, C., 2007. Recognising mental health problems in children and young people. Paediatr. Nurs. 19 (8), 38–44.

Hull, D., Johnston, D.I., 1993. Essential paediatrics. third ed. Churchill Livingstone, Edinburgh, p. 117.

Jellinek, M.S., Murphy, J.M., Robinson, J., et al., 1988. Paediatric symptom checklist: screening school-age children for psychosocial dysfunction. J. Paediatr. 112 (2), 201–209.

Johnson, J., 2008. The gynecologic system and the child. In: Greydanus, D.E., Feinberg, A.N., Patel, D.R., Douglas, N.H. (Eds.), The pediatric diagnostic examination. McGraw Medical, New York.

Iyriboz, Y., Hearon, C.M., Edwards, K., 1994. Agreement between large and small cuffs in sphygmomanometry: a quantitative assessment. J. Clin. Monit. 10 (2), 127–133.

Mackay-Jones, M.J., Molyneux, E., Phillips, S., Wieteska, S., 2001. Advanced paediatric life support, A practical approach, third ed. BMJ Books, Bristol.

McEwing, G., 2007. Physical growth and measurement. In: Glasper, A., McEwing, J., Richardson, J. (Eds.), Oxford Handbook of Children's & Young People's Nursing. Oxford University Press, Oxford.

McQueen, S., 2001. Clinical benefit of 3M Tempadot thermometer in paediatric settings. Br. J. Nurs. 10 (1), 55–58.

NICE, 2000. Guidance on the use of inhaler systems (devices) in children under the age of 5 years with chronic asthma. National Institute for Health and Clinical Excellence, London.

NICE, 2002. Inhaler devices for routine treatment of chronic asthma in older children (5–15). National Institute for Health and Clinical Excellence, London.

NICE, 2007a. Corticosteroids for the treatment of chronic asthma in children under the age of 12 years. National Institute for Health and Clinical Excellence, London.

NICE, 2007b. Feverish illness in children. National Institute for Health and Clinical Excellence, London.

NICE, 2007c. UTI in children. National Institute for Health and Clinical Excellence, London.

NICE, 2008a. Maternal and child nutrition. National Institute for Health and Clinical Excellence, London.

NICE, 2008b. Surgical management of treatment with otitis media and effusion, (OME). National Institute for Health and Clinical Excellence, London.

National Mental Health Association, 2003. Positive parenting. Strengthening families factsheet. NMHA, London.

Office of National Statistics, 2005. Mental health in children and young people in Great Britain 2004. HMSO, London.

Patel, L., Dixon, M., David, T.J., 2003. Growth and growth charts in cystic fibrosis. J. R. Soc. Med. 96 (Suppl. 43), 35–41.

Perloff, D., Grim, C., Flack, J., et al., 1993. Human blood pressure determination by sphygmomanometry. Circulation 88 (5), 2460–2470.

Pickersgill, J., Fowler, H., Bootham, J., et al., 2003. Temperature taking: children's preferences. Paediatr. Nurs. 15 (2), 22–25.

RCN, 2001. Protection of nurses working with children and young people: guidance for nursing staff. Royal College of Nursing, London.

RCN, 2003. Restraining, holding still and containing children. Royal College of Nursing, London.

RCN, 2007. Standards for assessing. measuring and monitoring vital signs in infants, children and

young people. Royal College of Nursing, London.

RCPCH, 2002. Growth reference charts for use in the UK. Royal College of Paediatrics and Child Health, London.

Rush, M., Wetherall, A., 2003. Temperature measurement: practice guidelines. Paediatr. Nurs. 15 (9), 25–28.

Rushforth, H., Warner, J., Burge, D., et al., 1998. Nursing physical assessment skills: implications for UK practice. Br. J. Nurs. 7 (16), 965–970.

Sims, J., 1996. Making sense of pulse oximetry and oxygen dissociation curve. Nurs. Times 92 (1), 34–35.

Thomas, D.O., 1996. Assessing children – it's different. RN 59 (4), 38–45.

Uzelac, P.S., Moon, R.W., Badillo, A.G., 2004. SOAP for internal medicine. Blackwell Publishing, Oxford.

Vessey, J.A., 1995. Developmental approaches to examining young

children. Pediatr. Nurs. 21 (1), 53–56.

Weed, L.L., 1964. Medical records, patient care and medical education. Ir. J. Med. Sci. June 271–282.

Weed, L.L., 1968. Medical records that guide and teach. N. Engl. J. Med. 278, 593–600, 652–657.

Weed, L.L., 1969. Medical records, medical education and patient care: the problem-oriented medical record as a basic tool. Case Western University, Cleveland.

Wong, D.L., 1995. Paediatric Quick Reference, second ed. Mosby, St Louis.

Wong, D.L., 1997. Whaley and Wong's essentials of pediatric nursing, fifth ed. Mosby, St Louis.

Wong, D.L., 2003. Essentials of paediatric nursing. Mosby, St Louis.

Yernault, J.C., Bohadana, A.B., 1995. Chest percussion. Eur. Respir. J. 8 (10), 1756–1760.

Further reading

Bee, H., 1997. The developing child, eighth ed. Addison-Wesley, New York.

Frisch, N.A., Coscarelli, W., 1986. Systematic instructional strategies in clinical teaching: outcomes in student charting. Nurse Educ. 11 (6), 29–32.

Hanning, C.D., Alexander-Williams, J.M., 1995. Pulse oximetry: a practical review. Br. Med. J. 311, 367–370.

Hazinski, M., 1992. Nursing care of the critically ill child, second ed.

Mosby Year Book, St Louis, inside cover.

http://medicine.ucsd.edu/ clinicalmed/together.htm.

http://www.chiro.org/ documentation/ABSTRACTS/ Maximizing_the_Effectiveness. html.

Langlois, J.P., Thach, S., 2000. Managing the difficult learning situation. Fam. Med. 32 (5), 307–309.

McPhee, A., 1987. Teaching students how to chart. SOAP notes. Nurse Educ. 12 (4), 33–36.

Stoneham, M.D., Saville, G.M., Wilson, I.H., 1994. Knowledge about pulse oximetry among medical and nursing staff. Lancet 344, 1339–1342.

Welk, D., 2001. Teaching students a pattern of reversals eases the care plan process. Nurse Educ. 26 (1), 43–45.

Chapter 7

Caring for the child who has died

Bernadette McCormick

CHAPTER CONTENTS

Introduction   81
    Learning outcomes   81
    Rationale   82

Family care when death is expected and planning can take place   82
    Other family members   82
    Family care when a dying child has to undergo resuscitation   83

Family care when parents are not present when their child dies   83
    Retention of organs and postmortem (PM)   83
    Organ donation   84

Special religious needs of the dying child and the care of the child's body after death   85
    Christian families   85
    Jewish families   86
    Muslim families of the Islamic faith   86
    Hindu families   86
    Sikh families   86

Guidelines   87
    Bereavement care after a child has died   87
    Equipment needed for caring for a child after death   87
    Method   88
    Observations and complications   90
    Dos and don'ts   92

INTRODUCTION

Nurses are at the forefront of delivering needs-led healthcare in a changing society. Advances in maternal and child health have influenced patterns of illness, promoting growth in community and palliative care services for children and young people with chronic and life-limiting illnesses (DoH 2008). Child health involves not only physical care but also religious and spiritual care (Scottish Executive Health Department 2002). The diversity offered by a multicultural society, incorporating an increasing number of asylum seekers and migrant workers, presents many challenges to nurses at all stages of life/death continuum.

Provision of effective and sensitive care to a child or young person who has died and their family is perhaps one of the most complex and demanding aspects of children's nursing. Nurses require knowledge of current legislation, an awareness of cultural preferences relating to preparation of the child's body and insight into the psychosocial effects of a child's death on the family. As the child is part of a family unit, the importance of the family role must be recognised not only in life but also in death (Clift 2006, Hindmarch 2000). While the importance of palliative care is alluded to in this chapter, the focus of the chapter is on care of the child after they have died.

LEARNING OUTCOMES

By the end of this section you should be able to:

- Be aware that a child and family may choose where the child dies and is cared for after death

- Describe the principles of caring for the child's body after death with reference to cultural and religious customs and legal requirements
- Help distressed relatives and staff to follow the procedures that are necessary when a child has died
- Identify resources, which may help family, and staff begin to accept the death of a child and understand and manage their own grief process
- Explain under which circumstances there may be a need for a postmortem and need for a Coroners referral.

RATIONALE

In the UK, childhood death occurs infrequently (Whittle & Cutts 2002) but the impact on the family is profound (Davies & Connaughty 2002). The nurse's professional experience of childhood death may be limited; however, when it does occur, compassionate, professional and effective management of the situation may positively influence the family's ability to grieve (Hindmarch 2000) and assist staff in obtaining a balance between professional and personal loss (Read 2002). Informing families that some choices are available to them which may allow them to feel in control of at least part of the process may offer some comfort at a time when the outcome is out of their hands.

FAMILY CARE WHEN DEATH IS EXPECTED AND PLANNING CAN TAKE PLACE

The child, young person and family should all be involved in the discussions about where the last days of life are spent (Freyer 2004). There should be several options from which they may choose the one most suitable to their individual needs including hospital, home or hospice. In some cases, despite the requirement for intensive care treatments to temporarily sustain life, the choice of dying at home has been facilitated (Longden & Mayer 2007). While a hospital ward may be too noisy, busy and lacking in privacy, some parents may find comfort in being in the hospital environment. This may be due to their fears about how their child will die: Will he be in pain? Will he bleed or choke to death? Careful discussion about

their reasons for wanting to be in hospital may uncover these fears. Explanation and reassurance will help to allay them. Parents may then decide that hospital is not their first choice. Some areas are fortunate to have children's hospices where it may be possible for the child and family to spend the last hours. This can be arranged days or weeks in advance where circumstances allow, but many hospices can be of assistance at very short notice. Some hospices will care for children who have already died (e.g. on a hospital ward). They take the child's body into the hospice so that the family may spend some time with the child in a setting, which is not part of a mortuary or Chapel of Rest but more like home.

In a non-emergency situation, choice of who should be present when the child or young person is dying should also be considered. Some families like to have the dying child surrounded by the whole family – parents, siblings and grandparents, uncles and aunts. Other parents may wish to be on their own with their child. The developmental age of the child or young person influences their level of understanding of their own death and may have reached the extent of the realisation of the impact upon others (Freyer 2004). Therefore, all attempts to integrate the child or young person's wishes with the parents' wishes about who should be present should be negotiated. The nurse may offer to tactfully refuse visitors if parents or dying children wish to have privacy. It can be difficult for parents to be assertive about numbers and timing of visits and visitors when their child is dying.

OTHER FAMILY MEMBERS

Siblings, grandparents and other relatives will also need a lot of support at the time of a child's death. This can be a particular issue for nurses if the parents are concentrating entirely on the dying child and dealing with their own grief. Sibling short- and long-term grief is influenced by individual, situational and environmental factors (Davies & Orloff 2004). These factors include the age of the grieving sibling, the circumstances of their brother or sister's death and also the closeness of the relationship between the child and their sibling. Nurses who recognise the individuality of each child or young person's death and adopt a flexible approach to care delivery at this time will help to provide emotional support not only leading up to and at the time of death, but also in the future. Other agencies may help provide support for family members, e.g. play therapists for siblings, religious figures to help grandparents.

FAMILY CARE WHEN A DYING CHILD HAS TO UNDERGO RESUSCITATION

The presence of the family in an emergency situation such as resuscitation has stimulated much debate. The right of parents to be present at a time when there is risk to their child's life seems unquestionable (Clift 2006). However, staff may be concerned about parents' presence hindering their attempts either through feeling intimidated as they may be being observed or by having to support distressed parents. Staff have expressed fears that witnessing resuscitation of their child may cause long-lasting psychological damage to parents and hinder their grieving process. Conversely, Hogg (2003) discovered that the imagined horror of the resuscitation attempt results in more damage to relatives who had not been present during resuscitation, than to those who had been. This supports earlier findings by Hallgrimsdottir (2000) who reported that parents felt that it brought a sense of reality to their loss and helped them in their grieving process. Parents also report that it was of some comfort to them that as they knew that everything possible had been done (Meyers et al 2000, Vanderbeek 2000). However, in order to effectively support families, a designated appropriate person should be identified to be with the parents (Meyers et al 2000). Parents must: (1) be given the choice of whether or not to stay; (2) not be left on their own to witness the events; (3) be supported by someone who can explain what is happening to their child.

FAMILY CARE WHEN PARENTS ARE NOT PRESENT WHEN THEIR CHILD DIES

If parents have not been present at the death of their child, they must be informed as soon as possible after death. Someone who has access to accurate information about the circumstances of the child's death and the experience and confidence to inform the relatives should perform this task. It is important to be gentle but direct. Using simple language such as 'she has died', rather than euphemisms such as 'she has passed away', will avoid misunderstandings and help parents to acknowledge their child's

death – the first step towards acceptance. Do not be afraid of silence once the news of the death has been given. In a study of bereaved parents, Soutter (1994) was told by them that 'words were not necessary because the pain was too great and could not easily be assuaged'. However, the same study also highlighted the comfort that was afforded to parents by the physical contact of an embrace. In some cultures, relatives are expected to show their grief by wailing and keening. This can be very noisy and possibly cause distress to staff and any other patients or relatives who may be nearby (in a hospital setting). Explanation that this is their way of expressing their grief should be given.

RETENTION OF ORGANS AND POSTMORTEM (PM)

Bereavement care includes determining the need for postmortem in discussion with the medical team and obtaining informed consent from the child's next of kin for the procedure. Obviously, this is a time of great stress and sadness for everyone and detailed discussions should be handled with sensitivity. Following the Royal Liverpool Children's Inquiry (2001) into the retention of organs, changes in the whole concept of communicating with families and gaining consent have taken place and have shaped the current process (DoH 2003).

- The possibility of a coroner's PM must only be mentioned if the death is reportable to the coroner.
- If the coroner declines a PM, but the clinician wishes a hospital PM to be undertaken, the next of kin must be made aware that this is a consented procedure to which they have a right to decline. No compulsion exists for this to be carried out.
- The full procedure must be explained to the next of kin including the opening of the body, removal and weighing of organs and if any organs or tissue will be retained and what will subsequently happen to these (Human Tissue (Scotland) Act 2006, Human Tissue Act 2004).

Box 7.1 details some of the major categories relating to the death of a child which indicate that the case must be referred to the coroner, by law (Regulation 51 of the Registration of Births, Deaths, and Marriages Regulations 1968). In these circumstances, the coroner will sometimes order a postmortem.

BOX 7.1   Deaths to be referred to the coroner

- When there is an element of suspicious circumstances or history of violence
- Where the death may be linked to an accident (whenever it occurred)
- Where the death is linked with an abortion
- Where the death may be related to a medical procedure or treatment
- When the death occurred during an operation or before full recovery from the effects of anaesthesia, or was in any way linked to the effects of anaesthesia
- When the actions of the deceased may have contributed to his or her own death, e.g. self-neglect or drug or solvent misuse
- An unknown cause of death
- A fostered or adopted child.

BOX 7.2   Religious/spiritual perspectives on postmortem

- Religions which absolutely forbid postmortem: Jews, Muslims, Zoroastrians (Parsees)
- Religions which strongly object to postmortem: Christian Scientists
- Religions which would prefer postmortem not to occur if at all possible: Rastafarians
- Religions which do not have specific views on the postmortem examination: Christians, Jehovah's Witnesses, Mormons, Buddhists, Hindus, Sikhs.

Written guidance detailing required reported deaths is available on the government website, at: www.dh.gov.uk

Sometimes local practice requires a postmortem to be performed in additional circumstances to those required by law, for example, if the death was within 24 h of admission to hospital or if the deceased was detained under the Mental Health Act. It is important to establish what local policy and practice require. Ethically, medical staff should always obtain consent for a postmortem from parents, but it is not legally required for a coroner's postmortem (Henderson 2006).

Seeking consent for a postmortem is a very emotive subject for families and nurses may play an integral role in ensuring that the approach is sensitive and positive (Henderson 2006). Careful explanation of the need for the examination and the actual procedure should be given. It must be stressed that the body will be treated with the utmost respect and the same care as for a living patient. Parents may be concerned that the body will be disfigured by the procedure and should be reassured that suture lines on the torso and above the hair line will be the only evidence of the postmortem and will not be unduly disfiguring. Parents should be given the opportunity to view the body afterwards. It is generally accepted that having this opportunity helps families to grieve (Haas 2003). However, evidence exists which suggests that this may not be the case in the neonatal death experience (Skene 1998). Therefore, caution should be shown

and each case treated as individual (Davies & Connaughty 2002).

The inability to stop a coroner's postmortem may cause extreme distress to some families, particularly those whose religion expressly forbids such a procedure (Box 7.2). These parents may need a lot of support, and advice should be sought from their religious or spiritual advisors concerning special procedures for handling the body during postmortem and returning organs to the body. Jewish and Islamic faiths require that any organs removed from the body during a legally required postmortem examination be returned to it for burial (Green & Green 2006). When a postmortem is required, any cannulae, drains or tubing should not be removed from the body without discussion with medical staff (Green & Green 2006).

ORGAN DONATION

In some cases, the question of organ donation may arise. Suitability for organ donation will depend on the child having no evidence of major untreated systemic infection, malignancy (excepting primary brain tumour), chronic severe hypertension or positivity to Australia antigen (hepatitis B) or human immunodeficiency virus antibodies (Browne & Waddington 1993). A child who is maintained on mechanical ventilation must have met the brain stem death criteria before organ donation can occur.

Browne and Waddington (1993) suggest approaching parents when the first set of tests has been completed and the criteria met. It may be possible to broach the subject earlier than this if someone who is experienced in discussing the subject with parents, e.g. a transplant coordinator, handles it sensitively. Ensure that when parents are approached regarding organ donation, someone with whom they have been able to build a relationship, for example a member of the medical or nursing staff, is present. Organ donation must always be broached sensitively and by someone who has a positive attitude towards transplantation but is not seen as biased.

If parents agree to organ donation, the transplant coordinator will help support them and explain forthcoming procedures. Parents should be aware that they can see their child after donation. They should be warned that their child will be white, cold and, depending on which organs have been retrieved, may have large scars.

Religious objection to organ transplantation is not the inevitable consequence of the laws and beliefs of the different faiths (Ethnicity Online 2004). However, the following examples illustrate how some find it a very difficult issue:

- Jehovah's Witnesses because other transfused blood will circulate through the organ
- Christian Scientists because they prefer the body to be inviolate and to rely on the healing power of prayer
- Orthodox Jews because of their beliefs in the sanctity of the body and physical resurrection.

Once parents have consented and the coroner has agreed, organ donation can take place. Table 7.1 lists the organs which can be used.

SPECIAL RELIGIOUS NEEDS OF THE DYING CHILD AND THE CARE OF THE CHILD'S BODY AFTER DEATH

Information contained within this section pertaining to religious customs and death is taken from About.com 2009, Green & Green (2006), Bull (2004) and Ethnicity Online (2004). There are several common themes between some religions relating to rituals after death. These are summarised in Box 7.3. Other special considerations are as detailed below.

CHRISTIAN FAMILIES

Many Christians will want their child to be baptised if death is imminent. If this is not possible before death, a priest may conduct a naming and blessing ceremony after death. In an emergency, any Christian may conduct a baptism. Baptism is important to

Table 7.1 Organs which can be donated from children

ORGAN	MINIMUM AGE OF DONOR	SPECIAL REQUIREMENTS OF DONOR'S CONDITION	TREATMENT NECESSARY TO MAINTAIN ORGAN IN GOOD CONDITION PRIOR TO REMOVAL
Kidney	2 years	No renal disease, good renal function	Inotrope infusion and intravenous fluids to maintain perfusion of kidneys
Liver	3 months	No liver diseases, drug abuse or alcoholism. Good liver function	–
Heart	6 months	No cardiac defect or disease. Donor's condition should be stable without excessive inotropic support	–
Heart and lung	6 months	No cardiac defect or disease or pulmonary dysfunction. No heavy smoking. Good arterial blood gases and lung compliance. Ventilation should not have been prolonged	–
Pancreas	14 years	No history of diabetes. If the liver is also being retrieved, patient must have spleen still intact	–
Cornea	Any age	No corneal scarring. No infectious eye disease	Eye care extremely important. Eyes must be closed and protected after death
Heart valves	6 months	–	Can be retrieved up to 72 hours after death

Reproduced with the permission from Browne J, Waddington P 1993 Care of the dying child. In: Carter B (ed.) Manual of paediatric intensive care nursing. Chapman and Hall, London, p 299

> **BOX 7.3 Rituals surrounding care of the body after death common to the Jewish, Muslim, Hindu and Sikh religions**
>
> It is important of discuss this with the family and not to make assumptions based on religion.
> - The child will not be left unattended while dying, nor must the body be left unattended after death
> - Cleansing of the child's body after death is only to be performed by special individuals:
>   a. Specially-trained members of the community of the same sex as the dead child perform Jewish last offices
>   b. A non-Muslim must not touch the body of a Muslim child, but if it is unavoidable, a non-Muslim should wear disposable gloves
>   c. A non-Hindu should preferably not touch the body of a Hindu child
>   d. Family members of the same sex as the child care for the body of a Sikh child
>
> - Therefore, the body of a child of any of these religions should simply be straightened, limbs straightened and the eyes closed, then covered with a clean sheet until further instructions can be obtained from the family. If a family member is not able to be present, it may be appropriate to ask if they wish a member of staff to remain with the body
> - It is important that the funeral should take place within 24 h of death. It can be possible to arrange this, even if there has to be a postmortem
> - Any religious emblems (bracelets or necklets made from Holy thread) and jewellery on the body of a Hindu or Sikh child must be left in place on the body.

Roman Catholics to the extent that they will allow even a non-believer to conduct an emergency baptism if a priest is not available. Roman Catholic families may also want a priest to perform the Sacrament of the Sick and Sacrament of the Dying (extreme unction). Holy Communion will be important if the child has taken their first Holy Communion.

JEWISH FAMILIES

Traditionally, the body is not to be touched for 20 min after breathing has stopped. After 10 min, a feather is then placed over the mouth and nose to ensure that breathing has stopped. The body should be touched as little as possible and gloves should be worn to do so. Close the child's eyes and straighten out the body, lying flat with feet together and arms by the sides. The body should be covered in a plain white sheet and should never be left alone or in the dark. A light should be left on as a mark of respect.

MUSLIM FAMILIES OF THE ISLAMIC FAITH

The dead child's extended family are likely to visit to pay respects and support the immediate family. Close the child's eyes and cover it with a clean sheet. The parents may wish the body to be placed with the face facing towards Mecca (south-east).

The family will usually wash the child's body. If the child has reached puberty, the child's body will be washed and prepared by family members who are the same gender as the child. Muslims believe that flexing the elbows, shoulders, knees and hips before straightening will help delay the onset of stiffening. Often Muslim families do not wish their child to go to the hospital mortuary but arrange for the body to go straight to the mosque for cleansing or to a Muslim undertaker.

HINDU FAMILIES

A Hindu family is likely to prefer that their child die at home and may wish a priest to be present at the child's bedside to perform holy rites. In addition to Holy thread (Yagyopavit) around the child's limbs or body, the skin may be marked with paste or a sacred leaf (Tulsi) or ghee (butter) placed in the mouth. Gloves should be worn if the child's body is touched. A light is often left on near the child's head as a mark of respect and to comfort the soul. Children under 5 years are buried and not cremated.

SIKH FAMILIES

It may be inappropriate to remove underclothing as this may have religious significance. If the child wears a turban, this must also be left in place after death. The face may be cleansed if it is dirty.

Touch the body as little as possible. Wear gloves if the body is touched. Wrap the child's body in a plain white sheet.

GUIDELINES

BEREAVEMENT CARE AFTER A CHILD HAS DIED

Parents

Invite parents and family to help with washing and dressing their child after death. This need not be rushed. Some parents will not want to be involved; others may welcome the opportunity (Browne & Waddington 1993). When parents wish to be involved, be sensitive as to whether or not your presence is required. Gentle explanation should be given to parents who choose to be involved. They should know that as their child is moved, air may escape from the lungs and result in a noise which may sound like a groan. They should also be aware there may be leakage of body fluids and that blood will pool according to gravity and may make their child's skin appear a strange colour.

Support beyond the time immediately following death

Davies and Orloff (2004) stress the vital importance of advice, counselling and support from appropriately trained staff for bereaved parents. Care and ongoing support for bereaved parents is becoming more widely available with ever-increasing numbers of bereavement groups established. Examples of national groups are those such as the Compassionate Friends, SANDS (the Stillbirth and Neonatal Death Society), the Child Bereavement Trust, The Child Death Helpline and CRUSE. There are also many groups related to specific illness such as the Children's Liver Disease Foundation and SPOCC (Society of Parents of Children with Cancer). It is useful to have a resource which lists all the available agencies, for example the Contact-a-family Directory. Parents should be given information as to how to access counselling and allowed to make a choice as to when or if it is appropriate for them. In the early stages of grief, they may not yet feel able to address counselling. They should also be informed that access to counselling can be something they can do at any time, even many years after the death of their child.

Staff

Pattison (2008) and Davies and Orloff (2004) highlight the fact that staff who are involved in caring for a dying child may also be affected emotionally and suggest that all nurses involved in the death of a child should be offered support from their colleagues and given the opportunity to reflect upon the event or undertake some sort of counselling, if only to evaluate the impact of the event. However, as the whole multidisciplinary team cares for a child, all members of that team will be touched by the child's death Therefore, the possibility of a multidisciplinary forum, facilitated by a trained counsellor, to discuss feelings surrounding the child's death should be considered. Suitable facilitators may be found from the clinical psychology department, the clergy or occupational health service. It is also important to be aware of any members of the team who might require individual support.

EQUIPMENT NEEDED FOR CARING FOR A CHILD AFTER DEATH

- Warm water for washing the child
- Soap
- Towels
- Clean nappy (if child still in nappies)
- Clean clothing which can be day or night-clothes according to the parents' preference
- Dressings if necessary (if there are cannulae, percutaneous lines or drains to be removed), e.g. small adhesive, waterproof plasters and gauze swabs or padding in case of leakage of body fluids from any wounds
- Spigots or plugs to cap the end of cannulae, drainage tubes, etc. if they are to be left *in situ* for a postmortem
- Gauze swabs in case the child's eyes need to be covered to help them remain closed
- Clean bed linen
- Linen skip for dirty linen
- Brush or comb
- Identity band with child's name and hospital registration number or labels which concur with local policy, e.g. Notice of Death Certificate and tape or safety pin to secure it to the sheet covering the body

- Clean sheet, big enough to wrap around the child's body
- Toy to place with the body if parents request it
- Flowers, if available, may be placed in the child's hand or nearby if suitable to the child's age and sex.

The following may also be needed:

- Documentation to list and record the child's belongings
- Scissors and a suitable container for obtaining and keeping a lock of the child's hair
- Equipment for taking hand and feet prints or casts
- Camera for photograph.

Photographs taken after death can be very important. Hawley (1997) describes that 'photographs taken at that time are among our most precious reminders [of the dead child]'. If it is a neonate who has died, it may be the only picture of their child that the parents will ever have.

Note: Some hospitals provide bereavement packs. They may include prompts to provide mementoes such as footprints, photographs, and information about how to register the death, people who could offer help and support groups. Some hospitals have special Moses baskets, cots or prams in which to place an infant's body.

A body bag made of heavy, waterproof plastic with zip, of a size suitable to contain the body, will be necessary if the child was suffering from hepatitis B, AIDS or was HIV-positive.

METHOD

1. Washing and laying out of the body should be considered within 2–3 h of death. This is because rigor mortis can begin as soon as 2 h after death, especially if the child's temperature was high at the time of death (Green & Green 2006). This may not always be the case, however, but it may be aesthetically more pleasing if the child has been washed. It is much more difficult to handle a body when rigor has commenced. Once washed, the child can be given back to parents to cuddle if they wish.

2. Remove the bedclothes and straighten the body as far as possible without using force. This may not be possible if the child has a physical deformity such as severe scoliosis, or severely retracted limbs. Support the head with one small pillow. If the cot is too small for a pillow, consider using a folded, soft towel. Cover the body with a sheet to preserve the child's privacy and dignity.

3. Remove the child's clothing; observe the body for any bruising or signs of injury. Any findings should be noted in the nursing documentation. Cover the body with the sheet.

4. Clean the child's eyes if necessary and close them. If they will not close of their own accord, it may be necessary to place dampened gauze swabs over each eye to help keep them shut. Sometimes a small piece of tape can be used, but it must be of a type which will not cause trauma to the skin when it is removed. Micropore tape is ideal for this.

5. Clean the child's mouth carefully. Often the jaw may be slack and leave the mouth gaping. This can be distressing for parents and presents a risk of leakage of body fluids. If it is gaping, it may be necessary to support the jaw (temporarily) with a small pad (e.g. a rolled face towel) under the chin. It may be acceptable to use a piece of cotton bandage tied gently around the head, but again be careful not to cause any trauma to the skin. Usually, once rigor starts to establish, the mouth will remain closed, unsupported.

6. Leakage of body fluids represents a potential hazard to those who have to handle the body after death (Green & Green 2006). Therefore, empty the bladder by applying gentle pressure to the lower abdomen. If there is a lot of leakage from the bowel or vagina, ensure that a nappy or incontinence pad is used. In any child who wore nappies when alive, the parents will find nothing odd in seeing them in a nappy after death and this will cope with most leakages. An incontinence pad may be more appropriate for an older child.

7. If there is to be a postmortem, in accordance with instructions from medical staff, lines, drains, catheters and cannulae should be left *in situ* (Green & Green 2006). Any

drainage bags, infusion tubing, etc. must be removed and the lines, drains, catheters and cannulae spigoted to prevent leakage of body fluids.

8. If there is no postmortem, then everything except tunnelled intravenous catheters should be removed and carefully disposed of according to local policy. Removing tunnelled catheters would cause significant trauma, which is why they should be left *in situ*. Any wounds left by removing cannulae, drains, etc. should be covered with waterproof tape. Any stoma or wound which could continue to leak should be covered with padding and then waterproof tape to prevent leakage. Any removable sutures or clips should be left in place.

9. If required, cut a lock of hair from the back of the child's head (where it will not be obvious that it has been removed). Take plaster casts or foot and handprints from the child's hands and feet. Consent should be obtained for these; many families do not wish their child's hair to be cut.

10. The child's body should then be washed all over and carefully dried. Applying a little petroleum jelly to the lips will help prevent the skin drying out and prevent any corrosion from gastric juices (Green & Green 2006).

11. If there is jewellery on the body, it is usual to remove it unless it has religious significance. If a nurse removes jewellery, it must only be done in the presence of a witness and its removal must be recorded in the documentation.

12. Make up the bed or cot with fresh linen and dress the child. Comb the hair. Place the child in the bed or cot and add a toy and/or flowers as appropriate. Cover the child with a sheet. Some areas will require that a child who has to be put into a body bag must be placed in it as soon as possible after death. If this has to be done, it is possible to leave the zip part way down so that parents may view the body, but it should be argued that there is no need for the body to be placed in the bag until it has to go to the mortuary or funeral parlour. The child is no more infectious after death than before and so parents should have the right to hold and cuddle their child in death as they did in life.

13. If parents are unsure whether or not to have photographs of their child, it may be a good idea to take them now. Explain to parents that even if they feel they do not want photographs now, they may subsequently change their minds. Explain that it is possible to take them and place them in the child's medical records so that they may be retrieved for the family at a later date if they do change their minds. You may not take photographs without the parents' consent.

14. Ensure that the child has a clearly legible identity name band *in situ* on the wrist or ankle. Some areas require there to be a name band on both wrist and ankle.

15. Tidy up. Dispose of linen, sharps and clinical waste carefully and safely to prevent injury or cross-infection and in accordance with local policy.

16. Document the child's property, noting if any jewellery was removed and reserve the property for the family to take home if they wish.

17. If parents have not been involved in the laying out of their child, it is at this point that it would be appropriate to ask them to return to spend time with their child. Encourage them to hold and cuddle their child. Do not be afraid to cry in front of the relatives, but ensure that they do not feel that they have to support you. Be aware that in some cultures it is a mark of respect to grieve loudly and obviously after a death.

Parents should be allowed to spend as much time with their child as possible. If circumstances (e.g. on a busy ward) make this difficult, explain to them beforehand that at this stage they will have limited time. Offer them a private place where they may see their child. This may need to be the hospital chapel or holy room. Some hospitals have special viewing rooms which are decorated like a bedroom and the child's body is placed in a bed, crib or cot according to age. Once the child has gone to the funeral director, the parents should be able to see their child there without any problem. The only exception to this is if the child is in a body bag because of a potential risk of infection. Be aware that, in many cases, once a potentially infectious body has left the hospital, it can only be seen from a distance if at all, and it may be impossible for the parents to hold and cuddle their child again. In this case, it is kindest to hold the body as long as possible where the parents can still have access.

18. When it is time to take the child to the mortuary or the child is to be collected by the funeral director, the body should be wrapped securely in a clean, white sheet, unless the parents specifically request otherwise. If the body has to be placed in a body bag, it must be done before the body goes to the mortuary or funeral parlour. The sheet or bag should be labelled according to local policy.

19. The Notification of Death certificate must accompany the body to the mortuary and is commonly pinned to the sheet. Obviously, pins must not be used on a body bag, as this would damage the integrity of the bag. Sticky tape would suffice. Some areas require a name band label to be attached to the outside of the sheet. The Notification of Death certificate must state if the child has a pacemaker *in situ* (it must be removed if the body is to be cremated as it is liable to explode during cremation), or if the body is potentially infectious.

20. Ensure that the parents have clear, preferably written instructions about what they must do to register the death, organise the funeral and so on. Verbal instructions may not be assimilated when parents are distressed. If there is a bereavement pack for parents, give this to them. If there is a bereavement counsellor, they will be able to support the parents through this process and will be able to help parents access support from other agencies such as bereavement groups.

21. Finally, check who has to be informed about the child's death and who is responsible for doing so. Again, bereavement counsellors may do this as part of their role. A checklist such as that illustrated in Table 7.2 may be utilised.

OBSERVATIONS AND COMPLICATIONS

Observations

As previously described, the nurse should observe the child's body for unusual marks and bruising

Table 7.2   Checklist of those who may need to be informed of the death of a child

PERSON/AGENCY TO BE INFORMED	TO BE INFORMED BY
Named nurse	Nursing staff
Medical records	Nursing staff
General practitioner	Medical staff
Health visitor	Nursing staff
Paramedical staff (physiotherapist, play therapist)	Nursing or medical staff
Religious/spiritual advisor	Nursing staff
Social worker	Nursing staff
Liaison nurse	Nursing staff
Community nurses	Nursing staff
Bereavement counsellor	Nursing staff
School: head, form teacher and school nurse	Hospital school/ nursing staff
Siblings' school	Nursing staff
Hospice	Nursing staff

and these should be recorded. The presence of jewellery on the body or the removal of jewellery from the body should also be observed and recorded.

Complications

Complications should not arise in caring for the body as long as careful thought and preparation are exercised. Without thorough preparation, complications that could arise include:

- Inappropriate handling of the body in relation to legal requirements (postmortem), religious custom or the parents' own wishes
- Nurses inexperienced in managing the death of a child are left without support or resources to tell them what to do
- Additional distress caused to parents who were not made aware of the risk of vocal-type noises emitting from the body or leakage of body fluids
- Additional distress caused to parents who are not made fully aware of the procedures surrounding the death of their child, e.g. having to wait for a death certificate leading to a delay in the funeral.

CCNs are likely to have been involved with the families of children with life-limiting illnesses during their treatment phase and will have had the opportunity to develop a trusting relationship. They may have met members of the extended family and close friends and will therefore be aware of the family dynamics. They may also have had the opportunity to discuss the family's spiritual beliefs.

When a child enters the palliative stage of illness, the parents should be reassured that this does not mean that no active treatment will take place. Treatment options will change, but symptom control in palliative care is often active treatment. A multidisciplinary approach, involving the CCN, general practitioner and the health visitor will be of the greatest benefit to the family. The primary healthcare team will be dealing with the family for many years after the death of the child. It is also important for the CCN to liaise with school nurses and teachers involved with either the dying child or the child's siblings. School friends may also need help to deal with the situation. Discussion should take place within the family as to how and where the child will be cared for. If there is a children's hospice near the family they should be informed of the support available from the hospice. It is often helpful to ask the hospice team to visit the family to explain their services, but only if the family consent. So much control has been taken away from the family because of the child's illness that it is imperative that their wishes during the last period of life are valued. It is important to remember that no two families will cope with grief in the same way (ACT & RCPCH 1997).

The decision that the family reaches must be adhered to as closely as resources permit. It is not possible to guarantee that one particular team member will be present at the time of death and the family need to be aware of this. However, they can be reassured that they will, wherever possible, be supported 24 h a day should they decide to care for their child at home. The government has consistently advocated that children should be cared for in their own homes and that appropriate services are developed to facilitate this (Health Committee 1997, DoH 2003, 2004, 2008). In 1998 the Department of Health provided funding for community children's nursing teams in memory of Diana, Princess of Wales (DoH 1998a, b) and in 2003 the New Opportunities Fund provided £48 million of lottery money to expand home-based paediatric palliative care teams in selected primary care trusts across the country. Although these initiatives have greatly improved palliative care options, some small CCN teams may not be able to provide 24-hour cover all the time, depending on their caseload commitment and whether there is more than one child needing palliative care. Children's Hospices Community teams are usually able to support CCN teams caring for terminally children in their own homes often sharing the clinical input, changing syringe drivers and managing symptoms and nutritional needs. The care of the child at home may involve many organisations but there needs to ensure that there are multidisciplinary meetings to ensure a seamless approach to the care. The family need to have a list of contact numbers and be aware of who is on-call. They also need to know the available options for short breaks, should they feel unable to cope at any time. The CCN must be able to recognise that some families need time on their own, away from professional input. The CCN needs to be sensitive to this and to appreciate that, by visiting more than the family wish, the CCN may be answering personal needs, rather than the family's.

The CCN is ideally placed to empower the family to care for their child and maximise the quality of the child's life. This can be an important time for the family to collect mementoes, photographs, video-recordings, items made by the dying child, etc. It is a period of adjustment, during which the family may be able to address the reality of impending loss and decide how and what to tell younger children, including the dying child. The CCN plays a crucial role in providing emotional support to the family and in turn will need opportunities to off-load, be this in the form of peer support or more formal clinical supervision (ACT & RCPCH 1997, NHS Executive 1998).

During the final period of terminal care, ideally, the CCN team will be available to the family at all times. Short breaks in the home may be offered. Symptom management, including pain control, is vital and a team member or alternative appropriate cover needs to be accessible at all times, in case treatment regimes need changing or the family requires help with nursing care. Regular visits from familiar faces will help to reassure the family. The family should be made aware of the facilities available at children's hospices after a child has died. Their child's body can rest in a chilled room at the hospice, often until the funeral. The hospice staff will care for the child's body and advise whether embalming (a process to preserve the body), is necessary. Many families find it comforting to be able to spend time with their child's body before the funeral.

The CCN or Hospice Community nurse will be able to offer guidance on issues surrounding the actual death of the child and the days immediately following. She will be able to discuss:

- The likely manner of death
- The importance of involving siblings and preparing for the death (Dyregrov 1996)
- The long-term benefits of those closely involved seeing and holding the body after death (Dyregrov 1996)
- That parents can wash and dress their child in favourite clothes following death, if they wish
- Where the child's body should rest before the funeral: the child's body may remain at home providing certain procedures have been undertaken by the funeral director; alternatively the body can be taken to a chapel of rest or a hospice
- How to register the death
- Funeral arrangements and what form this important ritual will take. The parents can be encouraged to allow the siblings some choice. Older children who have come to terms with their impending death may have had strong views on funeral arrangements.

In the months following death, many families need to maintain contact with the professionals involved in their child's care (Goldman 1998). Children's hospices are able to provide counselling services and family support leading up to and after the death of a child. Bereavement support should continue for as long as both parties feel necessary. Work with siblings can be undertaken, for example collecting together items which remind them of the child and putting them in a memory box. It may be years before the family is ready to place the lid on that box and it is important for them to realise that this is perfectly acceptable. This is something over which they do have control.

CCNs may be involved where children die unexpectedly, for example as a result of major surgery. The CCN may have been involved with the family prior to the hospitalisation which resulted in death. In this situation, bereavement visiting and maintaining contact may be appropriate.

DOS AND DON'TS

- Do consult the parents about their wishes for their child after they have died.
- Do remember to maintain the privacy and dignity of the child at all times after death.
- Do establish whether there is to be a postmortem.
- Do establish if there are any special religious, spiritual or cultural needs associated with care of the child after death.
- Do remember that the parents may not be the only family members who require support.
- Do remember to warn parents helping to wash and dress their child after death of how the child may appear, possible noises the body may make and leakage of body fluids.
- Do be aware if there are other staff who may be adversely affected and require support because of the death of a child.
- Do not remove lines, cannulae, etc. if there is to be a postmortem.
- Do not be afraid to show grief and cry with parents after a child has died, but do not allow your own grief to overshadow any situation or make parents feel that they must comfort and support you.

References

About.com, 2009. Online. Available: www.about.com.

Association for Children with Life Threatening or Terminal Conditions and their Families (ACT) and Royal College of Paediatrics and Child Health (RCPCH), 1997. A guide to the development of children's palliative care services. ACT, Bristol.

Browne, J., Waddington, P., 1993. Care of the dying child. In: Carter, B. (Ed.), Manual of paediatric intensive care nursing. Chapman and Hall, London, p. 299.

Bull, A., 2004. Culture and belief system information manual. Yorkhill Division, Greater Glasgow NHS, Glasgow.

Clift, L., 2006. Relatives in the resuscitation room: a review of benefits and risks. Paediatr. Nurs. 18 (5), 14–18.

Davies, B., Connaughty, S., 2002. Pediatric end-of-life care: lessons learned from parents. J. Nurs. Adm. 32 (1), 5–6.

Davies, B., Orloff, S., 2004. Bereavement issues and staff support. In: Doyle, D., Hanks, G., Cherny, N.I., Calman, K. (Eds.), Oxford textbook of palliative medicine, third ed. Oxford University Press, Oxford, pp. 831–839.

Department of Health, 1998a. Diana, Princess of Wales Memorial Committee. Preliminary advice. TSO, London.

Department of Health, 1998b. A proposal to develop a national children's community nursing service. DoH, London.

Department of Health, 2003. Every child matters. DoH, London.

Department of Health, 2004. National Service Framework for children, young people and maternity services. DoH, London.

Department of Health, 2003. Families and postmortems: A code of practice. Online. Available: www.dh.gov.uk.

Department of Health, 2008. Better care: better lives. DoH, London.

Dyregrov, A., 1996. Children's participation in rituals. Bereavement Care 15 (1), 2–4.

Ethnicity Online, 2004. Cultural awareness in healthcare. Online. Available: www.ethnicityonline.net.

Freyer, D.R., 2004. Caring for the dying adolescent: Special considerations. Pediatrics 113 (2), 381–388.

Goldman, A., 1998. Palliative care for children. In: Fauld, C., Carter, Y., Woof, R. (Eds.), Handbook of palliative care. Blackwell Science, London.

Green, J., Green, M., 2006. Dealing with death. A handbook of practices, procedures and law, second ed. Jessica Kingsley, Suffolk.

Haas, F., 2003. Bereavement care: seeing the body. Nurs. Stand. 17 (28), 33–37.

Hallgrimsdottir, E., 2000. Accident and emergency nurse's perceptions and experiences of caring for families. J. Clin. Nurs. 9 (4), 611–619.

Hawley, R., 1997. Seasons of grief. Nurs. Times 93 (8), 24–26.

Health Committee, 1997. House of Commons Select Committee. Health services for children and young people in the community: home and school. Third Report. TSO, London.

Henderson, N., 2006. Communicating with families about postmortems: practice guidance. Paediatr. Nurs. 18 (1), 38–40.

Hindmarch, C., 2000. On the death of a child. Radcliffe Medical Press, Oxon.

Hogg, C., 2003. Emergency Health Services for Children and Young People. A guide for commissioners and providers. Action for Sick Children, London.

Human Tissue (Scotland) Act, 2006. Scottish Executive, Edinburgh.

Human Tissue Act, 2004. HMSO, London.

Longden, J.V., Mayer, A.P., 2007. Family involvement in end-of-life care in a paediatric intensive care unit. Nurs. Crit. Care 12 (4), 181–187.

Meyers, T., Eichhorn, D.J., Guzzetta, C.E., et al., 2000. Family presence during invasive procedures and resuscitation: the experience of family members, nurses and physicians. Am. J. Nurs. 100 (2), 32–43.

NHS Executive, 1998. Evaluation of the pilot project programme for children with life threatening illnesses. TSO, London.

Pattison, N., 2008. Care of patients who have died. Nurs. Stand. 22 (28), 42–48.

Read, S., 2002. Loss and bereavement: a nursing response. Nurs. Stand. 16 (37), 47–55.

Registration of Births, Deaths and Marriages Regulations, 1968. HMSO, London.

Royal Liverpool Children's Inquiry, 2001. TSO, London.

Scottish Executive Health Department, 2002. Guidelines on chaplaincy and spiritual care in the NHS in Scotland. Scottish Executive Health Department, Edinburgh.

Skene, C., 1998. Individualised bereavement care. Paediatr. Nurs. 10 (10), 13–16.

Soutter, J., 1994. A strategy for caring for families in bereavement. Nurs. Times 90 (30), 37–39.

Vanderbeek, J., 2000. Till death do us part. Am. J. Nurs. 100 (2), 44.

Whittle, M., Cutts, S., 2002. Time to go home: assisting families to take their child home following a planned hospital or hospice death. Paediatr. Nurs. 14 (10), 24–28.

Chapter **8**

Cardiopulmonary resuscitation

Fiona Clements

CHAPTER CONTENTS

Introduction   94
   Learning outcomes   95
   Rationale   95
   Factors to note   95

Basic paediatric life support   96
   Method   96
   Dos and don'ts   98

Advanced paediatric life support   98
   The emergency trolley   98

Maintenance of airway   98
   Equipment   98
   Method   98

Vascular access   100
   Equipment   100
   Method   100

Drugs and fluid therapy   100
   Drug therapy   101

Defibrillation   101
   Dos and don'ts   102

Summary   102

INTRODUCTION

While few resuscitation situations involving children arise without warning, it remains imperative that children's nurses are skilled in the area of basic life support (Simpson 1994, Carter & Dearmun 1995). Paediatric basic life support (BLS) is described as the provision of cardiopulmonary resuscitation (CPR) with no devices or with bag-valve-mask ventilation or barrier devices, until advanced life support (ALS) can be provided (International Guidelines 2000). However, 'if basic life support is not effectively delivered to the child, attempts at advanced life support are likely to prove futile' (Simpson 1994, p 39).

As accidents remain the commonest cause of death in children and as the life expectancy of children with a variety of chronic illnesses is increasing, the need for parents, and also other members of the general public, to learn basic paediatric life support is becoming increasingly important (Carter & Dearmun 1995, Whitton 1995).

It is important to recognise that practising CPR using a baby or child manikin is the most effective way of ensuring that children's nurses have appropriate skills to help an infant or child in need. In addition, these skills, in order to be fresh, require to be updated regularly.

All nurses must be aware of the emergency call telephone number and procedure for their individual clinical areas.

Sudden cardiac arrest is a rare event in the paediatric population; most children will show signs of physiological deterioration, sometimes hours prior to the event (Tibballs et al 2005). As outcome from cardiac arrest is poor, it is important that deteriorating patients are recognised and appropriate interventions made. A number of early warning systems to detect clinical deterioration have been developed and are now used within adult medicine (Parr et al 2001, Hodgetts et al 2002). Early warning systems are now being developed throughout paediatric medicine (Tibballs et al 2005, Duncan et al 2006, McCabe et al 2009). Most paediatric hospitals are now using or developing early warning systems, it is important that the nurse is familiar with their format and use.

LEARNING OUTCOMES

By the end of this section, and following further reading and simulated practice, the nurse should be able to:

- Assess responsiveness in infants and children
- Use appropriate airway opening techniques
- Assess respiration by looking, listening and feeling for expired breath
- Provide rescue breathing using both mouth-to-mouth techniques and use of a bag-valve-mask system
- Pulse check using appropriate sites
- Provide chest compressions
- Identify priorities in advanced life support.

RATIONALE

Commentators on both sides of the Atlantic acknowledge the importance of resuscitation as a nursing skill (AHA 2000, Resuscitation Council (UK) 2005).

Cardiac arrest in children is often the terminal event of progressive shock or respiratory failure; early signs of shock or respiratory failure must be recognised and treated to prevent cardiac arrest (International Guidelines 2000, Resuscitation Council (UK) 2005).

Many children die or suffer permanent neurological impairment each year because of respiratory failure, sudden infant death syndrome, sepsis or trauma (CDC at: www.cdc.gov/injury/wisqars/index.html). Appropriate prompt action can help avoid many of them.

Advanced life support will be futile if basic life support is not delivered effectively.

FACTORS TO NOTE

Babies and children differ from adults in a number of ways:

- The causes of their cardiopulmonary arrest are different, with adults tending to suffer from *primary* cardiac arrest, whereas children, who predominantly have healthy hearts, tend to have *secondary* cardiac arrest following a period of hypoxia, often associated with an airway or breathing emergency. This fact suggests that cardiac arrest in children may be preventable if appropriate measures are taken to deal with the airway or breathing problem. The presence of hypoxia also explains why children fare so poorly following cardiopulmonary arrest. If the heart is deprived of oxygen to the point where it can no longer function, then similar effects must be seen in the brain and other vital organs (Hampson-Evans & Bingham 1998).
- Respiratory infection and sepsis are the primary causes of cardiopulmonary arrest in children under 5 years of age, with trauma being the major cause in the 5- to 14-year age group (Williams 1994).
- Babies and children differ from each other in resuscitation terms. The term 'infant' refers to the under 1-year-old, including the neonatal period; the term 'child' is defined as being from the age of 1 year through to puberty (ERC 2005, Resuscitation Council (UK) 2005, AHA 2005).
- The paediatric larynx is funnel shaped, not cylindrical. This renders the larynx more susceptible to impaction of foreign objects.
- The larynx of the child is soft and the trachea is short. The tongue of the infant or child is large in comparison and, as such, increases airway obstruction and obscures the view of the glottis (Williams 1994, Bishop-Kurylo & Masiello 1995).
- Infants have poorly developed accessory muscles and an immature bronchial tree, the diaphragm being the major muscle of respiration (Hazinski 1992).
- Chest compressions should be initiated in children if the pulse is absent or the heart rate is less than 60 beats/min, with signs of poor perfusion (ERC 2005, Resuscitation Council (UK) 2005)
- Basic life support should be initiated before the administration of any drugs, or other intervention, is considered.

- Cardiac arrest is defined as the absence of palpable central pulses. Four cardiac arrest rhythms may be identified on electrocardiograph (ECG) monitoring in children: asystole, pulseless electrical activity (PEA), ventricular fibrillation (VF) and pulseless ventricular tachycardia (VT).
- The presenting rhythm in most paediatric cardiac arrests is asystole or extreme bradycardia (Sirbaugh et al 1999, Young & Seidel 1999).
- Ventricular fibrillation (VF) and pulseless ventricular tachycardia (VT) has been reported in 10–20% of paediatric cardiac arrests (Mogeyzel et al 1995, Young & Seidel 1999). It is most likely to occur in children who are hypothermic, have structural cardiac disease or have taken an overdose of tricyclic antidepressants.
- Defibrillation takes precedence in the treatment of VF and VT. One shock at 4 J/kg should be delivered every 2 min in VF/VT cardiopulmonary arrest. Paediatric paddles should be used in children below 10 kg (ERC 2005, Resuscitation Council (UK) 2005).

BASIC PAEDIATRIC LIFE SUPPORT

METHOD

If the lone rescuer has been taught adult basic life support then they may use the adult sequence with the addition of providing five initial breaths and performing 1 min of basic life support prior to going for help (Resuscitation Council (UK) 2005).

The following recommendations should be used by those who have a duty of care to respond to paediatric emergencies.

1. Ensure that both the rescuer and child are in a safe environment leaving the child in the position you find him unless he would be in further danger.
2. Assess the level of responsiveness by gently shaking or pinching the child's fingers or toes. Tactile and verbal stimulation should be used. Do not shake children with suspected spinal injuries.
3. If the child is unresponsive, call for help but do not leave the child alone. It is possible that this unconsciousness may cause airway obstruction. Opening of the airway may be the only resuscitative action that is required.

Opening the airway

- The airway can be opened in either of two ways:
  - *Head tilt/chin lift* – one hand is placed on the child's forehead, and a finger of the other hand is placed on the bony tip of the chin. The head is then tilted back and the chin lifted upwards and forward (Fig. 8.1). It is important to avoid overextension of the neck and compression of the soft tissues under the chin as either of these can cause obstruction of the air passages.
  - *Jaw thrust* – this technique is the preferred choice where neck injury is suspected as it allows the airway to be opened without moving the neck. In this instance the index fingers of both hands are placed behind the angles of the jaw and the mandible is lifted upwards carrying the tongue forward. This manoeuvre may close the mouth, if so the thumbs should be placed on the tip of the chin to open the mouth (Hampson-Evans & Bingham 1998).
- If impaction of the airway by a foreign body is suspected or witnessed, and is visible in the mouth, it should be removed.
- Once the airway is open, assess breathing.
- Assess breathing by looking for the rise and fall of the chest, listening for breath sounds at the child's mouth and nose, and feeling for evidence of expired breath with your cheek, taking no more than 10 seconds. Care should be taken to differentiate effective breathing from ineffective gasping respiratory effort (Poets et al 1999).
- If there is no breathing, artificial ventilation should be commenced without delay.

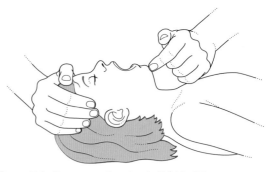

Figure 8.1 Airway opening: head tilt/chin lift.

- For infants, place the head in the neutral position and deliver breaths by covering the mouth and nose. It has been suggested that in some infants it is not possible for an adult to effectively cover both mouth and nose for ventilation (Tonkin et al 1995). If the nose and mouth cannot be covered by the rescuer's mouth, breaths could be delivered by covering either the nose or the mouth (if the nose is used, the mouth should be closed to prevent air escaping) (ERC 2005, AHA 2005).
- For the child, breathing should be by the mouth-to-mouth route using a head tilt, chin lift.
- Maintain the airway in an open position throughout ventilation.
- Deliver breaths slowly, 1–1½ seconds each, to minimise the possibility of gastric distension and optimise filling of lungs (McCrory & Downs 1990, Resuscitation Council (UK) 2005).
- Observe the chest during rescue breathing to ensure that it rises and falls. This movement confirms the patency of the airway.
- Deliver five initial rescue breaths (ERC 2005, Resuscitation Council (UK) 2005). If chest movement is not witnessed, reposition the airway. If this is unsuccessful, the possibility of a foreign body should be considered.

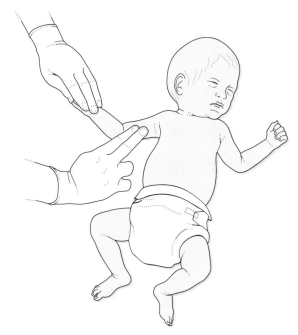

Figure 8.2 Palpation of the brachial pulse.

Checking the pulse

- Assess circulation by palpation of the pulse and observing for any other signs of life, e.g. swallowing, moving, breathing (Resuscitation Council (UK) 2005).
- For the child, the carotid artery should be palpated.
- For the infant, palpation of the brachial artery on the inside of the middle section of the upper arm (Fig. 8.2) is indicated as the carotid artery is difficult to locate owing to the short nature of the neck.
- If signs of circulation are detected within 10 seconds, continue rescuing breathing at a rate of 12–20 breaths/min, reassessing frequently. If the child starts breathing on his own, place in recovery position and seek help (AHA 2005).
- If no pulse is palpated or the pulse rate is less than 60 beats/min, with signs of poor perfusion, chest compressions should be commenced.
- For both infants and children, the lower-third of the sternum should be compressed in the midline.

- For infants, where only one rescuer is present, chest compressions should be delivered using two fingers to compress the chest by one-third of its anterior–posterior diameter, taking care not to compress over the xiphisternum (Clements & McGowan 2000). Healthcare providers should use the two-thumb encircling technique if two rescuers are present (both hands encircle the chest with fingers placed around the infants back and two thumbs are placed side by side on the lower third of the sternum) (ERC 2005, Resuscitation Council (UK) 2005).
- In the child, compressions may be delivered using one or two hands to enable the rescuer to compress the chest by one-third of its anterior-posterior diameter (ERC 2005, AHA 2005, Resuscitation Council (UK) 2005).
- In both the infant and the child, 15 chest compressions of the chest should be followed by two breaths. (Where lone rescuers find the transition between airway and breathing difficult, a compression ventilation ratio of 30:2 could be used) (ERC 2005, Resuscitation Council (UK) 2005).

DOS AND DON'TS

- Do practise locating brachial and carotid pulses.
- Do attend to the needs of the child before telephoning. The cause of the emergency is probably airway or respiratory in nature and quick attention to this may prevent the heart from stopping.
- Do not assume that you are competent in life support because you have read about it. It is imperative that you take time to practise using appropriately sized manikins.
- Do not blindly sweep fingers around an infant's, or child's mouth. Remember that the paediatric larynx is not cylindrical but funnel shaped and it is possible that blind finger sweeps may impact on an object in the larynx, causing harm.

ADVANCED PAEDIATRIC LIFE SUPPORT

Effective basic paediatric life support is a prerequisite for advanced life support, which aims at providing continued perfusion of the coronary and cerebral arteries with oxygenated blood through the use of additional equipment and medication, thus enabling the heart to regain its effectiveness as a pump (ERC 1994, Hampson-Evans & Bingham 1998).

Advanced paediatric life support inevitably will be performed and continued within the clinical setting where it is important that all staff involved is updated frequently on the techniques that are used in both types of life support, thus being familiar with paediatric practice (Williams 1994, Bishop-Kurylo & Masiello 1995).

What must be remembered is that basic life support techniques will continue despite the introduction of advanced life support.

THE EMERGENCY TROLLEY

Emergency equipment for use during advanced life support should always be readily available within all clinical areas. Although the type and style of emergency trolley will differ between clinical and community areas, the basic contents of the trolley should be similar. In comparison to emergency trolleys used within the adult setting, the trolley within the paediatric setting will carry a wide range of equipment in order to meet the needs of the wide age range and corresponding differences in body proportions of children. Box 8.1 identifies the basic requirements of the paediatric emergency trolley.

The contents of the emergency trolley should be checked on a regular basis, as per local policy, to ensure that all equipment is functional. Expiry dates should be checked on all drugs, intravenous fluids and disposable equipment; batteries and spare bulbs for the laryngoscope should also be checked.

MAINTENANCE OF AIRWAY

A secure and effective airway is essential if ventilation is to be maintained.

EQUIPMENT

- Face masks
- Self-inflating bag mask ventilation device with reservoir attached
- T-piece anaesthetic circuit
- Oxygen supply
- Oxygen tubing
- Selection of oropharyngeal airways
- Selection of endotracheal tubes
- Laryngoscope
- Blades for laryngoscope
- Zinc oxide tape for securing endotracheal tube
- Water-based lubricant jelly
- Scissors
- Suction source and catheters
- Stethoscope.

METHOD

1. Effective ventilation should be provided using a self-inflating bag mask ventilation device with reservoir. This is connected to the oxygen supply, thus providing a higher concentration of oxygen, which is preferential in advanced life support (ERC 1994).
2. The face mask should provide a good seal around the nose and mouth to enable optimal ventilation. A mask of an appropriate size should be chosen, the mask should fit snugly around the child's nose and mouth avoiding pressure on the eyes. A mask that is too large will allow carbon dioxide to accumulate and be

---

BOX 8.1   Basic contents of the paediatric emergency trolley

Airway maintenance

- Selection of oropharyngeal airways: variety of sizes ranging from infant to adult
- Endotracheal tubes: variety of sizes from infant to adult
- Laryngoscope with selection of blades straight and curved, spare handle, spare batteries and bulbs; McGill forceps
- Ventilation face masks: variety of sizes and types
- Self-inflating bag mask ventilation device with reservoir
- Re-breathing set
- T-piece/anaesthetic circuit
- Oxygen tubing, high concentration oxygen face masks, nasal prongs and portable oxygen supply
- Suction tubing, catheters and portable suction unit
- Oxygen saturation monitoring equipment.

Cardiac monitoring

- Cardiac monitor electrodes
- Cardiac monitor
- Defibrillator readily available
- Blood pressure cuffs.

Drugs and intravenous fluids

- Emergency drugs immediately available: adrenaline, atropine, amiodarone; other drugs agreed locally should be readily available.
- Sodium chloride 0.9% or balanced salt solution
- Dextrose 10%
- Protein plasma solution.

Other equipment

- Intravenous infusion equipment
- Selection of intravenous cannulae
- Intraosseous needles
- Selection of syringes and needles
- Splints
- Nasogastric tubes
- Stethoscope
- Scissors
- Alcohol wipes
- Lubricant gel (water-based)
- Surgical tape
- Blood specimen bottles, labels.

---

delivered back to the child (McCrory & Downs 1990, Williams 1994).

3. Where the child's airway cannot be maintained adequately, an oropharyngeal airway should be inserted.

4. The size of the oropharyngeal airway is determined by positioning the airway next to the child's face. A correctly sized airway should extend from the centre of the mouth to the angle of the jaw (ERC 1994, MacNab 1996).

5. In children, insert the airway with the convex side upwards. The tongue should be guided out of the way using a tongue depressor or the blade from a laryngoscope (MacNab 1996).

6. In the larger child, insert the airway with the concave side upwards; when the tip reaches the soft palate rotate the airway through 180° and slide over the tongue.

7. Oropharyngeal airways should be used with caution. Airways that are too small will cause additional obstruction, while those that are too large may damage the posterior pharyngeal wall (Williams 1994).

8. Once the airway has been inserted, bag mask ventilation should be continued.

Endotracheal intubation

Performed by experienced medical staff, endotracheal intubation remains the most effective method of securing and maintaining the airway. This should be performed as soon as possible when effective ventilation cannot be otherwise obtained (Williams 1994, International Guidelines 2000). However, it must be remembered that oxygenation is the priority.

- The size of the endotracheal tube is very important. This can be estimated by a number of methods:
  - In infants: the size of endotracheal tube usually required is 3.0–3.5 mm for the newborn, while infants from 6–9 months require size 4.0 mm (MacNab 1996)
  - In the child: the size of the endotracheal tube can be estimated by use of the following equation:

$$\text{Size of endotracheal tube in mm} = \frac{\text{Age in years} + 4}{4}$$

- The Broselow tape is a specifically designed tape measure, which can be used to identify the correct size of endotracheal tube (Begg 1995)
- These measurements provide an estimate of the internal diameter of the tube
- When preparing for intubation ET tubes 0.5 mm smaller and 0.5 mm larger should be readily available
- Before intubation, the child is oxygenated with 100% oxygen
- In infants and young children, a straight blade laryngoscope is normally used during insertion
- In older children, a curved-blade laryngoscope is normally used
- The endotracheal tube is frequently inserted via the nasal route within the intensive care setting; the laryngoscope and McGill forceps are used to help visualise and direct the insertion of the tube. Once inserted, the tube is fixed in place using zinc oxide tape. This route of insertion is technically more difficult in the emergency situation
- Once the tube has been inserted, oxygenation can be performed by attaching the re-breathing equipment directly to it, or by the use of a mechanical ventilator
- Symmetrical chest movement and equal lung air entries should be observed and heard.

VASCULAR ACCESS

Speed is vital when administering fluid or drugs in the advanced life support situation. The method and equipment used for administration will vary with the type of access that is used.

EQUIPMENT

- 70% isopropyl alcohol-impregnated swabs (Mediwipes) and/or antiseptic solution appropriate to local area
- Intravenous cannulae (varying sizes)
- Syringes (varying sizes)
- Central venous cannulae
- Intraosseous cannula
- Intravenous administration sets
- Sterile latex-free gloves
- Sterile dressing pack.

METHOD

Venous access

1. Where possible, peripheral venous access should be attempted; however, this is often difficult to achieve in the critically ill child.
2. If central venous access is already established, this should be used, but if it is not, only peripheral access should be attempted, as attempting central access is hazardous in the emergency situation (ERC 1994).
3. As establishing vascular access in paediatric cardiac arrest is difficult, immediate insertion of an intraosseous cannula may be preferable (International Guidelines 2000).

Intraosseous access

1. This is a safe, simple, rapid means of access in all children.
2. An intraosseous cannula is a fine screw-like needle which is inserted into the anterior tibial bone marrow; alternative sites include the distal femur, medial malleolus or anterior superior iliac spine (International Guidelines 2000).
3. Fluids and drugs can be rapidly infused using this type of access; however, it is not for long-term use.

If access is impossible to obtain, some drugs, e.g. adrenaline (epinephrine) and atropine, can be given via the endotracheal tube. The drug should be injected via a narrow-bore suction catheter beyond the tracheal end of the tube and then flushed in with 1–2 mL normal saline (Resuscitation Council (UK) 2000). The endotracheal dose of adrenaline (epinephrine) is 10 times that of the intravenous dose; the endotracheal dose of atropine is 0.02 mg/kg (International Guidelines 2000). This route is not suitable for fluid administration.

DRUGS AND FLUID THERAPY

Artificial ventilation with oxygen and fluid replacement therapy may re-establish cardiac output without the need for drug therapy. Paediatric emergency resuscitation trolleys should include a variety of crystalloid and colloid intravenous fluids. These would include saline solution in varying concentrations, Ringer's lactate solution, access to human albumin and plasma. The type of solution used is dependent on the cause of the arrest. These drugs and intravenous fluids should be available within the emergency resuscitation trolley.

DRUG THERAPY

The action of drugs used in resuscitation, and their metabolism, is poorly understood in children. The following examples are those recommended in the guidelines produced by the Resuscitation Council (UK) 2005.

Adrenaline

This is the first-line drug of choice in paediatric resuscitations. Adrenaline will cause an increase in peripheral vascular resistance without constricting coronary or cerebral vessels. This raises systolic and diastolic pressures during cardiac compressions.

The recommended dose in resuscitation is 10 µg/kg.

Sodium bicarbonate

Sodium bicarbonate had been routinely used in paediatric resuscitations for many years. The rationale for its use is the reduction of the metabolic acidosis, which occurs during cardiac arrest. However, a concern with the use of bicarbonate is that it produces more carbon dioxide, because of its buffering action, and thus acidosis is increased. Routine use is no longer recommended, however it may be considered where cardiac arrest has been prolonged or is thought to be associated with tricyclic antidepressant overdose.

The dose of sodium bicarbonate is recommended as 1–2 mL/kg of the 8.4% solution via the i.v. or i.o. route.

Atropine

Although there is no clear evidence that atropine is a useful drug in paediatric resuscitation, it may be considered as part of the ongoing management of haemodynamically significant bradycardia and after adequate oxygenation (International Guidelines 2000).

The recommended dose is 20 µg/kg with a minimum recommended dose of 100 µg and a maximum single dose of 600 µg (Resuscitation Council (UK) 2005).

Amiodarone

This is used in shock resistant VF and pulseless VT with its use considered prior to the 4th defibrillation shock. The recommended dose is 5 mg/kg via rapid intravenous bolus.

Glucose

Sick children and especially infants may develop hypoglycaemia. Blood glucose should be assessed as soon as possible and treated promptly with glucose solution (Williams 1994).

DEFIBRILLATION

Defibrillation is not commonly required in paediatric resuscitation. It is the term used for the stimulation of the heart muscle using electric currents and is normally performed by experienced medical staff and appropriately trained registered nurses. Used for ventricular fibrillation and pulseless ventricular tachycardia, the energy recommended is paediatric resuscitation is 4 J/kg (ERC 2005, Resuscitation Council (UK) 2005). A single 4 J/kg shock should be delivered every 2 min where VF/VT persists; ensuring basic life support is only interrupted briefly to deliver the shock.

Defibrillators are either manually or automatically (such as an AED) operated. Manual defibrillators must be available within healthcare facilities caring for children (ERC 2005). In areas where only AED are available they can be used in children over 8 years; in children younger than this specifically designed pads to reduce the energy delivered are recommended (Resuscitation Council (UK) 2005).

If using manual defibrillators with paddles or pads, the largest available should be chosen to provide good contact with the wall of the chest ensuring that they do not touch. The recommended sizes are 4.5 cm diameter for weights of <10 kg and 8–12 cm diameter for weights of >10 kg (ERC 2005).

Equipment should be readily available to all clinical areas. Often, however, the defibrillation equipment is shared between areas.

Equipment should be checked on a regular basis to ensure that it is charging and discharging properly. This should be performed by appropriately trained registered nurses. Bioengineering departments should check defibrillator equipment regularly as per local policy.

DOS AND DON'TS

- Do familiarise yourself with the location of the emergency trolley and equipment within your clinical area.
- Do ensure that you know the emergency call number for cardiac arrest.
- Do ensure that you attend a regular resuscitation update. A minimum of yearly is essential.
- Do familiarise yourself with the layout and contents of the emergency resuscitation trolley.
- Do ensure that parents are supported.

- Do not exclude parents and relatives from the resuscitation room unless it is at their request.

SUMMARY

Resuscitation must begin immediately and not wait until equipment arrives. All personnel working with children require education on both basic and advanced life support. It is imperative that the children's nurse is aware of the different techniques for both basic and advanced support and is competent in both.

It remains vital that basic life support skills and techniques are well taught and updated, as ineffective delivery of basic life support will render advanced life support futile. With further scientific evidence, resuscitation guidelines will continue to change and it is important that nursing staff continually update and revise their practice in resuscitation techniques.

References

American Heart Association, 2000. Supplement to Circulation 102 (8).

American Heart Association, 2005. Supplement to Circulation December.

Begg, J.E., 1995. A pediatric care and resuscitation cart: one community hospital's ED experience. J. Emerg. Nurs. 21 (6), 555–559.

Bishop-Kurylo, D., Masiello, M., 1995. Pediatric resuscitation: development of a mock code program and evaluation tool. Pediatr. Nurs. 21 (4), 333–336.

Carter, B., Dearmun, A.K., 1995. Child health care nursing – concepts, theory and practice. Blackwell Science, Oxford.

Centers for Disease Control and Prevention, WISQARS™ (Web-based Injury Statistics Query and Reporting System). Centers for Disease Control and Prevention, Atlanta, GA. Online. Available: www.cdc.gov/injury/wisqars/index.html.

Clements, F., McGowan, J., 2000. Finger position for chest compressions in cardiac arrest in infants. Resuscitation 44, 43–46.

Duncan, H., Hutchison, J., Parshuram, S., 2006. The pediatric early warning system score: A severity of illness score to predict urgent medical need in hospitalized children. J. Crit. Care 21, 271–279.

European Resuscitation Council, 1994. Guidelines for paediatric life support. Br. Med. J. 308, 1349–1355.

European Resuscitation Council, 2005. ERC Guidelines. Resuscitation 67 (Suppl. 1), S1–S189.

Hampson-Evans, D.C., Bingham, R.M., 1998. Paediatric resuscitation. The European Resuscitation Council Guidelines 1998. Care of the Critically Ill 14 (6), 188–193.

Hazinski, M.F., 1992. Nursing care of the critically ill child, second ed. Mosby, St Louis.

Hodgetts, T.J., Kenward, G., Vlachonikolis, I.G., et al., 2002. The identification of risk factors for cardiac arrest and formulation of activation criteria to alert a medical emergency team. Resuscitation 54, 125–131.

International Guidelines, 2000. International Guidelines for CPR and ECC – a consensus on science. Resuscitation 46 (1–3), 301–333.

MacNab, R., 1996. Paediatric life support. Paediatr. Nurs. 8 (4), 28–33.

McCabe, A., Duncan, H., Heward, Y., 2009. Paediatric early warning systems: where do we go from here? Paediatr. Nurs. 21 (1), 14–17.

McCrory, J.H., Downs, C.E., 1990. Cardiopulmonary resuscitation in infants and children. In: Blumer, J.L. (Ed.), A practical guide to pediatric intensive care. third ed. Mosby, St Louis.

Mogeyzel, C., Quan, L., Graves, J.R., et al., 1995. Out-of-hospital ventricular fibrillation in children and adolescents: causes and outcomes. Ann. Emerg. Med. 25, 484–491.

Noc, M., Weil, M.H., Sun, S., et al., 1994. Spontaneous gasping during cardiopulmonary resuscitation without mechanical ventilation. Am. J. Respir. Crit. Care Med. 150, 861–864.

Parr, M.J., Hadfield, J.H., Flabouris, A., et al., 2001. The medical emergency team: 12 month analysis of reasons for activation, immediate outcome and not-for-resuscitation orders. Resuscitation 50, 39–44.

Poets, C.F., Meny, R.G., Chobanian, M.R., et al., 1999. Gasping and other cardiorespiratory patterns during sudden infant deaths. Pediatr. Res. 45, 350–354.

Resuscitation Council (UK), 2005. Resuscitation guidelines 2005.

Resuscitation Council (UK), London.

Simpson, S.M., 1994. Paediatric advanced life support – an update. Nurs. Times 90 (27), 37–39.

Sirbaugh, P.E., Pepe, P.E., Shook, J.E., et al., 1999. A prospective population-based study of the demographics, epidemiology, management, and outcome of out-of-hospital pediatric cardiopulmonary arrest. Ann. Emerg. Med. 33, 174–184.

Tibballs, J., Kinney, S., Duke, T., et al., 2005. Reduction of paediatric in-patient cardiac arrest and death with a medical emergency team:

preliminary results. Arch. Dis. Child. 90, 1148–1152.

Tonkin, S.L., Davis, S.L., Gun, T.R., 1995. Nasal route for infant resuscitation by mothers. Lancet 45, 1353–1356.

Whitton, H., 1995. Infant resuscitation in parenthood education. Health Visit. 68 (11), 454–455.

Williams, C., 1994. Paediatric cardiopulmonary resuscitation. Br. J. Nurs. 3 (15), 760–764.

Young, K.D., Seidel, J.S., 1999. Pediatric cardiopulmonary resuscitation: a collective review. Ann. Emerg. Med. 33, 195–205.

Chapter 9

Hygiene

Emma Moore, Beryl Pearson

CHAPTER CONTENTS

Introduction   104
   Learning outcomes   104
   Rationale   104
   General factors to note   105
   Risk assessment   105
   Prevention of cross-infection   106
   Developmental needs   106
   Guidelines   107

Specific hygiene needs of the baby   107
   Baby bath   108
   Equipment   108
   Method   108
   Specific factors to note   109

Bathing a baby   109
   Nappy area care   110
   Umbilical cord care   111
   Nail care   111

Specific hygiene needs of the toddler
and pre-school child   111

Specific hygiene needs of older children   112
   Bed bath   112
   Toileting   114
   Hair care   114
   Oral and dental care   114
   Eye care   115
   Ear care   117
   Dos and don'ts   118

INTRODUCTION

This section will introduce general principles of care practices for the baby or child who is unwell, and being cared for either at home or in hospital. It will then address specific care in relation to developmental age groups. More specific care of problems common in sick children can be found in other sections.

LEARNING OUTCOMES

By the end of this section you should be able to:

- Explain the generic principles of hygiene practice for the healthy child
- Be aware of the necessity of prevention of cross-infection through good hygiene practice and be aware of the nurse's role in the maintenance and use of universal precautions
- Understand the specific needs related to the developmental stage and abilities of the child
- Explain the adaptation of techniques to meet the specific needs of the ill child
- Understand the specific aspects of hygiene management for the infant, child and adolescent.

RATIONALE

Personal hygiene is an essential component in maximising physical well-being and is vital for a healthy future; therefore meeting the child's hygiene needs is an integral aspect of nursing care, which enhances comfort, promotes self-esteem and prevents infection. As the child grows physically, and becomes more independent, their hygiene needs change.

GENERAL FACTORS TO NOTE

Safe practice

To maintain safe practice in any environment, the nurse undertaking the activity must be aware of local policy guidelines, which must be followed as for any nursing procedure.

- The safety of both the child and nurse are paramount when performing any aspect of hygiene care.
- No baby and child should ever be left unattended in a bath or with water even momentarily.
- Hold and closely supervise the baby who is unable to sit unsupported and, where used, place a slip mat in the bath.
- The ambient temperature of the environment needs to be maintained between 22°C and 25°C to reduce heat loss during hygiene care (Bailey & Rose 2000, Rudolf & Levene 2006).
- When running a bath for a child it is essential to run the cold water first and add the hot water to it or run both via a mixer tap – this helps to prevent hot water scalds (CAPT 2008) in any event water should be no hotter than 46°C.
- The water temperature should be maintained, appropriate to the needs/size/age of the child; however, there is no evidence of a specific recommendation and therefore assessment is needed on an individual basis. In a clinical situation, all water temperature should be thermostatically controlled.

RISK ASSESSMENT

Consent and participation

The consent of the child and family needs to be sought in all circumstances (see also Ch. 1), and family-centred care needs to be considered an integral aspect of the care of children in any environment (Smith 1999, Kirk et al 2005). Basic hygiene needs are considered fundamental to the child receiving nursing care; however, consent still needs to be sought from the child and family irrespective

of the expectation that it may be provided as a basic requirement. Prior to the activity, the nurse needs to negotiate with the child and the family the level of their interaction and participation during the personal care time (Coleman 2003, Corlett & Twycross 2006). Full explanations of what actions are being taken should be given, and these should be reinforced during the interaction.

In general, the preparation and consent of children decreases their anxiety, promotes their cooperation, supports their coping skills and helps them to more fully understand what is happening to them (Wong et al 1999, Mansson & Dykes 2004).

Family inclusion

The child and family need to be fully involved throughout the child's care and encouraged to be partners in care (Casey 1988, Smith et al 2002, DoH 2004). Education of the child and family and the sharing of information are important areas that are the nurse's responsibility (NMC 2008a,c). This involves the promotion of partnership and informed consent to develop the empowerment of the child and family in any given situation.

Family/carer presence and their involvement in the child's care will increase feelings of security, and decrease the anxieties of the child. Encouragement will need to be given to the family to promote their active inclusion in even the most basic of care activities, as often the stress of being a parent of a sick child can reduce the parent's ability to communicate effectively (Fleitas 2003). Their level of participation needs to be assessed early on, and then reassessed frequently to ensure opportunities are given for their involvement in the child's care. Nurses need to help find specific ways in which family members can support their child (NMC 2008a).

The child needs to be encouraged to develop their independence and positive feelings of control by being able to choose the desired level of activity and participation (Hallstrom & Elander 2004). The nurse needs to be aware of all aspects of communication, including the use and observation of verbal and non-verbal body language during the activity (Bannister 1997). Active communication may help the nurse, child and family to develop a rapport and provide assessment opportunities (Thomas 1996). Active communication is also combined with the use of play and humour during stressful situations (Wong et al 1999) (see also Ch. 10).

Documentation and safe practice

All care should be documented in the nursing notes, in accordance with the Nursing and Midwifery Council *Record-keeping guidance for Nurses and Midwives* (NMC 2009). Any changes resulting from assessment and reassessment should be noted and reported.

PREVENTION OF CROSS-INFECTION

Good hygiene represents an important defence against infection. A child's ability to fight infection will depend on their age, health and immunological status. The overprotection of children from contact with micro-organisms may render them unable to develop a natural immunity, but allowing children to develop preventable illness because of poor hygiene practice and infection control is unacceptable.

Universal precautions to prevent infection should be taken (see also Ch. 4). Hands should be washed thoroughly before and after handling any baby or child, in the home or in hospital (Lawson 2001). When handling any body fluids, and especially before any procedure requiring intimate contact, such as feeding or bathing, the nurse should wear gloves and other protective clothing (e.g. an apron) appropriate to the level of contact.

Hand washing is important for all carers and siblings. It is especially important in hospital due to potential contact with unusual or highly infectious diseases and to prevent cross-infection or spread of disease. Therefore the use of universal precautions and good hand washing techniques are essential to reduce cross-contamination (Lawson 2001, RCN 2004a). Older sibling children should be told to wash their hands after using the toilet, and before and after meals, especially if they want to hold or touch the baby, or share toys. Younger children should be encouraged to wash their hands aided by an adult.

DEVELOPMENTAL NEEDS

- Each child is a unique individual with their own routine, temperament and personality.
- Guidelines of developmental age and ability are helpful but each child must be respected as an individual. This can be acknowledged by calling the child by their name.

- Care and support given should provide the child with encouragement and confidence to retain their level of independence in self-care activities.
- Personal hygiene forms an important element of the healthy child's normal everyday routine.

These routines and practices should be maintained as much as possible while the child is sick, either in hospital or at home, and details should be recorded in the nursing notes or health records. Keeping to established routine provides comfort and reassurance to the child and family, especially during periods of stress.

Privacy and dignity

The nurse should respect the child's changing needs for privacy at different stages of development and well-being. In the older child or adolescent, a need for privacy emerges as sexual awareness develops. Illness and disability require that intimate tasks, which would normally be performed by the child or young person, may need to be performed by nurses and parents. Assessment of the usual practices for intimate and personal care should be established, and care should then be negotiated between the nurse, parent/carer and child. It is vital that the child is consulted at all stages of the interaction and that their needs and requests become paramount in the achievement and maintenance of personal hygiene (Needham 1997). The nurse should involve parents, where appropriate, and same-sex nurses and carers should be allocated if possible (RCN 2003).

Cultural needs

Nurses need to be aware of the individual family cultural background. Consideration must be given to family lifestyle and specific cultural values and norms, including cultural rituals and/or rites of passage – especially related to health and personal care. Nurses should also be sensitive to the need for 'same gender' care delivery for all children regardless of age, sex, ethnic background or culture (NMC 2008b).

The intimate nature of many nursing interventions, if not practised in a sensitive and respectful manner, could lead to misinterpretation. Care should be negotiated between the nurse, parent/carer and child. Assessment is the key to ensuring effective nursing care. Usual practices for intimate, personal care should be established and form the basis for care (RCN 2003).

Health promotion

The provision of personal care and the maintenance of hygiene provide an ideal opportunity for health education and promotion. The child and family may have concerns regarding their health and choose these times to raise concerns or discuss current/preventative practice. Aspects such as teeth cleaning, weight management, exercise, smoking and contraception are just some of the topics that may be discussed (DfES 2004).

Play

Personal care time and the maintenance of hygiene are ideal times to utilise age-appropriate play strategies. Play has a number of specific functions; as well as promoting learning and development, it can also be a coping strategy and distraction for the child (Crawford & Raven 2002, Chambers & Jones 2007).

Observation

Performing hygiene tasks for a baby or child gives the nurse an ideal opportunity to observe and monitor the health and general well-being of a child. As each element of hygiene care is performed, there is an opportunity for detailed assessment of the condition of a particular area (e.g. ears or eyes). The nurse may observe, for example:

- Signs of malnutrition
- Chest recession in a child with respiratory distress
- Bruises or bite marks on a child who may have been abused
- Skin infections such as impetigo or ringworm.

GUIDELINES

Before commencing any hygiene task, consider:

- Is the task really necessary? Children who are sick, or babies who are premature, should be left in peace with minimal disturbance unless there is a good reason to do otherwise. The clustering of care may be considered to be of benefit and limit the negative effects of continuous interaction (Young 1996).
- Could any other aspect of care be combined with hygiene needs? Examples include observations of vital signs, topical drug administration and specimen collection.
- Consider family-centred care: Could the parents be involved or undertake the task with supervision, or would they prefer the nurse to do it?
- What can the child do independently? Or what can the child begin to learn to do on their own? If a child is able to learn a basic skill or develop their independence, for example hair brushing, tooth cleaning or dressing, it may encourage a sense of achievement and a feeling that something positive has occurred.
- The developmental stage of the child and the appropriate level of activity and interaction.
- How can you make the experience fun? Can you introduce play or toys into the experience?
- Have you collected all necessary equipment together?

SPECIFIC HYGIENE NEEDS OF THE BABY

Birth is a traumatic, exhausting experience for mother, father and baby. The newborn baby is covered with both a protective substance called vernix caseosa, white grease that protects the skin *in utero* from the amniotic fluid that surrounds the infant, and blood from the mother. The adaptation of the skin from intrauterine life, where the skin has been surrounded by amniotic fluid, to the predominately dry cool extrauterine life takes about 14 days. At birth, the mean pH of skin is 6.34, which decreases to 4.95 by 4 days as the skin colonises with normal flora. The acidic quality of newborn skin provides a defence against harmful microorganisms (Medves & O'Brien 2001). After birth, excess moisture is wiped away and the infant is placed naked on the mother's abdomen or breast, covered perhaps by a clean towel to maintain warmth. Positive skin-to-skin contact at this stage can provide an ideal opportunity for the mother, father and child to familiarise themselves and bond. However, babies can lose heat rapidly and therefore specific attention needs to be paid to the ambient temperature in the room (Bailey & Rose 2000, Rudolf & Levene 2006).

A full-term healthy infant may be bathed within a few hours of birth, once the body temperature has stabilised (Trotter 2002). Newborn babies do not get especially dirty, and daily bathing of newborn babies is unnecessary as frequent bathing may disrupt the natural pH of the skin. It may also be unwise if the umbilical cord is still *in situ* (Skale 1992, Guala et al 2003). For the first 2–4 weeks baths should be carried out using only plain water (NICE 2006) and gauze or muslin cloths for cleansing, then gradually introduce tiny amounts of baby bath product. These should be of a neutral pH, contain minimal dyes and perfumes, and be used only two to three times a week (Trotter 2002).

For any baby, bathing is not only for skin cleansing, but is also a time for contact and interaction. The timing of hygiene activities should be planned for when the baby will enjoy them, when awake and content, however bathing after a feed is to be avoided as this may induce vomiting (Lee & Thompson 2007).

Maintaining a clean environment for the baby is an equally important part of their hygiene care. Newborn babies have very little defence against microorganisms; once the placental transference of immunity has worn off at 3 months, or if breast-feeding has stopped, babies must develop their own defences (Lawson 2001). Likely sources of contaminants are feeds, feeding bottles or pacifiers. If formula feeds are to be used, they must be made up under sterile conditions. Feeding bottles and pacifiers should be sterilised after each use. Weaning foods must be prepared using food hygiene guidance (see also Ch. 39).

Once the child is older and can reach for toys and put them in their mouth (usually at about 3 months), toys should be kept 'socially' clean, and sterilising them is not necessary. Reinforcing and teaching hand washing techniques before and after contact with the baby are important for all carers and siblings. For older children this is especially important when sharing the baby's toys.

The environment around a baby whether at home, in a hospital cubicle or ward, should be clean and as free as possible from excessive build-up of dust and dirt. Once a child is crawling, the floor and other surfaces should be kept 'socially' clean. Staff and visitors who have coughs or colds or other infections should not have close contact with a baby.

Any episode of ill health can interrupt the family bonding processes. Hygiene activities can form a useful way for the mother or father and baby to bond. During the activities the contact can give an opportunity for face-to-face contact, touch and 'talking'. For example, if the newborn baby is in a neonatal intensive care unit, inviting the family to help with these activities can encourage bonding when they can no longer fulfil other caring functions (see also Ch. 5).

BABY BATH

There are two ways of bathing a baby: to 'top and tail' or to give a baby bath. Babies, as mentioned above, do not need bathing daily unless they are sick or have very dirty nappies. Older babies who are more active, for example crawling, may require a daily bath. A baby bath may be too stressful for a sick child, for example a child with breathing difficulties or neurological disturbance. If this is the case, a top and tail can be performed instead.

Top and tail wash

Topping and tailing is a useful alternative to bathing. Top and tail is to wash the baby's face, hands and their nappy area. A bowl of clean water is required for both the top and the tail (bottom).

EQUIPMENT

- A small dish of warm clean sterile water for the baby's eyes
- A bowl of warm clean water for the face
- A bowl of warm clean water for the nappy area
- Non-sterile swabs for eye care (or at home a clean soft cloth)
- Muslin cloths/wash wipes/clean soft flannel for the rest of the baby's body
- A clean nappy
- Disposal bag or bucket for soiled nappy and clothes
- Soft baby hairbrush
- Clean clothes
- Clean warmed towels.

METHOD

1. Ensure that the environment is warm and comfortable, with no cool draughts. Wash your hands before approaching the baby.
2. Place the baby, dressed, on the towel.

3. Clean the baby's eyes. Clean the corners and outside the eye; do not attempt to clean under the lids. Use a different swab for each eye and discard after each use to prevent cross-infection.

4. Gently wash the rest of the face and around the mouth and nose with a clean cloth or swabs, and gently pat dry.

5. Do not attempt to clean inside any orifice, be it nose, eye, ear or mouth. All body orifices clean themselves naturally by production and secretion of mucus or fluid.

6. Wash the baby's hands with a wet washcloth, and dry. If nails are long, snip very carefully with blunt-ended baby scissors (preferably baby's own to maintain individual use and prevent cross-infection).

7. Gently brush the baby's scalp and hair with a soft baby brush to help prevent the occurrence of cradle cap.

8. Put on non-sterile gloves. Undress the baby so that the nappy area is accessible. With most babies' clothing this is possible without undressing the baby fully.

9. Take off the nappy. If the baby is wet, just clean with warm water. If the baby is soiled, wipe excess faeces away with swabs, the nappy or wipes and dispose of these in the appropriate bin along with your gloves. Observe for nappy rash. Always clean from front to back, thus avoiding contaminating the urethra with faeces. Wash the baby's bottom with a washcloth and dry.

10. Only the visible surface of genitalia should be cleaned: Do not retract a boy's foreskin (which will not fully retract until the boy is 18 months to 2 years) or clean inside the labia in a girl.

11. Ensure that all creases of skin and crevices are dry to prevent the development of a rash or infection.

12. Put on a clean nappy (underneath the umbilicus if the cord is still attached) and dress the baby in clean clothes.

SPECIFIC FACTORS TO NOTE

- Before and after carrying out any baby care it is important to wash hands thoroughly. Gloves should be worn when dealing with body fluids or excrement.

- Cotton wool balls should not be used for eye care as, if small cotton strands enter underneath the eyelid, they can damage the cornea (Marsden & Shaw 2003).

- The internal aspect of the ears and nose should not be cleaned unless really necessary and the use of cotton buds should be avoided.

- Alkali soaps should not be used as they can potentially damage the 'acid mantle' of the skin and the skin's barrier function (Garcia-Gonzalez & Riviera-Rueda 1998). The 'acid mantle' is the skin's protector that takes between 2 and 8 weeks to develop, depending on gestational age (Trotter 2002).

- Many parents use talcum powder, but the hygiene benefits of this are unclear. Powder tends to cling and cake to moist areas, can cause skin irritation and can be inhaled by the baby (Skale 1992, Campbell & Glasper 1995).

- Baby soap or baby bath solution is not necessary unless the baby's nappy area is very soiled (Brennan 1996). Use cleansing solutions that are mild and free from alcohol and perfume.

- If the baby is changed regularly, nappy creams are not necessary under normal circumstances (Brennan 1996). However, if a baby is prone to nappy rash, a protective barrier cream may be useful to reduce friction, wetting and contact with urine and faeces (Atherton 2004).

BATHING A BABY

Equipment

As for top and tail, plus a baby bath and stand.

Method

1. The baby bath itself should be prepared, adding cold water first, and then warm, to reduce the risk of the water not mixing properly and hotter water remaining at the base of the tub. The water temperature should be comfortable and appropriate to the size, age, health and preference of the child. The Child Accident Prevention Trust (CAPT 2008) and the Health and Safety Executive (2003) advocate that water should come out of bath taps at no more than 46°C to prevent the risk of serious scalding.

2. It is essential that the temperature of the water is tested at intervals as a scald can occur if the water is too hot. The traditional method of assessing the temperature of the bath is to dip one's elbow into the water. The water should be no deeper than 10 cm (4 inches) and should feel just warmer than tepid.

3. Water thermometers are available – but should be for individual use.

4. Make sure that the bath is placed at a comfortable height, preferably on a stand. Kneel or sit, whichever is easier. Stooping while holding the baby can lead to back problems, and will mean that the person bathing the baby will not relax and enjoy the occasion.

5. Undress the baby. If the nappy area is very soiled, clean off the faeces with cotton wool balls, the nappy or wipes. Wrap the baby securely in a towel.

6. Before commencing, clean the baby's eyes, face and mouth with a clean cloth or swabs. Start with the eyes and use a different swab for each eye to prevent cross-infection (see Eye care, below, for technique).

7. While the baby is still wrapped in the towel, hold the head over the bath and gently wash water over the hair, avoiding the eyes. Although not necessary, a mild shampoo or a small quantity of baby bath solution can be used. Use a corner of the towel to dry the hair, this helps reduce heat lost during the remainder of the bath through the wet head of the baby.

8. Unwrap the towel. Hold the baby securely, with one hand grasping the farthest upper arm, and the baby's neck and shoulders supported on the forearm (Fig. 9.1).

9. Place the baby gently in the water, allowing them a little time to get used to the sensation. If the baby is learning to sit, support them sitting in the water with a hand around their back, but never leave a baby unsupported. It can only take a moment for a baby to topple over. This may put the baby off baths for some time or, in the worst scenario, the baby may drown. A non-slip mat or seat cradle should be used to prevent an accidental slip.

10. If bathing an active baby in an adult-size bath, make sure they cannot accidentally touch the hot tap.

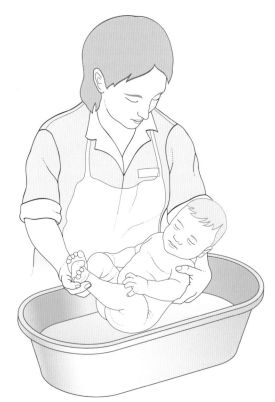

Figure 9.1 Holding the baby safely for a bath.

11. Gently wash the baby with the free hand, under the arms, back and the nappy area. Pay particular attention to skin creases. Allow the baby to kick and splash, exploring the weightless sensation. This should be fun for both carer and baby, but if the baby is clearly distressed, bring them out of the bath as soon as possible.

12. Do not let the baby become cold. Wrap the baby in the towel. When dry, dress in clean dry clothes. The room should be warm enough for older babies to play naked for a while, to kick and wriggle, free from the constraints of a nappy.

13. Ensure that all creases of skin and crevices are dry to prevent the development of a rash or infection.

NAPPY AREA CARE

Nappy rash – irritant diaper dermatitis (IDD) – is frequently seen in babies and younger children. It is caused by prolonged and repetitive contact with an irritant, primarily urine and/or faeces, but *Candida* infections also cause excoriation of the nappy area. Underlying skins conditions, medical conditions and medication may be contributory factors (Turnball 2001). IDD is unusual before 3 weeks of age, usually developing between 3 weeks and 2 years (Atherton 2004), and could be linked with decreased nappy area changes, increased mobility or dietary changes. Any factor which changes the acidity of urine and faeces can cause IDD and consequent associated discomfort (Scowen 1995).

Nappies should be changed immediately after defecating, and at reasonably frequent intervals to prevent IDD (Atherton 2004). Timing will depend on circumstances such as the developmental age of the baby, and therefore the volume of urine passed. On balance, changing a nappy immediately before a feed is preferable, although it can be frustrating for the baby, who may be crying with hunger. Changing the nappy immediately after a feed may either make the baby vomit or interrupt the progression to a sleep or resting time. If the baby has defecated during feeding, the nappy should be changed. When changing nappies, a cotton washcloth, mild soap and warm water are adequate to clean the area. Parents may prefer to use wash wipes, and there is some evidence to suggest that the modern types (gentle and non-alcohol based) may be gentler on both unbroken and broken skin (Odio et al 2001). Wipes should be avoided for babies less than 2–4 weeks old, as there may be potential to harm the 'acid mantle' in the skin of a newborn (Trotter 2002).

UMBILICAL CORD CARE

In the newborn, the umbilical cord should normally separate within 2 weeks of birth, and usual recommendations are to allow the cord itself to naturally air dry, and not to apply or use any special treatment (NICE 2006). Care of the cord should be undertaken according to local policy guidelines. The umbilical area must be observed for infection and swabbed for microbiological culture if any signs of infection are present (raised temperature, generally unwell, redness, inflammation, swelling of umbilicus or surrounding skin). If there is evidence of infection this must be reported immediately. If an umbilical catheter is *in situ*, care should be as for an intravenous or arterial line: the line must be secured carefully and the entry site kept clean and dry and aseptic technique should be used if handling is necessary.

NAIL CARE

Babies have fingernails and toenails that are usually soft and flexible but that can cause injury. Nails that are 'ragged' or extend beyond the tip of the finger can cause scratches to the face and possibly eyes. Clean the baby's hands and nails during regular bathing. Nails should be carefully trimmed using only baby's own baby nail scissors that have blunt rounded tips, and specially made baby clippers are now available. Baby's nails grow quickly and should be inspected regularly.

SPECIFIC HYGIENE NEEDS OF THE TODDLER AND PRE-SCHOOL CHILD

Due to the developmental and play experiences of this age group a daily bath or shower will become essential. Frequent washes of face and hands before, after and between meals will also be necessary.

Children being toilet trained should be taught and encouraged to wash their hands following toileting, as routine experience. Nappies where still worn should be changed every few hours.

Even if a child is ill, make hygiene activities fun and develop a comforting routine; encourage the child's independence and learning. Most toddlers and pre-school children enjoy a bath, and will happily play in the water; either a soapy bath solution or soap can be used, although soap in the eyes can sting badly. If the child has any skin condition such as eczema, then special bath solutions and creams may be necessary. Some children will dislike baths and may prefer spraying themselves with the showerhead or having a sponge bath. At this stage of development, toys and the environment should be kept socially clean. Attention will also need to be paid to hair, teeth and nails, continuing routines that should start as a baby.

Safety is paramount and small children must not be left alone in the bath even for a moment.

They should be warned not to touch the hot tap, and the temperature of the hot water should be controlled so it cannot scald if turned on accidentally. Water temperatures above 46°C can cause injury, and at 60°C can cause second-degree burns in 3 s and third-degree burns in 5 s (CAPT 2008). Water temperature in clinical settings is thermostatically controlled, but in other areas a risk assessment may need to be made.

SPECIFIC HYGIENE NEEDS OF OLDER CHILDREN

As school children grow older they become more independent. Hygiene needs alter as the body changes in adolescence: problems with acne, greasy hair or body odour may emerge; the menarche will occur as well as other sexual changes of puberty. Such changes can be disturbing even for the best-prepared teenager, especially when they manifest themselves outside the safety and reassurance of home or school. Teenagers can be very embarrassed if they cannot manage their own hygiene needs independently (Atmarow et al 1993). Sensitivity is needed if the adolescent requires assistance with hygiene activities in hospital (Horne 1999). When work is of a personal or intimate nature all nurses and healthcare staff, whether male or female, should follow the principles of good practice as outlined by the Royal College of Nursing (RCN 2003).

Some children, particularly adolescent girls and those from non-Christian backgrounds, are likely to prefer a female carer. This reflects social, religious and cultural preferences, and should be respected and accommodated.

For both the toddler and older child, a bed bath is usually given only when a child for whatever reason is too sick or disabled to get into a proper bath, and when a 'top and tail' wash is insufficient. Critically ill or unconscious children, children who have high temperatures and are sweating profusely, or children in traction after orthopaedic surgery may all need bed baths.

Parental involvement in bed bathing should be discussed with both the child and parent. Some children and parents prefer the nurse to perform the bed bath. For example, for some parents of chronically ill children it can be a welcome relief to have someone take over this aspect of care, whereas to parents of children who are acutely ill, continuing to care for their child's hygiene needs can be a way of maintaining control and feeling useful. The child may much prefer the parents to give the care, and their views and competence should be respected (Kristensson-Hallstrom 2000); however, as children get older their wishes and expectations may, at times, conflict with those of their parents (DoH 2003).

BED BATH

All children require similar basic equipment whether requiring a bath, a top and tail wash or a bed bath.

The basic principles of a bed bath are as follows:

- Ensure the time for the bath/bed bath is appropriate to the individual needs of the child.
- Gathering the equipment together and being well organised will save time and effort.
- Prepare the environment ensuring privacy and that it is safe, draught free and warm.
- Prepare the child.
- Consider other care interventions that can or could be planned into this activity, for example specimen collection, wound care, pain assessment and management.

The child may have their own individual preferences as to choice for personal cleaning lotions and materials. Allow the child as much independence as is safe to do so and, if the child wishes, involve the parents/carers. Their safety must also be considered, for example if they are using hospital-based equipment.

Many children prefer the option of a shower, if available, and if possible.

Equipment

- Washbowl with warm water
- Flannels or washcloths: at least two, one for the face and one for the genital area
- Soap or bath solution
- Hairbrush or comb
- Toothbrush and toothpaste

- Nail scissors
- Clean towel
- Clean clothes or nightclothes
- Clean bed linen
- Appropriate bags/receptacles for equipment disposal.

Method

1. Discuss the need for a bed bath with the child and parents and explain what will occur.
2. Other preparation may be necessary, e.g. toileting.
3. Prepare the environment: clear a surface, either a trolley or bedside table, for washing equipment. Draw the curtains/blinds to ensure privacy.
4. Ensure that the water remains hot enough; it may need changing.
5. Raise the bed to a comfortable working height. Ensure that you are comfortable and safe; you may need assistance from colleagues or parents with turning or lifting. Use manual handling aids where possible. Do not stretch over the bed, but walk around to the other side if necessary.
6. Strip the bed and bed area of any non-essential items or bedclothes.
7. Undress the child and leave covered with a sheet and/or gown.
8. Wash the child's eyes, using a different corner of the washcloth for each eye. Use more specific eye care if indicated (see below).
9. Wash the child's face, paying special attention to mouth and ears (see below).
10. Help the child to clean their teeth.
11. Before washing each body part, place a dry towel beneath it to prevent water dripping onto the sheets.
12. Cover the upper body with a sheet or towel, but leave the arms exposed. Using soap and water, or bath solution or special lotion, wash the child's hands, and trim and clean the nails if necessary. Wash each arm, paying particular attention to hands and nails, and the underarm area. Rinse the flannel and rinse off the soap. Rinsing may need to be repeated.
13. Gently remove the cover from the upper body, leaving genitalia covered, and wash and rinse the chest and abdomen.
14. Cover the upper body again, and wash the front of the legs and feet. Check for pressure sores on heels or ankles (see Ch. 23).
15. With a different washcloth or flannel, wash the 'front' genitalia and rinse. Where possible, children and young people may prefer to do this for themselves. *Note:* For post-pubertal boys, the foreskin should be pulled back and the penis washed underneath (Campbell & Glasper 1995).
16. With assistance, turn the patient onto one side.
17. Wash back, legs and finally buttocks, and dry.
18. Position the patient comfortably.
19. Brush or comb the hair, and check behind the head for skin lesions or sores. If hair washing is necessary and the child can tolerate the procedure, wash the hair by holding the child's head over the end of the bed (help will be needed) over a washbowl, using a jug to rinse. Equipment may be available to assist with water collection.
20. Dress the patient in clean clothes as appropriate.
21. Tidy away the bowl of water and wash things.
22. Ensure the child is comfortable and any equipment moved is returned.

At the same time as doing a bed bath there may be an opportunity to:

- Slide in a clean sheet to replace the old bottom sheet; change top sheet and pillowslips
- Change the position of leads from monitoring equipment, or of catheters or tubes taped to the skin, to avoid skin irritation or damage due to prolonged adhesion or pressure (some units will have their own local policies on frequency of repositioning); clean off any remaining adhesive with a gentle adhesive remover
- Perform passive limb exercises if indicated
- Perform other nursing care, e.g. observations, topical skin treatments
- Talk with the child; this may be an opportunity for the child to express their fears and thoughts about their illness, or just to have a good chat

- Use play and make the bed bath fun. The more alert child will enjoy toys and games appropriate for their age; if the child has learning or sensory disabilities they may enjoy the touch, smell and feel of the experience.

TOILETING

Ensure privacy. All children should have access to hand washing facilities after using the toilet, and this should be proactively encouraged for all children. This practice should be maintained when a child is confined to bed.

Ensure the toileting facilities are to an acceptable standard, and that toilet paper, hand washing and drying equipment are accessible.

HAIR CARE

- Children's shampoo should be used and, where appropriate, hair conditioner.
- With ingenuity, hair washing can be made fun and painless.
- Help children to brush or comb their hair at least once daily; they may require help to keep their usual style.
- Babies should have their hair washed when having a bath. For older children, follow their usual routine but they may require hair washing more frequently than usual. Babies may develop cradle cap, characterised by yellow scales on the scalp.
- Use the child's own hair toiletries, unless any specific prescribed care is required.
- If the child is unable to have their hair washed when bathing, then it may be necessary to wash this in their bed. This requires additional protection and equipment.
- Seek specific guidance from the child and their family regarding needs and preferences.
- Provide specific hair care for children with particular religious observances.
- Provide specific hair care for children who have kinky hair and require the use of special combs with wide teeth, and application of necessary hair products and toiletries.
- For children with long hair who are confined to bed, braiding or plaiting can help reduce knots or matting in their hair.

- Hair should not be cut without parental permission, although shaving of an area may be required for insertion of an intravenous cannula.

Head lice

Anyone can catch head lice, but pre-school children, primary school children and their families are most at risk.

There are three forms of head lice:

1. Nits are head lice eggs. The oval, yellowy-white eggs are hard to see and may be confused with dandruff. They attach themselves to the hair shaft and take about a week to hatch. The eggs remain after hatching and many nits are empty egg cases.
2. Nymphs hatch from the nits. The baby lice look like the adults, but are smaller. They take about 7 days to mature to adults and feed on blood to survive.
3. Adults are about the size of a sesame seed. They have six legs and are tan to greyish-white. The legs have hook-like claws used to hold onto the hair. Adults can live up to 30 days and feed on blood.

Head lice cannot jump, hop or swim and are transmitted through direct, prolonged head-to-head contact with an infested person. This is especially common during play or sport at school and with close contacts at home. Transmission is possible through infected clothes, combs, brushes or towels, but extremely unlikely. The lifespan of a louse is very short once detached from the hair so fumigation is not necessary.

If head lice are found then medical advice should be sought for the appropriate current method of treatment (Health Protection Agency 2008).

ORAL AND DENTAL CARE

It is important to promote dental and oral hygiene to preserve the development of healthy teeth and gums. Studies show that levels of tooth decay are a good predictor of oral health in later life (Powell 1998). Dental hygiene should begin as the primary teeth erupt. Parents/carers should ensure children develop good dental habits from an early age.

Babies are obviously not able to clean their own teeth. For the baby it is often easier to use a foam sponge. As more teeth appear, use a baby toothbrush. For the younger child (under 7 years), effective positioning should facilitate carers' access to the child's mouth. One way of doing this is to stand with the child's back towards the adult, using one hand to cup the chin and the other to brush the teeth. In the case of an ill child, find a position that is most comfortable and reassuring. Good practice is to clean teeth at least twice a day, preferably after meals (British Dental Association: www.bda.org). The more frequently and the longer teeth are cleaned the greater the probability of effective plaque removal. Children often have their own preferred type of toothpaste, and many now use electric toothbrushes (these have been shown to achieve a modest reduction in plaque and gingivitis compared with manual tooth brushing). Advice from local health visitors should be sought about whether additional fluoride is necessary as the benefits of fluoride toothpastes are firmly established. Even when the child is not eating, such as when they are unconscious, regular and thorough mouth care is vital. There are occasions when an optimum oral hygiene regimen may be sacrificed for patient comfort.

In ill health, children may become more prone to dental and gum diseases, and medication may affect oral status. Children may also become susceptible to oral infections such as oral *Candida* (thrush), which can cause pain and discomfort in the mouth, and this in turn may affect eating and drinking. Children receiving chemotherapy or radiotherapy may experience specific problems. In addition to normal oral care, these children may require the use of antifungal agents and/or an antibacterial mouthwash.

Younger children will require encouragement and supervision, and this is an ideal opportunity for health education such as avoiding giving prolonged bottled feeds of milk or juice, prevention of injury, avoidance of sugary foodstuffs and other dietary needs, e.g. calcium intake.

Nurses should perform mouth care for children who, for whatever reason, are unable to do so for themselves. Encourage children to visit the dentist from an early age. Regular dental checks should include prophylactic teeth cleaning.

General conditions that may compromise oral well-being include the following:

- Cerebral palsy
- Epidermolysis bullosa
- HIV
- Combined immune deficiency
- Metabolic disorders requiring high intake of oral carbohydrates
- Glycoprotein storage disease (some types)
- Downs syndrome and other mentally handicapping conditions
- Measles
- Anorexia
- Dehydration
- Chronic constipation
- Effects of chemo/radiotherapy
- Post-cytotoxic therapy
- Fever
- Grinding of teeth
- Thumb sucking
- Habitual licking or biting of lips
- Accidents or other illness causing:
  - Neurological damage
  - Unconsciousness
  - Loss of a limb
  - Maxillofacial injury
- Restricted oral access due to:
  - Orthodontic or maxillofacial surgery
  - Enlarged, protruding tongue
  - Respiratory problems
  - Restricted movement of tongue due to surgery or pain
  - Cleft palate (may have a prosthesis)
- Medication, e.g.:
  - Antibiotics
  - Antihistamine
  - Atropine
  - Diuretics
  - Insulin
  - Iron supplements
  - Long term, high sucrose content medication, e.g. lactulose
  - Morphine.

EYE CARE

Visual/structural problems for children range from the minor to the profound. It is essential that any nursing care ensures the child's comfort and does not cause problems that may worsen the child's eyesight.

Ensuring that the eyes are clean is part of the general care of any child. Equally, the nurse may see serious eye conditions where good eye care is part of the essential treatment. These may include common infections of the newborn, including, for example, *Chlamydia* infection, tear duct abnormalities and postoperative care.

The following groups of children will be particularly at risk of complications, which may include corneal damage, and infection:

- Unconscious children, especially those receiving muscle-relaxing drugs
- Children whose eyes are not properly shut (*Note*: incomplete eye closure of 1–2mm can go undetected but may still result in exposure keratitis)
- Immunosuppressed children
- Low-birth-weight infants, who are at increased risk of retinopathy of prematurity (Fleming et al 1996)
- Newborn babies under 6 weeks old, who do not produce tears, which contain a natural antibiotic agent, lysozyme (McQuaid et al 1996)
- Children undergoing eye surgery
- Children who cannot blink.

General hygiene and eye care

In the well child, it is unlikely that invasive eye care is required due to the natural self-regulation processes in the eye, which include the production of tears and the blinking mechanism (Rhee & Pyfer 1999). However, as with all nursing procedures, assessment is the vital first step. Early detection of eye problems can prevent further damage.

Eye care may be a distressing experience for any child. Explaining what will happen and building it into games, for example with dolls, may help the child to cooperate. Eye care may be performed by the parent or carer, or the children themselves, if they are happy to do so and have been taught any special techniques.

As eye care can require specialist knowledge, links with specialist ophthalmology colleagues should be developed by any children's unit.

Frequency of eye care

This will be variable. Healthy children may only need the area of skin around their eyes cleaned once or twice a day as part of their general hygiene routine; a sick or vulnerable child may need more frequent specific care. In other circumstances, e.g. if a child's eyes are discharging, they may require hourly treatment.

Purpose of eye care

- To maintain cleanliness of the eyes, thereby promoting comfort and preventing cross-infection
- To keep the mucosa moist
- To treat existing infection
- To administer medication.

Equipment

- Warm sterile saline/water
- Sterile gauze swabs. Cotton wool balls or material should not be used, as wisps of cotton may scratch the cornea (Laight 1996, Marsden & Shaw 2003)
- Eye swab if infection is suspected and cause unknown
- Gloves (preferably sterile)
- Disposal bag.

Technique and assessment

- Prior to any intervention the nurse should undertake a thorough hand wash and wear gloves to reduce the possibility of cross-contamination (RCN 2004a).
- Observe the eyes for redness, inflammation and swelling, and the presence of any discharge, foreign body or eyelash defect. Each eye should be assessed independently (Marsden & Shaw 2003).
- If there is any concern that the eye is infected, swab the eye using an appropriate swab.
- In the well child, a clean face flannel or wash wipe can be used, and the eyes cleaned first with a different section of the flannel. Wipe from the external inside aspect to the outside aspect of the eye. Do not use soap, which is unpleasant if it gets into the child's eyes.
- If the eye is infected, or the child particularly vulnerable to infection, use sterile swabs and sterile water/saline. To avoid cross-infection, clean the non-infected eye first, then the infected eye. Always wipe from the inside aspect to the outside aspect, and use a different swab for each eye.

- In a child who is at risk of corneal drying and ulceration, eyes should be kept moist using approved, prescribed artificial tear drops (e.g. hypromellose).
- Eye protection may be useful in such children if they are unconscious. This may be a simple eye dressing or a gelatine-based product such as Geliperm (Laight 1996).

EAR CARE

Caring for the ear should be part of routine hygiene care for all children. Occasionally the child will require clinical care of the external or middle ear; however, specialist knowledge is required to treat these conditions.

The ear has two important functions: hearing and balance. If either of these functions is disturbed, the child's normal sensations and perceptions can be altered, causing anxiety and confusion. Ear infections can also cause severe pain in children and attention should be paid to pain-relieving methods (RCN 2004a).

Ear problems experienced by children include:

- Deafness
- Otitis media or externa
- Foreign bodies
- Wax or 'glue'
- Perforated eardrum
- Conditions requiring surgery.

General hygiene and ear care

The external ear is covered by skin and needs daily care. Children often forget to clean behind their ears; however, daily ear cleansing should form part of the child's personal care routines. As with other areas of skin, the ear can become itchy, dry or eczematous; in this case, skin creams, drops or ointments may be needed (Wong et al 1999, RCN 2004a).

Never insert anything into the ear canal other than an auriscope or tympanic thermometer (and even in these cases, care must be taken). Cotton buds, hairgrips and fingers all have been known to cause inner ear damage (Martin 1994, Wong et al 1999). The outer aspects of the ear (pinna) and the area behind the ear can be washed with warm water. Special attention needs to be paid to the drying of the ear, but avoid the use of talcum powders due to the drying, allergic and other potential problems associated with this product.

Observation and examination of the ear

The nurse or parent should observe the outer ear during general hygiene care of the child. If the nurse observes inflammation, this may indicate infection. Ear infections may be extremely painful, therefore close observation of the child's behaviour may aid in the assessment and treatment. Small children especially may be distressed, clearly in pain. Some may be able to locate the pain to the ear; others may try to rub their ear or rub it against something to gain relief.

It is quite normal for a small amount of wax (cerumen) to be seen at the entrance to the ear canal (RCN 2004a). Cerumen is normally honey coloured, becoming darker as it is exposed to air. However, if the exudate is clear, this could indicate cerebrospinal fluid leakage, which may indicate a serious condition, for example head injury. If the exudate is green and/or offensive, this could indicate infection. The presence of blood may indicate haemorrhage, for example after surgery or trauma.

Foreign bodies

Foreign bodies, such as buttons, small toys, ends of cotton buds, even batteries, are not uncommon reasons for children to attend A&E departments. The presence of a foreign body will sometimes go unnoticed for some time, but may be indicated by signs of infection, hearing loss, bleeding, otorrhoea (discharge) or pain.

Removal of a foreign body must only be undertaken by an experienced practitioner. The use of syringing, speculums and aural clamps may be attempted in a specialist department but surgery may be necessary in order to remove the item and observe for signs of damage or infection (RCN 2004b).

In rare instances, an insect will enter the ear canal, and may still be alive, causing an incessant buzzing and tickling of the ear. If a light is shone into the ear, the insect may be drawn out.

Alternatively, a small amount of oil can be inserted into the ear to drown the insect, which is then syringed away.

DOS AND DON'TS

- Do assess the child's eyes carefully, especially if they fall into one of the risk groups.
- Do not confuse eye care as part of general hygiene with clinical eye care. This can over-hospitalise the child. Most children will just need a clean wet flannel.
- Do not attempt to insert anything into a child's ear.

- Do not attempt to undertake any task for which you have not received training.

References

Atherton, D.J., 2004. A review of the pathophysiology, prevention and treatment of irritant diaper dermatitis. Curr. Med. Res. Opin. 20 (5), 645–649.

Atmarow, G., Blomfield, J., Brady, S., 1993. The clean gang: the health education teaching package designed for schoolchildren. Nurs. Times 89 (45), 30–32.

Bailey, J., Rose, P., 2000. Temperature measurement in the preterm infant: a literature review. J. Neonatal Nurs. 6 (1), 28–32.

Bannister, A., 1997. Listening to children. Wiley, Chichester.

Brennan, G., 1996. Opinion: care of the new born baby's skin. Midwives 109 (1303), 240.

British Dental Association. Frequently asked questions: Children's teeth. Online. Available: www.dentalhealth.org.uk/faqs/leafletdetail.php?LeafletID=3#faq731.

Campbell, S., Glasper, E.A. (Eds.), 1995. Whaley and Wong's children's nursing. Mosby, London.

Casey, A., 1988. A partnership with child and family. Sr. Nurse 8 (4), 8–9.

Chambers, M., Jones, S., 2007. The surgical nursing of children. Elsevier, London.

Child Accident Prevention Trust, 2008. Bath water scalds. CAPT Fact sheet. CAPT, London.

Coleman, V., 2003. Enhancing consumer participation using the practice continuum tool for family-centred care. Paediatr. Nurs. 15 (8), 28–31.

Corlett, J., Twycross, A., 2006. Negotiation of Parental Roles within Family Centred Care: a review of the research. J. Clin. Nurs. 15, 1306–1308.

Crawford, C., Raven, K., 2002. Play preparation for children with special needs. Paediatr. Nurs. 14 (8), 27–29.

Department of Health, 2003. Getting the right start. National Service Framework for children: standard for hospital services. DoH, London.

Department of Health, 2004. The National Service Framework for children, young people and maternity services. DoH, London.

Department for Education & Skills, 2004. Every child matters. DfES, London.

Fleitas, J., 2003. The power of words: examining the linguistic landscape for pediatric nursing. Am. J. Matern. Child Nurs. 28 (6), 384–388.

Fleming, P.J., Speidal, B.D., Marlow, N., et al., 1996. A neonatal vade-mecum, second ed. Arnold, London.

Garcia-Gonzalez, E., Riviera-Rueda, M., 1998. Neonatal dermatology: skin care guidelines. Dermatol. Nurs. 10 (4), 274–275.

Guala, A., Pastore, G., Garipoli, V., et al., 2003. The time of umbilical cord separation in healthy full-term newborns: a controlled clinical trial of different cord care practices. Eur. J. Pediatr. 162 (5), 350–351.

Hallstrom, I., Elander, G., 2004. Decision-making during hospitalization: parents' and children's involvement. J. Clin. Nurs. 13, 367–375.

Health and Safety Executive, 2003. Scalding risks from hot water in health and social care: local authority circular. Health and Safety Executive, Caerphilly.

Health Protection Agency, 2008. Headlice. Online. Available: www.hpa.org.uk/web/HPAwebFile/HPAweb_C/1194947368754.

Horne, S., 1999. Phenomenology: understanding the life experience of long-term ventilated adolescents. Paediatr. Nurs. 11 (6), 37–39.

Kirk, S., Glendenning, C., Callery, P., 2005. Parent or nurse? The experience of being a parent of a technology-dependent child. J. Adv. Nurs. 51 (5), 456–464.

Kristensson-Hallstrom, I., 2000. Parental participation in pediatric surgical care. AORN J. 71 (5), 1021–1029.

Laight, S., 1996. The efficacy of eye care for ventilated patients: outline of an experimental research pilot study. Intensive Crit. Care Nurs. 12 (1), 16–26.

Lawson, L.G., 2001. Handwashing: a neonatal perspective. J. Neonatal Nurs. 7 (2), 42–46.

Lee, L., Thompson, K., 2007. Parental survey of beliefs and practices about bathing and water safety and their children: guidance for drowning prevention. Accid. Anal. Prev. 39, 58–62.

Mansson, M., Dykes, A., 2004. Practices for preparing children for clinical examinations and procedures in Swedish pediatric wards. Pediatr. Nurs. 30 (3), 182–187.

Marsden, J., Shaw, M., 2003. Correct administration of topical eye treatment. Nurs. Stand. 17 (30), 42–44.

Martin, R.L., 1994. Nuts and bolts: how to care for the external ear. Hearing Journal 47 (2), 43–44.

McQuaid, L., Huband, S., Parker, E., 1996. Children's nursing. Churchill Livingstone, Edinburgh.

Medves, J., O'Brien, B., 2001. Does bathing newborns remove potentially harmful pathogens from the skin? Birth 28 (3), 161–165.

NICE, 2006. Clinical Guideline 37 Postnatal Care – Routine postnatal care of women and their babies. Online. Available: www.nice.org.uk/Guidance/CG37.

Needham, J., 1997. Teenage quality circles: not just a paper exercise. Paediatr. Nurs. 9 (7), 15–17.

NMC, 2009. Record Keeping: Guidance for nurses and midwives. NMC, London.

Nursing and Midwifery Council, 2007. Advice sheet on record keeping. NMC, London.

Nursing and Midwifery Council, 2008a. Advice for nurses working with children and young people. NMC, London.

Nursing and Midwifery Council, 2008b. Chaperoning. NMC, London.

Nursing and Midwifery Council, 2008c. The Code: Standards of conduct, performance and ethics for nurses and midwives. NMC, London.

Nursing & Midwifery Council, 2009. Record Keeping: Guidance for Nurses and Midwives. NMC, London.

Odio, M., Streicher-Scott, J., Hamsen, R., 2001. Disposable baby wipes: efficacy and skin mildness. Dermatol. Nurs. 13 (2), 107–121.

Powell, L., 1998. Caries prediction: a review of the literature. Community Dent. Oral Epidemiol. 26, 361–371.

Rhee, D., Pyfer, M., 1999. The Wills eye manual. Williams and Wilkins, Philadelphia.

Royal College of Nursing, 2003. Protection of nurses working with children and young people. RCN, London.

Royal College of Nursing, 2004a. Good practice in infection control. RCN, London.

Royal College of Nursing, 2004b. ENT/Maxillofacial Nursing Forum. Action on ENT: guidance on ear care. RCN, London.

Rudolf, M., Levene, M., 2006. Paediatrics and child health. Blackwell, Oxford.

Scowen, P., 1995. Skin care and nappy rash. Prof. Care Mother Child 5 (5), 138.

Skale, N., 1992. Manual of pediatric nursing procedures. JB Lippincott, Philadelphia.

Smith, L., 1999. Family centred decision-making: a model for parent participation. J. Neonatal Nurs. 5 (6), 31–33.

Smith, L., Coleman, V., Bradshaw, M., 2002. Family-centred care: concept, theory and practice. Palgrave, Basingstoke.

Thomas, D.O., 1996. Assessing children – it's different. RN 59 (4), 38–45.

Trotter, S., 2002. Skincare for the newborn: exploring the potential harm of manufactured products. RCM Midwives J. 5 (11), 376–378.

Turnball, R., 2001. Treatment approaches to some childhood skin conditions. Community Nurse 6 (12), 15–16.

Wong, D.L., Hockenberry, M., Wilson, D., et al., 1999. Whaley and Wong's nursing care of infants and children, sixth ed. Mosby Year Book, St Louis.

Young, J., 1996. Developmental care of the premature baby. Baillière Tindall, London.

Chapter 10

Play

Joyce Stebbings

CHAPTER CONTENTS

Introduction   120

Sick child at home   121

Types of play   122

Preparation   122
    Preparation guidelines   123
    Pre-admission programmes/preop clubs   124
    Guided imagery and visualisation   126

Adolescents   127

Siblings   128

Praise and rewards   128

Play and the way forward   129

INTRODUCTION

'Children's natural and instinctive medium of expression is play' (Cattanach 2003). Play facilitates communication between the child and their carers, thereby providing a sense of control, trust and understanding. 'Hospitalisation, medical procedures and surgery are a source of anxiety for children/young people and their families' (Lansdown 1996).

There are a variety of different types of play applicable to children according to their age and stage of development. These will be described, citing examples from practice of children who have successfully used play to help them understand and cope with their illness. Play programmes designed for the hospitalised child, taking into account the child's individual needs, age, cognitive understanding and illness, can provide a positive introduction to the ward environment, thus aiding the nurse in the holistic care of the child. The core of this text is designed to explore the importance of play in the life of the sick child. It is hoped that those who use this book will find this section a useful addition. When children are provided with an environment where play occurs naturally, they are able to express feelings, indulge in fantasy and work through difficult situations if appropriate. This last aspect is one where the intervention of skilled and trained adults may be needed. Hospital play specialists (HPS) are people who have undergone an appropriate training and have the in-depth knowledge and skills to work with children when they are sick, to help them cope with their illness through play. As play is a pleasurable activity, its normality helps to promote confidence in an unfamiliar environment, thus aiding the recovery process. Alison Webster (2000) felt that if play was:

> Viewed as a language and not just activities (then) play becomes an important child-centred communication tool. It can be used to build up support strategies and understanding between children and the adults caring for them.

The use of play was initially introduced into paediatric wards in 1963, when consultant paediatrician, Dr Morris, noted how withdrawn and unnatural children appeared to be when admitted to hospital (Morris 1989). He believed that just because a child was in hospital, opportunities for play should not be taken away. Save the Children Fund set-up play schemes with the aim of reducing stress and anxiety and encouraging normal play.

Play is an activity that we are all involved in, often without realising it. From waving to a baby in a cot, which involves eye contact and communication, to a more involved imaginative play session with an older child; both are forms of play. The involvement and cooperation of the child with the adult has healing potential for the child. Some people may think that they have forgotten how to play, or have never experienced play themselves. To those of you in this situation, just relax and do what comes naturally; let the children take the lead, copy them, laugh with them, get down to their level physically as well as spiritually. The child's uncomplicated mind will easily show us how to enjoy play, but sometimes our expectations and inhibitions get in the way. Once the child's trust has been obtained, the ability to play becomes one of the greatest assets of a children's nurse.

SICK CHILD AT HOME

With the introduction of the National Service Framework and the advancements in medical technology the number of children with complex medical needs being treated at home is on the increase. Although the need for play specialists in the community is still relatively low, the need for play interventions is still essential in the care of the child at home. Children with a terminal illness can often enjoy those play sessions as a way to bring some normality into their day and be a child or young person again and not someone with an illness.

Although we use play as a means to help them express how they are feeling it is important not to forget the child inside. Helen Langton (2000) writes:

> The child enjoys having one-to-one attention from somebody with whom they have established a relationship of trust. It is often during these sessions the child will feel able to discuss their fears and beliefs, particularly while using play as a means of communication.

Listed below are some pointers for the community nurse:

- Information given using a child-centred approach such as preparation using play techniques can help a child reduce the experience of pain. For those with severe anxiety or other additional problems, preparation in the community is more effective.
- For children experiencing difficulty with injections such as methotrexate, an injection plan can be made. It is a little bit like a child's contract. With the child you draw up a list of things that everyone agrees to, usually in the order they happen. For example, does the child want cream or not, how do they want to sit, do they want to shout? These are all choices that can be made in advance and it is a good tool to use to get the child talking about the situation in question. If there are some choices that cannot be made then these also have to be discussed. Afterwards, the child can decorate the list. When it is all finished, the child and nurse sign and date it. The child and nurse both keep a copy. As each injection is due this can be looked at and followed. If things change it can be renewed. For older children, this has been an effective tool that can work both in the hospital and at home.
- When you go out for a visit always take something with you for the child to look at or play with. This could even be some stickers that the child can choose from before you go.
- I used to work with an oncology nurse specialist. When he went out into the community, I would create some special stickers for him to take with him. This became something special for two boys who were collecting the different Power Rangers stickers. Each time he went out to take some blood from their port-a-cath he would make sure he left them a sticker. The boys looked forward to his

visits just for the stickers and not the blood-taking. This was exactly what we were trying to achieve.

● Always try and leave on a positive note. When any treatment is done to a child they can often get upset; this is normal. Staff shortages or increases in workload mean having no excess time available and it is not always easy, but try to spend a short time with them doing something they like. If the nurse hurries out of the door after a procedure, the child will associate them with that unpleasantness. In my experience, if you leave on a positive note, the child will remember and welcome you back another time.

TYPES OF PLAY

Play in hospital can be based around the work of Sylva (1993) who describes two main categories of play: normative and therapeutic.

The purpose of normative play is to establish norms and rules. This sort of play, which children use most often, engages others, including friends and siblings and uses the toys around the child. Normative play helps to bring familiarity to an unfamiliar situation such as an experience in hospital. Normative play is undertaken voluntarily and is pleasurable. Very rarely does it have any goals and the child is in control. In a safe, relaxed and inviting environment, children can feel able to carry out their play.

Therapeutic play is structured by adults and followed through by the child. Its purpose is to help the child to achieve 'emotional and physical well-being' by means of various activities, in order to achieve therapeutic ends. Through play, a child is given the opportunity to overcome fears and anxieties by bringing unconscious feelings to the surface. This play also incorporates desensitisation. A child who developed a needle phobia was able, with great pleasure, to work through his feelings of anxiety by handling and familiarising himself with the properties of a syringe, first without a needle, and then progressed to using a needle and injecting into an orange. The mother was also present during this session and felt comfortable handling the syringe and working through her own anxieties relating to her son's treatment.

Puppets allow children to talk about their illness through the third person and are very simple and quick to create, e.g. draw a face on your finger and bring the child into conversation.

A 5-year-old with cystic fibrosis was able to express to a puppet how he was feeling about being in hospital far easier than to a member of staff. To him it felt safe and it was like talking to a friend.

Another 4-year-old with arthritis expressed her anger at her consultant by using 'play-mobile' people. She positioned the characters in such a way that the one she had decided was to become the consultant was in a bed and she was the nurse inflicting pain on him; she squealed with delight when he cried. The most favourite activity postoperatively is 'gunging' the imaginary doctor or nurse with cornflour mixture.

After an uncomfortable procedure has been carried out, silent play or simple discussion using any of the above examples can allow the child to be angry about the invasion of their body in a secure and non-threatening environment.

PREPARATION

Play in hospital aims to inform children about the unusual situation in which they find themselves and thereby allay fears and increase confidence. It will also provide a much-needed link with home and normality. Using play preoperatively, or prior to other frightening procedures (venepuncture, radiotherapy, nasogastric feeding), goes a long way in helping children to express their real feelings. This is supported by Sutherland (2003) when she wrote that:

> Children who are properly informed and prepared for surgery are less anxious and experience a shorter and less psychologically traumatic recovery and discharge adjustment.

Before preparing a child for a procedure or operation, various factors have to be taken into consideration. These are the age of the child or adolescent, cognitive development, emotional maturity, previous experiences, cultural differences, coping strategies and parental anxiety. Where possible, a trusting relationship should be formed before any preparation begins. It is also important that whoever is leading the session is fully aware of the implications of the operation or procedure for the child. During preparation, the use of real hospital equipment is vital. The use of syringes, masks, anaesthetic cream, clear plasters, stethoscopes, etc. will allow children to familiarise themselves with equipment that may be used during their own procedure or operation. Picture books, photographs and DVDs may help a child by clarifying images and thoughts. 'Good preparation can help children organize their thoughts, actions and feelings about an event prior to it happening' (Oner-Ozkan & Ercan 2005). During preparation sessions the child must be given physical and emotional space to express feelings and fears. The session should not be rushed as this may add to the child's feeling of loss of control. The whole hospital experience tends to remove control from the child. If the child can be given space to think through and explore the forthcoming procedure through play, they can be given back some control over the situation, and this will help boost their confidence. In some cases it may be appropriate to include sessions for the parent/carer and siblings, as the child being treated may pick up their feelings towards the procedure. Nancy Browne (2007) also agrees with this point when she wrote that, 'preoperative anxiety in parents directly influences the anxiety of their child'.

It is really important that you do not miss out those children with additional needs. It is easy to think that just because their understanding or communication is different from that usually seen, they will not see the potential procedure as frightening. 'Changing a child's routine can cause them anxiety especially if their understanding is limited in any way. Children can be supported to manage changes if the adults around them take time to prepare them in a way the child can understand' (Warner 2006). In these cases, adapting aids is necessary. Consulting other colleagues or the child's school for ideas on doing this may be the solution.

Using photographs with children with autism is very effective. But it is important that these photographs just show what it is you want them to see. For example if you are telling them about sitting on some weighing scales prior to coming in for surgery and your picture is with another child or teddy sitting on those scales, then it is extremely difficult for them to rationalise. They cannot see themselves sitting on scales that a child or teddy is already on.

If at all possible, it is always a good idea to have a visit to the ward prior to admission. This will cut down on any excess stress that a new environment may cause.

Note: The child should *always* be warned if the procedure is going to hurt as this will help build up a trusting relationship.

PREPARATION GUIDELINES

1. Always be honest with the child.

2. It is important that everyone dealing with the child is as relaxed as possible, as this will give confidence to both child and family.

3. Most children benefit from individual preparation.

4. Give information that is child-friendly, using words and phrases that the child and family will understand, ensuring that it is consistent and allows time for questions. It is important to use the correct names of equipment to avoid confusion

5. Timing: Young children who have limited or no understanding of time cannot manage their anxiety about a future event if told far in advance. Where possible, discuss with parent/carer.

6. Avoid using phrases such as 'We will give you medicine to put you to sleep'. This can be confused with when a pet dies and is 'put to sleep'. 'Can I take your temperature?' may evoke anxiety as to where you are taking it: 'Will I get it back?'

7. Stress sometimes results in the child being unable to fully absorb what is being said. Be aware of non-verbal indications that the child may no longer be listening. Remember to acknowledge feelings and give reassurance and further explanations when needed.

8. Children often regress while in hospital and may require repetitive explanations and information about their procedures.

9. Some parents may be anxious that telling their child about a procedure will cause more anxiety. It is worth explaining that a child who is not given accurate information may fantasise and fear something worse.

10. Be aware of the implications for children, especially when procedures are performed on vulnerable body parts such as the eyes, genital or anal areas. They may have anxieties about this.

11. All children and families are different, with a variety of previous experiences. The preparation must be tailored to fit the particular situation.

12. If siblings are present, then find out from parents what their understanding of the procedure is so that, if necessary, time can be spent with them.

Emergency admissions and procedures often do not allow for effective preparation; it is worth ensuring that a preparation book (a book with a series of descriptive photographs about procedures) is always available (see Box 10.1).

PRE-ADMISSION PROGRAMMES/PREOP CLUBS

Pre-admission clubs are usually run about 1 week before a child is to be admitted for surgery. They have been established to help inform and reduce the anxiety felt by the child and their families about coming into hospital. When they arrive, the child and family will be met by a member of staff who will show them a photograph book depicting what will happen on the day. This usually includes pictures of the anaesthetic room and staff they may meet. Hospital equipment is also available for the child to play with and become familiar with.

The benefits of these clubs is that paperwork can be filled in, in advance, and children who have difficulty with coming to hospital or those with hospital-related phobias can be picked up in advance. The child can then be given additional support by a play specialist if required. If a play specialist is present sometimes a parent is more likely to talk to them about their child's fears rather than feel they are wasting a nurse's time. If you are a nurse or student admitting or pre-clerking a child for surgery, it is important to ask these questions. Having all the information means you are more ready to be able to help the child. Include the parents and siblings as well in the photograph book or tour, as this will help them too. Around 93% of all children's fears are picked up from other family members.

Needle play

This type of play is used to help children who have fears with any procedure that involves needles of any kind. This is done on a one-to-one basis with the child using real needles in a controlled manner. It leads to a better understanding of the procedure and provides an opportunity for feelings to be discussed. A needle plan can be drawn up depicting how the child wants to sit or whether to have cream or not, etc. This gives the child a feeling of control where they previously felt they had none. As the child psychologist Richard Lansdown wrote in his pamphlet *Helping Children Cope with Needles* (1987), 'the aim is to help all children cope by reducing the sensation of pain to one of pressure'. He went on to say that it would be ideal to 'enable all children to keep still (most important for medical and nursing staff) and to come away from the experience without anxiety about the next time'. A qualified play specialist or staff who have attended a 'needle play' workshop should carry out this type of play. In extreme cases, a referral to a child psychologist may be necessary.

Some points to consider to help minimise the distress for the child are:

- Have everything ready in the treatment room before the child enters. This then shortens the time a child has to spend there and their distress
- It can often be difficult for the parents to distract their child and hold them. So if no play specialist is present make sure you have an extra person available who can take on this role. Also have plenty of toys available for distraction; you never know how long it might take. Better to be prepared

---

BOX 10.1 Examples of how play can allay fears in children

A 5-year-old newly diagnosed diabetic was getting increasingly scared about having her injections, so she was given a friendly teddy called Toby. She was told the story that Toby was also diabetic and that he needed his injections too. But only diabetic children could give them. She looked unsure but then asked some questions about what medicine he had. The pen injector was the same as the one she used, so she liked that. She practised getting it ready. When she was due for her own injection the nurse asked if she would get Toby's ready, which she did. The nurse asked if she wanted hers before Toby's and she said that she did. She said that she had to show Toby that he did not have to be scared. The little girl then did Toby's injection, talking to him as she did so. Afterwards she gave him a hug.

The little girl saw Toby as a friend and helped him have his injection. She saw herself in the parent role, and she took to it well. She was given the opportunity to play with the injector pen, which she had not done. It then became something familiar and not something to be feared. By introducing Toby, he became the one who was scared, not her, and so she could act her feelings through him.

- It only takes one bad experience to make a child so fearful that it reaches panic, so we have to try and get it right first time. For some, the experience of the Tegaderm plaster is enough – just the thought of peeling it off their skin with the anaesthetic cream sends them into a panic. Something we use in these cases is cling film. If you tear off a large piece of cling film and fold it into a bandage like strip, then put it over the cream in a figure of eight motion it will hold the Emla or Ametop cream in place. I call it a 'hand/arm sandwich'. The child can then unwind as they would a sandwich. No stress involved

- For those who need a finger prick test and have become fearful, fill a rubber glove with some diluted red food colouring and tie a knot in the end. Prick the top of the glove finger and the child can pretend to be a nurse. The blood should drip from the finger. It is a bit messy but fun. Role play is a good technique to get the child talking about his or her fears. Remember to try it first to make sure it works

- Syringe painting is also messy but fun

- Guided imagery and visualisation can also be a good technique to use with older children to help them work through difficulties they may be experiencing with needle procedures.

Messy play

Messy play is an activity that allows children to be as messy as they wish:

> ... giving considerable pleasure and satisfaction to the sick child. The finished work is admired, bringing self-esteem and a good self image, helping the child to gain confidence and to cope with situations. (Play Focus 2002)

This is very beneficial in the clinical environment of the hospital. It is a great kick against the system and an outlet for expression of emotion, be it frustration, anger, despair, loneliness or isolation. Playdough, cornflour and water, and syringe painting all provide therapeutic opportunities for expressive play. A young sibling showed great pleasure in thumping the play dough very hard when her sister was readmitted to the children's ward on her birthday, which was seen as a reflection of her inner feelings.

The use of paintings and drawings may also allow children to express how they are feeling about a situation.

Distraction

Distraction therapy is a non-pharmacological method used to enable a child to reduce anxiety and pain by focusing on something other than the procedure. If there is time, preparation is important before the proceduce, but if not, some things that should be considered before you consider any distraction include:

- How long is the procedure?
- What choices can be made, both about the procedure and the distraction technique? If you are going to use breathing exercises or guided imagery it may be appropriate to practise beforehand
- Where possible establish a relationship with the child or young person
- Previous experiences
- Does the child like to look?
- Giving permission to cry, shout, etc.
- Childs interests, hobbies
- Attention span
- Who is coming with the child, young person?

Introduce the toy at the correct time, where it will have the most benefit. Timing is important. From experience it is always ideal to take a selection of toys with you during the procedure. It is better for the child to be prepared for unexpected delays than having to leave the room to go and get something different.

In order for the distraction to be effective the child has to be open to it. Should the child become so distressed that it is no longer of any benefit then withdraw the toy but stay in the room. If they would like to, then the child can play with it afterwards. Remember to use praise and encouragement to reward how well they did. Make your own bravery or star patient certificates to give out to the children as appropriate.

A selection of distraction tools that can be used are listed in Table 10.1. Remember to think about what method would work best for the individual child. The items used for distraction must not be readily available for normal play, as this will reduce the attention span of the child. Leave the box in the treatment room for easy accessibility.

Bubbles

Encourage the child to blow the bubbles high and low. Look at colours and shapes within them.

Table 10.1	Distraction tools
AGE-GROUP	**APPROPRIATE TOYS**
Babies	Musical toys, rattles, dummy, cuddling, blowing bubbles
Toddlers	Blowing bubbles, pop up toys, control and response toys, finger puppets, musical toys, songs or rhymes, aqua draw mini mats
Pre-school	Interactive noisy books, *Where's Wally* book, counting, sticky bubbles, shouting, *1001 Things to Find* (Usborne Books)
School age children/ adolescents	*Where's Wally* book, mazes, *1001 Things to Find* (Usborne Books), joke books, puppets, counting, games consoles, guided imagery, sticky bubbles, controlled breathing, shouting, 20Qs, Game boys, MP4 players

Sticky bubbles

These bubbles can be made into a game of trying to catch them on your finger or how many you can cover the doctor in.

Counting

Use number games; count up and down.

Puppets

Encourage the child to talk about procedures, using the puppet.

Imagination

Talk with the child about their favourite activity or hobby.

Breathing

During venepuncture, some children will be helped by getting them to breathe in; then, as the needle is inserted, they can be asked to breathe out. This may help them feel that they have more control over the situation.

Relaxation tapes

Play the tape during a procedure. Gently talk the child through the forthcoming procedure.

Shouting

Allow the child to shout. Shout with the child, if appropriate.

Squeezing

In stressful situations, give the child a ball to squeeze.

(*Distraction Boxes can be applied for by contacting the Starlight Children's Foundation; Tel. 020 7262 2881; for more information go to: www.starlight.org.uk/menu_pages/page_details.asp?t=distraction_boxes*)

GUIDED IMAGERY AND VISUALISATION

'Guided imagery provides relaxation and distraction and allows the child to maintain control', said Burgess (2001). Visualisation exercises are helpful when undertaken by those familiar with the procedure. They should be used with caution and not by inexperienced practitioners.

Guided imagery is using the child's imagination to take them to a place where they feel safe and in control. This is a good distraction tool when used appropriately. There are many different techniques that can be used to start off a guided imagery/visualisation session but I have detailed below just one of the relaxation induction techniques that can be used with a child. Remember to take your time. Before starting get to know a little about the child you are working with. For example if the child likes football, then you can use the image of going to a football match or playing in the game.

To begin:

- Ask the child to close their eyes. Tell them that they can open them again later if this is distressing them.
- Get the child to rest their arms by their side and feel their body supported by the chair or bed (wherever they are resting).
- Start off by telling them you are going to start counting from 1 to 20. As you count you could ask them to imagine slowly walking along the beach to get to the football match. Each time they breathe out they can feel all the energy flow away (breathe nice and slowly). Remember to reduce the tone of your voice as you count down, when you get to the end you should be almost whispering.
- Bring in the use of their senses as you count down. Feeling the sand beneath their feet or listen to the noise of the ocean – can they feel the

heat of the sun on their face? Each out-breath means that they are deeper relaxed, wash the cares away. Feel their body float like a cloud as it catches all the fears they may be feeling.

- Once you reach about 18, start to slowly bring in where it is you are going, e.g. a football match. You can say that they are almost at the match – can they hear the noise of the fans? What colour of shirts are they wearing, etc? Make some suggestions about what to look for with an occasional question. To bring them back out you have to let them know it is time to go now – in relation to the football match you could say that the 90 minutes are up and it's time to go.
- Let them know that you are counting backwards 20–1 (20 being the start and 1 when they will have woken up).

Note: This is just a simple technique, practice is essential before using it on a child. Training is recommended.

BOX 10.2 Example

A young teenager was coming into hospital for an injection. She had got herself into such a fearful state that she was beginning to vomit. When she had calmed down a little, she was asked if she would like to try some guided imagery to help her through what was going to happen. She agreed, as it was something different. She was asked about things she liked doing and she said she liked making things for a new dolls house she had been given for her birthday. She collected dolls houses. I asked her if she wanted me to let her know when the injection was ready; she said No. Using a relaxation technique, she became a character in the dolls house. We went around the dolls house making sure that she noted every intricate detail. At this time, the injection was ready. I took her out to the house garden where there were flowers and some were a bit prickly. By incorporating the scratch she felt from the injection into her vision, she was not aware that it had taken place. After a few more minutes of looking, I said it was time to leave now and began to count down so that she could come back to the present. When she realised that the procedure was done she was shocked and did not believe it had taken place. It took her a little while to take it all in. This was a technique that worked well for this young lady and something she could use herself in the future; a very positive experience for her.

For younger children, you can ask them to imagine a feather blowing in the breeze. Their job is to keep it in the air. Something simple like a feather is an easier concept for a younger child to recognise. You can use the counting technique as a way of controlling the child's breathing and how hard they are trying to blow. As the procedure begins to start you can always say that the feather is falling and they may need to blow just that little bit harder to keep it in the air.

ADOLESCENTS

This is a particularly difficult age-range to cater for with regards to their play needs. Adolescents do not like the word play, so social activities or just activities to stop you feeling bored are the best phrases to use. Listening to them and valuing what they have to say is one of the most important things. Information should be appropriate and medical staff should be honest about their treatment, using words that they understand. Although this is similar for younger children too, this age range are more able to take on board more detailed explanations. Communication and facilities are also high on their list of essentials. As technology advances, most teenagers have access to PCs, mobiles and games consoles and these are almost expected when they come into hospital. Keeping up-to-date with friends and what is happening outside is also important and therefore having this facility available on the wards is essential. Most adolescent units will have this already but some other hospitals do not have it readily available except in the school room. What about the rest of the time…?

Choices

Adolescents feel that they have little choice or involvement with regard to decisions about treatment, include them whenever possible. Their cooperation is far more effective than refusal.

Example
When a new adolescent room was being set up on the ward, I consulted the adolescents on what rules there should be for its use. Both the nursing staff and the adolescents were asked to write what their expectations were. The result was really interesting, as the adolescents were much stricter on themselves than the nursing staff. By working together, we came up with a set of adolescent rules that everyone agreed to.

Privacy

I am mentioning this, as sometimes it is forgotten. Although they like having a chat they also like their privacy too. Give them the space and knock before entering their cubical or bed space, especially if the curtains are closed. After all, this would be what you would want as well in the same situation.

Appointments

If it is possible, give the adolescent time to meet with the doctor individually. This can be tricky as some parents like to be present with their child. Adolescents do not always want to share everything in front of them. This means a change in hospital policy but there are ways around it. It is worth considering, especially as young people may be changing to adult services and they will be expected to go on their own. This could be part of getting young people ready to move from paediatric to adult services:

> Adolescents are often not ready for adult services but they feel patronized by a system that makes no distinction between children and the 12 to 18 age-range.
> (Lindon 2007)

Resources

Within each area where adolescents are treated, there should be sufficient resources which are age appropriate to them, e.g. chess, playing cards, magazines, etc. Games consoles and game boys are excellent but actually making sure they are kept up-to-date and safe from theft can be very difficult and pricy in a hospital environment, so looking at other facilities can be more resourceful. There should also be leaflets available which they may find helpful such as those on smoking, drinking and drugs, etc.

Routine

The routine of most adolescents is stay up late and wake up late. In a hospital environment this can pose a problem, especially if you are trying to get them to do school work. If this is the case then you will need to have a routine in place much the same as if he/she were at home. Some hospitals have contracts with adolescents especially regarding behaviour and sleeping and awake times. I have drawn up individual contracts for specific issues, such as inappropriate behaviour.

This point was also raised by Jennie Lindon (2007) regarding adolescents and their involvement in healthcare:

> Adolescents do not appreciate being told off by health professionals and cease to listen or attend under those circumstances. Any kind of health education or service needs to recognize that some level of risky behaviour is within the norm for adolescents. Health education and care will not work to control young people, any more than it does with adults.

Interactive websites

There are many websites where children and young people can access health information. A web address where you can access some of these websites is: www.equip.nhs.uk/groups/kids.html

Children and young people are all very knowledgeable about how to find things out on a computer. Check with them that they have the correct information. Or make a list for them of good places to look. It is better if it comes from the people who know their condition best.

SIBLINGS

Siblings often experience feelings of abandonment, guilt, loss and uncertainty. Introducing play that includes the sibling will go a long way to encourage harmony within the family during an unfamiliar experience of hospitalisation.

Those who are well informed, and who assume a helping role, seem more able to accommodate the changes in the family and to perceive the experience in positive terms (Whitaker 2002).

PRAISE AND REWARDS

It is really important to give praise to the children when they have done well. It makes them feel good about themselves. This can be done with a reward of a certificate or a sticker. It is a good idea to call them star patient awards as bravery implies that one child is braver than the other.

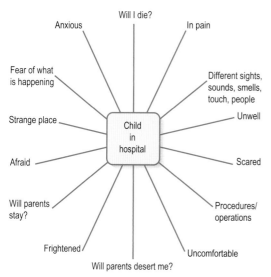

Figure 10.1 What a child may experience during their stay in hospital.

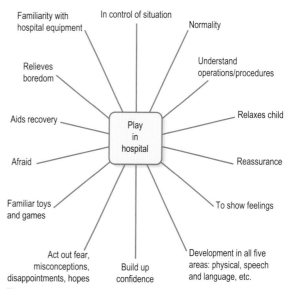

Figure 10.2 Benefits of play in hospital.

PLAY AND THE WAY FORWARD

Play specialists should be employed on most children's wards across the country. The introduction of a team member who works regular hours and is responsible for creating a safe, fun and non-threatening environment gives the child some normality in an abnormal situation, but with money restraints being placed on many NHS Trusts, play specialists and play are not always seen as essential by some managers (Fig. 10.1). This point was raised recently by the Healthcare Commission (2007) when it wrote, 'Trusts need to recognise the benefits of play and communication'. They go on to write, 'As staff who specialise in play do not deliver clinical care, they may not be seen as a priority in some trusts. However, their work directly with children or through other staff can greatly improve the experiences of children in hospital. Trusts need to recognise the impact this has and give it a much higher priority'. This can only be achieved by working together with the nursing staff, and other members of the multidisciplinary team to promote the benefits of play (Fig. 10.2).

The ability to understand the importance and value of play will add a vital component to the skills of the children's nurse, not only on the ward but also en route to theatre, in the anaesthetic room and in all other areas where children are nursed.

References

Browne, N.T., 2007. Nursing care of the paediatric surgical patient. Jones and Bartlett, Sudbury, p. 6.

Burgess, C.A., 2001. Complementary therapies: guided imagery and infant massage. Paediatr. Nurs. 13 (6), 37–41.

Cattanach, A., 2003. Introduction to play therapy. Routledge, London, p. 43.

Healthcare Commission for Audit and Inspection, 2007. Improving services for children in hospital. Healthcare Commission, London, p. 4, 33.

Langton, H., 2000. The child with cancer: family-centred care in practice. Harcourt, Edinburgh, p. 365.

Lansdown, R., 1987. Helping children cope with needles – a guide for parents and staff. Department of Psychological Medicine, Great Ormond Street Hospital, London, p. 2.

Lansdown, R., 1996. Children in hospital. Oxford University Press, London.

Lindon, J., 2007. Understanding children and young people – development from 5–18 years. Hodder Arnold, London, p. 286, 287.

Morris, D., 1989. Hospital – a deprived environment for children. A case for hospital play schemes. Save the Children Fund, London.

Oner-Ozkan, B., Ercan, S., 2005. Relationship between preparatory information, preoperative and postoperative anxiety, and coping strategies in children and adolescents undergoing surgery. In: Velotis, C.M. (Ed.), Anxiety disorder research. Nova Science, New York, p. 265.

Play Focus, 2002. Messy play for children in hospital. National Association of Hospital Play Staff, Beaconsfield, Bucks, p. 1.

Sutherland, T., 2003. Comparison of hospital and home base preparation for cardiac surgery. Paediatr. Nurs. 15 (5), 13–16.

Sylva, K., 1993. Play in hospital – when and why it's effective. Current Paediatrics 3, 247–249.

Warner, H.K., 2006. Meeting the needs of children with disabilities – families and professionals facing the challenge together. Routledge, Abingdon, Oxon, p. 157.

Webster, A., 2000. The facilitating role of the play specialist. Paediatr. Nurs. 12 (7), 24.

Whitaker, J., 2002. Making connections: play and siblings. In: NAHPS Journal. Summer edn. National Association of Hospital Play Staff, London, p. 12.

Further reading

Cohen, D., 2006. The development of play, third ed. Routledge, Abingdon, Oxon.

Cook, P., 1999. Supporting sick children and their families. Baillière Tindall, Edinburgh.

Dell Clark, C., 2003. In sickness and in play – children coping with chronic illness. Rutgers University Press, New Jersey.

Edwards, M., Davis, H., 1997. Counselling children with chronic medical conditions. British Psychological Society Books, Blackwell Science, Oxford.

National Association of Hospital Play Staff, 2002. Guidelines for professional practice. NAHPS, Beaconsfield, Bucks.

Shuttleworth, A., 2003. Children first: a health website for children. Nurs. Times 99 (44), 18–19.

Wilson, K., Ryan, V., 2005. Play therapy a non-directive approach for children and adolescents. Elsevier, London.

Chapter 11

Skin care

Jacqueline Denyer, Rosemary Turnbull

CHAPTER CONTENTS

Introduction   131
    Learning outcomes   131
    Rationale   132
    Factors to note   132
    Equipment   132

Guidelines for performing skin care   132
    Cradle cap/seborrhoeic dermatitis   132
    Nappy rash   133
    Eczema herpeticum   133
    Impetigo   133
    Dos and don'ts   133
    Atopic eczema   134
    Dos and don'ts   135
    Psoriasis   135
    Dos and don'ts   136

The pre-term infant   136

The child with fragile skin   136
    Bathing   137
    Method   137
    General care of the child with fragile skin   137

INTRODUCTION

The skin is the largest organ of the body and has many functions, the most important being:

- Thermoregulation
- Protection: from physical and mechanical injury
- Waterproofing
- Synthesis of vitamin D
- Transmission of sensation (Gawkrodger 2003).

In the absence of disease it is important to maintain the skin in good condition to minimise infection and dry skin. In many cultures, this can be achieved through regular bathing and drying (Denyer & Turnbull 1996). Often underestimated in their effects on general health and well-being, childhood skin disorders may reduce quality of life through pain and irritation. Although rare, some skin conditions can prove to be life threatening. Appropriate skin care is essential in those with healthy or diseased skin in order to maintain the functions of the skin as far as possible.

LEARNING OUTCOMES

By the end of this section you should be able to:

- Maintain good skin care in the presence of health and disease
- Develop an understanding of children who require additional skin care
- Apply topical treatments as prescribed in the correct way
- Adapt such treatments to the individual child.

RATIONALE

Children's nurses are frequently involved in the care of children with many skin conditions, including atopic eczema; in general wards when the child is admitted for another condition; in out-patient departments and in the dermatology ward.

The healthy child may suffer from dry skin conditions or infections. The majority of dermatological conditions can be exacerbated by the dry hot atmosphere of the hospital ward. A hospital admission, whether for management of the skin condition or for another reason, provides an ideal opportunity for intensive skin care and for assessment and review, enhancing parental education, and building on and reiterating knowledge.

Painful and irritated skin has a profound effect on the child's self-image, mood and peer acceptance. Those who will require additional skin care over and above routine cleansing include:

- Infants with cradle cap and dry skin
- Infants with nappy rash
- Children with skin infections
- Children with eczema or psoriasis
- The pre-term infant whose skin is thin and delicate
- Children with serious inherited skin disorders.

FACTORS TO NOTE

- Children can develop a range of skin conditions, many of which are transient, e.g. contact dermatitis, and cause few ill-effects, while others can develop into more persistent serious conditions.
- Dry skin is a common problem and its management can be incorporated into the regime of daily hygiene.
- Children enjoy bubble baths but these may have a drying effect and may necessitate restriction. After bathing, the skin should be checked for any signs of dryness or irritation and moisturisers applied as necessary.
- Children's skin is often sensitive and an unscented preparation should be chosen.
- Use of coconut and olive oils features in Asian and Afro-Caribbean cultures as a part of daily skin care. Caution must be exercised in using nut oils in view of the increasing awareness of the risk of anaphylaxis in response to such products.

- It is crucial that a detailed history and examination of the skin is made in order to plan, implement and evaluate an individualised treatment plan for the child.
- Where possible, the child and parents should be encouraged to participate in the care. Children may be afraid or fractious and adolescents may rebel against lifelong daily treatments.
- It should be remembered that treatments are often time-consuming and monotonous.
- Preparations can stain all clothing and soft furnishings, and can make carers reluctant to pick up or cuddle the child.

EQUIPMENT

- Plastic aprons to protect clothing/uniform
- Gloves, for use when applying medicated creams/ointments or when dealing with children whose skin is infected
- Bath situated in a warm private environment
- Soft towels
- Prescribed bath additive
- Soap substitute
- Prescribed cream/ointment
- Emollient
- Foil bowls and spatula (for decanting creams/ointments not in pump dispensers)
- Selection of toys for distraction
- Clothing
- Nappies if required.

GUIDELINES FOR PERFORMING SKIN CARE

CRADLE CAP/SEBORRHOEIC DERMATITIS

This is characterised by erythema and a yellow scale on the scalp, which can spread to eyebrows. Generally affecting infants under 3 months of age, occurring on the scalp (cradle cap), eyebrows, face and limb flexures, it can also favour the nappy area. Unlike atopic eczema, it is not itchy or painful but can look unsightly, causing distress to parents. It will generally clear on its own with mild emollient therapy such as an emollient bath daily and a light emollient cream. If it does not clear, the infant should be referred to a dermatologist/paediatrician for further assessment.

For cradle cap, olive oil can be applied to the scalp and gently massaged in to loosen the scales and encourage them to separate. The oil can be left in for 30 min to overnight, depending on the severity of the cradle cap. A soft baby brush can then be used to gently remove the loosened scales. Temptation to remove adherent scales by picking must be resisted as hair loss may result (Gill 2003).

The oil should not be left on the scalp, so a medicated or mild infant shampoo can be used to remove it.

NAPPY RASH

Nappy rash is a relatively common condition of infancy. It can be caused by irritation from faeces and urine or fungal contamination. Infant skin is generally more fragile and therefore more prone to physical and chemical injury/irritation as the dermis is immature due to decreased collagen and elastic fibres, as well as immature blood and nerve supply. The normal pH of skin is acidic; moisture in the nappy area increases the pH, making the skin more permeable (Turnbull 2003). Children suffering from gastroenteritis or malabsorption syndromes frequently pass watery stools, which may be acidic and cause damage to the nappy area. These children may require more frequent nappy changes and application of occlusive ointments such as petroleum jelly; this will go some way to reducing contact with irritants. Exposure of the excoriated skin will help minimise nappy rash (Turnbull 2003).

The carer must be educated on prevention of nappy rash by frequent changing and gentle cleansing followed by application of a barrier cream/ointment, such as zinc and castor oil cream or petroleum jelly. The use of fragranced cleansing wipes should be discouraged in the presence of nappy rash, as they will only serve to irritate the skin.

When there is no improvement using simple measures, secondary infection such as with *Candida albicans* (thrush) should be suspected and a swab obtained for culture before commencing prescribed treatments (Turnbull 2003). If nappy rash is severe and persists despite all measures, the infant should be referred to a dermatologist/paediatrician for diagnosis.

ECZEMA HERPETICUM

This is caused by the herpes simplex virus (HSV) and many eczematous children have an abnormal response to HSV, which can result in dissemination of the herpes and subsequent toxaemia (Harper 1990).

It is recognised as small clusters of clear fluid-filled vesicles, which can take on a punched-out appearance. The child may be generally unwell with pyrexia and malaise.

This is a dermatological emergency and the child should be seen by a GP or emergency department immediately and all parents should be alerted to this condition and advised to keep the child away from those with cold sores. Healthcare workers with cold sores should not care for the child with eczema and should refrain from work until clear. The child will require adjustment to the topical therapies and treatment with antiviral medication.

IMPETIGO

This is a highly infectious disorder caused by *Staphylococcus aureus* and/or group A streptococci. It is characterised by small blisters that burst easily, releasing a yellow exudate, which in turn forms a pale honey-coloured crust.

The infectious nature of this condition necessitates the child being kept off school or nursery. Sites around the nose and mouth are most commonly affected (Doherty 2001). If the infection is extensive, then systemic antibiotics are indicated and they should be prescribed immediately and not withheld until microbiology results are available.

Topical antibiotics are only of use if the infection is identified early enough and the impetiginised area is localised; however, one must be aware that in some instances such as eczema the possibility of multiresistant strains should be a consideration.

Crusts can be removed by the use of warm saline soaks or a weak solution of potassium permanganate as per pharmacy instruction.

DOS AND DON'TS

- Do isolate the child from others. If in hospital, universal precautions are indicated against infection. At home, the child should have their own towel and avoid using a flannel. Bed linen such as pillowcases should be changed daily to minimise reinfection.

- Do cut the child's fingernails to minimise damage if the skin is scratched. The wearing of mittens/gloves will minimise skin damage.
- Do introduce distraction methods to stop the child scratching or picking at crusts and so spreading the infection.

ATOPIC ECZEMA

Eczema is a chronic inflammatory disorder of the skin. The condition is erratic and varies somewhat in severity. It generally presents in infancy from 3 months of age and there is often a genetic predisposition, i.e. family history of asthma, eczema and allergy. Any area of the body can be affected and education on factors that may exacerbate the condition is crucial in order to give optimum care to the child and promote an adequate quality of life. There is no cure for this condition but several of these factors can assist in the reduction of exacerbations (McHenry 1995). There has been a recent development from NICE (2007) recommending a staged approach to management of eczema in children 0–12 years. This document includes precise instruction on all aspects of care of a child with atopic eczema.

Factors to note

- Eczema results in intense pruritus (itching) which makes the child irritable and fretful; this in turn results in sleep disturbance.
- The skin becomes red (erythematous) and small blisters (vesicles) occur which, when scratched, result in weeping, bleeding areas of skin.
- There is no cure and the aim is to control the condition and minimise exacerbations. A basic regime may be enough to maintain control of the skin.
- The aim of treatments is to replace moisture and reduce inflammation. This is achieved through regular use of emollients, and application of prescribed topical therapies depending on severity of the skin at any given time.
- If frequent exacerbations are common, reassessment will be necessary to rule out anything that may be a contributing factor. It may also be useful to establish who does the skin care and how it is carried out. Are the parents or carers applying adequate amounts of topical therapies? It may be necessary to re-educate the carer and, where appropriate, the child, and together negotiate achievable goals.

- One must constantly assess and reassess the child's progress and treatment and alter the treatment accordingly. There are many triggers believed to cause eczema flare-ups and reducing contact with them may minimise exacerbations. Attention to the following may serve to improve the child's eczema:
  - Avoid any known aggravating factors
  - Wear 100% cotton clothing; as wool can irritate the skin
  - Sleep in a well-ventilated room
  - Reduce dust-mite activity through the use of special mattress covers to minimise the harbouring of the house dust mite (HDM). Daily vacuuming of the house and mattress, and damp dusting of the room will also reduce HDM
  - Avoid contact with and handling of all hairy/furry animals
  - Keep finger- and toenails short to minimise damage caused by scratching
  - Encourage the child to rub on the skin instead of scratching it
  - Develop distraction techniques and help parents to develop these to minimise anger and frustration
  - To ensure adequate rest and sleep, a prescribed sedative, antihistamine, may be administered early enough to allow a good sleep period before the child is due to rise
  - Also allowing adequate time for application of topical therapies.

Method

1. Bathing in warm/tepid water at least once daily with added emollient oil and use of a soap substitute cream will serve to remove surface debris and hydrate the skin.
2. To minimise irritation use a soft towel and pat, not rub, dry.
3. Prescribed topical steroids if used should be applied twice daily after bathing (unless medical advice differs) to all areas of eczema; there should be enough to show a fine visible film.
4. Emollients should be applied liberally and in a downward direction to minimise plugging of hair follicles which could result in infection. (The use of regular emollients serves to soften the skin and therefore reduce pruritus and the need for more potent topical steroids.)

5. The topical immunomodulators tacrolimus and pimecrolimus are a second-line treatment when eczema is not controlled on the first-line. These act differently from topical steroids and advice on each differs so application guidelines *must* be checked.

If it is not possible to control the child's eczema with this basic regime, it may be necessary to use wet wraps for a short time. NICE (2007) suggest 7–14 days. These increase steroid absorption as well as cooling the skin and reducing pruritus (Lawton 2002). Wet wraps must be used under the direction of the dermatologist/paediatrician. Wet wraps are lengths of tubefast cut to make a full body suit with normal clothing worn on top. They are relatively time-consuming to apply and should be seen not as a maintenance treatment, but as a means of regaining control of the child's eczema. The length of time wraps are required will depend on the child's response to treatment; once control is achieved, then the strength of topical steroids should be reduced to achieve maintenance. There are now several brands of tubefast available as well as wet wrap garments; choice generally depends on what is available to carry out the procedure competently. The parent/carer will need additional support during this treatment.

Lichenification is a thickening of the skin as a result of repeated damage through scratching and is visible in knee and elbow flexures. Limbs may respond to application of Ichthopaste/Viscopaste bandages overnight, but the bandages can be left *in situ* for up to 3 days. They are useful to soften the skin as well as producing a cooling effect. A low-potency topical steroid can be applied under the bandages if need be; the paste bandage is then covered with Coban elasticated dressing (Robinson 2003).

Note: Occlusive bandages create a warm humid environment which encourages bacterial growth and therefore spread infection; they must not be used in the presence of infection. This also applies to infectious diseases.

Observations and complications

The skin of most children with eczema will be colonised with *Staphylococcus aureus*. Infection should be considered when there is deterioration in the skin. Symptoms may include:

- Weeping/wet areas of eczema
- Areas of crusting

- Enlarged lymph nodes
- Pyrexia
- Irritability.

Streptococcal infection should be considered if there is family history of sore throats, and the child may be unwell.

DOS AND DON'TS

- Do educate parents in the management and treatment of the condition and regularly assess and reassess their techniques.
- Do be aware of the side-effects of prolonged or incorrect use of topical steroids. Preparations used in children tend to be mild and should not cause problems. Misuse of stronger steroids can result in thinning of the skin.
- Do monitor growth, as prolonged use of topical steroids, especially moderate and potent types, can inhibit normal growth. Growth should be monitored at each clinic appointment by measuring the child's height and weight and recording the results on a growth chart.
- Do ensure that the school receives education on the child's eczema and conditions that may aggravate the skin, e.g.:
  - Avoid sitting in the centre of the room or next to radiators
  - Use a soap substitute at all times
  - Identify an area where the child can apply emollients.
- Do not bathe in hot water as heat causes vasodilatation and will increase irritation.
- Do not use scented bath oils, creams, laundry powders or fabric softeners as they include fragrance which will irritate the skin.
- Do not dip fingers into pots of cream or ointments as this will increase the risk of contamination and cause infection. The preparation should be decanted onto a saucer each time it is used.
- Do not sit in hot, dry environments.

PSORIASIS

Psoriasis is a chronic relapsing non-infectious inflammatory disease characterised by recurrent flares and remissions (Lawton 2003). There are various types of psoriasis affecting people in different ways; therefore, treatments are tailored to meet individual needs. Psoriasis can affect any age but is uncommon in children and rarely seen before 3 years of age (Harper 1990). There are many factors that can trigger or exacerbate the disease process.

Factors to note

- Trauma – lesions appear at the site of injury
- Infection – beta haemolytic streptococcal tonsillitis
- Stress/emotional upset
- Sunlight – the majority will improve but a small percentage will become worse.

There are several treatments for psoriasis depending on severity at any one time. The most common treatments for psoriasis are mainly topical and can only be used when the disease process is active and not as preventive measures.

Method

1. Coal tar preparations: the exact mode of action is unclear but they are known to inhibit DNA synthesis, therefore reducing cell proliferation and inhibiting the psoriatic process.
2. Keratolytic agents are creams and ointments that reduce scaling by reducing thick plaques.
3. Bathing daily in a prescribed tar-based preparation or emollient bath oil and application of the prescribed keratolytic cream or ointment to affected areas may help to regain control of the disease process.
4. The application of emollients regularly throughout the day will promote skin softening and so reduce scaling and flaking of skin.

Care of the scalp

- Cocois or olive oil is massaged into the scalp and left *in situ* for the prescribed length of time; the hair is then combed out to remove loosened plaques
- Shampoo using a prescribed tar-based solution
- Comb again to remove plaques and then allow hair to dry naturally
- The procedure should be performed separately from the bath to minimise irritation to the skin of the body.

DOS AND DON'TS

- Do remove the preparation immediately and notify medical staff if irritation during treatment occurs.

- Do inform the parent and child that many preparations are messy and will stain clothing and sometimes skin. It should be stressed that any skin discoloration from treatments will fade.
- Do encourage the wearing of pale clothing to minimise the visibility of shed skin scales.
- Do avoid stressful situations.
- Do inform the child's school and arrange to chat with teachers, which will help reduce teasing; it is also crucial to refer the child to someone who will help them develop coping mechanisms.
- Do not allow the child to see this as a handicap but try to promote positive aspects of body image.
- Do not omit any prescribed treatments or use products prescribed for other people as treatment for psoriasis is individualised.

THE PRE-TERM INFANT

The skin of the pre-term infant is thin and there is absence of subcutaneous fat. Often, pre-term infants receive intensive therapy which involves the use of intravenous cannulae and monitoring with sticky equipment such as cardiac electrodes. Endotracheal tubes are sometimes secured with sticky tapes. Wherever possible, use of such tapes should be avoided and silicone or hydrocolloid dressings used in their place. Where use of adhesive tape is essential, care must be taken on removal to ensure no tearing of the skin results. A Silicone Medical Adhesive Remover (SMAR) should be used to destroy the adhesive properties of the tape prior to removal, or use petroleum jelly or liquid paraffin if a SMAR is not available.

THE CHILD WITH FRAGILE SKIN

Skin fragility may be a feature of prematurity or a genetic defect such as epidermolysis bullosa (EB). EB is a group of rare genetically determined mechano-bullous disorders affecting the skin and mucous membranes (Fine 2008). Defects arise from protein defects leading to skin loss and blistering resulting from minimal everyday friction and trauma. In its severe form EB occurs in 1:175 000 live births. The effects vary from minor blistering of the hands and feet in warm weather to death in early infancy in its most severe form. At present, gene therapy is not available for those affected, although work is progressing towards this. Children with a severe form of EB require multidisciplinary care at a specialised centre, but day-to-day care is carried out at home with the support of community nurses. Its aim is to:

- Maintain skin integrity
- Minimise damage
- Control critical colonisation and treat infected wounds
- Control pain
- Optimise nutrition
- Provide psychological support.

BATHING

Prior to bathing, the nurse must consider whether it is an appropriate procedure – if the child is very sore, then bathing is likely to cause added distress and should be deferred. Cleansing of unaffected areas may be a more suitable alternative (Lin & Carter 1992). Severely affected children often develop large chronically unhealed wounds which make handling difficult and such children are unable to tolerate exposure of all their wounds at any one time. Rotational dressings are then carried out and bathing is not advisable.

Bathing is a clean, rather than a sterile procedure. Prescribed analgesia must be given and replacement dressings prepared in advance of bathing to avoid delay in re-dressing the wounds.

Observation should be made of the site, size and condition of any wounds and the general condition of the skin. Particular care must be taken to identify infection and wound swabs taken if appropriate. Assessment should be made as to the efficacy of the analgesia and the suitability of prescribed dressings. Observations should be recorded and consented photographs taken as necessary in order to monitor progress or deterioration.

METHOD

1. Line a baby bath with a towelling sling or soft towel to prevent skin damage from the base or sides of the bath by avoiding shearing forces from a hard surface.
2. Add prescribed emollient(s).
3. Use a second person if necessary to assist and minimise trauma.
4. Pat rather than rub the child dry using a soft non-shedding towel to avoid leaving fibres

in the wound which may result in over-granulation.

5. Apply prescribed non-adherent dressings to promote a warm moist environment in order to encourage wound healing.

Note: Avoid prolonged bathing, which may result in a fall of temperature and result in delayed wound healing.

GENERAL CARE OF THE CHILD WITH FRAGILE SKIN

- Ensure that all who are in contact with the child are aware of the skin fragility and appropriate method of handling.
- Remove cord clamp in the newborn and replace with a ligature.
- Avoid the use of plastic identification bands which could rub and cause skin damage.
- Avoid the use of adhesive tapes.
- Use alternative fabrics to secure intravenous cannulae and electrodes, such as silicone tape or hydrocolloids. Use silicone medical adhesive removers (SMAR) to safely remove adhesive products (Mather & Denyer 2008).
- Choose soft cotton clothing. Turn underclothes inside out to avoid seams rubbing.
- Educate theatre and anaesthetic staff prior to any procedures.

COMMUNITY PERSPECTIVE

The health visitor and GP are likely to be the first community healthcare professionals to become aware of skin problems in the younger child. Depending on their level of knowledge of dermatology, health visitors may be confident to manage conditions such as atopic eczema in partnership with the GP. If the eczema is severe, the child should be referred to a consultant dermatologist. The amount of involvement CCNs have with families of children with eczema will vary according to local policies.

When a child has been admitted to hospital with infected eczema or a severe exacerbation, and has been discharged, home visits to check the child's progress and assist the family with time-consuming treatments have been shown to be beneficial. Home visits also enable the CCN to identify factors which may be exacerbating the eczema, e.g. pets or high levels of house-dust mite. The CCN will also gain insights into the nature of the condition at its most severe and how exhausted the families may become.

The CCN is in an ideal position to liaise with schools concerning the care of pupils with eczema, thus giving the teachers additional insight into problems that may occur.

Families who give a high input of care to their child with eczema may be entitled to Disability Living Allowance. The CCN may be asked to assist in filling in the application forms.

A multidisciplinary approach to the care of children with eczema has been proved to work well (Masini et al. 1997, unpublished work). Health visitors, CCNs and dermatology nurses, together with their medical colleagues, can develop a service to support the many families who struggle to cope with the demands of a badly affected child.

References

Denyer, J., Turnbull, R., 1996. The skin. In: McQuaid, L., Huband, S., Parker, E. (Eds.), Children's nursing. Churchill Livingstone, Edinburgh, Ch. 17.

Doherty, C., 2001. Infections and infestations. In: Hughes, E., Van Onselon, J. (Eds.), Dermatology nursing: a practical guide. Churchill Livingstone, Edinburgh, Ch. 13.

Fine, et al., 2008. The classification of inherited epidermolysis bullosa (EB). Report of the third International Consensus meeting on diagnosis and classification of EB. J. Am. Dermatol. 58 (6), 931–950.

Gawkrodger, D., 2003. Dermatology, an illustrated text. third ed. Churchill Livingstone, Edinburgh.

Gill, S., 2003. Infantile seborrhoeic dermatitis and cradle cap. In: Barnes, K. (Ed.), Paediatrics: a clinical guide for nurse practitioners. Butterworth-Heinemann, Edinburgh, Ch. 9.

Harper, J., 1990. Handbook of paediatric dermatology. Butterworth-Heinemann, London.

Lawton, S., 2002. How to wet wrap. Br. J. Dermatol. Nurs. 3 (1), 8–9.

Lawton, S., 2003. Psoriasis. In: Barnes, K. (Ed.), Paediatrics: a clinical guide for nurse practitioners. Butterworth-Heinemann, Edinburgh, p. 79.

Lin, A.N., Carter, D.M. (Eds.), 1992. Epidermolysis bullosa: basic and clinical aspects. Springer-Verlag, New York.

Mather, C., Denyer, J., 2008. Removing dressing in epidermolysis bullosa. Nurs. Times 104 (14), 48.

McHenry, P.M., 1995. Management of atopic eczema. Br. Med. J. 310, 843–847.

NICE, 2007. National Institute for Health and Clinical Excellence, Clinical Guideline, December 2007, Management of atopic eczema in children from birth to 12 years. London.

Robinson, J., 2003. Atopic eczema. In: Barnes, K. (Ed.), Paediatrics: a clinical guide for nurse practitioners. Butterworth-Heinemann, Edinburgh, Ch. 9.

Turnbull, R., 2003. Nappy rash. In: Barnes, K. (Ed.), Paediatrics: a clinical guide for nurse practitioners. Butterworth-Heinemann, Edinburgh, p. 11.

Useful addresses

Dystrophic Epidermolysis Bullosa Research Association (DEBRA)
DEBRA House
Wellington Business Park
Dukes Ride
Crowthorne
Berkshire RG11 6LS

National Eczema Society
Hill House
Highgate Hill
London N19 5NA
Online at: www.eczema.org

Psoriasis Association
Milton House
7 Milton Street
Northampton NN2 7JG

SECTION 3

Organisational aspects of care

SECTION CONTENTS

12. Bowel care   141

13. Central lines   152

14. Chest drainage   163

15. Incubator care   170

16. Lumbar puncture   175

17. Neurological observations and coma scales   182

18. Phototherapy   195

19. Cast care   200

20. Positioning, handling and exercises   211

21. Postoperative care   222

22. Preoperative care   228

23. Pressure area care   234

24. Radiography   240

25. Removal of drains and packs   251

26. Seizures   257

27. Stoma care   265

28. Suctioning   274

29. Temperature control   280

30. Tracheostomy care   284

31. Traction   299

32. Urine testing and urinary catheterisation   308

33. Venepuncture and cannulation   320

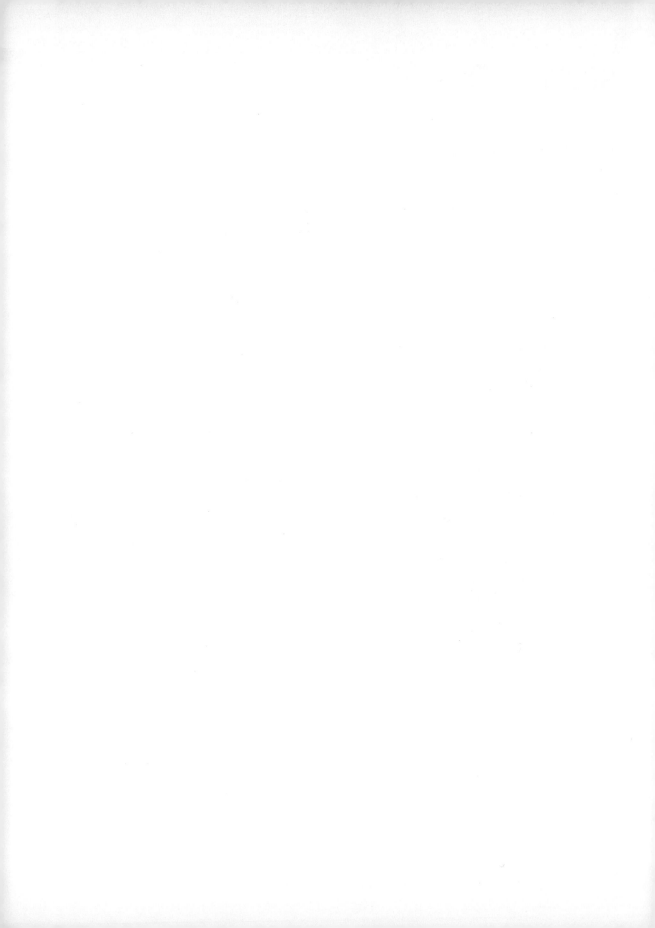

Chapter 12

Bowel care

Louise Ford

CHAPTER CONTENTS

Introduction   141
   Learning outcomes   141
   Rationale   142
   Definitions of terms   142
   Factors to note   142

Normal bowel movements   143
   Infants   143
   Children   144
   Children with developmental delay   144

Potential changes in bowel movements   144

Constipation   144
   Implications for nursing practice   145
   Principles in managing functional
   constipation   145
   Factors to note   146

Diarrhoea   147
   Management of diarrhoea in infants
   and young children   147
   Factors to note   147
   Assessment of dehydration   148
   Dos and don'ts   149

INTRODUCTION

The concept of what a 'normal' bowel movement is varies considerably between individuals. Some parents may become concerned if their child has not had a bowel movement every day (Thompson 2001b). There is now a growing body of literature indicating that nurses have an important role in the prevention and management of constipation in children and young people (Rogers 2000, Day 2001, Thompson 2001b, Burnett et al 2004, Sullivan et al 2006); the RCPCH Joint Advisory Committee on Children's Nursing (RCPCH 1996) highlighted the need for studies to evaluate the use of nurse-led clinics and associated outcomes. In spite of these recommendations being 12 years old, Burnett et al in 2004 have suggested that poor health outcomes could still be attributed to lack of management of care and subsequent follow-up.

LEARNING OUTCOMES

By the end of this section you should be able to:
- List the potential causes of constipation/diarrhoea
- Identify the role of the children's nurse in preventing constipation
- Discuss health promotion strategies used to promote normal bowel habits
- Identify the potential consequences of abnormal bowel habits for the child and family.

RATIONALE

The RCN (2003a) guidelines on digital rectal examination (DRE) highlight the fact that many nurses are concerned about DRE and the manual evacuation of faeces. These are invasive procedures that do not form part of the normal assessment and delivery of care for infants, children and young people with bowel problems. However, for some children and young people, especially those with spinal injuries, these procedures can become an important part of their bowel management (RCN 2003a). The RCN (2003b) also recommend that all trusts/hospitals develop a strategy to ensure that when DREs are required, care is delivered by those on the children's nurse's registers (Part 8 or Part 15 of the Nursing and Midwifery Council's register). Carrying out a DRE and other related procedures requires the skill and expertise of an expert practitioner; this is not a procedure that should be considered as a part of routine practice (RCN 2003a). The DRE guidelines (RCN 2003a) also clearly outline the need to listen to children and young people and the importance of informed consent from them and their family members before carrying out all such invasive procedures; this includes all aspects of bowel care.

DEFINITIONS OF TERMS

- The word *constipation* has Latin origins and means 'constipare' or to crowd together (Rogers 2003); constipation is now generally defined as difficulty or a delay in the passage of stools that may not necessarily be hard in consistency (Rogers 2000). It can also be defined based on a number of characteristics that includes the frequency of passing stools (Bosch et al 2002) or one or more episodes of faecal incontinence (Loening-Baucke 2007).
- *Encopresis* is referred to as the movement of stools in a place that is not considered to be socially acceptable and that the underlying reason is not one of constipation (Rogers 2000).
- *Diarrhoea* is referred to as a change in bowel habit that results in frequent and/or loose(er) stools (Armon et al 2001).
- *Soiling* is the passage or leaking of fluid or semi-solid stool into the underclothing; this is usually as a result of overflow from a rectum that is loaded with faeces (ERIC 2001, Burnett & Wilkins 2002).

The above terminology is now mainly superseded by the term faecal incontinence; however, soiling and encopresis are terms that are used interchangeably (Weaver et al 2007, Rubin & Dale 2006); the Paris Consensus on Childhood Constipation Terminology Group (PACCT) have published working definitions and criteria for defining what is chronic constipation and its diagnosis (Hyman et al 2006, Rasquin et al 2006, Benninga et al 2005).

FACTORS TO NOTE

Growth and development issues

The daily frequency of defecation of infants and children varies with age and often carers/parents are not able to report their children's bowel habits (Scaillon & Cadranel 2006). The issue of what is normal in terms of defecation is further compounded by the fact that very little is known about the normal bowel habits of children, particularly those of school age because of the negative consequences of having poor toilet facilities at school (Vernon et al 2003). This is further compounded when the infant or child has disabilities (Bosch et al 2002, Rogers 2002).

Patel et al (2000) reported that children's attendance at A&E departments complaining of acute abdominal pain is frequently caused by constipation. Murphy (2001) notes that, for community children's nurses, infants and children with constipation can represent 36% of their caseload. Therefore nurses and other healthcare professionals have an important role to play in terms of promotion of healthy bowel habits (Farell et al 2003). For this to occur it is essential that the children's nurse understands the need for a healthy diet balanced with adequate fluid intake, together with an understanding of the normal physiology of the bowel and the mechanisms of defecation.

There is a clear relationship between dietary fibre intake and constipation which implies there is some parental control or lack in terms of the dietary fibre that children and young people consume, thus suggesting a lack of parenting skills. This may result in feelings of guilt and the expectation that healthcare professionals will blame the parents for the child's condition and burden the health services with a condition that is preventable (Day 2001, Farell et al 2003, Burnett et al 2004). Constipation can often begin with a period of acute illness when the child has become dehydrated. When pain has been experienced on defecation the child may retain that learned experience and begin to hold and retain faeces adding to the problem. If this is not addressed this can become a long-term issue.

Often constipation arises at potty training time, especially if not ready to be trained. They can develop an aversion to the potty because of over enthusiastic or punishing parents.

Psychosocial issues

Constipation in children can result in significant levels of stress for the family and can cause families to blame themselves or feel guilty because their child is constipated (Rubin & Dale 2006). Consequently, this needs sensitive, effective treatment and management (Elshimy et al 2000, Rubin & Dale 2006). Farell et al (2003) report that healthcare professionals can underestimate the impact of childhood constipation on all members of the family; if left untreated, this can be significant and can impact upon the relationships between parents and within families (Farell et al 2003). Joinson and Heron (2007) as a part of the Avon Longitudinal Study of Parents and Children (ALSPAC) identified other psychological problems associated with constipation in children of 7 years old, including social isolation, which may result in a negative impact upon the child's self-confidence and a subsequent lack of self-esteem (Goh et al 2001). This can result in failure to achieve at school and has the potential for being a precursor to mental ill health (Murphy 2001).

Vernon et al (2003) highlight the importance of the need of children to use the toilet regularly while at school in order to encourage normal processes of elimination. The findings of this pilot study demonstrated that a significant number of children deliberately avoid the use of the school toilets and resist the need to have a 'poo'. The children cited a lack of privacy, poor hygiene of the actual toilets, a lack of hand washing facilities and the threat of being bullied as the reasons for avoidance of use of school toilets. Improvements in standards of toilets in schools would be cost-effective, not only in terms of preventing infectious diseases but also in the prevention of urinary tract infections and bowel problems (Barnes & Maddocks 2002, Vernon et al 2003). These issues are a cause for concern, not only for those that set the standards for school toilets but also for those healthcare professionals working with children in schools; Barnes and Maddocks (2002) advocate that the standards set for toilets in the workplace should also be applied to schools. The Bog Standard Campaign called for minimum standards in both drinking water and toilet facilities in schools, as a prerequisite to child health (further information can be accessed directly from the ERIC website: www.eric.org.uk). There are now guidelines available to help address these issues and to assist staff develop good practices for both children and staff in schools and for assisting children with continence problems (Rogers 2006).

Evidence-based care

The management of childhood constipation must follow an evidence based algorithm and care pathway, written by experts that are preferably practitioners working with these families on a day-to-day basis (Bell & Wall 2004).

NORMAL BOWEL MOVEMENTS

INFANTS

- Within the first weeks of life, the infant produces approximately four stools a day. This reduces to two per day when the infant reaches 4 months of age (Felt et al 1999).
- There are also differences between stools of breast-fed and formula-fed babies (see Ch. 39); for example, breastfed babies may have twice as many stools as formula-fed babies; with constipation in formula-fed infants more likely to occur (Chao & Vandenplas 2007).
- In infants under 6 months, episodes of straining and crying may be mistaken by parents to mean the infant is constipated even if passing an otherwise soft stool (Rubin & Dale 2006).
- Infants are more prone to loose stools than to constipation and it is possible that primary care-givers or parent(s) may not always be aware of the number of times an infant defecates or the consistency of stools (Scaillon & Cadranel 2006).
- Loening-Baucke (2005) reviewed 4000 charts of children younger than 2 years and identified 2.9% were constipated in the first year of life.

CHILDREN

- Most children achieve bowel control before or simultaneously with bladder control (Brazelton 1962).
- The average age for toilet training to be completed is approximately 28 months of age (Tobias et al 2008).
- The highest incidence of constipation occurs during toilet training and is the second most reported event that leads to constipation in children (Borowitz et al 2003).
- It is generally accepted that if a child defecates less than three times a week; and the stools are hard and painful to pass, they are at risk of being deemed constipated (van Ginkel et al 2003).
- According to Tobias et al (2008) constipation is the most common reason for attending paediatric out-patients, with 20–25% of those visits to a gastroenterology consultant (Limbos 2005).
- Loening-Baucke (2007) identified in her study that boys with constipation had higher rates of faecal incontinence than girls with constipation.

CHILDREN WITH DEVELOPMENTAL DELAY

- The most common form of spina bifida occurs in the lumbosacral region (Tinkle & Sterling 1997). Because of motor and sensory deficits, this results in damage to nerves to the bladder and bowel and causes problems with incontinence (Tobias et al 2008).
- For some children with developmental delay, bowel and bladder control may not occur simultaneously (Bosch et al 2002).
- Tse et al (2000) identified that 50% of children with developmental delay had chronic constipation.
- Children with Down syndrome are also prone to constipation (Buie & Flores Sandoval 1995).

POTENTIAL CHANGES IN BOWEL MOVEMENTS

According to Rubin and Dale (2006), there are three stages of childhood that are associated with a child presenting with problems with defecation: in infancy at the time of weaning; in toddlers when acquiring toileting skills and in children at school.

CONSTIPATION

Possible causes of constipation include:

- *Diet* – a lack of fibre can result in a lack of agents to bulk the faeces, causing a decrease in peristaltic movement; this is often found to be a direct consequence of being a 'faddy eater' and/ or having a poor appetite (Rogers 2003, Burnett et al 2004)
- *Fluid intake* – drinking too much milk and inadequate solid food consumption (Burnett et al 2004). Poor fluid intake or excessive loss through diarrhoea/vomiting or a high temperature, therefore causing stools to harden (Clayden & Keshtgar 2003)
- *Lifestyle changes* – many children have lifestyles that are sedentary in nature because of the increased popularity of computer and video games (Burnett & Wilkins 2002)
- *Physiological problems* – for example Hirschsprung's disease (congenital megacolon). This occurs in 1:5000 infants and is diagnosed by rectal biopsy, which will indicate a lack of parasympathetic ganglion cells in the wall of the large bowel (Tobias et al 2008). In all cases, treatment involves a surgical resection of the affected gut, usually in the first year of life (Tobias et al 2008). Approximately 3–10% of children with Down syndrome also have Hirschsprung's disease (Buie and Flores Sandoval 1995)
- *Drug-induced constipation* – some medication can cause constipation, for example antihistamines, some anticonvulsants and pain medication (opiates) (Di Lorenzo 2000, Nurko et al 2001)
- *Metabolic disorders* – for example hypothyroidism, hypercalcaemia and hypokalaemia (Nurko et al 2001)
- *Perineal or rectal pain when defecating* (Borowitz et al 2003) – for example an anal fissure or possible child sexual abuse (Rogers 2003)
- *Delays in defecation* (Taylor 2000) – can be due to associated pain on defecation; for example ignoring the need to have a 'poo' because of the poor provision of facilities at school (Vernon et al 2003)
- *Familial tendencies* – constipation in parents may result in constipation in one child or siblings (Burnett et al 2004).

IMPLICATIONS FOR NURSING PRACTICE

Treatment and/or bowel management for children and their families should take place in the community with healthcare professionals that are appropriately qualified; it is also important to have the needs of the child and family central to delivering care (Farell et al 2003, Rogers 2003). Health promotion and the care of children and families in the community is central to the development and delivery of future services (DoH 2004). Burnett et al (2004) acknowledge that clinical nurse specialists have an important role in the management of constipation and should also involve the development of nurse-led clinics (Burnett et al 2004).

Families need to be reassured that their needs and concerns are taken seriously and interventions are planned to meet their actual, not perceived, needs. Most children that suffer from faecal soiling benefit from well-managed supportive interventions; it is important to note that constipation is a symptom and not a disease (Tobias et al 2008); when the family understands the problems that have resulted in constipation then treatment and other therapeutic interventions become more effective (Tobias et al 2008). In order to provide effective care an initial assessment that is detailed and traces the child's history of bowel habits is therefore essential (Rogers 2003, Baker et al 2006, Weaver et al 2007).

PRINCIPLES IN MANAGING FUNCTIONAL CONSTIPATION

- *Soften and clear any impacted faecal matter* – this may involve the use of a hypertonic phosphate enema and is best given in a clinic by an appropriately qualified healthcare professional. These hypertonic enemas are poorly absorbed by the colon, resulting in water retention, adding bulk to the stool and promoting evacuation of stool from the lower part of the colon and rectum (Bulloch & Tenebein 2002). If the child has retained a large faecal mass, then the only option possible is to carry out an evacuation in the hospital setting under general anaesthetic (Rogers 2000, Philichi 2008). Enemas are not the first-line treatment; oral preparations are tried first.
- *Dietary and fluid advice* – children should be encouraged to take regular water-based drinks throughout the day, with extra fluid taken when the weather is hot; if the child is reluctant to take extra fluids an alternative could be ice lollies or jellies. While there is no recommended daily intake of fibre for children, there is a general consensus that this is calculated using the given formula (Rogers 2003, p 552):

Child's age + 5 = daily amount of fibre intake in grams (up to age 13 years).

- Dietary fibre increases water retention and any increase in intake must be accompanied by an increase in fluid intake (Rogers 2003). The increased consumption of high-fibre, insoluble foods is more effective than advocating the increase of fluid intake on its own, e.g. fruits, vegetables and wholegrain cereals should be seen as a part of a balanced diet in the treatment of constipation (Burnett & Wilkins 2002, Baker et al 2006). Care should be taken not to introduce large quantities of fibre when the child is impacted as this can make the problem worse.
- *Establish regular pain-free patterns of defecation* – encourage the child to sit on the toilet with legs well supported (Rogers 2003, Weaver & Dobson 2007) for 5 min up to three or four times a day. Attempts to defecate should follow meals to maximise the use of the gastric-colonic reflex (Rogers 2003, Weaver & Dobson 2007).
- *Maintenance of regular bowel movements* – this may require the use of laxatives that should be based on individual assessment of need and may include softening agents such as lactulose or a stimulant such as senna (Rogers 2000). There is general consensus that laxative use may have to continue for at least six months to a year (Rogers 2003, Philichi 2008). The correct dose is established when the child has daily soft stools and no adverse effects (Benninga et al 2004).
- *Ongoing support* – this is vital and some studies have indicated that children can have ongoing problems with constipation and encopresis; consequently ongoing management and follow up may be protracted (Philichi 2008). Procter and Loader (2003) have reported in their study that some children had persistent problems with constipation 6 years later, suggesting that constipation is not something that children can 'grow out of'. It is imperative to demystify and educate the child and family in order to gain cooperation and understanding.

- *Exercise* – while there is little scientific evidence to support the benefit of exercise as a means of reducing the incidence of constipation, it is known that exercise increases motility and therefore aids the passage of food through the digestive system. Exercise is useful in reducing obesity and other diseases, e.g. type 2 diabetes (Burnett & Wilkins 2002); the increase in non-sedentary play activities should therefore be encouraged; particularly after meals and before sitting on the toilet (Weaver & Dobson 2007).

FACTORS TO NOTE

Medication used to treat constipation

Within the UK, the treatment of constipation is well established; with the development of algorithms and care pathways (Rogers 2008, Galal et al 2007) to inform treatment protocols and the use of pre-parations to treat constipation in children. At the time of going to publication the National Institute for Clinical Excellence (NICE) were working on guidance for childhood constipation. It is also important to remember that many of the drugs that are prescribed are not licensed for use for children or are used in doses that exceed manufacturers' recommendations (Price & Elliott 2004); always check and refer to the BNF for up-to-date information on all medicines (Galal et al 2007). For further discussion of drug licencing, see Ch. 42 and the NMC Standards for Medicines Management (2008).

Rectal examination is an invasive procedure and should only be used for infants and children when a part of a prescribed regime of treatment (RCN 2003a). Enemas should therefore only be used with a high degree of caution and administered by an appropriately qualified nurse specialist (RCN 2003a). The preferred choice of medication is the use of oral preparations (Thompson 2001b).

Softening agents

- *Docusate sodium* (Dioctyl) is available as a suspension for children and helps to reduce the surface tension of the hard stools, therefore allowing water to be absorbed to soften the stool (Burnett & Wilkins 2002).
- *Lactulose* is an osmotic laxative, which can be given up to three times a day and over long periods of time and can be given to infants and young children (Galal et al 2007).

- *Liquid paraffin* use is debatable because of side-effects and it is rarely used as it can cause interference with the absorption of fat soluble vitamins, therefore it would need to be given to children at least 30 min before or after meals (Galal et al 2007); other problems can include absorption into the circulatory system and it is not recommended for children under 12 months of age (Sharif et al 2001). The main problem associated with the use of liquid paraffin is the potential of oil leaking through the anal sphincter (Burnett & Wilkins 2002).

Agents used for the evacuation of the bowels

- *Senna* stimulates the contraction of smooth muscle in the colon and the transport of fluids and electrolytes and leads to defecation (Burnett & Wilkins 2002, Rogers 2003) and is useful when trying to re-establish regular bowel functioning (Galal et al 2007). Senna is often used as an alternative when the child refuses other medication, such as lactulose or sorbitol. The laxative dose should be adjusted to a maintenance dose that avoids potential side-effects such as abdominal pain or stomach cramps (Galal et al 2007).
- *Movicol®* is a glycol preparation with added electrolytes known as polyethylene glycol 3350 (PEG) (Rogers 2003). Movicol has been found to be a safe and effective treatment and is generally well tolerated by children (Vincent & Candy 2001, Thomson et al 2007). Unlike some medication, Movicol has been licenced for use for children aged 2 years and older since 2003 (Rogers 2003, Hanson & Bansal 2006) and found to be more effective than using lactulose as a preventative or maintenance regimen for faecal impaction (Candy & Edwards 2002). Polyethylene glycol without electrolytes is also licenced for use for children aged 8 years and older and can be used to manage care for children with constipation in the long term; it can be dissolved in any clear liquid drink of the child's choice (Pashankar & Bishop 2001, Loening-Baucke 2002).
- *Bisacodyl* (Dulco-lax) is often preferred for older children if they are able to easily swallow the 'perles' (Burnett & Wilkins 2002).

Administration of enemas and suppositories

The administration of medications via the rectum is a procedure frequently performed by nurses and does carry with it potential risks, which can be fatal (Higgins 2007, Addison et al 2000). Consequently, any nurse undertaking these procedures must have the relevant knowledge and skills to carry out these procedures safely and effectively following training and supervised practice in accordance with trust/hospital policies and procedures (Higgins 2007, Addison et al 2000, Dowse & Mackender 2000, Willis 2000); and in accordance with NMC Guidelines on the administration of medicines (2007).

Suppositories

There still remains much debate regarding the correct way to insert a suppository (base or apex first) (Higgins 2007). Moppett (2000) maintains that recommendations from manufacturers either suggest apex (pointed end) first insertion or make no recommendations at all. According to a small study, by Abd-el-Maeboud et al (1991), suggested that suppositories inserted apex first cause distension of the anus and the possibility of the sphincter not closing. Higgins (2007) suggests that the lack of evidence to currently inform these practices highlights deficits in the research-based literature and more studies are needed to advocate either blunt end or pointed end insertion.

Enemas

Historically, the administration of enemas was considered to be a first-line phase of treatment for the management of disimpaction of the bowel. The advent and development of oral medications means that this line of intervention can be replaced with the use of oral medications (Tobias et al 2008). The use of milk and molasses enemas, once considered to be safe have been reported to be associated with cardiovascular failure (Tobias et al 2008).

DIARRHOEA

Diarrhoea can be defined as a change in bowel movements that are often very watery, increased in volume and frequency (Cheng et al 2005). According to Kosek et al (2003), each child under 4 years old has approximately 3.2 episodes of diarrhoea per annum.

Possible causes of diarrhoea include:

- Infections: enteral infections, e.g. viral (commonest cause), bacterial, parasitic; non-enteral infections, e.g. otitis media, pneumonia, urinary tract
- Appendicitis, intussusception, short bowel syndrome
- Malabsorption syndromes: coeliac disease, cystic fibrosis
- Constipation with overflow
- Drug induced, e.g. antibiotics
- Food allergy/intolerance (of lactulose or cow's milk protein)
- Child abuse: Münchausen by proxy, sexual (Armon et al 2001)
- Eating contaminated foods or water (undercooked or raw foods) (Jones 2002)
- Faecal/oral route – as a consequence of poor hand washing technique and contaminated toys (Jones 2002)
- Chronic non-specific diarrhoea (CNSD) or toddler diarrhoea (Thompson 2001a)
- Environmental sources (Elliott 2007).

MANAGEMENT OF DIARRHOEA IN INFANTS AND YOUNG CHILDREN

Guidelines published by the World Health Organization in 2003 highlight the fact that preventative measures are important when combating infectious diarrhoea. This needs to include the support for the promotion of breastfeeding, coupled with safe weaning, adequate nutrition; safe, clean water and good sanitation and measles immunization – these are all measures that can be taken in an attempt to prevent and reduce infectious diarrhoea and infant mortality rates globally (King et al 2003). What is important to note is the fact that hand washing is the first and foremost way of preventing diarrhoeal infections (Curtis & Cairncross 2003).

FACTORS TO NOTE

- Diarrhoea is defined as a change in bowel habit that results in the child having more frequent and/or looser stools; acute diarrhoea is often caused by infectious intestinal disease (IID) (Armon et al 2001).
- In the developed world, infectious diarrhoea is still a cause for concern in terms of morbidity, mortality and economic cost (Gracey et al 2004, Cheng et al 2005).

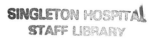

In developed countries, it is the most common cause for attendance at the GP or the A&E Department (Elliott 2007).

Fluids, such as cola, apple juice and sports drinks may exacerbate diarrhoea, due to their high sugar content and therefore should be avoided, breastfed infants should continue and have oral rehydration supplements if needed (Guerrant et al 2001, Elliot 2007).

ASSESSMENT OF DEHYDRATION

Historically, dehydration has been classified as mild, moderate or severe and children rarely fall into one category or another (Table 12.1), with the categories developed in an *ad hoc* way (see Friedman et al (2004) for discussion of the development of a clinical scale to assess dehydration in children between 1 and 36 months old). For the management of dehydration and gastroenteritis in infants and children, see Cheng et al (2005) and Elliott (2007).

COMMUNITY PERSPECTIVE

The CCN has a vital role in the management of children with constipation. The CCN is ideally placed to support the child and family in the community with home visits and telephone calls to provide holistic advice and support for the child and family (Rogers 2005). The child's home is an ideal venue to assess their feelings surrounding toileting.

Although disimpaction can occur fairly quickly, a child 'may need maintenance therapy for up to 24 months and may suffer a number of relapses before their constipation is resolved' (Cross et al 2005). It is extremely important that the child and family have open access to advice during this period to enable early recognition of potential problems or relapse, facilitating a prompt response. CCNs are in an ideal position to offer this support.

The CCN will liaise with the child's school or school nurse with the child's approval to ensure that the toilet facilities are satisfactory and to promote the importance of the child being allowed access to fluids and a private toilet when required. Play specialists can enhance the community support for the child and family. Involvement of the child and adolescent mental health service (CAMHS) may also be useful.

The role of the CCN is expanding in some areas. Nurse-led clinics are being developed in hospital and in the community, with the CCN receiving direct referrals from GPs, paediatricians health visitors and school nurses. There are some nurses undertaking nurse prescribing courses, enabling nurse-led clinics to function efficiently.

Table 12.1   Symptoms associated with dehydration

SYMPTOM	MINIMAL OR NO DEHYDRATION (<3% LOSS OF BODY WEIGHT)	MILD TO MODERATE DEHYDRATION (3–9% LOSS OF BODY WEIGHT)	SEVERE DEHYDRATION (>9% LOSS OF BODY WEIGHT)
Mental status	Well, alert	Normal, fatigued or restless, irritable	Apathetic, lethargic, unconscious
Thirst	Drinks normally	Thirsty, eager to drink	Drinks poorly, unable to drink
Heart rate	Normal	Normal to increased	Tachycardia, with bradycardia in most severe cases
Quality of pulses	Normal	Normal to decreased	Weak, thready or impalpable
Breathing	Normal	Normal, fast	Deep
Eyes	Normal	Slightly sunken	Deeply sunken
Tears	Present	Decreased	Absent
Mouth and tongue	Moist	Dry	Parched
Skin fold	Instant recoil	Recoil in <2 s	Recoil in >2 s
Capillary refill	Normal	Prolonged	Prolonged, minimal
Extremities	Warm	Cool	Cold, mottled, cyanotic
Urine output	Normal to decreased	Decreased	Minimal

Adapted from King et al 2003.

DOS AND DON'TS

- Do take the concerns of the family regarding changes in bowel movement of their child seriously.
- Do consider the child's school environment, the locality and the standards of school toilets as this may inhibit defecation.
- Do complete a full assessment of the child including dietary habits and patterns of defecation.

- Do check trust/hospital policies and procedures for digital rectal examination and the administration of medications per rectum.
- Do not undertake a digital rectal examination as a student; this must be undertaken by a qualified competent practitioner – and they are rarely performed.

References

Abd-el-Maeboud, K.H., el-Naggar, T., el-Hawi, E.M., et al., 1991. Rectal suppository: commonsense and mode of insertion. Lancet 338 (8770), 798–800.

Addison, R., Ness, W., Abulafi, M., et al., 2000. How to administer enemas and suppositories. NTPLUS 96 (6), 3–4.

Armon, K., Stephenson, T., MacFaul, R., et al., 2001. An evidence and consensus based guideline for acute diarrhoea management. Arch. Dis. Child. 85 (2), 132–141.

Barnes, P.M., Maddocks, A., 2002. Standards in school toilets – a questionnaire survey. J. Public Health Med. 24 (2), 85–87.

Baker, S., Liptak, G., Colletti, R., et al., 2006. Evaluation and treatment of constipation in infants and children: Recommendations of the North American Society for Pediatric Gastroenterology, Hepatology and Nutrition. J. Pediatr. Gastroenterol. Nutr. 43 (3), 405–407.

Bell, E.A., Wall, G.C., 2004. Pediatric constipation therapy using guidelines and polyethylene glycol 3350. Ann. Pharmacother. 38 (4), 686–693.

Benninga, M., Candy, D.C., Catto-Smith, A.G., et al., 2005. The Paris consensus on childhood constipation terminology (PACCT) Group. J. Pediatr. Gastroenterol. Nutr. 40, 273–275.

Benninga, M., Voskuiji, W., Taminiau, J., 2004. Childhood constipation: Is there new light in the tunnel? J. Pediatr. Gastroenterol. Nutr. 39 (5), 448–464.

Borowitz, S.M., Cox, D.J., Tam, A., et al., 2003. Precipitants of constipation during early childhood. J. Am. Board Fam. Pract. 16, 213–281.

Bosch, J., Mraz, R., Masbruch, J., et al., 2002. Constipation in young children with developmental disabilities. Infants and Young Children 15 (2), 66–77.

Brazelton, T.B., 1962. A child-orientated approach to toilet training. Pediatrics 29, 121–128.

Buie, T.M., Flores Sandoval, A.F., 1995. Down syndrome and the gastrointestinal tract. In: Van Dyke, D.C., Mattheis, P., Eberly, S.S. et al., Medical and surgical care for children with Down syndrome. Woodbine House, Bethesda.

Bulloch, B., Tenebein, M., 2002. Constipation: Diagnosis and management in the pediatric emergency department. Pediatr. Emerg. Care 18 (4), 254–258.

Burnett, C., Wilkins, G., 2002. Managing children with constipation: a community perspective. J. Fam. Health Care 12 (5), 127–132.

Burnett, C.A., Juszczak, E., Sullivan, P.B., 2004. Nurse management of intractable functional constipation: a

randomised controlled trial. Arch. Dis. Child 89 (98), 717–722.

Candy, D.C.A., Edwards, D.A., 2002. Study of Movicol for the treatment of faecal impaction in children. J. Pediatr. Gastroenterol. Nutr. 34, 462.

Chao, H., Vandenplas, Y., 2007. Therapeutic effect of Novolac-IT in infants with constipation. Nutrition 23 (6), 469–473.

Cheng, A.C., McDonald, J.R., Thielman, N.M., 2005. Infectious diarrhea in developed and developing countries. J. Clin. Gastroenterol. 39 (9), 757–773.

Clayden, G., Keshtgar, A.S., 2003. Management of childhood constipation. Postgrad. Med. J. 79, 66–621.

Cross, J., Elbadri, A.M., Emery, R., et al., 2005. Impact paediatric bowel care pathway. Norgine Ltd, Harefield, Middlesex.

Curtis, V., Cairncross, S., 2003. Effect of washing hands with soap on diarrhoea risk in the community: a systematic review. Lancet Infect. Dis. 3, 275–281.

Day, A., 2001. The nurse's role in managing constipation. Nurs. Stand. 16, 41–44.

Department of Health, 2004. National Service Framework for Children, Young People and Maternity Services – Core Standard. DoH, London.

Di Lorenzo, C., 2000. Childhood constipation. J. Pediatr. 136, 4–7.

Dowse, J., Mackender, J., 2000. Back to basics: continence. Nurs. Times 96 (30), 7–9.

Elliott, E.J., 2007. Acute gastroenteritis in children. BMJ 334, 35–40.

Elshimy, N., Gallagher, B., West, D., et al., 2000. Outcome in children under 5 years of age with constipation: a prospective follow-up study. Int. J. Clin. Pract. 54, 25–27.

Enuresis Resource and Information Centre, 2001. Childhood soiling: minimum standards of practice for treatment and service delivery: benchmarking guidelines. ERIC, Bristol.

Farell, M., Holmes, G., Coldicutt, P., et al., 2003. Management of childhood constipation: parents' experiences. J. Adv. Nurs. 44 (5), 479–489.

Felt, B., Wise, C., Olson, A., et al., 1999. Guideline for the management of pediatric idiopathic constipation and soiling. Arch. Pediatr. Adolesc. Med. 153 (4), 380–385.

Friedman, J.N., Goldman, R.D., Srivastava, R., et al., 2004. Development of a clinical dehydration scale for use in children between 1 and 36 months of age. J. Pediatr. 145, 201–207.

Galal, N., Chong, S.K.F., Williams, J., et al., 2007. Constipation in childhood: a multidisciplinary approach to management in the community. Paediatr. Nurs. 19 (7), 20–22.

Goh, J., Bryne, P., McDonald, G., et al., 2001. Severe juvenile chronic constipation. Ir. Med. J. 94, 81–82.

Gracey, M., Lee, A.H., Yau, K.K., 2004. Hospitalisation for gastroenteritis in Western Australia. Arch. Dis. Child. 89, 768–772.

Guerrant, R.L., Van Gilder, T., Steiner, T.S., et al., 2001. Practice guidelines for the management of infectious diarrhea. Clin. Infect. Dis. 32, 331–351.

Hanson, S., Bansal, N., 2006. The clinical effectiveness of Movicol® in children with severe constipation: an outcome audit. Paediatr. Nurs. 18 (2), 24–28.

Higgins, D., 2007. Bowel care part 6 – administration of a suppository. Nurs. Times 103 (47), 26–27.

Hyman, P.E., Milla, P.J., Benninga, M.A., et al., 2006. Childhood functional gastrointestinal disorders: neonate/toddler. Gastroenterology 130, 1519–1537.

Joinson, C., Heron, J., 2007. The psychological effects of incontinence in children. Continence UK 1 (3), 59–63.

Jones, S., 2002. A clinical pathway for pediatric gastroenteritis. Gastroenterol. Nurs. 26 (1), 7–20.

Kosek, M., Bern, C., Guerrant, R.L., 2003. The global burden of diarrhoeal disease, as estimated from studies published between 1992–2000. Bull. World Health Org. 81, 197–204.

Limbos, M., 2005. Approach to the child with constipation. In: Osborn, L., DeWitt, T., First, L. et al., Pediatrics. Elsevier, Philadelphia.

Loening-Baucke, V., 2002. Polyethylene glycol without electrolytes for children with constipation and encopresis. J. Pediatr. Gastroenterol. Nutr. 34 (4), 372–377.

Loening-Baucke, V., 2005. Prevalence, symptoms and outcome of constipation in infants and toddlers. J. Pediatr. 146 (3), 359–363.

Loening-Baucke, V., 2007. Prevalence rates of constipation and faecal and urinary incontinence. Arch. Dis. Child. 92, 486–489.

Moppett, S., 2000. Which way is up for a suppository? NTPLUS 96 (19), 12–13.

King, C.K., Glass, R., Bresee, J.S., et al., 2003. Managing acute gastroenteritis among children. Oral rehydration, maintenance, and nutritional therapy. MMWR Recomm. Rep. 52 (RR-16), 1–16.

Murphy, W., 2001. Constipation and soiling: a community approach. Paediatr. Nurs. 13 (8), 31–35.

Nurko, S., Baker, S., Colletti, R., et al., 2001. Managing constipation: evidence put to practice. Contemp. Pediatr. 18 (12), 56–65.

NMC, 2008. Standards for medicines management. NMC, London.

Pashankar, D., Bishop, W., 2001. Efficacy of optimal dose of daily polyethylene glycol 3350 for treatment of constipation and encopresis in children. J. Pediatr. 139 (3), 428–432.

Patel, H., 2000. Predictive factors for short-term symptom persistence in children after emergency department evaluation for constipation. Arch. Pediatr. Adolesc. Med. 154 (12), 1204–1208.

Philichi, L., 2008. When the going gets tough. Pediatric constipation and encopresis. Gastroenterol. Nurs. 31 (2), 121–130.

Price, K.J., Elliott, T.M., 2004. Stimulant laxatives for constipation and soiling in children (Cochrane Review). In: The Cochrane Library, Issue 3. Wiley, Chichester.

Procter, E., Loader, P., 2003. A 6-year follow-up study of chronic constipation and soiling in a specialist paediatric service. Child Care Health Dev. 29 (2), 103–109.

Rasquin, A., Di Lorenzo, C., Forbes, D., et al., 2006. Childhood functional gastrointestinal disorders: child/adolescent. Gastroenterology 130, 1527–1537.

Rogers, J., 2000. The causes and management of constipation in children. Community Nurse 6, 39–40.

Rogers, J., 2002. Solving the enigma: toilet training children with learning disabilities. British J. Nurs. 11 (14), 956–958.

Rogers, J., 2003. Management of functional constipation in childhood. Br. J. Community Nurs. 8 (12), 550–553.

Rogers, J., 2005. Reducing the misery of constipation in children. Pract. Nurs. 16 (1), 12–16.

Rogers, J., 2006. Managing bowel and bladder problems in schools and early years settings – Guidelines for Good Practice. Promocon, Manchester.

Rogers, J., 2008. The IMPACT paediatric bowel care pathway. Nurs. Times 104 (18), 46–47.

Royal College of Nursing, 2003a. Digital rectal examination. Guidance for nurses working with children and young people. RCN, London.

Royal College of Nursing, 2003b. Preparing nurses in the care of children and young people. RCN, London.

Royal College of Paediatrics and Child Health and the Joint Advisory Committee on Children's Nursing, 1996. Developing roles of nurses in clinical child health. Royal College of Paediatrics and Child Health, London.

Rubin, G., Dale, A., 2006. Clinical review of chronic constipation in children. BMJ 333, 1051–1055.

Scaillon, M., Cadranel, S., 2006. Food allergy and constipation in childhood: how functional is it? Eur. J. Gastroenterol. Hepatol. 18, 125–128.

Sharif, F., Crushell, E., O'Driscoll, K., et al., 2001. Liquid paraffin: a reappraisal of its role in the treatment of constipation. Arch. Dis. Child. 85, 121–124.

Sullivan, P.B., Burnett, C.A., Juszczak, E., 2006. Parent satisfaction in a nurse led clinic compared with a paediatric gastroenterology clinic for the management of intractable, functional constipation. Arch. Dis. Child. 91, 499–501.

Taylor, P., 2000. Managing constipation in children. Drug Therapy Bulletin 38, 57–60.

Thomson, M.A., Jenkins, H.R., Bisset, W.M., et al., 2007. Polyethylene glycol 3350 plus electrolytes for chronic constipation in children: a double blind, placebo controlled, crossover study. Arch. Dis. Child 92, 996–1000.

Thompson, J., 2001a. Toddler diarrhoea. Community Pract. 74 (5), 195–196.

Thompson, J., 2001b. The management of chronic constipation in children. Community Pract. 74 (1), 29–30.

Tinkle, M., Sterling, B., 1997. Neural tube defects: A primary prevention role for nurses. J. Gynecol. Neonatal Nurses 26, 503–512.

Tobias, N., Mason, D., Lutkenhoff, M., et al., 2008. Management principles of organic causes of childhood constipation. J. Pediatr. Health Care 22 (1), 12–23.

Tse, P., Leung, S., Chan, T., et al., 2000. Dietary fibre intake and constipation in children with severe developmental disabilities. J. Paediatr. Child Health 36, 236–239.

Vernon, S., Lundblad, B., Hellstrom, A.L., 2003. Children's experiences of school toilets present a risk to their physical and psychological health. Child Care Health Dev. 29 (1), 47–53.

Van Ginkel, R., Reitsma, J.B., Büller, H.A., et al., 2003. Childhood constipation: longitudinal follow-up beyond puberty. Gastroenterology 125, 357–363.

Vincent, R., Candy, R.M., 2001. Movicol for the treatment of faecal impaction in children. Gastroenterol. Today 11 (2), 50–52.

Weaver, A., Dobson, P., 2007. An overview of faecal incontinence in children. Nurs. Times 103 (47), 40–42.

Willis, J., 2000. Bowel management and consent. Nurs. Times 96 (Suppl. 6), 7–8.

World Health Organization, 1995. The treatment of diarrhoea: a manual for physicians and other senior health workers. WHO, Geneva, Switzerland.

World Health Organization, 2003. The treatment of diarrhoea: manual for physicians and other senior health worker. Report No. WHO/FCH/CAH/03.7. Department of Child and Adolescent Health and Development. World Health Organization, Geneva.

Further reading

Avon Longitudinal Study of Parents and Children (ALSPC). Online. Available: www.bristol.ac.uk/alspac.

ERIC. Education and Resources for Improving Childhood Continence, Online. Available: www.eric.org.uk.

Promocon, Online. Available: www.promocon.co.uk/managingbowelandbladderproblems.shtml.

Thompson, J., 2001. Intussusception, pyloric stenosis and Hirschsprung's disease. Community Pract. 74 (8), 312–313.

Young, R., Beerman, L., Vanderhoof, J., 1998. Increasing oral fluids in chronic constipation in children. Gastroenterol. Nurs. 21 (4), 156–161.

Chapter 13

Central lines

Barbara Doyle

CHAPTER CONTENTS

Introduction   152
    Learning outcomes   152
    Rationale   152
    Factors to note   153
    General guidelines   154

Administration of bolus drugs into a heparinised central line via the cap   155
    Equipment   155
    Method   156

Connecting or changing an infusion set   156
    Additional equipment   156
    Method   156

Accessing a port for use   156
    Equipment   157
    Method   157

Routine heparinising of a port   157
    Equipment   157
    Method   157
    Central line dressings   158

Care of central venous line exit site   158
    Factors to note   158
    Equipment   158
    Method   158

Dressing a port in use   159
    Method   159

Dressing change on a long line   159
    Observations and complications   159
    Dos and don'ts   161

INTRODUCTION

A central line is inserted when a child requires frequent and/or long-term venous access. Reasons for insertion may include the administration of total parenteral nutrition, cytotoxic drugs or frequent intravenous antibiotics. These lines are usually inserted under general anaesthetic in theatre by experienced paediatric surgeons or by experienced anaesthetists. The use of ultrasound imaging is recommended to locate and assist in central venous access device insertion (NICE 2002).

LEARNING OUTCOMES

By the end of this section you should be able to:

- Be aware of the different types of central venous lines currently in use
- Understand the reasons for their use and all aspects of their care
- Understand the importance of asepsis in central venous line care
- Explain all aspects of the care to the child and family
- Recognise potential problems and deal with them appropriately.

RATIONALE

Central venous lines play a crucial role in the administration of treatment to many children with acute and chronic potentially life-threatening illnesses (see Table 13.1 for examples). They reduce the need for frequent venepuncture, which is

Table 13.1 Types of line used for various conditions

CENTRAL VENOUS LINES		PORT	LONG LINE
Single	*Double or triple*		
Solid tumours Chronic malabsorption for total parenteral nutrition	Bone marrow transplants Acute myeloid leukaemia Acute lymphoblastic leukaemia (ALL) Non-Hodgkin's lymphoma Neuroblastoma	Cystic fibrosis Haemophilia Beta-thalassaemia major and other transfusion-dependent haemoglobinopathies ALL (low risk) Solid tumours (low-intensity chemotherapy)	Critically ill, requiring inotropes, etc.

extremely distressing for all children, particularly the very young.

Nurses have a key role in the care of these lines. In addition to performing the practical procedures, they are responsible for the education of the child, family and those in the community who are unfamiliar with central lines (McInally 2005). A sound policy for line care, adhered to by all involved, will help to ensure that a line can safely remain in use for as long as required.

Central venous lines and ports will be encountered by community staff as most children will go home with these devices *in situ*. The amount of direct involvement by community staff in the care of these lines is variable, as in many instances, the parents will carry out all the care at home.

FACTORS TO NOTE

There are three types of central line used for children.

Tunnelled central venous line

Also known as a Broviac, or Hickman line, or often by the child as a 'wiggly'. These are skin-tunnelled silastic catheters which are inserted, under general anaesthetic, into the subclavian or internal jugular vein (Fig. 13.1). These lines can be single, double or triple lumen with each lumen having an external clamp. The type inserted depends upon the clinical requirements of the patient.

The Groshong catheter is a similar type of line, but it has an internal valve to prevent the backflow of blood, so does not require an external clamp.

Note: 10 mL or larger syringes are recommended, particularly when confirming patency.

Implanted port

Also known as a Port-a-Cath, Vascuport or TIVAD (totally implantable venous access device). This is a silastic catheter, inserted into the subclavian or internal jugular vein, which is attached to a metal or

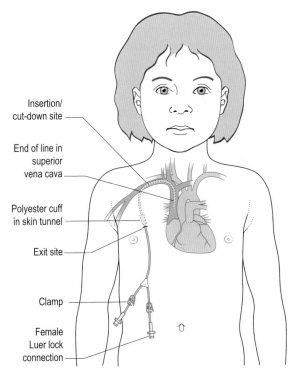

Insertion/
cut-down site

End of line in
superior
vena cava

Polyester cuff
in skin tunnel

Exit site

Clamp

Female
Luer lock
connection

Figure 13.1 Position of central venous line.

plastic chamber sealed at the top with a septum of self-sealing silicone. The port (chamber) is positioned under the skin on the chest wall. Access to this system is via straight or angled Huber non-coring needles through the septum of the port (Fig. 13.2).

Note: Always use 10 mL or larger syringes with the ports as recommended by the manufacturers.

Non-tunnelled long line

This is a short-term venous access device more commonly used in the intensive care or high-dependency setting. These lines are not skin-tunnelled and can be inserted under local anaesthetic. They are usually held in place with skin sutures. These lines can have a single, double or triple lumen. Peripherally inserted central catheters (PICC lines) are included in this category of central venous lines.

Note: 10 mL or larger syringes are recommended with PICC lines.

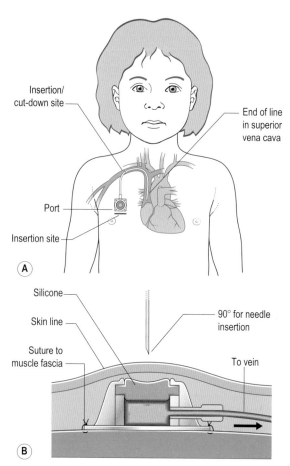

(A)

Insertion/cut-down site
End of line in superior vena cava
Port
Insertion site

Silicone
Skin line
Suture to muscle fascia
90° for needle insertion
To vein

(B)

Figure 13.2 (A) A port *in situ*. (B) Cross-section of a port.

The type of line used for a particular child will depend upon various factors:

● The age of the child
● The length of time it will be required
● What treatments it will be used for
● How often it will be used.

This is usually decided by the medical consultants in charge of the individual child's care and is often also dependent upon the treatment protocol. Full details of the line inserted, i.e. make, model and size, should be documented in the child's medical notes. This assists staff to obtain the correct repair kit in the event of a line break. Table 13.1 gives examples of conditions and the type of line used for each condition.

Preparation of the child and family for the insertion of any central line is essential (McInally 2005). This includes information from medical and nursing staff, plus preparatory work by the hospital play specialist if available. After discussion with the child and family, it may be useful to introduce them to another child with the same type of line.

Central venous lines can be *in situ* for months or even years, often in children who are immunocompromised (Cesaro et al 2004, Ewenstein et al 2004, McIntosh 2003, McInally 2005, Valentino et al 2004). As they provide direct access to the child's central venous system, the major risk is of infection either to the exit site or the line itself with the potential for septicaemia. For this reason alone, strict aseptic non-touch procedures need to be maintained when accessing all types of central line (NICE 2003, Pratt et al 2007).

Many children will go home with these lines *in situ* so they and their families need to follow the same procedures and be knowledgeable about potential problems and how to deal with them (McInally 2005, Pratt et al 2007). Community nursing staff may also be involved in their care.

GENERAL GUIDELINES

● All staff undertaking these procedures must be knowledgeable about, and adhere to, the relevant hospital policy.
● Thorough hand washing is the single most effective means of improving central line care (NICE 2003, Pratt et al 2007). In many centres, sterile gloves are worn when performing any procedures involving accessing the central venous system via these lines.

- Before accessing any line, it is important to check for any sign of damage to the line or attachments. It is also necessary to observe for signs of leakage of blood or fluids from the exit site or any attachments or connections when accessing a line.
- When drugs are administered via the system, it must first be flushed with an appropriate solution, i.e. 0.9% sodium chloride. The line must be flushed before and after each drug, and before heparinising the system to maintain patency (see below). The volume of the flush solution should be equal to at least twice the volume of the line and any add-on devices, usually 5–10 mL (INS 2000, NICE 2003, Pratt et al 2007). A small number of drugs are incompatible with 0.9% sodium chloride, e.g. amphotericin (AmBisome) and some cytotoxic drugs. In these cases the line must be flushed with an alternative, e.g. 5% dextrose, or as indicated by the pharmacist.
- Lines which are not in use must be heparinised, i.e. flushed with a heparin solution, to maintain their patency. The solution most commonly used is heparin 10 units/mL of normal saline (Coulthard and Skinner 2007, Pratt et al 2007).

Central venous lines require heparinising weekly when not in use, and daily if being used intermittently for drug administration. Heparinisation has been shown to significantly reduce bacterial colonisation of central venous lines (Pratt et al 2007). It has also been shown to have a strong non-significant trend towards a reduction in line-related bacteraemia. Some lines with very small lumens will require heparinisation more frequently. There is considerable variation in the frequency of heparinising lines, so local hospital policy must be adhered to.

Ports require a heparin flush every 4 weeks when not in use, as recommended by the manufacturers. Long lines are rarely not in use, being removed when no longer required. Follow individual hospital policy for heparinising these lines.

According to the manufacturer's instructions, Groshong catheters do not need heparinising. A 0.9% sodium chloride weekly flush is sufficient.

- The distal hub of a central venous line is capped with a Luer lock cap. Various systems are available and the type used will vary depending upon individual hospital preference. Needleless systems are commonly used to reduce the risk of needlestick injuries to the child, carers or staff.

The exact method of accessing the lines will therefore vary depending upon the system used. However, the basic principles will still apply.

- The Luer lock cap is changed using an aseptic procedure with the line clamped at all times. The frequency of cap changes will depend on the number of occasions the line is accessed, and the type of cap used, according to the manufacturer's guidelines (Pratt et al 2007).
- Cleaning solutions for caps and exit sites also differ between hospitals, usually being determined by the consultant microbiologist based on interpretation of current research. The recommended cleaning agent is 2% chlorhexidine gluconate in 70% alcohol (Pratt et al 2007).
- Guidance must be sought from experienced nursing or medical staff if there are any problems with a line, e.g. resistance when flushing a line, or inability to aspirate blood.
- Date of insertion of the Port-a-Cath needle, size of Gripper needle used and date when infusion lines require to be changed should all be documented in the nursing notes.

ADMINISTRATION OF BOLUS DRUGS INTO A HEPARINISED CENTRAL LINE VIA THE CAP

This applies to any type of central line.

EQUIPMENT

- Dressing pack and dressing trolley (already cleaned)
- Prescription chart
- Drugs and diluents (if not prepared by pharmacy)
- 0.9% sodium chloride
- Heparin/saline solution (10 units heparin/mL saline) if required
- Syringes (10 mL syringes required for ports)
- 21G needles
- Filter needle (for any glass ampoules)
- Cap-cleaning equipment, 2% chlorhexidine gluconate in 70% alcohol swabs
- Sterile latex-free gloves.

METHOD

1. Wash and dry your hands thoroughly to prevent spread of infection.
2. Open dressing pack, open all syringes and needles, drop onto sterile field. Check and draw up all the prescribed drugs (see Ch. 42), flushing solution and heparin/saline solution using appropriate syringes and needles. Discard needles, ensuring that the contents of each syringe are identifiable to prevent errors in administration.
3. Empty cleaning swabs onto sterile field.
4. Take the prepared equipment to the child and explain the procedure to the child and family. Expose the end of the line for easy access.
5. Open the pack of sterile gloves; wash and dry your hands thoroughly; put on gloves. (The sterile inner paper from packaging can be used as a drape if required.)
6. Ask the child or parent to hand you the end of the line.
7. Thoroughly clean the end of the cap with the cleaning swab; allow to dry.
8. Withdraw fluid from the line to observe backflow of blood, so ensuring patency.
9. Administer the drugs over the manufacturer's recommended time, flushing before and after each drug with 5 mL of the correct flushing solution.
10. Heparinise the line. Flush the line with 4–5 mL of heparinised saline, closing the clamp while administering the last 0.5–1 mL. Remove the syringe. Continuous positive pressure ensures that the whole line is filled with heparinised saline and has not allowed aspiration of blood into the proximal end of the line. This minimises the risk of a blood clot and subsequent line blockage.
11. Ensure that the child is comfortable and the line is secured (some children wear a wiggly bag, which is a drawstring bag made of washable fabric and worn around the child's neck).
12. Clear away and dispose of all used equipment, as per hospital policy, to maintain a safe environment.

CONNECTING OR CHANGING AN INFUSION SET

ADDITIONAL EQUIPMENT

- Intravenous fluid and prescription chart
- Intravenous administration set and filter if required (some centres use 96-h filters).

METHOD

1. Wash and dry your hands thoroughly.
2. Prime the administration set with the prescribed intravenous fluid.
3. Follow steps 2–6 of the previous procedure.
4. If the line is heparinised, clean the end of the cap and line thoroughly with cleaning solution and allow to dry. Withdraw 3–5 mL of solution from the line, observing for blood; flush with 5 mL 0.9% sodium chloride and attach the intravenous administration set.
5. If the line is already attached to an infusion, clamp the line, clean the cap, remove the old infusion set and attach the new set. Flush with 0.9% sodium chloride only if the fluid to be administered is different from the previous one.
6. Ensure that the whole system from the child to the intravenous fluid bag is complete and secure, and that the child is comfortable. Open the clamp, set the infusion pump to the prescribed rate and commence infusion.
7. Clear away and dispose of all used equipment.

ACCESSING A PORT FOR USE

This applies to ports only.

A variety of right-angled Huber needles (e.g. Gripper) are available with an integral extension for connection to infusion sets (Table 13.2). A foam pad or winged plastic section is attached to these needles at the right-angled bend. This section should lie flat against the child's chest when the needle is in place. A dressing is placed over this to keep the needle securely in place. The size of needle chosen will depend upon the viscosity of the fluids to be administered, while the length is determined by the size of the child and the amount of subcutaneous tissue over the port.

Table 13.2 Gripper needles with extension	
SIZE (G)	LENGTH
20 gauge (0.9 mm)	0.75 inch (19 mm)
20 gauge (0.9 mm)	1.00 inch (25 mm)
20 gauge (0.9 mm)	1.25 inch (32 mm)
22 gauge (0.7 mm)	0.75 inch (19 mm)
22 gauge (0.7 mm)	1.00 inch (25 mm)
22 gauge (0.7 mm)	1.25 inch (32 mm)

EQUIPMENT

- Dressing trolley
- Dressing pack
- Prescription chart
- Cleaning swabs of 2% chlorhexidine gluconate in 70% alcohol
- Sterile latex-free gloves
- Gripper needle of appropriate size and length
- Luer lock cap or needleless valve
- 10 mL syringe
- 21G needle
- 0.9% saline
- Occlusive dressing.

Local anaesthetic cream, e.g. EMLA or tetracaine (Ametop), should be applied to the skin over the port ½–1 h before the procedure to minimise discomfort.

When accessing a port, it may be necessary to hold the child securely, especially a young child. The parents and an additional nurse may be required. Preparation for this procedure by the play specialist is invaluable if available.

METHOD

1. Clean the dressing trolley with alcohol-based solution, e.g. Azowipes, and assemble the required equipment.
2. Explain the procedure to the child and parents; allow them time to ask questions.
3. Wash and dry your hands thoroughly.
4. Prepare a sterile field by opening the dressing pack and emptying other sterile items onto it. Empty 2% chlorhexidine gluconate in 70% alcohol swabs into a Gallipot within the sterile field.
5. Wash and dry your hands thoroughly and put on gloves.

6. Connect the Luer lock cap to the extension of the Gripper needle. Draw up 0.9% saline solution using a syringe and needle; prime the extension and Gripper needle; clamp the line; remove the syringe, retaining all items within the sterile field.
7. Ask an assistant or the child or parent to remove the anaesthetic cream.
8. Place a dressing towel over the child's abdomen below the port.
9. Clean the raised port access site and surrounding skin thoroughly with cleaning swab, working in a spiral from the raised centre outwards for at least 10 cm (4 inches). Repeat at least twice; allow to dry.
10. Palpate and locate the port, holding the outer edges through the skin with the fingers. Ensure that the port is secure and non-mobile. Visualise the centre of the port and insert the Gripper needle at an angle of 90° to the skin, through the silicone, until it meets the back-plate of the port (Fig. 13.2).
11. Via the cap, insert the syringe. Unclamp the line, withdraw the plunger until blood is aspirated, then flush with 0.9% saline clamping the line while administering the last 0.5–1 mL, i.e. under positive pressure.
12. Cover the Gripper needle with an occlusive dressing. It may also be necessary to pad the underside of the needle with sterile gauze if too long a needle has inadvertently been used.
13. Ensure that the child is comfortable and the line is well secured.
14. Clear away and dispose of all equipment.

Note: When a port is in long-term use, the needle must be changed every 2 weeks as recommended by the manufacturers; weekly if the child is neutropenic.

ROUTINE HEPARINISING OF A PORT

EQUIPMENT

As for accessing a port for use (above) with heparinised solution in place of 0.9% saline.

METHOD

1. Follow steps 1–10 of the method for accessing a port for use (above).

2. Via the cap, insert the syringe; unclamp the line; withdraw the syringe plunger until blood is aspirated. Flush with heparinised saline, removing the Gripper needle while still injecting the last 0.5 mL. Support the port with thumb and forefinger when removing the needle. (Another pair of hands is required, e.g. parent or another nurse.) This positive pressure manoeuvre prevents backflow of blood into the system, so preventing clot formation and potential occlusion.

3. Immediately wipe the puncture site with 2% chlorhexidine gluconate in 70% alcohol swabs; apply a plaster if requested by the child. Ensure that the child is comfortable.

4. Clear away and dispose of used equipment.

CENTRAL LINE DRESSINGS

There are many local variations in the method and frequency of dressings. A Cochrane review by Gillies et al (2003) found insufficient data on which to base a conclusion on which dressing to use to reduce infection rates. The conclusion was that the dressing of choice could be based on patient preference and cost. The epic-2 (Pratt et al 2007) guidelines recommend sterile, transparent semi-permeable dressings which should be changed aseptically every 7 days unless there is an indication to change them sooner.

Various cleaning solutions have also been compared for effectiveness in preventing infections. A metaanalysis by Chaiyakunapruk et al (2002) of many studies of different cleaning solutions showed that a chlorhexidine gluconate solution was more effective than povidone-iodine solutions for line site care. The current epic-2 guidelines (Pratt et al 2007) recommend the use of an alcoholic chlorhexidine gluconate solution preferably 2% chlorhexidine gluconate in 70% alcohol for skin cleaning around central venous line sites.

The main reasons for using a dressing on exit sites, especially for children are:

- To prevent contamination with extraneous matter
- To promote patient comfort
- To aid the secure fixation of the central line
- To prevent small children from interfering with the line.

CARE OF CENTRAL VENOUS LINE EXIT SITE

These lines are skin-tunnelled from the entry to a major vein to the exit site on the chest wall. A few centimetres up the line from the exit site, there is a Dacron cuff around the central line (Fig. 13.1). This helps to secure the line once the overlying skin has grown into it over the first couple of weeks from insertion, and may act as a partial barrier to ascending infective organisms from the exit site. This exit site is a potential site of infection as it is a long-term break in the skin's integrity. As a potential source of infection, the exit site requires careful monitoring and scrupulous hygiene.

FACTORS TO NOTE

Most children with central venous lines will go home with them *in situ* (McInally 2005). The child and parents need to be taught the importance of maintaining a clean exit site. Many parents want to learn how to do the dressing, so nursing staff need to teach them and assess their competency prior to the child's discharge. There will be some parents who do not wish to take on this responsibility, so alternative solutions need to be found. In these situations, dressings may be done on weekly clinic visits or in the home by community staff.

EQUIPMENT

- Dressing trolley
- Dressing pack containing sterile towels and swabs
- 2% chlorhexidine gluconate in 70% alcohol swabs
- OpSite IV3000 (10 × 12 cm)
- Bag for disposal of used equipment
- Additional tape, e.g. Mepore, for securing the line
- Sterile latex-free gloves (as per local policy)
- Swabs if infection at exit site is suspected.

METHOD

1. Assemble the equipment, take it to the child's bed and pull the curtains for privacy.

2. Explain the procedure to the child and family; allow time for questions and encourage the cooperation of all involved.

3. Wash and dry hands thoroughly, open the dressing pack and prepare all the equipment.
4. Remove the old dressing and discard it in the disposal bag.
5. Examine the exit site for any signs of infection, e.g. redness or exudate. Take swabs for culture if any signs of infection are present.
6. Wash and dry hands thoroughly. Put on sterile gloves if used.
7. Using 2% chlorhexidine swabs, wipe round the exit site in a circular movement, starting at the centre and working outwards for at least 5 cm. Repeat at least twice with a new swab each time; allow to dry.
8. Clean the line with another swab, from the exit site away from the child for at least 10 cm. Allow the cleaning solution to dry.
9. Coil the line and apply OpSite IV3000 over the exit site, ensuring good adhesion by applying gentle pressure over the whole dressing. If a child is sensitive to OpSite IV3000, another sterile dressing may be required.
10. Loop the hub end of the line up to the chest and secure it with another piece of tape or insert the hub into a wiggly bag if worn by the child. (If a wiggly bag is worn, we suggest that a clean bag is used each day.) Ensure that the child is comfortable.
11. Clear away and dispose of all used equipment.
12. Label swabs and appropriate microbiology forms if required.
13. Record appropriate information in the child's nursing notes.

DRESSING A PORT IN USE

A dressing is only required if a port is in use for treatment. When not in use, the skin's integrity is not broken, as no needle requires to be *in situ*, so normal personal hygiene is sufficient once the initial insertion wounds have healed.

The dressing on an accessed port need only be changed if it becomes soiled or there is a clinical indication, i.e. potential infection. The recommended weekly or 2-weekly needle change will obviously entail a dressing change as part of that procedure.

METHOD

The method is the same as for care of the central venous line exit site but extra care should be taken to prevent dislodging the needle.

DRESSING CHANGE ON A LONG LINE

A long line is generally sutured at the exit site at the time of insertion. The long line entry site is protected under OpSite IV3000 for ease of observation. This dressing can remain in place for up to 7 days, but can be changed sooner if required (NICE 2003, Pratt et al 2007). Care must be taken not to dislodge the long line. The hub(s) should be padded to ensure the child's comfort.

The procedure for cleaning the site is the same as for central venous lines.

OBSERVATIONS AND COMPLICATIONS

Infection and potential septicaemia

Of the central line during placement
Sterile conditions in theatre should prevent this, but if the child has a systemic infection at the time of insertion, the lumen of the line can become affected.

Via the infusion system during use
Aseptic handling of the line and any infusions or additives should prevent infection occurring via this route. Filters can also be used, specifically for total parenteral nutrition solutions, with different filters being used for the vitamin and lipid solutions. Pratt et al (2007) found no reliable evidence that the routine use of in-line filters prevented infection.

Of the exit site or skin tunnel
Scrupulous hygiene of the exit site is essential to block this route of infection. Indications of infection are redness and/or exudate at the exit site, and in some instances pain or swelling.

If an infection is suspected, i.e. the child has a fever, blood cultures and exit site swabs should be taken, and then intravenous antibiotics commenced. These can usually eradicate any infection. Only in extreme circumstances are lines removed because of infection, and then only after lengthy consideration by medical staff in consultation with the child and family. These lines are very precious, especially in the high-risk patients who have them, so prevention of infection is imperative (McIntosh 2003).

Occlusion

Fibrin clot within the line

This is prevented by regular heparinisation, but it is sometimes necessary to dissolve a clot by using an antifibrinolytic agent such as urokinase (5000 units) (Medicines for Children 2003, BNF for Children 2007).

A line that does not flush back or bleed back, and has had no obvious kinks in it, is most likely to have an occlusion caused by a fibrin clot.

Drug precipitate

This can occur if certain solutions are not infused correctly, for example etoposide, calcium, diazepam, phenytoin and total parenteral nutrition. Precipitates can be removed by using 90% alcohol or hydrochloric acid, depending upon the likely cause of the occlusion; this must be carried out *only* by experienced senior personnel (RCN 2007).

Kinking of the line

This may be either externally or internally within the child's venous system. Visually check all external parts of the line for kinks first, then try altering the child's position. If the line still appears to be blocked, a chest X-ray may be required to check for internal kinks.

Catheter misplacement

Perioperatively

If this occurs there is a potential for pneumothorax, haemothorax, perforation of a vein or dislodgement during surgery. Any of these complications could be apparent in theatre and would be rectified there. The use of ultrasound imaging in theatre during the placement of these lines should reduce the incidence of these complications.

Postoperatively, confirm the correct placement of the line with the medical staff before using the line. Observe the child for any signs of chest pain, dyspnoea, cyanosis or bleeding/haematoma. Notify medical staff if any adverse signs are present.

Line accidentally pulled by the child

Check the exit site for signs of trauma or external appearance of the cuff. If the cuff is not visible or partially visible, check that the line is capable of being aspirated and flushes with no pain or swelling along the tunnel site. Inform medical staff of the situation. A slight misplacement may just require a further restraining suture around the cuff, allowing continued use of the line. A major displacement may result in the line having to be removed.

Superior vena cava syndrome

This can occur at any time because of a thrombus causing obstruction of the venous return to the superior vena cava. Signs include engorgement of head and neck veins, oedema of the head and neck and potential respiratory distress. Medical intervention is required.

Air embolism

This can occur if the line is damaged or left unclamped during a cap change. Careful handling, strict procedures, good staff and family education should prevent this. All caregivers should be taught to clamp the line close to the exit site if it should become inadvertently split or cut. Report the incident immediately to senior medical or nursing staff.

Central line breakage

This can occur if, for example, the line is cut or bitten by the child. The line must be clamped above the break as explained above. Repair kits are available for all central venous lines. The repair is performed under aseptic conditions by experienced senior nurses or medical staff. Details of the child's central venous line should be documented in the medical notes so that the appropriate repair kit is used.

Potential complications are summarised in Table 13.3.

Table 13.3 Summary of potential complications	
OBSERVATION	**POSSIBLE CAUSE**
Fever	Line infection/septicaemia
	Exit site infection
Line not flushing or	Kink in line
bleeding back	Fibrin clot
	Drug precipitate
	Displacement of line
Chest pain, dyspnoea,	Pneumothorax
cyanosis	Haemothorax
	Superior vena cava syndrome
Fluid leaking out of line	Damage to line, e.g. split or tear
	Connections not correctly
	attached

The CCN is likely to be involved in the care of tunnelled central venous lines and implanted ports. Hospital visits can be minimised and in-patient time reduced if the CCN undertakes the administration of drugs and blood sampling at home or in school. Routine flushing of lines can also be undertaken by the CCN if the family do not wish to take on this responsibility.

Although cross-infection is less likely to occur in the home environment, there are other safety aspects that need to be addressed. The CCN may have difficulty in maintaining an aseptic field when there are other siblings or pets in the household. The CCN will also need access to an anaphylaxis kit (see Ch. 42).

The CCN is also in a position to educate the family about the central lines, enabling them to undertake more of the care themselves if they wish.

DOS AND DON'TS

- Do ensure that the line is clamped during cap changes.
- Do always wash and dry hands thoroughly.
- Do always maintain strict aseptic techniques.
- Do seek expert advice or help with any problems.
- Do educate the child and family in correct line care and how to clamp the line when it is cut or damaged.
- Do not carry out any procedure for which you have not been trained.
- Do not be afraid to seek help from experienced personnel. These lines are very precious, and with good care can last a long time, greatly aiding in the child's treatment.
- Do not use syringes smaller than 5 mL as they will produce a greater pressure than that of the central line and may result in a fracture if the line is blocked.

References

BNF for Children, 2007. The essential resource for clinical use of medicines in children. Online. Available: www.bnfc.org.

Cesaro, S., Corro, R., Pelosin, A., et al., 2004. A prospective survey on incidence and outcome of Broviac/Hickman catheter-related complications in pediatric patients affected by hematological and oncological diseases. Ann. Hematol. 83 (3), 183–188.

Chaiyakunapruk, N., Veenstra, D.L., Lipsky, B.A., et al., 2002. Chlorhexidine compared with povidone-iodine solution for vascular catheter-site care: a meta-analysis. Ann. Intern. Med. 136 (11), 792–801.

Coulthard, M.G., Skinner, R., 2007. Should paediatric central lines be aspirated before use? Arch. Dis. Child. 92, 517–518.

Ewenstein, B.M., et al., 2004. Consensus recommendations for the use of central venous access devices in haemophilia. Haemophilia 10, 629–648.

Gillies, L., et al., 2003. Gauze and tape and transparent polyurethane dressings for central venous catheters. Cochrane Database Syst. Rev. 3, CD003827.

INS Intravenous Nurses Society, 2000. Infusion nursing standards of practice. J. Intraven. Nurs. 23 (65) Suppl III.

McInally, W., 2005. Whose line is it anyway? Management of central venous catheters in children. Paediatr. Nurs. 17 (5), 14–18.

McIntosh, N., 2003. Central venous catheters: reasons for insertion and removal. Paediatr. Nurs. 15 (1), 14–18.

Medicines for Children, 2003. Royal College of Paediatrics and Child Health. Neonatal and Paediatric Pharmacists Group, London.

NICE National Institute for Clinical Excellence, 2002. Ultrasound imaging for central venous catheter placement. NICE, London.

NICE National Institute for Clinical Excellence, 2003. Infection control: prevention of healthcare associated infection in primary and community care. No. 4. Care of patients with central venous catheters. Clinical Guidelines 2. NICE, London.

Pratt, R.J., et al., 2007. Epic2: National evidence based guidelines for preventing healthcare associated infections in NHS hospitals in England. J. Hosp. Infect. 655, S1–S64.

RCN Royal College of Nursing, 2007. Standards for infusion therapy. RCN, London.

Valentino, L.A., Ewenstein, B., Navickis, R.J., Wilkes, M.M., 2004. Central venous access devices in haemophilia. Haemophilia 10 (2), 134–146.

Further reading

Royal College of Nursing, 2001. Administering intravenous therapy to children in the community setting – guidance for nursing staff. RCN, London

Chapter 14

Chest drainage

Michaela Dixon

CHAPTER CONTENTS

Introduction   163
  Learning outcomes   163
  Rationale   163

Pathophysiology   164

Pneumothorax   164

Haemothorax   164

Pleural effusion/empyema   164
  Factors to note   164

Chest drainage   165
  Equipment   165
  Method   166
  Observations and complications   166
  Care of the child   166
  Care of the equipment   167

Removing the drain   168

Nursing considerations   168
  Dos and don'ts   169

INTRODUCTION

Chest drainage may be observed in several practice placement areas, including intensive care, the neonatal unit and the emergency department, as well as the general paediatric ward. It is a relatively common practice that requires a thorough knowledge of research-based principles and pathophysiology to assist with clinical decision-making, to manage effectively and prevent complications (Lehwaldt & Timmins 2007).

LEARNING OUTCOMES

By the end of this section you should be able to:
- Explain why chest drainage is used
- Understand how chest drainage is set up
- Understand how the patient is assessed and the drainage monitored
- Explain why some traditional practices are controversial
- Know of complications that may occur.

RATIONALE

A systematic review of the nursing management of chest drains in 2001 found that there was lack of rigorous research in all areas of chest drain management, particularly in the under 18s (Charnock 2001). This review also noted that practices varied according to individual institutions and that there were often no written protocols to guide practice. After searching the Cochrane library and other relevant sources, it is evident that to date there has not been any further system-atic review of the area of practice undertaken. As a consequence of this lack of evidence, most of the information in this chapter remains based upon adult studies.

PATHOPHYSIOLOGY

Before learning about chest drainage, it is impor-tant to remember some key points relating to the anatomy and physiology of the chest:

- The lungs maintain expansion through diaphragmatic and intercostal contraction during inspiration, causing air to be drawn into the lungs by negative pressure, followed by expiration and elastic recoil of the lungs to their original state (Tortora & Derrickson 2009)
- The heart is positioned in the mediastinum. If blood builds up around the heart, or the lung is pushed over to the wrong side of the chest, the heart will become restricted and its function compromised. This is known as cardiac tamponade (Allibone 2003)
- The pleural cavity is a potential space, lying between the visceral and parietal pleura, the diaphragm and mediastinum. Pressure in the space is normally negative (−4 to −10 mmHg) (Ward et al 2002)
- A small amount of fluid is secreted into the space and acts as a lubricant to reduce possible shearing forces being exerted on each other by the pleura (Coughlin & Parchinsky 2006)
- Any injury, disease or surgical intervention that may cause accumulation of air or fluid in the pleural cavity may impair ventilation, through first reducing elastic recoil of the lung and second, by compression of the lung (Lazzara 2002, Allibone 2003).

The following conditions require chest drainage.

PNEUMOTHORAX

Air is present in the pleural space which limits the ability of the lung to expand during inspiration. A pneumothorax may be termed spontaneous (fre-quent in neonates who aspirate stomach contents, causing alveolar rupture); tension (the alveoli rupture and leak air into the pleural space – this may occur in critically ill children requiring positive pressure ventilation); or open (through trauma) (Lazzara 2002).

A tension pneumothorax is a life-threatening emergency, which requires immediate intervention.

HAEMOTHORAX

Blood is present in the pleural space and mediasti-num. This can occur after chest surgery such as tho-racotomy or sternotomy for repair of congenital heart lesions or as a consequence of trauma. If there is a mix of blood and air present in the pleural space then this is termed a haemopneumothorax.

PLEURAL EFFUSION/EMPYEMA

Secretions such as fluid or chyle from the thoracic lymph duct (chylothorax) fill the pleural space, often as a complication of surgery, or a pre-existing illness (e.g. cystic fibrosis, heart failure or oncological conditions). The collection of purulent material (pus) in the pleural space is known as an empyema and usually occurs as a consequence of infection such as pneumonia.

FACTORS TO NOTE

Insertion of a chest drain may be performed as an emergency by the doctor. If this is the case, there is little time to alert and prepare parents or the child for the procedure, but simple, brief explana-tions should be given. If the parents are not pres-ent, it is not usually possible to wait to gain their consent, as a delay could be life-threatening, but every effort should be made to contact them and inform them of the situation. If chest drains are expected as a result of surgery, children can be prepared through play, with verbal and visual explanation suitable for their conceptual under-standing. There will be more time to give parents and the child fuller information.

The procedure is painful and distressing. Co-operation is likely only in the older child; therefore, if time allows, sedation and analgesia should be given, usually by intravenous injection. Local anaes-thesia is normally used around the puncture site. If the child is ventilated, breathing against the venti-lator may worsen the condition, therefore the use of muscle relaxants may be indicated. It is important to ensure that the ventilator settings are adjusted, e.g. rate increased, to take into account a child who has received a dose of muscle relaxant.

Full monitoring of the child's respiratory rate and effort, heart rate and oxygen saturations should be in place prior to and for the duration of the procedure.

Resuscitation equipment including Ambu bag or T-piece bagging circuit, appropriately sized face mask, airway adjuncts (e.g. Guedel airway), suction equipment and oxygen must be available.

The child should have an intravenous line, although in an emergency the insertion of the chest tube may have higher priority (APLS 2005).

CHEST DRAINAGE

EQUIPMENT

Chest drain

The doctor will specify the size and type of drain dependent on whether air or serous matter needs draining.

For a child with suspected pneumothorax in a resuscitation situation, needle thoracocentesis may be performed using a large intravenous cannula and a 20 mL syringe – this is an emergency procedure and the child will require formal chest drain placement after the initial resolution of the pneumothorax (APLS 2005).

There are a number of proprietary chest drains available, ranging from 8 to 32 French gauge (Fg). These chest drains consist of a PVC catheter, with drainage eyes and radio-opaque markings (for visualisation on X-ray), and may include a trocar. Some are specifically designed for neonatal or emergency use. The use of a trocar when inserting chest drains in children is not recommended and indeed in adult practice it is also seen as no longer necessary, due to the potential for secondary trauma within the chest cavity (Tang et al 2002).

Chest drainage system

There are now many systems in use on paediatric units, including the traditional self-assembly sets and the ready-assembled proprietary closed versions (Fig. 14.1). All follow the underwater seal principle, and consist of tubing, a water chamber, collection chamber and suction chamber or connections (Fig. 14.2).

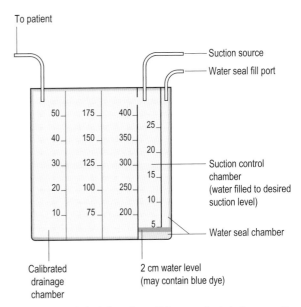

Figure 14.1 Principles of an all-in-one chest drainage unit. *Note* that it is the level of water in the suction chamber, not the level of suction at source that controls the level of suction in the patient.

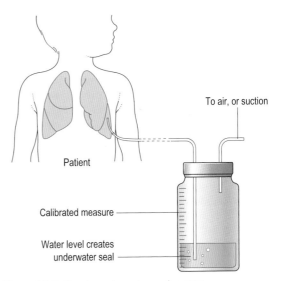

Figure 14.2 Simple underwater seal system.

Other equipment

- Large dressing trolley
- Medication as above: local anaesthetic, intravenous analgesia, sedation and muscle relaxants (ventilated children only)
- Sterile or distilled water

- Sterile gloves (latex free)
- Syringes and needles
- Dressing of choice
- Skin disinfecting solution
- A surgical dressing or cut-down pack may be helpful, and should contain the following:
  - Sterile drapes
  - Gauze swabs
  - Suture and needle, suturing forceps
  - Sterile scissors
  - Small scalpel
  - Two chest drain clamps (see below).

METHOD

Position

The child will be positioned either on the back or side, depending on the chosen site for the tube and the reason for chest drainage. Because fluid follows gravity, tubes to drain secretions or blood will normally be placed posteriorly, at the lung base. As air normally rises, a tube to drain a pneumothorax will be positioned anteriorly, at the apex of the affected lung (Tang et al 2002, Allibone 2003). Evidence suggests that in most circumstances the actual insertion of the drain within the pleural cavity is more important rather than the precise orientation of the drain (Tang et al 2002).

The nurse is responsible for preparation of the child and equipment, assisting the doctor with the procedure and maintaining asepsis, connecting the system, and comforting and observing the child.

The chest drain should be connected as soon as possible to the underwater seal drainage system. With the all-in-one systems, suction is regulated by the volume of water in the suction chamber (Fig. 14.1) (Smith et al 1995). The drainage system should at all times be at least 30 cm below the child's chest (Tang et al 2002, Allibone 2003).

The drain will be sutured to the skin by the doctor. Traditionally a purse-string suture was also used to ease removal; this type of suturing technique is used less often nowadays. It is important to note in the child's nursing records the presence or absence of a purse string suture as this will assist when preparing for the removal of the drain.

The tubing should be securely attached to the child's skin with adhesive tape to prevent pull on the insertion site. A dry keyhole dressing may be applied to the skin, and secured with tape, or a spray or occlusive dressing used, which allows for visual inspection of the wound.

The child should be positioned comfortably after the procedure, reassured and comforted. All used equipment should be disposed of according to local polices. The child should have a chest X-ray to check drain placement. The procedure and the result of the X-ray should be documented in both the nursing and medical notes.

OBSERVATIONS AND COMPLICATIONS

Complications of chest drain insertion (Allibone 2003, Coughlin & Parchinsky 2006)

- Traumatic perforation of the lung
- Traumatic perforation of the mediastinal structures including the heart and major blood vessels
- Traumatic perforation or damage to the diaphragm and intra-abdominal organs
- Trauma to the intercostal neurovascular bundle, which may lead to intercostal neuralgia or haemothorax
- Infection – either at insertion site or within the pleural space
- Subcutaneous emphysema (air collecting in the subcutaneous tissue).

Observations

The child's condition should be observed throughout the procedure and thereafter, especially in the first minutes and hours following insertion, when physiological changes may occur. The frequency of observation will depend on the child's condition, but in the first hour it may be quarter- to half-hourly.

Observation should be systematic, starting with the child and then the equipment. All observations should be recorded in the child's records.

CARE OF THE CHILD

Respiratory system

- Respiratory rate, colour, work of breathing, oxygen saturations
- Listen to the child's breath sounds, using a stethoscope. Listen to all areas of the chest using a side by side comparison, i.e. listen to the right upper area and then the left upper area, before

moving down to the middle area and then the bases. Remember to also listen into the axillary area as air from a pneumothorax may collect in this region. Observe the chest wall for equal movement to each side.

Cardiovascular system

- Heart rate and blood pressure – a fall in blood pressure or rising heart rate may indicate cardiac tamponade, or recurring pneumothorax, and should be reported immediately
- Skin colour and peripheral perfusion – these should improve after the chest drain is inserted and respiratory function improves.

General condition

- The child's general condition and responsiveness should be assessed
- Chest drains are uncomfortable (Gray 2000) and therefore frequent assessment of pain in the child is important with the administration of appropriate analgesia
- Temperature should be monitored regularly to identify infection.

CARE OF THE EQUIPMENT

- Identify and label the drains. The child may have more than one, especially after surgery, and it is important to understand their position and intended purpose.
- Observe the insertion site and dressing. There may be signs of fluid or air leakage, or the skin around the site may feel crackly. If so, surgical emphysema may be present and should be reported to the medical staff. The dressing should be left in place if clean and dry.
- Observe the chest tubes. The connections should be secure. Some units use adhesive tape to ensure that they do not become accidentally separated, though be aware that adhesive tape may actually conceal a loose connection.
- The tubing should be free and unkinked. Excess tubing should not hang in dependent loops from the bed, as this can increase resistance and lessen effective drainage; indeed a column of water accumulating in a loop of tubing may effectively seal the drain and prevent the effective drainage of air (Tang et al 2002,

Lazzara 2002); instead it should be positioned in flat loops on the bed (Avery 2000, Rushing 2007).

- Observe the colour of the drainage and presence of blood (some bloody drainage can be expected immediately after surgery or insertion of a chest drain). Check the volume of fluid drained. It is common practice to mark the level of fluid on the collecting chamber, along with the time and the nurse's initials. The level should be recorded on the fluid balance chart, in accordance with local policy, remembering that drainage represents serous fluid loss, and the doctor may wish to prescribe replacement intravenously, using clear fluid or blood or other blood products. Keep medical staff informed.
- If the drain is a pleural drain, look for the fluid level swinging within the tubing, as the pressures change when the child breathes. Positive pressure ventilation will cause a reverse swing to the negative pressure of spontaneous ventilation. If the fluid is no longer swinging, the air may have completely drained, or the chest drain may have become blocked. This should be reported and discussed with the medical staff as soon as possible.
- If the water is bubbling, this may indicate air draining. If the bubbling is continuous, and the child is not receiving positive pressure ventilation, this may indicate an air leak in the drainage system. The system will need to be checked by briefly clamping the chest tube near the patient; if the bubbling continues, there is an air leak (Lazzara 2002). If suction has been applied, the water will bubble gently, but excessive bubbling may indicate too high suction.
- Check the bottle. It should be well secured, approximately 30 cm below the child's chest.
- Check the fluid level in the drainage chambers; the system will need changing if the chambers are two-thirds full, as too much fluid will increase the resistance to drainage (Allibone 2003). There is little evidence available to be more specific about the frequency of bottle change.
- Check the suction level – suction may not be applied to some intercostal drains; however, if there is a persistent air leak or a large fluid collection, the application of low-pressure suction can expedite the drainage of excessive

air or fluid (Tang et al 2002). Drains placed after surgery are normally placed on 'low flow' suction for this reason. There is no definitive evidence about the pressure that should be used; however, the literature suggests that a pressure of 5 kPa or 20 mmHg is usually sufficient (Tang et al 2002). There are some potential problems associated with the application of suction to an intercostal drain – if there is too little suction, it may prevent lung expansion and contribute to infection and atelectasis (Tang et al 1999). If an excessive pressure is used, there is a risk of damage to the lung tissue (Allibone 2003).

REMOVING THE DRAIN

The medical staff will decide to remove the drain on the basis of clinical signs and/or chest X-ray, which will indicate whether the original problem has resolved.

Removing the drain is a painful and distressing experience for the child. In a review of studies into chest drain removal pain and its management, Bruce et al (2006) determined that the majority of studies indicated the presence of moderate to severe pain during the procedure even after the administration of morphine or the use of local anaesthetic agents. Careful consideration must therefore be given to the choice of a combination of analgesic agents for the procedure.

The tube is removed using an aseptic technique. Any tape holding the tube in position is removed. The tubing is clamped, and any suction discontinued. If the timing can be coordinated, the drain is removed on expiration as this is thought to minimise the risk of the reoccurrence of a pneumothorax, due to the positive pressure within the thoracic cavity during expiration. In a prospective study involving adult patients in 2001, Bell et al (2001) found no significant difference in the rate of post-removal pneumothorax when comparing end inspiration and end expiration removal. As there is little available evidence, it remains common practice to remove drains on expiration as detailed.

If a purse-string suture has been used, the suture is pulled tight to occlude the wound, while the drain is gently and firmly withdrawn. This prevents air being sucked into the pleural space on inspiration. An impermeable dressing is applied

to the skin until the wound has healed, so that air cannot enter the pleura through the open drain wound (Rushing 2007).

The child is made comfortable and observed for recurrence of the problem.

NURSING CONSIDERATIONS

Chest drain 'milking'

Chest drain 'milking, when the tubes are stripped with a roller or clamp, has been widely practised in many units and is identified frequently in literature published before the mid-1990s. It was believed to encourage drainage and prevent clots. Its practice is now discouraged, as the negative pressure created can be exceedingly high, up to −400 cmH₂O, causes trauma to the mediastinum or pleural space and has not been shown to significantly improve output from the drain (Lazzara 2002). It has also been shown that milking has no particular effect on preventing clot formation (Coughlin & Parchinsky 2006, Rushing 2007).

Clamping chest drains

Clamping chest drains when transferring or moving the child is another traditional nursing practice that has been shown to be potentially dangerous. If air is draining, clamping the chest drain can cause a build-up of pressure in the pleural space, leading to tension pneumothorax and sudden lung and circulatory collapse (Avery 2000, Tang et al 2002, Allibone 2003).

The only indications now accepted for possibly clamping underwater seal drains are:

- When changing chest drainage bottles (Allibone 2003)
- In children with pneumothorax, when reinflation of the lung is confirmed by chest X-ray but there is suspicion of an ongoing air leak, allowing for observation of a recurring pneumothorax before the drain is removed. There is a risk of tension pneumothorax developing in this situation and the child must be closely observed during this procedure (Tang et al 2002)
- On accidental disconnection of the chest drain, although it has been argued that a more appropriate response if this has occurred is to submerge the disconnected chest drain under water, while quickly reconnecting the drainage tubes, or reassembling a new drainage system if the previous one has been contaminated.

If the bottle is accidentally tipped over or raised above the child's head, it should be immediately returned to its proper position. It should not normally need replacing, as long as the contents of one chamber have not spilled into another.

DOS AND DON'TS

- Do ask if you are not sure about what you are doing.
- Do not milk chest drains.
- Do not clamp drains when moving children – except in specific circumstances.

References

Advanced Paediatric Life Support Group, 2005. Advanced paediatric life support: the practical approach, fourth ed. BMJ Publishing Group, London.

Allibone, L., 2003. Nursing management of chest drains. Nurs. Stand. 17 (22), 45–54.

Avery, S., 2000. Insertion and management of chest drains. NTPLUS 96 (37), 3–6.

Bell, R.L., Ovadia, P., Abdullah, F., et al., 2001. Chest tube removal: end inspiration or end-expiration? J. Trauma Inj. Infect. Crit. Care 50 (4), 674–677.

Bruce, E.A., Howard, R.F., Franck, L.S., 2006. Chest drain removal pain and its management: a literature review. J. Clin. Nurs. 15, 145–154.

Charnock, Y., 2001. The nursing management of chest drains: a systematic review. The Joanna Briggs Institute for Evidence Based Nursing and Midwifery, Adelaide, Australia.

Coughlin, A.M., Parchinsky, C., 2006. Go with the flow of chest tube therapy. Nursing 36 (3), 36–41.

Gray, E., 2000. Pain management for patients with chest drains. Nurs. Stand. 14 (23), 40–44.

Lazzara, D., 2002. Eliminate the air of mystery from chest tubes. Nursing 2 (6), 36–43.

Lehwaldt, D., Timmins, F., 2007. The need for nurses to have in service education to provide the best care for clients with chest drains. J. Nurs. Manag. 15, 142–148.

Rushing, J., 2007. Managing a water-seal chest drainage unit. Nursing 37 (12 Pt 1), 12.

Smith, R.N., Fallentine, J., Kessel, S., 1995. Underwater chest drainage: bringing the facts to the surface. Nursing 25 (2), 60–63.

Tang, A., Hooper, T., Hasan, R., 1999. A regional survey of chest drains: evidence-based practice? Postgrad. Med. J. 75 (886), 471–474.

Tang, A., Velissaris, T.J., Weeden, D.F., 2002. An evidence-based approach to the drainage of the pleural cavity: an evaluation of best practice. J. Eval. Clin. Pract. 8 (3), 333–340.

Tortora, G.J., Derrickson, B.H., 2009. Principles of anatomy and physiology, twelfth ed., vol. 2. Wiley, New York.

Ward, J.P., Ward, J., Wiener, C.M., et al., 2002. The respiratory system at a glance. Blackwell, Oxford.

Chapter 15

Incubator care

Susan Alexander

CHAPTER CONTENTS

Introduction 170
    Learning outcomes 170
    Rationale 171
    Factors to note 171
    Equipment 172
    Method 172
    Observations and complications 173

Transition from incubator to open cot 173
    Dos and don'ts 173

INTRODUCTION

The maintenance of a neutral thermal environment is of the utmost importance when nursing the pre-term, ill or cold infant. A neutral thermal environment is one which balances heat production and heat conservation and dissipation, thus enabling the infant to maintain a normal core temperature with minimal oxygen requirements and calorie expenditure (Amlung 1998).

The neutral thermal environment can be maintained in four main ways:

1. By the use of an open crib with blankets and clothing: the dressed infant covered with blankets has the ability to maintain body temperature within a wide range of environmental temperatures; however, observation is greatly diminished

2. By the use of a heated water-filled mattress: this has become a useful adjunct to care for the healthy pre-term infant in the nursery, making access easier than closed incubators (Gray & Flenady 2003)

3. By using radiant heaters, e.g. Baby Therms: infants can then be nursed naked allowing for improved observation of the ill infant

4. By using an incubator, where infants can be nursed naked (Fig. 15.1); however, the environment is enclosed.

LEARNING OUTCOMES

By the end of this section you should be able to:

- Develop an understanding of thermoregulation in the term and pre-term infant

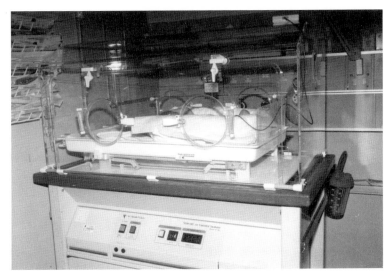

Figure 15.1 Infant being nursed in an incubator.

- Identify the infant who requires to be nursed in an incubator
- Prepare an incubator to receive an ill infant
- Demonstrate an understanding of temperature regulation devices used in the incubator
- Provide safe and effective care to the infant nursed in the incubator.

RATIONALE

Both term and pre-term infants have difficulty in maintaining body temperature owing to an inability to control their heat loss. A low admission temperature is an independent risk factor for morbidity and mortality in pre-term babies (Costeloe et al 2000). Prevention of heat loss in ill and distressed infants is crucial to their survival; thus the provision of a neutral thermal environment, when nursing the infant, is of the utmost importance (Amlung 1998). Environmental temperature, which maintains the infant's skin temperature between 36.5 and 37.5°C (rectal 37°C) is known to promote minimal metabolic rate and oxygen consumption (Merenstein & Gardiner 2006). This is defined as the neutral thermal environment.

FACTORS TO NOTE

Infants are at risk of poor temperature control caused by an immature hypothalamus resulting in poor control of heat loss and heat production (see Ch. 29). This is more marked in the pre-term

infant. Pre-term infants lack glycogen and stored fats, particularly brown fat which is important both as an energy source and for heat production. Brown fat is laid down in a variety of locations in the body between 26 and 28 weeks' gestation; infants born before this time may lack the ability to generate their own heat. Infants who do have brown fat have the ability to generate heat from birth (Mance 2008). Brown fat in infants differs from that in adults in that it has a higher number of mitochondria and an abundant sympathetic nerve supply. Brown fat accounts for 10% of the term infant's total adipose tissue (Flaherty 1996). Infants have a thin subcutaneous fat layer resulting in poor insulation (England 2003).

Term and pre-term infants do not have the ability to shiver to produce heat in response to cold and their metabolic response is limited. Changes in peripheral vascular tone, with constriction of skin vessels, occur in an attempt to reduce heat loss, thus keeping the blood in the central circulation. Non-shivering thermogenesis may occur where heat production is achieved from brown fat (Mance 2008). Heat loss in the infant is nearly four times greater, per unit of body weight, than in adults. This is primarily due to the higher ratio of surface area to body weight in infants (Lyon 2004).

Infants lose heat in four ways:

- *By conduction* occurring when the infant comes into direct contact with a cooler surface, thus losing heat to that surface (Fellows 2001)

- *By convection* when warmth is lost to the surrounding air or water; this necessitates the maintenance of room temperature between 24 and 26°C (Fellows 2001)
- *By radiation* heat loss from the infant to a surface nearby without direct contact; this may occur if the infant is placed near cold external walls (Lyon 2004)
- *By evaporation* caused by the evaporation of surface body water; this water is converted into vapour and is of particular significance in the newborn (Lyon 2004).

Exposed to extremes of temperature, infants will suffer from decreased lung surfactant, hypoglycaemia, increased oxygen consumption and decreased blood coagulability in cold conditions, and increased fluid loss, hypernatraemia and recurrent apnoea in heat. Both extremes of temperature may result in death (Mance 2008).

EQUIPMENT

- Incubator
- Temperature monitor
- Servo control skin probe (if required)
- Sterile water (if required).

METHOD

Incubators can be used to maintain a neutral thermal environment in two ways: skin servo control and air (non-servo) control. Skin servo control involves attaching a skin probe to the abdomen of the infant, normally over the liver. If the infant's temperature falls, additional heat is provided until the target temperature is reached. Recent incubators have a skin sensor detach alarm to prevent overheating in case the probe becomes dislodged (Lyon 2004). In the air (non-servo) control mode the air temperature of the incubator is raised or lowered depending on the measured temperature of the infant (Lyon 2004). (For detailed guidance on the use of individual incubators the nurse should refer to the manufacturer's operating guidelines.)

- Position the incubator in an area of the ward away from direct sunlight and draughts. Direct sunlight will cause the incubator to overheat.
- Fill the water reservoir with sterile water if additional humidity is required. The use of incubator humidity has increased over the past

Table 15.1 Neutral thermal environmental temperatures determined by age and weight

Weight (g)	Incubator temperature (°C)		
	Day 1	Days 2–7	1–2 weeks
<1000	35 ± 0.5	34 ± 0.5	33 ± 0.5
1000–1500	34 ± 0.5	33.5 ± 0.5	32 ± 0.5
1500–2500	33 ± 0.5	32 ± 0.5	30 ± 1

After Beischer et al. (1997).

two decades in response to the increasing number of very low birth weight and extremely pre-term infants within neonatal intensive care units (Sinclair & Sinn 2007). Ensure that the temperature of the incubator is maintained at a constant level, not in excess of the humidity, to prevent additional heat loss caused by evaporation.

- The room temperature should be maintained between 24 and 26°C (England 2003). This helps prevent heat loss through the incubator wall.
- The incubator heater should be switched on and temperature limits set (Table 15.1). The incubator should be warmed to between these temperature limits before the infant is transferred into it.
- Attach the servo control probe to the infant's abdomen, if required, and adjust temperature limits for skin temperature (as per local policy).
- Prevent heat loss from the incubator by keeping the portholes closed when the infant is not being attended to.
- Minimal handling and coordination of care to prevent constant disruption (clustered care) will not only allow the infant to rest but will also reduce heat loss.
- Warm your hands before touching the infant.
- Warm additional equipment before putting it into the incubator.
- Ensure that the infant is kept as dry as possible to reduce evaporative heat loss.
- Significant heat loss from the infant's head can be reduced by the use of a hat (Mance 2008).
- Clean the incubator in accordance with the manufacturer's instructions.
- Change the incubator as per local policy.

OBSERVATIONS AND COMPLICATIONS

- The infant's temperature should be checked on a regular basis, if not continuously monitored. Bailey and Rose (2000) recommend the use of the axilla for monitoring neonatal temperature.
- Routine care should be clustered to reduce heat loss from the incubator.
- The incubator temperature limits should be set to ensure that the infant does not overheat or become hypothermic.
- Incubator temperature should be monitored continually and maintained within set limits.
- Empty and replace the water in the reservoir fully every 24 h to reduce infection risk. The reservoir should be washed and dried every 24 h.
- Porthole access may be problematic if the infant is unstable. Under these conditions the infant should be transferred to a radiant warmer.

TRANSITION FROM INCUBATOR TO OPEN COT

Weaning from an incubator to an open cot is an important step in the discharge preparation of an infant. Practice will differ between units, with some units having detailed policies. These policies may be based on a combination of the following:

- The infant's condition should be stable
- The weight of the infant
- Steady weight gain demonstrated by the infant
- The temperature of the incubator being gradually reduced. This may be reduced over a 24-h period; however, the incubator should never be turned off as this will result in air not being circulated

- Monitoring the infant's temperature is important to ensure that they are maintaining their temperature
- The infant should be placed in a cot, in a draught-free position in the ward
- The infant should be clothed and wrapped. Special attention should be paid to the wearing of a hat because of the increased heat loss from the head. Clothing and wrapping may be commenced when the infant is in the incubator, with suggestions regarding clothing being the first stage of incubator weaning rather than decreasing incubator temperature (Medoff-Cooper 1994).

DOS AND DON'TS

- Do ensure that the care is clustered to decrease disturbance of the infant.
- Do encourage parents in the care of their infant. This will help enhance the parent–infant relationship.
- Do ensure that the infant is wrapped well and that the head is covered if the infant is being removed from the incubator for feeding or cuddling.
- Do ensure that sheets, etc. are warmed before putting them into the incubator.
- Do ensure that the sterile water in the reservoir, if used, is fully changed every 24 h.
- Do not leave the incubator in direct sunlight or draughts.
- Do not leave portholes or incubator doors open unnecessarily.
- Do not allow the infant's head to be covered by the Perspex heat shield as this may cause hypoxia (Fraser & Cooper 2003).
- Do not turn off the incubator while the infant is inside.

References

Amlung, S.R., 1998. Neonatal thermoregulation. In: Kenner, C., Lott, J.W., Flandermeyer, A.A. (Eds.), Comprehensive neonatal nursing: a physiologic perspective. second ed. W B Saunders, Philadelphia Ch. 16.

Bailey, J., Rose, P., 2000. Temperature measurement in the pre-term infant. J. Neonatal Nurs. 6 (1), 28–32.

Beischer, N.A., Mackay, E.V., Colditz, P.B., 1997. Obstetrics and the newborn, third ed. W B Saunders, London.

Costeloe, K., Henessay, E., Gibson, A.T., et al., 2000. The EPIcure study: outcomes to discharge from hospital for infants born at the threshold of viability. Pediatrics 106, 659–671.

England, C., 2003. The healthy low birth weight baby. In: Fraser, D.,

Cooper, J.K.H. (Eds.), Myles textbook for midwives. fourteenth ed. Churchill Livingstone, Edinburgh.

Fellows, P., 2001. Management of thermal stability. In: Boxwell, G. (Ed.), Neonatal intensive care nursing. Routledge, London, Ch. 4.

Flaherty, L., 1996. Neonates and premature infants: overview of differences and ED management. J. Emerg. Nurs. 22 (2), 120–124.

Fraser, D., Cooper, A., (Eds.), 2003. Myles textbook for midwives, fourteenth ed. Churchill Livingstone, Edinburgh.

Gray, P.H., Flenady, V., 2003. Cot-nursing versus incubator care for pre-term infants. The Cochrane Library, Oxford.

Lyon, A., 2004. Applied physiology: temperature control in the newborn infant. Current Paediatrics 14, 137–144.

Mance, M.J., 2008. Keeping infants warm: Challenges of hypothermia. Adv. Neonatal Care 8 (1), 6–12.

Medoff-Cooper, B., 1994. Transition of the pre-term infant to an open crib. J. Obstetr. Gynaecol. Neonatal Nurs. 23 (4), 329–335.

Merenstein, G.B., Gardiner, S.L., 2006. Handbook of neonatal intensive care, sixth ed. Mosby, St Louis.

Sinclair, L., Sinn, J.K.H., 2007. Higher versus lower humidity for the prevention of morbidity and mortality in pre-term infants in incubators (Protocol). Cochrane Database Syst. Rev. 2, CD006472.

Further reading

Flenady, V.J., Woodgate, P.G., 2003. Radiant warmers versus incubators for regulating body temperature in newborn infants. Cochrane Database Syst. Rev. 4, CD000435.

Laptook, A., Jackson, G., 2006. Cold stress and hypoglycaemia in the late pre-term ('near-term') infant: impact on nursery of admission. Semin. Perinatol. 30, 24–27.

Moore, J., 2003. From birth to neonatal unit: a cold journey. J. Neonatal Nurs. 9 (4) [4 page insert].

Chapter 16

Lumbar puncture

Gaynor Pettitt

CHAPTER CONTENTS

Introduction 175
   Learning outcomes 175
   Rationale 176
   Factors to note 176

Administration of intrathecal drugs 176
   Preparation of the child and family 176
   Risks and complications 177

Preparing for the procedure 178
   The nurse's role in the procedure 178
   Manual handling risks 178
   Positioning the child 178
   Equipment 178

The procedure 179
   Post-lumbar puncture activity 179

Summary 180

INTRODUCTION

Lumbar puncture is an invasive procedure in which a spinal needle is inserted into the subarachnoid space of the lumbar spine for diagnostic or therapeutic purposes. During the procedure, cerebrospinal fluid is obtained and analysed, for blood cells, white cells protein glucose and for the presence of bacteria, viruses or abnormal cells.

Lumbar puncture can be carried out in an emergency setting with an acutely unwell child when meningitis may be suspected. It may also be carried out as a planned or diagnostic procedure. Often oncology patients undergo this procedure in a day-care setting to have intrathecal medication administered. This is when medication is injected directly into the spinal fluid. The urgency of the procedure and condition of the child will be paramount in planning the preparation and timing of the procedure.

LEARNING OUTCOMES

At the end of this section you should be able to:

- Give a rationale for lumbar puncture
- Give a rationale for the preparation of the child and family
- Assess the risks associated with the procedure to both the patient and healthcare staff
- Give a rationale for post-procedure nursing care
- Understand the role of the multidisciplinary team members in the procedure
- Identify other policies that impact on this procedure.

RATIONALE

Lumbar puncture is performed to:

- Obtain a specimen of cerebrospinal fluid for diagnostic purposes
- Measure the pressure of the lumbar CSF
- Instil therapeutic drugs
- Instil contrast media during radiological investigations.

Health benefits include the speedy diagnosis and treatment of meningitis, and investigations for other neurological disease and treatments for oncology patients. While we consider the risks and complications of the procedure, it is worth noting that the benefits to health outweigh the possible side-effects in nearly all cases (Kneen et al 2002).

FACTORS TO NOTE

Lumbar puncture is an invasive procedure and should be performed aseptically following local guidelines.

ADMINISTRATION OF INTRATHECAL DRUGS

In general it is not safe to administer drugs via the intrathecal route and the inappropriate injection of vesicant drugs (particularly vesicant chemotherapy) via this route will inevitably cause necrosis of the spine and brain, leading to a painful and almost inevitable death for the patient. There are a limited number of drugs which are safe via this route and which are used in the treatment of childhood cancer, however their use is heavily regulated by the Department of Health to prevent any unsafe drugs being injected.

Readers should look at the most recent guidance on the Department of Health website (www.dh. gov.uk/en/Publicationsandstatistics/Lettersandcirculars/Healthservicecirculars/DH_086870). This guidance, 'Health Service Circular HSC 2008/001' is the basis for every Trust's policy on intrathecal chemotherapy administration and specifies which hospital staff are allowed to participate in the prescribing preparation, delivery checking and administration of intrathecal drugs (DoH 2008). All staff involved have to undertake an agreed training programme and be added to a Trust Intrathecal Register for their role in intrathecal chemotherapy. All hospital personnel who are not on one of these registers are not allowed to undertake any practice relating to intrathecal chemotherapy. Although drugs are occasionally administered via this route in specialities other than oncology, there is less regulation, and anyone involved in this is recommended to read the guidance for chemotherapy as a measure of good practice.

PREPARATION OF THE CHILD AND FAMILY

It is vital to prepare both the child and family, as this will help to:

- Minimise stress and discomfort
- Promote safety and aid recovery
- Contribute to a successful lumbar puncture
- Inform the child, young person and family so they can participate in the consent process (DoH 2001a).

A full explanation of the reasons for performing the lumbar puncture including benefits to health, potential complications and risks, must be given. This should be at an age-appropriate level so the child and family can fully understand. This information can also be supported with written information leaflets or information available on websites such as (Patient UK at: www.patient.co.uk). The sharing of information is emphasised in the NSF (2004) Standard 3 and Standard 4 which state that the child and family should receive information about diagnosis, treatments and services available to them.

Parents may wish to stay with their child during the procedure, and may help to reassure the child by talking, holding hands or head stroking. Optimising the parents' role reduces the child's anxiety during the procedure. Staff should be sensitive to parents who are unable to provide this support (Mackenzie 2006). Nurses should promote an environment that encourages full parental involvement as the benefits to the child are well documented (Dudley & Carr 2004).

Preparing the child for the procedure through the use of play is also well documented. This is beneficial, particularly for children who have to undergo repeated procedures, such as the child with leukaemia (Broome et al 1990).

The healthcare professional performing the lumbar puncture should obtain consent from both the parents and child as appropriate (DoH 2001b). This consent will also involve a discussion of options for analgesia and sedation appropriate to the clinical situation. A child who requires routine and repeated lumbar puncture will be given the option to have the procedure under general anaesthesia or sedation with local anaesthetic (Gajjar et al 2000).

Conscious sedation with local anaesthetic combined with psychological or behavioural techniques are also used (Pederson 1996). In an acute setting when a lumbar puncture needs to be carried out in a timely and safe manner, a topical anaesthetic followed by an injected anaesthetic is recommended (Ellenby et al 2006). The nurse can play a vital role in supporting both child and parent through this procedure: to hold the child and to assist the doctor in obtaining spinal fluid under aseptic technique.

RISKS AND COMPLICATIONS

Lumbar puncture is indicated for both diagnostic and therapeutic reasons. A nurse should have a knowledge of the indications and contraindications to performing a lumbar puncture, and also an understanding of the procedural technique and risks. The risks, although rare, can be potentially life-threatening. These risks can be minimised by following the correct procedural and post-procedural care (Ellenby et al 2006).

Pain distress and anxiety

Pain distress and anxiety will be interpreted and experienced differently between each child and family. These effects can be minimised by promoting parents to support and comfort their child throughout the procedure. The relationship between non-essential touch and children's distress during lumbar puncture has been clearly identified (Vannorsdall et al 2004). Gentle stroking, holding hands and touch can contribute to a safe and successful lumbar puncture.

Pederson (1996) also identified the effects of promoting non-pharmacological techniques (e.g. using distraction focusing on breathing, relaxation techniques and the use of imagery) with children during lumbar puncture. In an observational study, less verbal expressions of fear and resistance were reported as well as less muscular rigidity and less reports of post-procedural pain.

Adverse reactions to lumbar puncture

These can include:

- Herniation
- Cardiorespiratory compromise
- Local or referred pain
- Headache
- Bleeding
- Infection
- Leakage of CSF
- Sub-arachnoid epidermal cyst.

Herniation of the brain stem

Herniation of the brain stem is also known as coning, and is a rare complication in which the brain stem herniates through the foramen magnum leading to death (van Crevel et al 2002). With the advent of more sophisticated imaging techniques such as computerised tomography (CT scan) and magnetic resonance imaging (MRI), the need for lumbar puncture as a diagnostic tool has reduced (Joffe 2007). However, fatalities as a result of herniation are still reported (van Crevel et al 2002). Lumbar puncture is contraindicated in patients with raised intracranial pressure, signs of abnormal posturing, deteriorating levels of consciousness and Glasgow coma scale less than 13, pupillary changes, irregular respirations, or a history of recent seizures (Joffe 2007). A lumbar puncture should not be performed if there is obvious meningococcal disease (Advanced Life Support 2001) dehydration, or shock.

Post-lumbar puncture headache and backache

This is a recognised complication following a lumbar puncture. The incidents documented are relatively lower compared with adults. This may be because infants and young children cannot verbalise pain as well as adults and adolescents (Atabaki et al 1999). Studies have identified headache pain associated with movement and posture suggesting headaches are more reported with age increasing with adolescents and also with girls (Ebinger et al 2004a). Other studies have indicated that the complication is due to spinal fluid leakage at the puncture site (Atabaki et al 1999), while some suggest that post-lumbar puncture headache and backache may be caused by epidural fluid collections (Choi et al 2004). The headache may be aggravated with movement such as standing upwards, moving the head such as coughing and may subside while lying down in supine position (Atabak et al 1999).

There is also some evidence to suggest that the size of the needle (gauge) used and technique applied may also limit the risk of headache post-lumbar puncture (Baxter et al 2006). Robbins (1990) suggest treatment of prolonged headache with an epidural blood patch, although most studies in this area have been in the management of headaches in adults. Treatment of the symptoms recommend bed rest, hydration regular analgesia and antiemetic medication for nausea (Connolly 1999). Lower back pain is also treated with analgesia and rest.

Infection

There is a rare but recognised risk that infection can be introduced into the cerebrospinal fluid (CSF) at the puncture site. This risk is minimised by the procedure being performed under strict aseptic conditions. If the child was well before the lumbar puncture, signs of meningitis, fever, malaise, irritability, vomiting and drowsiness should be reported immediately, and antibiotics commenced. The lumbar puncture site should also be observed for redness, heat, discharge and swelling, a small swelling can be expected due to the insertion of the needle (Ellenby et al 2006).

Leakage of CSF

Occasionally CSF can leak from the puncture site after the procedure, a sterile gauze pad should be applied with pressure. It is unclear whether lying flat prone or supine will contribute to closing the dura (Wojner & Malkoff 2001). If leakage persists, the medical staff should be informed.

PREPARING FOR THE PROCEDURE

THE NURSE'S ROLE IN THE PROCEDURE

The nurse has a role to provide safety and support before during and following the procedure. During the procedure, the nurse will hold the patient in the correct position preventing sudden movement that could dislodge the needle. This procedure needs coordinating with the multidisciplinary team to ensure success. Sudden movement can be unsafe and cause damage to the spinal nerves. If a child is struggling excessively, alternative methods of analgesia and sedation should be considered. The nurse should ensure that the procedure is performed in a safe environment with emergency equipment checked and nearby. A pulse oximeter will be required for monitoring vital signs during the procedure. Continual observation should also be made of the child's neurological, respiratory and cardiovascular status. In the event of deterioration, the procedure should be abandoned and the appropriate action taken.

MANUAL HANDLING RISKS

1. Moving and holding the child needs to be thought out and planned carefully.
2. The procedure is normally carried out on a height-adjustable treatment couch, this enables both the nurse holding the child and the doctor performing the procedure to be in the correct position to prevent back strain (Owen 2000). It is also recommended that a height adjustable stool should be available for the doctor to work at the correct height. Some treatment couches have now been specifically designed for lumbar puncture with a removable curved side to enable easier holding.
3. The child should be transferred to the couch using the appropriate manual handling risk-assessment and technique, using a slide board or slide sheet if appropriate (Nelson et al 2005).
4. Both nurse and doctor should avoid twisting and bending forward and stooping, maintaining a neutral a position as possible (Owen 2000).

POSITIONING THE CHILD

The most important factor in performing an easy atraumatic tap is the correct positioning of the child (Patten 1998). If the operator is right handed, the child should be on their left side or vice versa. The child should be placed on the edge of the couch on a firm surface with knees flexed up to the chest and neck flexed forward. The plane of the back and shoulders should be perpendicular to the bed (Fig. 16.1). The nurse restrains the patient by placing one arm under the flexed knees and another arm around the shoulders (Ellenby et al 2006). The older child may be comfortable with a pillow between the legs; this provides support for the legs and prevents the patient from rolling forwards (Patten 1998). A pillow can also be used to support the right arm. The doctor and nurse need to repeatedly check that the back is vertical to the couch.

EQUIPMENT

- Height adjustable patient bed/couch
- Height adjustable chair
- Adequate lighting
- Dressing trolley prepared for a sterile procedure

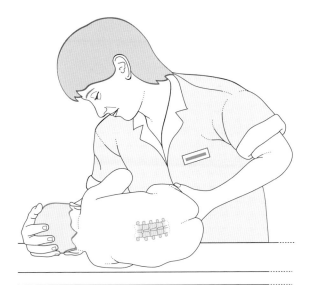

Figure 16.1 Positioning the child for lumbar puncture.

- Spinal needle 22 gauge 1.5 inches (3.8 cm) for infants
- Spinal needle 22 gauge 3.5 inches (6.3 cm) for older children
- Sterile dressing pack
- Sterile gloves
- Apron
- Antiseptic cleansing solution
- 2 mL syringes plus needle and local anaesthetic, e.g. lignocaine 1% (topical local anaesthetic should be applied beforehand and allowed to take effect)
- Specimen bottles (× 3) for bacteriology, virology and protein estimation
- 1 bottle for glucose
- Waterproof plaster or waterproof covering
- Rubbish bag.

Some hospital sterile supply departments will provide a lumbar puncture pack containing the above equipment.

THE PROCEDURE

1. The doctor will put on an apron and perform a clinical hand wash as per hospital policy. The second nurse will open the sterile pack and gloves onto the dressing trolley for the doctor. The doctor will dry his hands with the sterile towel and apply the sterile gloves. The second nurse will assist in pouring cleansing solution into the sterile container.
2. The first nurse will place the child into the lateral decubitus position placed curled on one side with the knees flexed up to the chest and neck flexed forward. The plane of the back and shoulders should be perpendicular to the bed. This position exposes the lumbar area to enable access to the spinal fluid (Fig. 16.1).
3. The doctor will cleanse the child's lumbar region at least three times in a circular manner, starting inwards then outwards. A further sterile drape will be applied to establish a sterile field. The doctor will establish a landmark for insertion of the lumbar puncture, drawing an imaginary line between the two posterior iliac crests and with insertion of the spinal needle below aiming for L3–L4 or L4–L5 (3rd, 4th and 5th lumbar vertebrae) interspaces. The doctor will inject a local anaesthetic following removal of the topical anaesthetic (if used). The doctor should wait approximately 5 min for the local anaesthetic to work.
4. The first nurse throughout this time will hold and comfort the child.
5. The doctor inserts the needle aiming for the umbilicus, the needle is advanced into the spinous ligament until a fall in resistance is felt. The stylet is then removed.
6. The second nurse assists in holding the bottles to catch 10 drops of CSF into each sterile container and 3 drops into the glucose bottle.
7. The doctor reinserts the stylet and removes the needle.
8. Pressure is applied with sterile gauze for a moment.
9. A waterproof plaster is then applied.
10. The nurses can now comfort the child and family and the child can now enjoy returning to the arms of his parents and to a more comfortable position.
11. The specimens should be labelled appropriately and sent to the laboratories. The equipment should be cleaned and tidied away appropriately using local guidelines.

POST-LUMBAR PUNCTURE ACTIVITY

There is no clear evidence that the duration of rest following a lumbar puncture has a role in preventing post-lumbar puncture headache (Evans 2000, Ebinger 2004b, McArthur 2002).

The nurse should be aware of local guidelines in place when advising children and families, following lumbar puncture.

SUMMARY

During a lumbar puncture the nurse can provide a vital role in preparing the child and family for the procedure. Holding the child correctly throughout the procedure and supporting the child and parents who may be present. The nurse also has a role to be aware of the risks associated with the procedure and to carry out nursing observations both before, during and following the procedure. The frequency of these observations will depend upon local policy, and also the dependency of the child. For example, an acutely unwell child may require constant pulse oximetry, cardiac monitoring and frequent neurological recording. A child having chemotherapy in an out-patient setting will need less frequent and intense monitoring. The Paediatric Early Warning System (PEWS) observation protocol should be followed if it has been implemented in the Trust/hospital that you are working in. The nurse should also have knowledge of the contraindications of lumbar puncture and should not allow the procedure to be performed if these signs are present (Box 16.1).

BOX 16.1 Relative contraindications to lumbar puncture

- Prolonged or focal seizures
- Focal neurological signs, e.g. asymmetry of limb movement and reflexes, ocular palsies
- A widespread purpuric rash in an ill child
- Glasgow Coma Scale score of less than 13
- Pupillary dilatation
- Impaired oculocephalic reflexes (doll's eyes reflexes)
- Abnormal posture or movement – decerebrate or decorticate posturing or cycling movements of the limbs
- Inappropriately low pulse, elevated blood pressure and irregular respirations
- Coagulation disorder
- Papilloedema
- Hypertension.

From Advanced Life Support Group (2001, p 134).

References

Advanced Life Support Group, 2001. Advanced paediatric life support: the practical approach, third ed. BMJ Publications, London, pp. 133–136.

Atabaki, S., Oschenschlager, D., Vezina, G., 1999. Post lumbar puncture headaches in paediatrics. Arch. Paediatr. Adolesc. Med. 153 (7), 770–773.

Baxter, A.L., Fisher, R.G., Burke, B.L., 2006. Local anaesthetic and stylet styles: factors associated with resident lumbar puncture success. Paediatrics 117 (3), 876–881.

Broome, M.E., Bates, T.A., Lillis, P.P., et al., 1990. Children's medical fears, coping behaviors and pain perceptions during a lumbar puncture. Oncol. Nurs. Forum. 17 (3), 361–367.

Choi, J.E., Chang, J.Y., Shin, J.Y., et al., 2004. CSF leakage after diagnostic lumbar puncture: case reports. Clin. Paediatr. 43 (8), 769–771.

Connolly, M., 1999. Postdural puncture headaches. Am. J. Nurs. 99 (11), 48–49.

Department of Health, 2001a. Consent. A guide for children and young people. DoH, London.

Department of Health, 2001b. Consent. What you have a right to expect a guide for parents. DoH, London.

Department of Health, 2008. Health service circular HSC 2008/1. Department of Health. Online. Available: www.dh.gov.uk/en/ Publicationsandstatistics/ Lettersandcirculars/ Healthservicecirculars/ DH_086870 Website.

Dudley, S.A., Carr, J.M., 2004. Vigilance: The experience of parents staying at the bedside of hospitalized children. J. Paediatr. Nurs. 19 (4), 267–275.

Ebinger, F., Kosel, C., Pietz, J., et al., 2004a. Headache and backache after lumbar puncture in children and adolescents; a prospective study. Paediatrics 113 (6), 1588–1592.

Ebinger, F., Kosel, C., Pietz, J., et al., 2004b. Strict bed rest following lumbar puncture in children and adolescents is of no benefit. Neurology 62 (6), 1003–1005.

Ellenby, S., Tegtmeyer, K., Lai, S., et al., 2006. Lumbar puncture. N. Engl. J. Med. 355 (13), e12.

Evans, R., 2000. Assessment: prevention of post-lumbar puncture headaches. Neurology 55, 909–914.

Gajjar, A., Harrison, P.L., Sandlund, J.T., et al., 2000. Traumatic lumbar punctures at diagnosis adversely affects outcome in childhood lymphoblastic leukaemia. Blood 96, 3381–3384.

Joffe, A.R., 2007. Lumbar puncture and brain herniation in acute bacterial meningitis. A review. J. Intensive Care Med. 22 (4), 194–207.

Kneen, R., Solomon, T., Appleton, R., 2002. The role of lumbar puncture in suspected CNS infection – A disappearing skill? Arch. Dis. Child 87 (3), 181–183.

Mackenzie, A., 2006. Management of procedure-related pain in children and adolescents. J. Paediatr. Child Health 42 (1–2), 14–15.

McArthur, J., 2002. Review: Longer bed rest does not prevent post puncture headaches than immediate mobilization or short bed rest. Evid. Based Nurs. 5 (3), 87.

National Service Framework for Children and Young People and Maternity Services, 2004. Core Standards. October.

Nelson, A.L., Fragel, G., Menzel, N.N., 2005. Myths and facts about back injuries in nursing. In: Nelson, A. (Ed.), Safe patient handling and movement. Springer, New York.

Owen, B.D., 2000. Preventing injuries using an ergonometric approach. AORN J. 72 (6), 1031–1036.

Patten, J., 1998. Neurological differential diagnosis, second ed. Springer, New York.

Pederson, C., 1996. Promoting parental use of non-pharmacological techniques with children during lumbar puncture. J. Paediatr. Oncol. Nurs. 13 (1), 21–30.

Robbins, K.B., 1990. Prolonged headache after a lumbar puncture. Clin. Paediatr. 29 (6), 350–352.

van Crevel, H., Hijdra, A., de Gans, L., 2002. Lumbar puncture and the risk of herniation: when should we first perform CT? J. Neurol. 249 (2), 129–137.

Vannorsdall, T., Dahlquist, L., Shroff Pendley, J., et al., 2004. The relationship between non essential touch and children's distress during lumbar puncture. Child Health Care 33 (4), 299–315.

Wojner, A.W., Malkoff, M., 2001. Lumbar puncture (perform). In: Lynn-McHale, D.J., Carlson, K.K. (Eds.), ACCN procedure manual for critical care. fourth ed. WB Saunders, Philadelphia, pp. 602–606.

Chapter 17

Neurological observations and coma scales

Alison Warren

CHAPTER CONTENTS

Introduction   182
   Learning outcomes   182
   Rationale   182
   Factors to note   183

Neonates   186

Sick children   186

Neurological assessment   187
   Guidelines   187
   Equipment   187
   Method   187
   Dos and don'ts   193

INTRODUCTION

Neurological observations enable the nurse to assess the neurological status of infants and children. A coma scale is a tool that instructs the assessor to perform and record a series of prescribed neurological and haemodynamic observations on a scaled chart. Results are plotted on each level of the scale and a corresponding number allotted. The numbers for the different observations are totalled to give an overall figure known as the coma scale rating, with a maximum score of 15 and a minimum score of 3. The lower the rating, the poorer the child's neurological status (James & Trauner 1985).

LEARNING OUTCOMES

By the end of this section you should be able to:

- Understand the importance of accurate neurological assessment
- List the different elements of neurological assessment
- Explain the significance of changes in the child's neurological status
- Understand how, when and why coma scales are utilised and appreciate their limitations.

RATIONALE

Deterioration in the level of consciousness can occur rapidly with devastating, sometimes fatal consequences which may only be averted with prompt action and treatment. Subtle changes in the neurological assessment may first be noted by a bedside nurse (Disabato & Burkett 2007). Therefore the ability to accurately assess the child's neurological status and interpret the results in order to detect promptly any alteration in conscious level is a vital skill for a children's nurse.

FACTORS TO NOTE

Rapid assessment

Initial management of an infant or child with a decreased conscious level is to support airway (immobilise cervical spine if trauma is suspected), breathing and circulation. A score (AVPU) has been introduced for rapid assessment of disability, particularly pre-hospital and in emergency departments. The score assesses neurological status as *alert* (A), responds to *voice* (V), responds to *pain* (P), or *unresponsive* (U) (ALSG, 2001). This scoring system, entitled the AVPU score, is simple to use and requires little training (Mackay et al 2000), allowing the observer to swiftly evaluate priorities of care without the need for additional charts or equipment. It does not, however, replace more accurate coma scales that are essential for serial assessment and evaluation of the patient's level of consciousness.

Coma scales

Coma scales were introduced in the early 1970s in a successful attempt to standardise nursing and medical approaches to neurological assessment (Teasdale & Jennett 1974). Coma scales cover the following five main assessment criteria:

- Eye opening
- Verbal response
- Motor response
- Equality, size and reaction of pupils to light
- Strength and spontaneity of limb movement.

The most commonly used coma scale is the Glasgow Coma Scale (GCS). Devised by Teasdale and Jennett (1974), this is an adult scale that has also been adapted for children in recognition of the fact that verbal and motor responses must be related to the child's age (Campbell & Glasper 1995).

There are various paediatric adaptations of the GCS, for example that of James and Trauner (1985), and its subsequent revision as the Birmingham Children's Hospital (BCH) model, as demonstrated in Table 17.1.

Another adapted GCS scale is known as the Paediatric Glasgow Coma Scale (PGCS) or Adelaide

scale. Physicians at Adelaide Children's Hospital first adapted it for use in paediatrics and their adaptations were to the verbal and motor responses. These were developed to correlate with expected developmental milestones of children of different ages. The adaptations themselves were minor. They expected nurses to be trained to use the tool and to be able to apply knowledge of normal development when assessing the verbal and motor components of the scale. Table 17.2 demonstrates how a nurse would be expected to interpret a score against normal, verbal developmental milestones.

The Advanced Life Support Group (ALSG, 1997) developed a simplified version of a children's coma scale for use in children under 4 years (Table 17.3).

Which scale to use is a matter of local choice according to the wishes of the multi-professional team. However, the nurse using the tool must have been given suitable tuition in how to use the tool and interpret the results, and be aware of the limitations of each scale. In addition, it must be remembered that the normal responses of a child who is developmentally delayed, or has an existing neurological deficit, may not fall within the specified age range, i.e. 'child over 5 years' and 'child under 5 years'. It has been suggested that age-related scales should be replaced with criteria that reflect patients' 'usual ability' to allow for infants/children who have not achieved recognised developmental milestones (Warren 2000).

Early warning systems

Many acute children's services are adopting Paediatric Early Warning Systems (PEWS) to assist in detecting children at risk of deterioration (Monaghan 2005). Most of these systems use age appropriate vital sign indicators to trigger intervention. PEWS scores have proved to identify patients at risk before a life threatening event occurs (Duncan et al 2006).

However, coma score evaluation is not always an integral part of PEWS documentation, therefore appropriate charting should be used in addition to detect neurological deficit according to local policy.

Applying a painful stimulus during neurological assessment

In a child who has a decreased conscious level, it is often necessary to apply a painful stimulus to evoke a response. The methods used to evoke a response

Table 17.1   BCH model, paediatric adaptation of Glasgow Coma Scale

	ADULT/CHILD ACCORDING TO USUAL ABILITY	CHILD/INFANT ACCORDING TO USUAL ABILITY	SCORE
Eyes open	Spontaneously – without stimulation	Spontaneously	4
	To verbal stimuli – when spoken to, not necessarily on command		3
	To pain – in response to any painful stimulus	To pain	2
	None – no eye opening at all		1
	Eyes closed due to swelling/bandage		C
Best verbal response	Oriented – able to give name and address in response to verbal question	Usual ability – alert, uses sentences if previously able; recognisable words if not yet able to make sentences; babbles and coos for child not yet able to make words	5
	Confused – able to converse but not oriented in person	Less than usual ability, confused or no longer able to talk in sentences/spontaneous irritable cry	4
	Inappropriate – recognisable words but not in an exchange	Cries to pain – cries only in response to painful stimuli	3
	Incomprehensible – grunts, groans, incomprehensible sounds	Only moans – but does not cry in response to painful stimuli	2
	None – no verbal response even to painful stimuli	None – no vocalisation, even to painful stimuli	1
Best motor response	Obeys commands – obeys verbal commands	Normal – normal play or voluntary or spontaneous movements	6
	Localises – hands move above chin in response to supraorbital pressure painful stimulus	Localises – as for adult/child or withdraws to painful stimulus	5
	Withdraws – movement of limb away from painful stimulus	Withdraws – as for adult/child	4
	Flexion abnormal – decorticate flexion at wrist and elbow, and abduction at shoulder to painful stimulus	Flexion abnormal – as for adult/child	3
	Extension abnormal – decerebrate extension to painful stimulus	Extension abnormal – as for adult/child	2
	None	None	1

C, closed. (Adapted from James & Trauner 1985).

differ according to Trust/hospital policies, personal preferences and expertise. Moreover, with a deteriorating conscious level, the necessity to accurately interpret a deficit in neurological status is of paramount importance so that the appropriate intervention can ensue. It is also essential that the choice of stimuli used, either peripheral or central, reflects the condition of the patient.

Frawley (1990) described the potential of damage to the nailbed following repetitive pressure assessments, thus advocating the use of side finger pressure. Following this article, many healthcare professionals adopted side finger pressure to avoid potential trauma, assuming peripheral pressure is advocated. However, many different modes of stimulus are regularly used in the paediatric setting, including squeezing the ear lobe, rubbing the sternum, pinching flesh under the arm,

squeezing the shoulder and supraorbital pressure, with the most common being either nailbed or side finger pressure. No method of painful stimulus is regarded as a gold standard in the assessment of infants and children and few of the above techniques have been validated in paediatric practice.

Side finger pressure is performed by placing the child's finger (third and fourth fingers are most sensitive) between the nurse's thumb and a pen or pencil and gradually increasing pressure until a response is obtained (Fig. 17.1).

Applying pressure to the nailbed is achieved in a similar way to that of side finger pressure but is contraindicated in patients with poor perfusion or reported coagulopathy. Moreover, nurses should also be aware of the limitations of 'peripheral' stimuli when assessing deeply comatosed patients.

Table 17.2   Paediatric Glasgow Coma Scale

	>1 YEAR	<1 YEAR	SCORE
Eye opening	Spontaneously	Spontaneously	4
	To verbal command	To shout	3
	To pain	To pain	2
	No response	No response	1
Best motor response	Obeys commands		5
	Localises pain	Localises pain	4
	Flexion to pain	Flexion to pain	3
	Extension to pain	Extension to pain	2
	No response	No response	1

	>5 YEARS	2–5 YEARS	0–2 YEARS	
Best verbal response	Orientated and converses	Appropriate words and phrases	Smiles and cries appropriately	5
	Disorientated and converses	Inappropriate words	Cries	4
	Inappropriate words	Cries	Inappropriate crying	3
	Incomprehensible sounds	Grunting	Grunting	2
	No response	No response	No response	1

Reproduced from Lloyd-Thomas (1990) by kind permission of the BMJ Publishing Group.

Table 17.3   Advanced Life Support Group children's coma scale: <4 years

RESPONSE	SCORE
Eyes	
Open spontaneously	4
React to speech	3
React to pain	2
No response	1
Best motor response	
Spontaneous or obeys verbal command	6
Reaction to painful stimulus	
Localises pain	5
Withdraws in response to pain	4
Abnormal flexion to pain (decorticate posture)	3
Abnormal extension to pain (decerebrate posture)	2
No response	1
Best verbal response	
Smiles, orientates to sounds, follows objects, interacts	5

CRYING	INTERACTS	
Consolable	Inappropriate	4
Inconsistently consolable	Moaning	3
Inconsolable	Irritable	2
No response	No response	1

Reproduced from Lawton (1995) by kind permission.

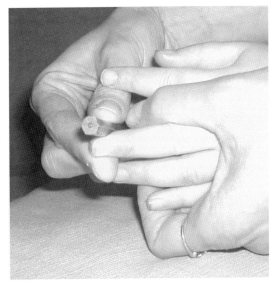

Figure 17.1 Side finger pressure.

Supraorbital pressure, or 'central stimuli', is regarded as a more accurate method of evoking response in patients in deep coma. It is particularly painful and should only be performed by staff aware of the contraindications of the procedure and who are competent and confident to do so safely. The advantage of this painful stimulus over 'peripheral' methods is to avoid eliciting reflex responses, particularly in the lower limbs, which could mislead the observer.

There are two factors of paramount importance when evoking a pain response in children with a diminished level of consciousness:

- That the mode of stimulus used is consistent, as variations can cause assessment anomalies. This can only be achieved by performing a full set of coma score observations at the bedside handover.
- That the assessing nurse is confident that the mode of painful stimulus used is sufficient to evoke a response. If there is any doubt, a senior nurse or doctor should be consulted.

NEONATES

Neonates are notoriously difficult to assess neurologically and certainly most existing coma scales, even those that are adapted for infants and children, are not sufficiently accurate when assessing a child under 6 months of age (Allan 1994). Tatman et al (1997) devised and tested a grimace score for infants and children unable to vocalise. It is an assessment of orofacial movement as opposed to a vocal response and has five elements (Table 17.4). Primarily aimed at intubated children in an intensive care unit, it has also proved effective for neonates and infants. Hazinski (1999) highlights the need to evaluate the baby's alertness and response to the environment, and Reeves (1989) highlights the importance of referring to the child's parents who are most cognisant of their child's normal behaviour. Palpation of the fontanelles is also beneficial when assessing for signs of elevated intracranial pressure (ICP) or volume status in an infant. The anterior fontanelle should feel firm and flat; however, it will bulge if pressure in the superior vena cava increases (a physiological sign of raised ICP or congenital heart failure). A sunken fontanelle is a sign of volume depletion and dehydration (Hazinski 1999). Measurement of head circumference and observing the shape of the skull can also be of significant value when assessing a neonate.

SICK CHILDREN

A decreased level of consciousness can be associated with a number of causes with the end result being alterations in cerebral blood flow causing hypoxia, ischaemia, cerebral oedema and raised ICP. Common causes of these conditions are listed in Box 17.1.

BOX 17.1   Possible causes of decreased conscious level in children

- Reduced cerebral blood flow caused by:
  a. Respiratory insufficiency
  b. Hypovolaemia
  c. Gross anaemia
  d. Poor cardiac output state
- Cerebral oedema caused by:
  a. Fluid overload
  b. Multisystem failure
  c. Seizures
  d. Hyperpyrexia
  e. Electrolyte imbalance
- Raised intracranial pressure due to:
  a. Hydrocephalus
  b. Space-occupying lesion
  c. Intracerebral bleeding (traumatic or spontaneous)
  d. Meningitis
  e. Trauma/head injury
  f. Arterial blood gas abnormality, e.g. raised PCO_2
- Encephalopathy due to:
  a. Infection, e.g. Chickenpox, herpes
  b. Sepsis
  c. Liver disease
  d. Renal disease
  e. Ingestion of toxins
  f. Hypo/hyperglycaemia
- Blood clots or air emboli caused by intravenous therapy, invasive monitoring or extracorporeal techniques.

Table 17.4   Grimace score

OROFACIAL RESPONSE	SCORE
Spontaneous normal facial/oromotor activity, e.g. sucks tube, coughs	5
Less than usual spontaneous ability or only responds to touch	4
Vigorous grimace to pain	3
Mild grimace or some change in facial expression to pain	2
No response to pain	1

After Tatman et al (1997).

It is worth noting that comatosed children require and respond to stimulation, both verbal and touch (Hendrickson 1987, Hobdell et al 1989).

In a review of major research studies, Chudley (1994) describes how some nursing interventions can cause an increase in ICP in patients with previously raised ICP. Suctioning of an endotracheal tube, repositioning/turning, moving the neck from the midline, clustering of care activities and invasive procedures, e.g. passing a nasogastric tube, are all mentioned. This highlights the importance of planning care to ensure minimal handling, with periods of rest to allow the ICP to stabilise or return to a baseline between care episodes, for any child with an actual or suspected raised ICP. However, decisions about timing of care must always be carefully balanced with the need to monitor closely in order to determine and act swiftly on any detrimental changes in the child's condition.

NEUROLOGICAL ASSESSMENT

GUIDELINES

The important role which parents play in the neurological assessment of a child must be further stressed. A frightened child is unlikely to cooperate, particularly if asked by a stranger to obey commands whether or not the child is physically able to do so. However, they may respond to requests made by their parents, rather than a nurse. Hazinski (1999) describes phrasing questions to the child around people and things that are familiar to them, for example using a popular children's television character. This information will of course be gained from the initial history taken from the child (if able) or family (see Ch. 6). It is also of value to remember that head injury in a child, or baby, could be non-accidental, therefore child protection procedures should be instigated according to local policy and the interactions between the child and parents monitored closely.

EQUIPMENT

- Thermometer
- Blood pressure monitor
- Pen or pencil
- Pen torch or ophthalmoscope
- Colourful and noisy toys if appropriate
- Paediatric neurological observation assessment tool/recording chart.

METHOD

Initial observations

Always ensure the child's airway (± cervical spine), breathing and circulation are stable.

- *Airway* – check the patency and maintenance of the airway (if cervical spine injury is suspected, ensure immobilisation)
- *Breathing* – evaluate respiratory rate, air entry, work of breathing and colour
- *Circulation* – evaluate heart rate, peripheral and central pulses, skin perfusion and blood pressure (Resuscitation Council (UK) 2004) (see also Ch. 8).

Appropriate emergency equipment should be available to monitor and support ABC before (D) disability (neurological status) is assessed.

1. Collect equipment together, approach the child, and try to gain their confidence. Remember a child may not be cooperative, particularly if they are frightened or in pain.
2. Before undertaking physical observations, assess the child's clinical signs and behaviour generally, taking into account pre-existing conditions, previous hospital admissions, past medical history and the knowledge gained from the initial history-taking assessment.
   a. Is the child asleep or awake, settled and peaceful or irritable and unhappy?
   b. Note their general colour – is there evidence of pallor, redness, mottling or cyanosis? All over or in specific areas?
   c. Do they appear bothered by bright lights (photophobia)?
   d. Do they seem reluctant to move their head or cry out if their legs are straightened?
   e. Is the child sleeping or unusually quiet? Note their effort and efficacy of breathing – is it regular and easy, or shallow, laboured or irregular? Are there any audible respiratory noises, e.g. wheeze, grunting, stridor, etc.?
   f. Observe the eyes – is there evidence of bulging, deviation, drooping of the eyelids or 'sun setting' (the sclera being visible above the iris)? Is there any discoloration of the sclera or pupils?
   g. Smell their breath – can the odour of alcohol, solvents or ketones be detected?
   h. Are there any rashes, skin lesions and/or discoloration? A purpuric rash (purple/red spots) which does not blanch white if the skin

is rubbed/depressed with a finger could be suggestive of meningococcal infection; café au lait spots (coffee-coloured patches on the skin) is an indicator of neurofibromatosis; jaundice is a sign of hepatic dysfunction and possible encephalopathy.

i. Is there evidence of seizure activity? If so, observe carefully, ensuring airway maintenance, record and report (see Ch. 26).

j. If the child is awake and conscious, utilise normal play to assess the conscious level, in particular, eye, motor and verbal responses in accordance with coma score documentation.

k. Does the child respond appropriately, both verbally and physically, according to age and expected developmental milestones? Remember that the effects of hospitalisation can cause psychological upset (Fletcher 1981), therefore behavioural changes could be associated with the fact that the child is in an unfamiliar and often frightening environment.

3. What sort of position has the child adopted? If mobilising, observe posture and gait – are the limbs flaccid or rigid when moved? In neonates and infants, a typical sign of cerebral irritation is back arching and muscle rigidity – opisthotonos – accompanied by a high-pitched cry.

4. Summarise the initial assessment. Is there any cause for concern such as unusual, unexplained irritability? Severe agitation in a child, or baby, can be a sign of cerebral irritation and deterioration of conscious level.

5. If any anomalies have been detected inform a senior nurse or doctor immediately and proceed with the coma score assessment to ascertain if there is any further evidence of neurological deficit.

Assessment

It is advocated that a full coma score assessment is performed at every nursing handover to reduce the potential discrepancy between observers.

Before commencing, always check if the child/infant is on medication or has a pre-existing condition that could affect 'normal' parameters or behaviour. Information should be gained from the parents/primary carer in regard to the child's normal behaviour and whether or not they have reached developmental milestones (access to the child's 'Red Book' may be helpful).

1. Explain to the child, if applicable, and parents, what you are about to do. Stress that the observations will not hurt.

2. Assess and record any observations which do not require physical intervention, e.g. respirations (see Ch. 6).

3. Then proceed to recordings of temperature, pulse and blood pressure.

a. *Temperature*: Observe for swings in temperature; hyperpyrexia can be indicative of raised ICP due to pressure on the hypothalamus disrupting thermoregulation (Sherman 1990). Hyperpyrexia also increases cerebral metabolic rate, cerebral blood flow and cerebral oxygen consumption which further increases ICP (Hall 1997). Hypothermia can affect haemodynamic values (cardiac arrhythmias are not uncommon) and conscious level due to decreased cerebral metabolism and cerebral blood flow (Dennis & Mayer 2001).

b. *Pulse rate*: Severe, raised ICP can be indicated by bradycardia caused by excessive pressure on the medulla; however, this is a late 'pre-terminal' sign in children and emergency assistance should be sought (Sherburne & Curtis 1990). Tachycardia could be attributed to a number of things including pain, infection, medications or blood loss.

c. *Blood pressure*: Hypertension again can be a late sign of raised ICP in children due to pressure on the medulla, particularly when associated with bradycardia; this is a life-threatening event requiring immediate intervention (Hazinski 1999). Increases in systolic arterial pressure also occur if ICP is high; this is a physiological response to maintain cerebral perfusion – a phenomenon called autoregulation (Hazinski 1999). Other causes such as pain and anxiety should also be taken into account if the blood pressure is elevated. The phenomenon described as Cushing's triad – hypertension, bradycardia and respiratory depression – is a very late sign of severe, acute, irreversible brain damage with a high risk of mortality (Sherburne & Curtis 1990).

d. *Respiratory rate*: An abnormal respiratory rate can be attributed to a number of factors, e.g. anxiety, pain, infection, pyrexia or hypovolaemia. However, with suspected raised ICP, pressure on the medulla depresses the respiratory centre; therefore respiratory insufficiency can be a sign of brain stem compression (Hazinski 1999).

4. Eye opening, verbal/grimace and motor responses should be assessed simultaneously; all scores should be recorded in the appropriate section of the assessment chart.

a. If the infant/child has their eyes open and is responding to the environment, is vocalising and moving all limbs, then they would score the maximum – 15 (Tables 17.1–17.3).

b. If the child is non-vocal or intubated then a grimace score is advocated (to maintain a maximum score of 15). In some cases neonates/infants are easier to score using this system as facial expression or grimace can ensure accuracy of neurological assessment (see Point 7 below).

5. Pupil reactions: Indicate 3rd cranial nerve (Oculomotor) function, and ICP, pupils should be of equal size and react briskly and equally to light. Any inequality of pupil size or reaction is indicative of a problem on the same side of the brain as the abnormal reaction. Fixed dilated pupils can be an ominous sign indicating brain stem herniation (coning). However, hypothermia and some drugs (e.g. large doses of atropine, some ophthalmic drugs) can cause dilated pupils. Similarly, certain pharmacological agents can cause pinpoint pupils (Fig. 17.2)

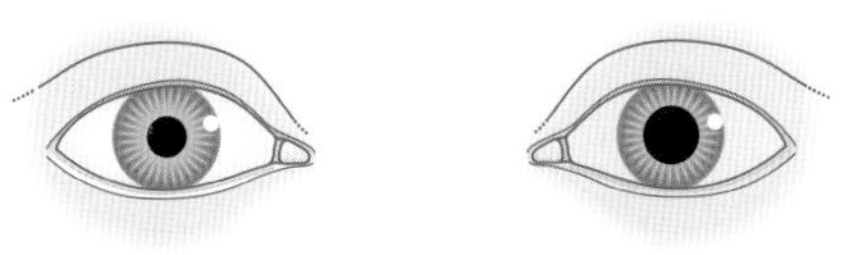	Unequal (anisocoria)	Compression caused by herniation
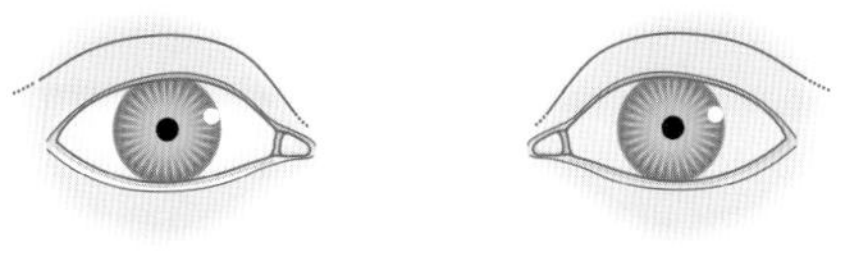	Constricted (miosis)	Pontine haemorrhage, carotid injury, ischaemia Consider pharmacological agents, e.g. opiates
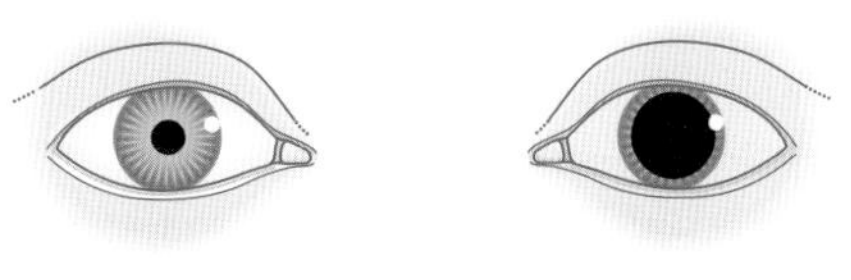	Unilateral dilated (unilateral mydriatic)	Third cranial nerve (oculomotor) damage, damage to mid brain ICP, severe anoxia-ischaemia. Often a pre-morbid sign (coning)
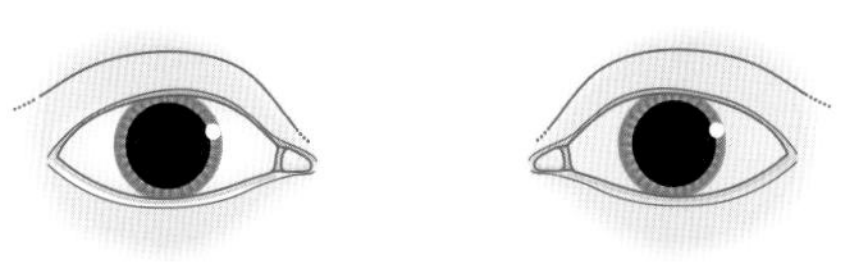	Bilateral dilated (bilateral mydriatic)	Third cranial nerve (oculomotor) damage, damage to mid brain ICP, severe anoxia-ischaemia. Often a pre-morbid sign (coning)
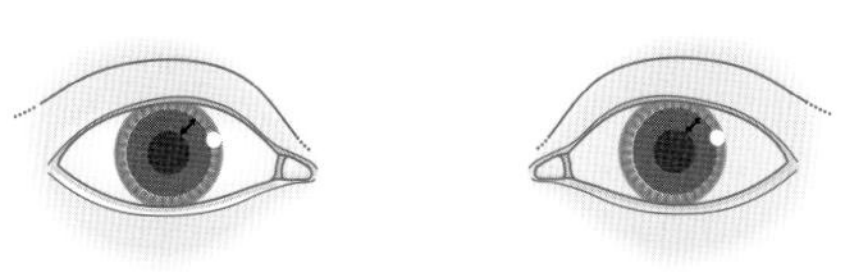	Spasmodic changes (Hippus)	Pressure on third cranial nerve, transtentorial brain herniation
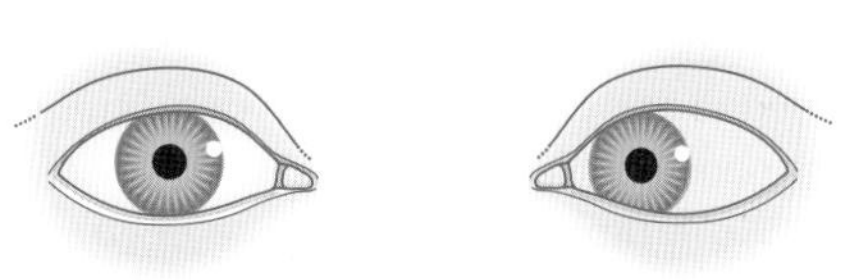	Squint	Compression of fifth cranial nerve (abducens) may indicate brain stem lesion
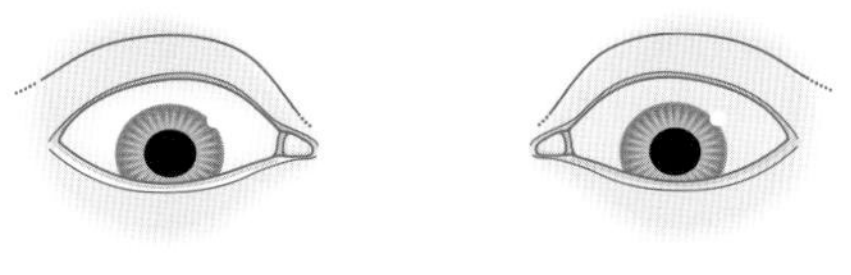	Depressed eyes – 'sun setting'	Pressure on the orbital roof of third ventricle may indicate hydrocephalus

Figure 17.2 Guide to abnormal pupillary response.

a. It is important to assess and record the size and equality of the child's pupils *before* shining light into them.

b. Is there any evidence of a squint or deviation which was previously unreported?

c. If the child is asleep, try and rouse them first. If they cannot open their eyes, it may be necessary for the nurse to lift the eyelids. It is important that both lids are lifted simultaneously; this may require two people.

d. Ideally, pupil reactions should be tested by turning off the main overhead lights and shining a bright, narrow beam directly onto the pupil.

e. Note the size of the pupil and observe whether the pupil reacts to light. Does it contract briskly (+), is it sluggish (S) or non-reactive (−)?

f. A child who has been deeply asleep or sedated may be reluctant to open their eyes and, likewise, pupils may be a little sluggish to react at first.

g. With a child unwilling to cooperate, give them the torch to play with and observe what happens from a short distance away; flick the lights on and off until you observe pupillary response.

h. Be aware that pupil reactions can be affected by pre-existing conditions and pharmacological agents.

i. Coma score documentation should incorporate a scaled guide to pupillary response to ensure consistency of the observer's recordings (Fig 17.3).

6. Verbal response: (for verbal scores in the child/infant, see Tables 17.1–17.3).

a. Is the child alert, vocalising and able to concentrate on what is being said to them? Listen – are they chatting apparently normally, aware of their surroundings and parents?

b. Is a baby babbling or cooing?

c. Is the toddler making words and noises which are normal for them? (Check with parents.) They may appear confused due to unfamiliarity with the surroundings.

d. Is any crying appropriate and can it be consoled by parents or with distraction techniques? Is it associated with pain, fear or hunger?

e. If an infant is crying, does it sound particularly high pitched? An abnormally

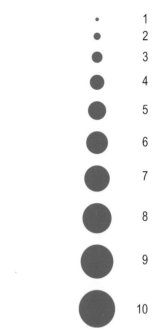

Figure 17.3 Pupillary sizing.

high-pitched cry in a baby can be due to raised ICP or cerebral irritation.

f. Grunting noises in any child/infant are a sign that something is seriously wrong.

g. The child who makes no noise or facial expression could be deeply unconscious.

7. Grimace score: As previously mentioned, the grimace score is recommended as a verbal score alternative and is commonly used in the assessment of children/infants who have an endotracheal or tracheostomy tube *in situ* (in the absence of muscle relaxants) (Tatman et al 1997). However, this score has proved to be useful and less susceptible to observer error in neonates and infants where definition of vocal response can be misleading, particularly to a novice. Moreover, anecdotal evidence demonstrates that children who are uncooperative, postictal, receiving sedation/analgesia, have documented learning or sensory disability or are experiencing a language barrier have been neurologically evaluated with greater reliability using this scoring method. The grimace score is a 5-point scale that corresponds to the verbal score, but reflects cerebral function by the assessment of oromotor or facial responses (Fig. 17.4, Table 17.4).

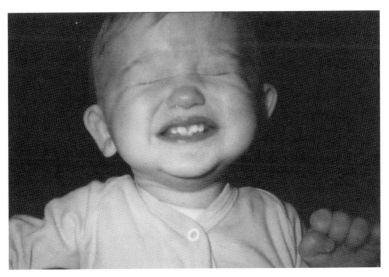

Figure 17.4 Vigorous grimace to pain.

8. Motor response: Assess the child's movements (for motor response scores in the child/infant, see Tables 17.1–17.3). A decreasing conscious level can be determined by abnormalities in motor response.

a. Is the child playing with toys or feeding from a bottle using both hands?

b. Can they grasp your fingers equally in strength with both hands? Can they push your hand away?

c. Do the legs move normally – kicking or reacting if their feet are tickled?

d. If the child is not moving, can a response be elicited by asking them to move, e.g. 'Can you lift your arm for me?' Are the movements equal? What about symmetry of movement?

e. Does the infant reach towards a noisy toy or move lower limbs if tickled?

f. Pay particular attention to the muscle tone – are the limbs stiff (hypertonia) or flaccid/floppy (hypotonia)?

g. Decorticate posturing (abnormal flexion) is an indication of neurological deterioration. The child displays involuntary flexion of the limbs with adduction to the midline (Fig. 17.5A).

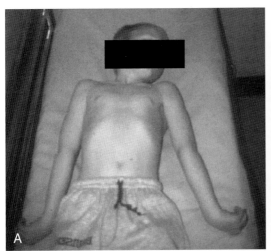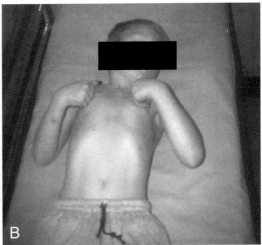

Figure 17.5 Posturing: (A) decorticate; (B) decerebrate. *(Courtesy of APLS.)*

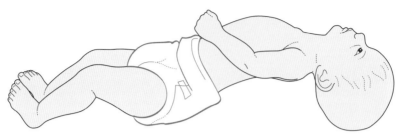

Figure 17.6 Opisthotonos.

If deterioration continues, decerebrate posturing (abnormal extension) ensues, the limbs increase in tone, straighten and are abducted away from the midline (Fig. 17.5B). A child can alternate between decorticate and decerebrate posturing as a result of fluctuating cerebral blood flow to the brain stem and cerebral hemispheres. Opisthotonos is a sign of cerebral/meningeal irritation, particularly in neonates and infants; it also occurs with depressed brain function and injury to the brain. Rigid body spasms cause the back to arch and the head and limbs to hyper-extend. Opisthotonos is an ominous neurological sign (Fig. 17.6).

h. If there is no movement, a sufficient painful stimulus must be used to evoke a response.

i. For a child to localise they must physically try to remove the person or object causing the pain, for example, grasping or pushing away the assessor's hand. Babies cannot localise but should withdraw the limb from the painful stimuli.

j. If the child is old enough/developmentally capable, ask them to close their eyes and touch their nose with the tip of their finger; this tests proprioception, the awareness of parts of the body in space without looking.

9. Strength and spontaneity of limb movement: Limb strength/power should be recorded for both the right and the left side of the body. Any notable inequality of the two sides can indicate a problem occurring in one side of the brain. If hypo or hypertonia is present, is it evident in all limbs equally or just affect one side of the body?

a. Is one or more of the limbs weaker than the others?

b. Observe the conscious child at play – are all limbs being used equally?

c. Is the child sitting straight or showing a tendency to lean to one side?

d. In an infant, check their grasp – do they reach for toys, kick their legs?

e. Request the older child to wiggle their fingers and toes, kick with their legs and wave their arms.

The spontaneity of movements should be recorded independently to the strength/power. A child may display involuntary spontaneous movements but show no reaction to command or painful stimuli; this is a significant neurological indicator requiring documentation and reporting.

Observations

- All observations must be recorded on coma scale, neurological chart or PEWS documentation (a modified paediatric coma scale is preferable but not essential).

- Total the score for all observations (maximum 15, minimum 3). Interpret, compare with previous observations (if recorded), evaluate and report findings.

- Is the child improving or deteriorating? Are there any observations which cause concern?

- Assess when subsequent observations should be performed. Generally, in the acutely unstable child/infant, a repeat set should be carried out within 15 min. As the condition stabilises, observations can be reduced; however, assessments used to determine deterioration in neurological status should not be performed any greater than hourly.

- Some paediatric centres have additional documentation to record 'significant events' and 'special instructions' that are facilitated to record additional information pertinent to the patient's neurological status and management, thus assisting in the evaluation of coma score and neurological status in children and infants (Warren 2000).

- For the intensive care child, if muscle relaxants are infusing, pupillary reaction is the only definitive observation that can be performed, although there are other indicators that can assist with neurological assessment. However, once paralysing agents are discontinued, regular observations should be recommenced. Accepting that sedation and analgesia will alter conscious level, the child should respond to tactile or painful stimuli and much can be gained from 30-min to 1-hourly monitoring of pupil, grimace and motor responses.

Complications

There are no procedural complications associated with neurological assessment. However, hazards lie in user error:

- The inexperienced practitioner inaccurately undertaking observations without adequate supervision/training
- Misinterpretation of observational results: if a nurse is unsure of the implications of the neurological observation results, the advice of a senior colleague or doctor should be sought.

COMMUNITY PERSPECTIVE

Neurological assessment is a procedure that would not often be undertaken in the home. However, there will be occasions when carers and professionals involved in the child's care will need to be aware of altering levels of consciousness, for example in a child with a life-limiting condition or needing palliative care. It is unlikely that formal recording of observations will be appropriate and admission to hospital should be an option if the carers are concerned or unable to cope at home.

The role of the CCN would be to raise the awareness of the carers without causing apprehension, showing them how to undertake any monitoring required. During visits routine assessment of the child's neurological status should be performed and compared with the carers' observations. Findings will then be documented and liaison maintained with medical staff as necessary.

DOS AND DON'TS

- Do ensure that airway, breathing and circulation are stable and maintained.
- Do remember that a child's neurological status can deteriorate rapidly; be alert for signs of raised intracranial pressure.
- Do remember to gain as much information about the child's/infant's usual activities and capabilities: observe movements, vocal ability and reaction to the surroundings prior to neurological assessment.
- Do remember that the child's parents are invaluable when trying to ascertain what is normal or abnormal for their child; this information will aid evaluation of neurological status.
- Do report any abnormalities, however trivial as they could be a sign that the child's condition is altering.
- Do ensure that painful stimuli are adequate to evoke a response. If in doubt, consult a senior nurse/doctor.
- Do be aware of the limitations and contraindications of peripheral stimuli and be knowledgeable of other methods of evoking a pain response.
- Do perform a bedside handover to reduce the risk of misinterpretation of the same physical signs.
- Do not omit neurological observations. If the child/infant is sleeping, a sleeping child could be comatosed.

References

Advanced Life Support Group, 1997. Advanced paediatric life support: the practical approach. second ed. BMJ Publications, London, p. 119.

Advanced Life Support Group, 2001. Advanced paediatric life support: the practical approach. third ed. BMJ Publications, London, p. 17.

Allan, D., 1994. Paediatric coma scale. Surg. Nurs. 7 (3), 14–16.

Campbell, S., Glasper, E.A. (Eds.), 1995. Whaley and Wong's

children's nursing. UK ed. Mosby/Times Mirror International, London, pp. 660–679.

Chudley, S., 1994. The effect of nursing activities on intracranial pressure. Br. J. Nurs. 3 (9), 454–459.

Dennis, L.J., Mayer, S.A., 2001. Diagnosis and management of increased intracranial pressure. Neurol India 49 (Suppl 1), S37–S50.

Disabato, J., Burkett, K., 2007. Nursing care of the pediatric neurosurgery patient. Springer Berlin, Heidelberg, pp. 1–27.

Duncan, H., Hutchison, J., Parshuram, C.S., 2006. The pediatric early warning system score: A severity of illness score to predict urgent medical need in hospitalized children. J. Crit. Care 21 (3), 271–278.

Fletcher, B., 1981. Psychological upset in posthospitalized children: a review of the literature. Matern. Child Nurs. J. 10, 185–195.

Frawley, P., 1990. Neurological observations. Nurs. Times 86 (35), 29–34.

Hall, C.A., 1997. Patient management in head injury care: a nursing perspective. Intensive Crit. Care Nurs. 13, 329–337.

Hazinski, M.F., 1999. Manual of pediatric critical care. Mosby Year Book, St Louis.

Hendrickson, S.L., 1987. Intracranial pressure changes and family presence. J. Neurosci. Nurs. 19 (1), 14–17.

Hobdell, E.F., Adams, F., Caruso, J., et al., 1989. The effect of nursing activities on the intracranial pressure of children. Crit. Care Nurse 9 (6), 75–79.

James, H.E., Trauner, D.A., 1985. The Glasgow Coma Scale. In: James, H.E., Anas, N.G., Perkin, R.M. (Eds.), Brain insults in infants and children. Grune and Stratton, Orlando, pp. 179–182.

Lawton, L., 1995. Paediatric trauma – the care of Anthony. Accid. Emerg. Nurs. 3 (4), 172–176.

Lloyd-Thomas, A.R., 1990. Primary survey and resuscitation – II. Br. Med. J. 301, 380–382.

Mackay, C.A., Burke, D.P., Burke, J.A., et al., 2000. Association between the assessment of conscious level using the AVPU system and the Glasgow coma scale. Pre-hospital Immediate Care 4, 17–19.

Monaghan, A., 2005. Dectecting and managing deterioration in children. Paediatr. Nurs. 17 (1), 32–35.

Reeves, K., 1989. Assessment of pediatric head injury. J. Emerg. Nurs. 15 (4), 329–332.

Resuscitation Council (UK), 2004. European paediatric life support course, provider manual. Resuscitation Council (UK), London.

Sherburne, D., Curtis, B., 1990. Disorders of brain function. In: Porth, C. (Ed.), Pathophysiology: concepts of altered health states. Lippincott, New York, pp. 929–968.

Sherman, D., 1990. Managing acute head injury. Nursing 90, 47–52.

Tatman, A., Warren, A., Williams, A., et al., 1997. Development of a paediatric coma scale in intensive care clinical practice. Arch. Dis. Child 77 (6), 519–521.

Teasdale, G., Jennett, W.B., 1974. Assessment of coma and impaired consciousness. A practical scale. Lancet 2, 81–84.

Warren, A., 2000. Paediatric coma scoring researched and benchmarked. Paediatr. Nurs. 12 (3), 14–17.

Further reading

NICE, 2003. Head injury. Triage, assessment and early management of head injury in infants, children and adults. National Institute for Clinical Excellence, London. Online. Available: www.nice.org.uk.

SIGN, 2000. Early management of patients with a head injury. Publication 46. Scottish Intercollegiate Guidelines Network, Edinburgh. Online. Available: www.sign.ac.uk.

Westbrook, A., 1997. The use of a paediatric coma scale for monitoring infants and young children with head injuries. Nurs. Crit. Care 2 (2), 72–75.

Chapter 18

Phototherapy

Susan Alexander

CHAPTER CONTENTS

Introduction   195
   Learning outcomes   195
   Rationale   195
   Factors to note   196

Phototherapy   196
   Equipment   196
   Method   197
   Dos and don'ts   198

INTRODUCTION

Hyperbilirubinaemia, commonly referred to as jaundice, is a condition wherein the production of bilirubin is greater than its elimination (Boyd 2004). Management of this condition is dependent on the cause and can be either by phototherapy or in extreme cases, by exchange transfusion. This chapter will review the use of phototherapy which consists of the application of fluorescent light to reduce the serum bilirubin level of an infant. This light is normally a mixture of blue and white radiant light and is not in the ultraviolet range (Metherall 2003).

LEARNING OUTCOMES

By the end of this section you should be able to:

- Identify the infant with a raised serum bilirubin level
- Initiate phototherapy, as directed by medical staff, safely and appropriately
- Understand the needs of the infant undergoing phototherapy
- Recognise any adverse reactions
- Explain the need for phototherapy to the parents/primary care-givers.

RATIONALE

The primary aim of phototherapy is to prevent kernicterus, i.e. severe, permanent neurodevelopmental handicap caused by persistent raised serum unconjugated bilirubin (Stokowski 2006, Boyd 2004).

FACTORS TO NOTE

Normal red blood cell life in the adult human is approximately 120 days. In the neonate this is reduced to a lifespan of between 40 and 70 days (Boyd 2004).

Red blood cells are broken down in the spleen (by the reticuloendothelial system) and to a lesser extent in the liver. Bilirubin is one of the end-products of red blood cell breakdown, being derived from the haem part of haemoglobin (Fig. 18.1). Bilirubin, unconjugated, is not water soluble and is toxic to the body at high levels. If not converted to the water-soluble (conjugated) bilirubin, the unconjugated bilirubin will be deposited in the brain cells, which will lead to a condition called kernicterus (Stokowski 2006).

Unconjugated bilirubin is transported in the bloodstream bound to albumin, a plasma protein, to the liver where, following a complex process of enzyme actions, it is converted to conjugated bilirubin (Stokowski 2006).

Conjugated bilirubin is water soluble and is excreted by the liver via the biliary system into the intestine (Stokowski 2006).

In the intestine the bilirubin is converted to urobilinogen, some of which is absorbed by the enterohepatic circulation and is eventually excreted in the urine. The majority of the urobilinogen is oxidised in the colon to a brown pigment, urobilin,

which is excreted in the stool (Merenstein & Gardner 2006). An increase in serum bilirubin causes jaundice, a yellow/amber discoloration of the skin, also seen in the sclera of the eyes and mucous membranes (AAP 2004). This is seen when the serum bilirubin rises above 80 micromoles (µmol) per litre. Approximately 60% of normal newborns will be clinically jaundiced sometime during the first week of life (Maisels & McDonagh 2008). Often, the nurse who notices the infant's jaundice initiates the checking of the serum bilirubin level (Truman 2003). In the majority of cases this is relatively benign; however, close monitoring of the serum bilirubin level is important because of the risk of kernicterus (Maisels & McDonagh 2008).

An early high level of serum bilirubin, normally within the first 24 h of life, may indicate ABO or Rhesus incompatibility. Persistent jaundice after the first week of life must be fully investigated to determine the cause. Biliary atresia is one condition where the prognosis is improved with an early diagnosis (Merenstein & Gardner 2006, Kelly & Davenport 2007).

Breast milk jaundice is a benign condition, which may persist up to 3 months after birth and is thought to be caused by a factor within the breast milk which inhibits bilirubin conjugation (Percival 2003, Alex & Gallant 2008).

Estimations can be made using a transcutaneous bilirubin monitor; however, the serum level should always be obtained before phototherapy is commenced (Truman, 2003). Phototherapy is ineffective before the infant is jaundiced; hence it cannot be used prophylactically. However, early use in infants with known haemolytic disease is indicated as a means of control of the serum bilirubin level. Initiation of therapy is dependent not only on the serum bilirubin, but also the gestational age at birth of the infant (Percival 2003). Pre-term and sick infants are more prone to the complications of jaundice; hence phototherapy is initiated at lower serum bilirubin levels.

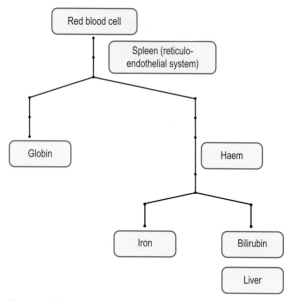

Figure 18.1 Breakdown of red blood cells.

PHOTOTHERAPY

EQUIPMENT

- Open cot, baby therm or incubator
- Phototherapy unit(s)
- Eye shield/cover.

METHOD

Commencement of phototherapy is determined by the serum unconjugated bilirubin level (Metherall 2003, Truman 2003, Nurse 2009). The following guidelines refer to the use of a phototherapy unit (Fig. 18.2). Some neonatal units, however, use fibreoptic blankets, known as 'bili blankets', which are wrapped around the infant (Mills & Tudehope 2001, Nurse 2009).

1. The infant is placed naked, with gonads protected, into an open cot, baby therm or incubator.

2. The phototherapy unit is placed over the infant, approximately 45 cm above the body. *Note:* The units are normally fixed onto stands at this height. More than one unit may be used.

3. The infant's eyes are covered to prevent retinal damage (Ostrowski et al 2000).

4. The phototherapy unit is switched on; treatment can be given continuously or intermittently.

5. The infant should be turned on a regular basis, every 2 h, to ensure that all of the skin is exposed. However, it must be noted that some authors advocate that changing position frequently has no effect on the efficacy of phototherapy (Chen et al 2002, Shinwell et al 2002).

6. The phototherapy unit should be switched off when the infant is being fed or the eye shields are removed.

7. The duration of treatment will be determined by the level of serum unconjugated bilirubin.

8. In some areas, the nursing staff may be responsible for checking the serum bilirubin level by capillary heel stab.

9. Where the infant is being constantly observed, protective glasses should be available for staff use.

10. Care should be coordinated (clustered care) to ensure minimal disruption to the infant.

Observations and complications

- Check the infant's temperature regularly as infants are prone both to hypothermia (due to being naked) and to hyperthermia because of heat radiated from the phototherapy unit (Walker et al 2007)

- Cyanosis can be missed – if the infant's condition is unstable, monitor oxygen saturations continuously or as condition determines (Nurse 2009)

- Increase fluid intake by 25–30% (or as determined by local policy) to maintain

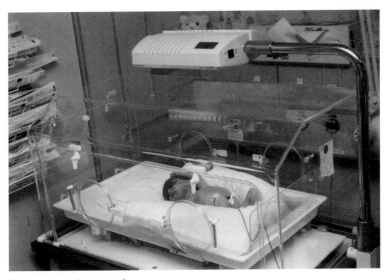

Figure 18.2 Infant under the phototherapy unit.

hydration, as the infant's insensible losses are known to rise (Boyd 2004). Weigh the infant daily to determine fluid requirements (Nurse 2009)

- Cover the gonads of the very and extremely low birth weight infants; this has to be balanced with maximum skin exposure. DNA mutations and breaks have been reported with the use of phototherapy (Edwards 1995).
- Check skin colour using daylight, as assessment of jaundice is often difficult under artificial light (Blackwell 2003).
- Loose green stools are common during treatment. Stools should be monitored, as fluid loss may increase as a result of frequent loose stools.
- Ensure that the infant's eyes remain closed when shields are in place, as corneal abrasions may occur. The shields should be removed and the eyes checked on a regular basis (Ostrowski et al 2000).
- The effect of phototherapy on the eyes is uncertain. However, animal studies indicate that retinal degeneration can occur if there is continuous exposure (Sisson 1970).
- The infant may become lethargic, irritable and develop poor feeding.
- Tanning and rashes are common. This is referred to as 'bronze baby syndrome' (Watchko & Maisels 2003).

DOS AND DON'TS

- Do encourage parents to be involved in care.
- Do ensure that care is clustered.
- Do encourage mothers to continue with breastfeeding.
- Do ensure that the position of the infant is changed to ensure maximum exposure.
- Do not use creams, lotions or oils on the infant's skin, as they may cause burning.
- Do not remove the eye shields while the phototherapy unit is in operation.

References

American Academy of Pediatrics, 2004. Management of hyperbilirubinemia in the newborn infant of 35 or more weeks of gestation. Pediatrics 114, 297–316.

Alex, M., Gallant, D.P., 2008. Toward understanding the connections between infant jaundice and infant feeding. J. Pediatr. Nurs. 23 (6), 429–438.

Blackwell, J.T., 2003. Management of hyperbilirubinaemia in the healthy term newborn. J. Am. Acad. Nurse Pract. 15 (5), 194–198.

Boyd, S., 2004. Treatment of physiological and pathological neonatal jaundice. Nurs. Times 100, 40–43.

Chen, C.M., Liu, S.H., Lai, C.C., et al., 2002. Changing position does not improve the efficacy of conventional phototherapy. Acta Paediatr. Taiwan. 43, 255–258.

Edwards, S., 1995. Phototherapy and the neonate: providing safe and effective nursing care for jaundiced infants. J. Neonatal Nurs. 1 (5), 9–12.

Kelly, D.A., Davenport, M., 2007. Current management of biliary atresia. Arch. Dis. Child. 92, 1132–1135.

Maisels, M.J., McDonagh, A.F., 2008. Phototherapy for neonatal jaundice. N. Engl. J. Med. 358 (9), 920–928.

Merenstein, G.B., Gardner, S.L., 2006. Handbook of intensive care, sixth ed. Mosby, St Louis.

Metherall, J., 2003. Phototherapy for neonatal hyperbilirubinaemia: delivering an adequate dose. J. Neonatal Nurs. 9 (6), 182–186.

Mills, J.F., Tudehope, D., 2001. Fibreoptic phototherapy for neonatal jaundice. Cochrane Database Syst. Rev. 1, CD002060.

Nurse, S., 2009. Neonatal jaundice and phototherapy. In: Kelsey, J., Ewing, G. (Eds.), Child health practice. Churchill Livingstone, Edinburgh.

Ostrowski, G., Pye, S.D., Laing, I., 2000. Do phototherapy hoods really protect the neonate? Acta Paediatr. 89, 874–877.

Percival, P., 2003. Jaundice and infection. In: Fraser, D., Cooper, M. (Eds.), Myles textbook for midwives. fourteenth ed. Churchill Livingstone, Edinburgh.

Shinwell, E.S., Sciaky, Y., Karplus, M., 2002. Effect of position on bilirubin levels during phototherapy. J. Perinatol. 22 (3), 226–229.

Sisson, T., 1970. Retinal changes produced by phototherapy. J. Paediatr. 77, 251.

Stokowski, L.A., 2006. Fundamentals of phototherapy for neonatal jaundice. Adv. Neonatal Care 6 (6), 303–312.

Truman, P., 2003. Jaundice in the preterm infant. J. Neonatal Nurs. 9 (1), 22–26.

Walker, L., Vroman, L., Becker, J., et al., 2007. Open crib phototherapy: using evidence to change practice. Nurs. Women's Health 11 (4), 402–404.

Watchko, J.F., Maisels, M.J., 2003. Jaundice in low birthweight infants: pathobiology and outcome. Arch. Dis. Child Fetal Neonatal Ed. 88, 455–458.

Further reading

Romagnoli, C., Zecca, E., Papacci, P., et al., 2006. Which phototherapy system is most effective in lowering serum bilirubin in very preterm infants? Fetal Diagn. Ther. 21, 204–209

Chapter 19

Cast care

Lynne Chadburn

CHAPTER CONTENTS

Introduction   200
   Learning outcomes   200
   Rationale   200
   Factors to note   201

Application of the cast   204
   Equipment   204
   Method   204
   Observations and complications   205

Advice to carers   206
   Hygiene and skin care   206
   Positioning and safety   207
   Eating and drinking   207
   Sleeping   207
   Mobility   207

Removal of a cast   207
   Equipment   207
   Method   207
   Dos and don'ts   209

INTRODUCTION

Casts are used to obtain immobilisation, protection and correction of bone, tissue damage, deformity and pain relief. Correct care is essential to prevent complications arising. Stone (2000) acknowledges that casting which includes the application, adaptation and the removal of casts, requires skill, knowledge and judgement to care for patients safely.

LEARNING OUTCOMES

By the end of this section you should be able to:
- Understand the principles of plaster care
- Develop an understanding of the factors which predispose to common complications
- Recognise common complications
- Explain nursing interventions required when complications arise
- Advise carers and their children on future plaster care.

RATIONALE

Newman & Fawcett (1995) and Smith (2004), endorse the importance of effective communication and information to allow children and carers to be adequately prepared and understand the necessity for the application of the cast, its subsequent care and the recognition of possible complications. It is therefore necessary that the nurse has the required skills of cast application and knowledge of the principles involved, including possible complications which may arise (BOA 1998, RCN 1999).

FACTORS TO NOTE

Casting materials

Plaster of Paris, fibreglass, flexible polyester based and semi-rigid materials are the most commonly used materials today. Each has its own advantages and disadvantages for use (Miles et al 2000).

Plaster of Paris

This is a high-quality gypsum impregnated onto an open weave fabric material. It has been the most common choice for immobilisation for many years. It is relatively inexpensive, pliable and easy to mould, smoothing to conform almost exactly to the extremity (Cutler 2007).

However, despite starting to set in 5–7 min, it may take up to 48 h for the plaster cast to dry completely (Prior & Miles 1999a, Altizer 2004). During this time, the wet cast should be supported by a pillow and handled with the palms of the hands to prevent denting the cast (Pifer 2000, Altizer 2004). Walking on a cast before it is fully set will cause the same problem.

Fibreglass

A fibreglass cast is usually a knitted fibreglass fabric impregnated with a polyurethane resin, which hardens on exposure to water in a matter of minutes. It only takes a few seconds in water to initiate the chemical reaction.

It comes in a variety of colours, is radiolucent, lightweight and is stronger than Plaster of Paris (McRae & Esser 2002). However, it requires five to eight layers for weight-bearing casts (Cutler 2007) and, although more resistant to damage, it can be brittle and crack from repetitive use and can leave a sharp edge, potentially causing excoriation of the skin (Cutler 2005).

It takes approximately 30 min to dry completely, making weight-bearing and use of the casted limb possible much sooner (Prior & Miles 1999a). Fibreglass casting materials have water-resistant properties. However, the underlying padding if not waterproof can pose a problem if exposed to water and may result in excoriation of the skin or formation of a pressure sore.

The resilience of the material makes it more difficult to conform well to the extremity and, unlike Plaster of Paris, it does not mould specifically. The extremity must be in the correct position before application; if not, wrinkles may develop which cannot be smoothed out and can result in pressure sores (Miles et al 2000).

The resin becomes tacky when in contact with water and may make the material resist coming off the roll. If pulled too hard on application, it may compromise the circulation. It is essential that healthcare professionals applying casts are familiar with the products they are using and read the manufacturers' advice and instructions for use (Miles et al 2000, Cutler 2007).

Fibreglass is more expensive than Plaster of Paris, and for this reason is often not the initial cast of choice following trauma or surgery, when removal may be necessary because of swelling or wound inspection. Fibreglass casts can leave sharp edges and, as noted by Prior and Miles (1999a), may cause breakdown of the skin.

Polyurethane–based materials

Polyurethane-based materials that incorporate a flexible polyester were introduced early in the 1990s and are used in some areas. It is radiolucent, lightweight, durable, flexible and conforms to the limb shape very easily and it can be removed with a serrated scissor edge or with the oscillating saw. Fewer layers are required for weight-bearing purposes. This type of casting material lends itself well to focused rigidity casting (FRC). The main concept of FRC is the stabilisation of a fracture with maximum support at the fracture site but less support targeted above and below the fracture site. This allows a degree of functional movement and micro-motion that encourages the stimulation of blood flow and therefore promotes the healing process. FRC is achieved by using four layers of material at the fracture site and two layers elsewhere. The application is very specific and moulding of the material is paramount to its success. A single cast can be used throughout a treatment episode because it can be adjusted to accommodate swelling or muscle atrophy. This method of casting was developed in Germany and evaluated in the UK by Petty and Wardman in 1998. Their study looked at the safety and effectiveness of this new technique, the effect on patients living with a cast, patient satisfaction and cost-effectiveness of the materials, and concluded that FRC application is beneficial to the patient allowing early mobilisation and better function with less impact on daily living and although the initial cost of the material is more expensive, it is more cost-effective because less material is required. Munshi et al (2000) used FRC for treatment of a stable forearm greenstick fracture in children and highlighted similar results.

Semi-rigid materials

At first glance, this material looks like fibreglass. However, the composition is slightly different and combines flexibility with resilience after the final curing stage. A semi-rigid cast is more commonly used in conjunction with a fibreglass membrane (combination casting) to add strength and stability to the finished product. It is versatile, lightweight, radiolucent, flexible, mouldable and leaves a soft edge. The application of this material is again quite specific. It can be removed using a serrated edge scissor or by unwrapping it like a bandage, therefore making it beneficial to children by reducing the trauma of removal especially in the pre-verbal child or a child with learning difficulties. Schuren 1998 provides a full guide to this material, its application and how to use it.

All materials generate heat initially; therefore it is advisable to use cool or tepid water for dipping the tape, otherwise the patient may sustain a plaster burn (Prior & Miles 1999b).

Allergic skin reactions can sometimes be caused by certain paddings and casting materials. Parents and children should be advised on what to look for (Miles et al 2000).

Effects of application on the patient and family

The cast is most often applied following trauma. However, it can also be applied to correct bony or tissue deformities which may be present at birth, e.g. developmental dysplasia of the hip and congenital talipes equinovarus.

Irrespective of the reason for a cast being applied, nurses must be aware that, although the procedure may be routine for them, it can be very stressful for both child and carers. This is why a clear explanation of the reasons behind the application and its subsequent care are essential.

Very often, carers are not prepared for the frustrations, fears and difficulties associated with the child's cast confinement (Prior & Miles 1999b). Preparation of the family for the reality of home care could help to make what may be a difficult recovery period more acceptable to all concerned. Problems may not be eliminated fully but prior warning enables the carers and child to deal with them in whatever way is convenient to their circumstances (Miles et al 2000). What makes these problems overwhelming is learning about them after discharge when lack of knowledge, equipment and support

becomes apparent. Smith (2004) concurred that families with children in hospital require information about their illness, treatment and subsequent care and that families caring for children living with casts on may require the information to be more specifically related and to be supported with information in a written format and upon discharge telephone contact details for help if needed.

A simple explanation of what is normal and what is not can be very helpful, for example the psychological aspects of cast confinement may mean that a once independent child may now be totally dependent, causing insecurity, frustration, tantrums and demanding behaviour, as highlighted by Clarke and Dowling (2003). Educating the family will help to eliminate this.

Casting can be used over a prolonged period. This is often age and disease related and may be for a number of years rather than weeks or months. This can cause major disruption to family life at home.

Types of cast

There are many different types of cast which can be altered as dictated by the orthopaedic medical staff to meet the individual's needs.

The most common casts used for children are:

- Below-elbow: distal radius and ulna fractures (Fig. 19.1)
- Above-elbow: proximal radius and ulna fractures; supracondylar fractures (Fig. 19.2)
- Scaphoid: scaphoid bone injuries (Fig. 19.3)
- Below knee: fibula and tibial fractures, metatarsal fractures, ligament and tendon injuries (Fig. 19.4)

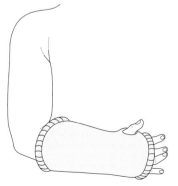

Figure 19.1 Below-elbow cast.

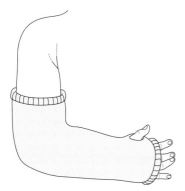

Figure 19.2 Above-elbow cast.

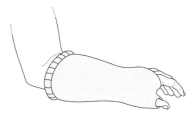

Figure 19.3 Scaphoid cast.

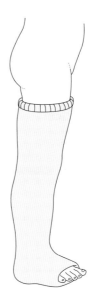

Figure 19.5 Above-knee cast.

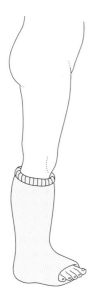

Figure 19.4 Below-knee cast.

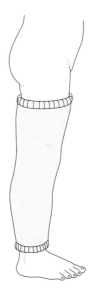

Figure 19.6 Cylinder cast.

- Above-knee: fibula and tibial fractures, patella fractures, tendon and ligament injuries, talipes equinovarus (Fig. 19.5)
- Cylinder: patella fractures, ligament and tendon injuries (Fig. 19.6)
- Hip spica: femoral fractures, developmental dysplasia of the hip (Fig. 19.7)
- Broomstick: developmental dysplasia of the hip (Fig. 19.8).

The multidisciplinary team

The child in a cast may require input from various members of the multidisciplinary team while in the hospital and in the community.

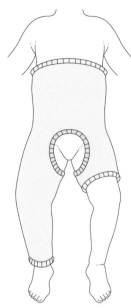

Figure 19.7 Hip spica cast.

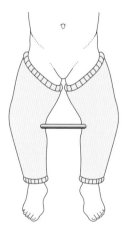

Figure 19.8 Broomstick cast.

Physiotherapists
Advice can be given to the carers on lifting techniques, sitting, turning and carrying of the child, especially those whose needs prevent them doing it themselves. Many carers experience low back pain as a result of not being taught how to lift correctly (Newman & Fawcett 1995). Physiotherapists may also provide wheelchairs (reclining or ordinary), leg extensions and extra-wide pushchairs. Teaching the correct method and use of crutches may also be carried out by physiotherapists.

Occupational therapists
Occupational therapists may be required to assess the home circumstances and provide various aids to caring for the child at home, e.g. a wheelchair ramp, plastic bedpans, etc.

APPLICATION OF THE CAST

EQUIPMENT

Whatever the type of cast or reason for application, there is usually little variation in the equipment used.

- Stockinette
- Conforming undercast padding
- Plaster of Paris or fibreglass/polyurethane-based material/semi-rigid
- Disposable apron
- Disposable latex-free gloves
- Protective sheet
- Plaster bucket and stand
- Plaster sink
- Limb support
- Tepid/cool water.

METHOD

The nurse applying the cast needs to understand the medical prescription, identify the patient and the affected limb to be cast, inspect the child's skin and assess the necessity for appropriate prescribed analgesia prior to application, e.g. oral or inhalational (Entonox) (Pickup et al 2000).

1. Prepare the child and carer for the procedure, explaining why the cast is being applied and what the equipment is for. This is to minimise anxiety and gain cooperation.
2. Ensure that any administered analgesia has taken effect. This is also to reduce anxiety and gain cooperation.
3. Ensure privacy and protect the child's and carer's clothes using a protective sheet.
4. Position the child comfortably, using a limb support, if necessary, to facilitate progress of the procedure.
5. Apply the stockinette first. Stockinette is supplied in different sizes; choose the one that when applied will be smooth and close fitting, avoiding any wrinkles or pleats. Apply a

conforming undercast padding, a single layer application, 50% coverage on each turn. Do not protect bony prominences with extra padding, as this creates space between cast and limb, allowing movement of the cast and potential plaster sore development. If concerned about bony prominences, use a suitable undercast felt. The undercast padding will protect the skin during the period of immobilisation, and from the plaster saw when the cast is being removed.

6. The person applying the cast should wear a plastic apron to protect clothing and use disposable gloves, especially if a synthetic cast is to be used as it may be an irritant to the skin.

7. Position the affected limb correctly or as directed by the orthopaedic medical staff. Persuade children to achieve the position themselves if possible. The application of above-elbow and lower limb casts should only be applied using a minimum of two members of staff to hold and maintain the position from the outset to the completion of the cast.

8. Unwind the cast bandage for approximately 10 cm before immersing it in the water. This prevents the end of the bandage becoming lost in the roll. If a synthetic material is used, immerse totally in the water for 10–15 s to initiate the chemical reaction of the resin, allowing the material to be applied and to eventually become rigid. Please refer to the manufacturer's instructions on all materials.

9. Withdraw the bandage from the water, gently compressing it to remove excess water. Do not wring out the bandage, especially if Plaster of Paris is being used, as this will result in a loss of the plaster cream.

10. Apply the wet cast bandage with even pressure around the correctly positioned limb, taking care not to pull too tightly, as this may compromise circulation. Apply the next cast bandage to the previous before it begins to dry. This will ensure good lamination between layers and an even finish. Warn the child that the bandage may feel warm and explain that it is the chemical reaction which will eventually harden the cast.

11. Turn back the ends of the stockinette and apply the casting material, allowing enough padding to remain visible at each edge. This will ensure patient comfort and reduce the risk of the cast rubbing against the skin and causing a sore. During application, cut the casting material around digits to ensure correct fit. Use undercast felt to protect the skin. Check the edges of the cast upon completion and trim if necessary.

12. When handling a wet cast, use the palms of the hands and not just the fingers. Supporting the cast thus will minimise the risk of indentations, which may cause pressure sores and the development of cracks in the cast, which will weaken the support it provides.

13. The limb should be elevated for the first 24–48 h and circulation checks maintained. This will minimise swelling of the limb and aid early detection of any possible circulatory problems.

14. On discharge, all carers must be given written as well as verbal instructions about the cast to ensure continuity of care.

OBSERVATIONS AND COMPLICATIONS

Frequency of observations varies from centre to centre depending on the reason for the application of the cast and the severity of the injury.

Circulatory, motor and sensory checks are essential, as trauma to a limb can affect the circulation, muscles and nerves. These checks may be performed every 30 min to 1 h initially for up to 24–48 h, depending on the severity of the injury.

Circulation

Indication of a problem in the circulation to the limb is noted by a change in colour to a blue or pale appearance, a change in the temperature of the peripheries from warm to cool and by the absence of a distal pulse. (*Note:* It may not be possible to feel the distal pulse as it may be covered by the cast.)

Muscle

Damage to muscle following injury, if neglected, may be irreparable, especially if a condition known as compartment syndrome develops. Compartment syndrome is an orthopaedic emergency and if appropriate action is not taken the patient may face surgery (fasciotomy) to relieve the pressure or amputation of the affected limb (Miles 2004).

Observations to detect this are referred to as the five Ps:

1. *Pain*: increasing in nature and extreme pain, made worse on flexion of the digits of the affected limb
2. *Pallor*: of the extremities with swelling
3. *Pulse*: diminished or absent
4. *Paraesthesia*: altered sensation, often tingling
5. *Power loss*: inability to move the associated extremities (Prior & Miles 1999b, Miles et al 2000).

Nerves

Damage to nerves is indicated by altered sensation, pins and needles or numbness.

- Any of the above changes must be reported immediately to the senior orthopaedic medical staff.
- If a compartment syndrome is suspected then the cast can be split through to the skin immediately and, if necessary, supported with a loosely applied crepe bandage. Do not wait for the orthopaedic medical staff to arrive.
- Do not elevate the limb as this could compromise the circulation further.

Swelling

Swelling usually peaks in 24–48 h, which is why elevation is important during this period. This helps to prevent venous pooling and oedema (McConnell 1993).

Wound infection and pressure sores

Assess for the following signs and symptoms:

- Drainage/seepage at the ends of the cast or over the wound site
- Foul odour
- Tingling or burning sensation under the cast
- Pain under the cast, particularly over bony prominences or pins.

If wound infection or a pressure sore is suspected, a window may be cut out of the cast. If a sore or infection has developed, this enables dressings to be changed and the window can be replaced and held in position with tape or a bandage.

Too tight/loose

Too tight a cast will lead to circulatory problems. If it is too loose, it will not support the limb and may cause friction and potential cast sore development. In both circumstances, the cast should be removed and replaced.

Skin

Assessment of the skin prior to cast application should be undertaken routinely and findings documented (Altizer 2004). Ensure that adequate padding at the distal and proximal ends of the cast will reduce the risk of irritation and the cast rubbing, causing the skin to break down. If the cast is rubbing, then it can be trimmed to below the affected area and protected with more padding (Prior & Miles 1999a).

ADVICE TO CARERS

HYGIENE AND SKIN CARE

Information about keeping a cast clean, particularly around the perineal area for those in a hip spica, is very important. Excreta can seep inside the cast and cause skin and odour problems (Newman & Fawcett 1995).

Miles et al (2000) suggested using a smaller-sized nappy than usual, tucking it between the skin and the cast and ensuring that the plastic backing is next to the cast's inside surface. Observation of the area immediately under the cast is needed to ensure that the nappy is not causing any pressure sores. However, this very much depends on whether adequate space has been left around the perineal area to allow for this. Where possible, do not place the nappy over the cast, as excreta will be absorbed into the cast causing odour and softening. Also suggested by Miles et al (2000) is the use of a smaller nappy inside a larger nappy to absorb more urine, particularly at night, specifically for those children in hip spicas. Carers are also advised to check and change the nappy more frequently and as necessary.

For the older child in a hip spica, the use of a bedpan and urinal is recommended. Carers need to be made aware that they will require these items before discharge home. Waterproof tape (sleek) can be placed around the edges of the cast and replaced as necessary.

A thorough wash from head to toe may replace normal bathing. Hairwashing may be a problem and require two people – one to hold the child's head over the sink/bath, the other to wash. An alternative is to use dry shampoo.

Waterproof cast covers available from different companies can now be purchased to aid with personal hygiene. They are extremely useful to use on holiday, especially in hot countries.

POSITIONING AND SAFETY

The affected limb should be positioned on cushions or pillows initially when at rest. A hip spica cast often extends up to the diaphragm, so enabling the child to sit up requires special consideration. The use of pillows and cushions or a bean bag may assist in achieving this (Sparks et al 2005). Turn the child from front to back several times a day to prevent pressure sores. The change in position also encourages different play activities. Some children may develop a 'commando crawl' when placed on their abdomen allowing them to move more freely (Sparks et al 2005). Safety straps on pushchairs and highchairs, and side rails on cots/beds, will be required as children soon learn how to manoeuvre themselves. A car seat may require alterations to ensure safe transportation.

EATING AND DRINKING

The extension of a hip spica cast may cause eating and drinking to be awkward, and the child may experience discomfort after meal times because of the restriction caused by the rigid cast. It is better to ask carers to give smaller, more frequent meals to avoid discomfort, than let them discover this through experience. If the cast reduces mobility, it may be necessary to increase the fibre content in the diet and give more fluids to prevent constipation. A closed cup or the use of a flexible straw may be the best method for drinking to prevent too many accidents and spillages on to the cast.

SLEEPING

Sleeping may be affected as a result of the effects of trauma and/or hospitalisation. Cramp can be caused by the inability of the child to turn over in bed so they need turning during the night. If itching occurs underneath the cast, due to the weight and heat from the bed covers, lift the bed clothes off the cast using extra pillows at the bottom of the bed. Faced with these difficulties, the child may be restless and may only sleep for short periods.

MOBILITY

Balance may be affected by lower limb casts. If a weight-bearing cast has been applied, crutches may be advised initially, but the child must not be discharged home until shown the correct use of crutches by an appropriately trained person, e.g. a physiotherapist.

The ability to get out of the house is important for both the carers and the child to prevent social isolation. Input from the physiotherapist and occupational therapist is necessary for the provision of ramps, wheelchairs, wide pushchairs, etc. Transportation may be a problem, especially with hip spica casts. A hospital taxi or ambulance may be required for discharge and follow-up appointments. If the child cannot safely be strapped into a car seat, a seat belt extension may need to be obtained.

Clothing

Shirts, shorts, dresses and skirts can usually be worn normally. However, a larger size may be necessary for those in a spica cast. Underwear, trousers, etc. for lower limb casts, spica and broomstick casts can be split at a side seam and Velcro strips, poppers or zips inserted for ease of access.

Advice for parents is available from national associations, such as Action for Sick Children, STEPS (National Association for Children with Lower Limb Abnormalities) and the Scoliosis Association.

REMOVAL OF A CAST

EQUIPMENT

Tools for removal of a cast:

- Plaster saw – used only for removing dry casts
- Plaster shears – for removing wet casts
- Plaster spreaders
- Bandage scissors.

METHOD

1. Ensure that the equipment you require is available and clean.
2. Assess the cast before attempting to remove it. Ask questions about its origin, look for evidence of pin sites, was the cast applied in theatre, is there swelling present? Once you are

satisfied with the assessment you can decide the most appropriate way to remove the cast (Miles et al 2000).

3. Explain to the child and carer what you will be doing, and give reassurance regarding the use of the saw and the noise it makes (Altizer 2004). The blade oscillates, so an explanation is needed to reassure the child that the blade will not cut through the protective padding. Children should also be told that they may experience a vibrating or tickling sensation and slight warmth, especially during the removal of a large cast. This will help minimise anxiety and gain cooperation for the procedure to continue.

4. If necessary, mark the cast with a pen for exact lines to be cut avoiding bony prominences and fracture/wound sites. This will minimise the possibility of trauma. The cast should be bivalved, i.e. the cast is cut in two on both sides, lengthways to allow safe removal of the limb from the cast.

5. Position the child comfortably, enabling easy access to the cast on a secure and steady surface. Remove any clothing covering the cast and protect other clothing with an apron, or protective sheet, if necessary.

6. The cast saw has an oscillating circular blade that creates a vibration that rubs against the hard surface of the cast in order to remove it. It should be held with both hands using an in and out technique keeping the machine moving along the length of the cast at all times to minimise the heat that is generated during this procedure (Miles et al 2000). The saw can cut the skin and become hot enough to cause a burn if used inappropriately (Miles 2004, Miles et al 2000).

7. Avoid using the saw on the extreme edges of the cast. These areas should be cut with a pair of scissors.

8. When cutting is complete, open the cast with care using the plaster spreaders, avoiding too much disturbance to the limb.

9. Use the bandage scissors to cut the padding.

10. Note any signs of pressure from the cast on the skin or damage from the saw. If any, notify the doctor and document in the child's care plan/progress notes.

11. It is important to remember that for:
    a. Lower limb plasters – the child should not weight bear until seen by a doctor
    b. Upper limb plasters – arms should be supported until seen by a doctor.

12. Carers and child should be advised that once the cast is removed it may take some time for life to return to normal. A rehabilitation period may be necessary as muscles and joints have been inactive for some time (Altizer 2004).

COMMUNITY PERSPECTIVE

The CCN will liaise with the family on the ward to ensure that they feel confident to take the child home. Home visits may be arranged to advise on adaptations in the home, e.g. moving the child's bed downstairs. Discharge planning should ensure that there is sufficient equipment at home, e.g. pillows, vacuum cushions, bedpans/urinals. Referral to the physiotherapist may be needed for advice about seating, mobilising and appropriate use of a buggy or wheelchair.

The family should be given information concerning the charity STEPS (National Association for Children with Lower Limb Abnormalities), which may be able to provide additional equipment such as pushchairs or a low table with an attached seat for a child with a hip spica.

The CCN will need to visit to ensure that the parents are coping with the physical care as well as the frustrations of restricted mobility and changed pattern of family life. The CCN may be required to trim casts and apply sleek plaster to the edges.

Where there is a community play specialist, visits may be helpful in showing parents ways in which to occupy the child and the use of play techniques to relieve frustration and encourage normal development. School-age children will need the involvement of the education department to supply a home tutor.

Results of findings by STEPS showed that 'high levels of emotional distress associated with diagnosis and treatment were often exacerbated by lack of information and equipment at the point of discharge' (Hinde 1996). The provision of equipment for children with hip spicas and splints was found to be both uncoordinated and patchy. Often the first problem for parents is that of safety in the car, which is likely to occur immediately on discharge. They require access to appropriate harness devices or car seats. The problems for children with hip spicas are ongoing, as there appears to be a national lack of suitable equipment. Even where families are able to acquire a suitable pushchair, there may be a problem of access to the home, as adaptations such as ramps are not usually available because this is not a long-term need.

DOS AND DON'TS

- Do carry out observations for complications.
- Do exercise extremities as well as joints proximal to the cast. This will encourage venous return and thus help to reduce swelling. It will also help to prevent muscle wasting and joint stiffness.
- Do use the palms of the hands when moving a newly casted limb, for the first 24 h if Plaster of Paris is used, and for 30 min if fibreglass material is used.
- Do elevate the limb whenever possible, especially during the first 24–48 h after application.
- Do instruct the patient and carers to return to the hospital if:
  - Pain is experienced that is disproportionate to the injury
  - There is marked swelling or discoloration of the peripheries
  - There is altered sensation or inability to move fingers or toes
  - The cast cracks, becomes soft, loose or uncomfortable.
- Do inspect the skin around the edges of the cast.
- Do advise the patient to use the crutches as instructed.
- Do give written cast care instructions.
- Do not allow the patient to weight-bear until the cast is completely dry, or as instructed by orthopaedic medical staff.
- Do not permit any writing on the cast until it is completely dry, and advise the use of felt tip pens only, as ballpoint pens may cause cracks to develop in the cast.
- Do not allow the cast to get wet.
- Do not encourage anything to be poked down inside the cast such as pencils, knitting needles, etc., as sores may develop as a result.
- Do not allow the cast to become too hot, e.g. sitting too close to a fire or radiator. Once hot, the cast will take some time to cool down and may cause a burn beneath the cast.

References

Altizer, L., 2004. Casting for immobilization. Orthop. Nurs. 23 (2), 136–141.

BOA, 1998. The British Orthopaedic Association advisory book on consultant orthopaedic and training services. British Orthopaedic Association, London.

Clarke, S., Dowling, M., 2003. Sica cast guidelines for parents and health professionals. J. Orthop. Nurs. 7, 184–191.

Cutler, S.W., 2005. The art of casting: A thesis on cast immobilization. Body Cast 20 (4), 13–14.

Cutler, S.W., 2007. Understanding the handling characteristics of casting material. Body Cast 22 (2), 7–9.

Hinde, S., 1996. Provision and availability of equipment for children in hip spicas and splints. STEPS, Lymm, Cheshire, UK.

McConnell, E.A., 1993. Providing cast care. Nursing 23 (1), 19.

McRae, R., Esser, M., 2002. Practical fracture management, fourth ed. Churchill Livingstone, Edinburgh.

Miles, S, Members of the Royal College of Nursing and the Society of Orthopaedic Nursing, 2000. A practical guide to casting, second ed. BSN Medical, Hull.

Miles, S., 2004. Accountability in casting and splinting in the A&E department. J. Orthop. Nurs. 8, 114–116.

Munshi, P., Neale, G., MacLellan, G., 2000. Detachable functional forearm focused rigidity cast. A 'one off' definitive treatment for stable forearm greenstick fractures. Injury 31 (4), 239–242.

Newman, D., Fawcett, J., 1995. Caring for a young child in a body cast: impact on the care giver. Orthop. Nurs. 14 (1), 41–46.

Petty, A., Wardman, C., 1998. A randomized, controlled comparison of adjustable focused

rigidity primary casting technique with standard plaster of paris/ synthetic casting technique in the management of fractures and other injuries. J. Orthop. Nurs. 2, 95–102.

Pickup, S., Pagdin, J., 2000. Procedural pain: Entonox can help. Paediatr. Nursg. 12 (10), 33–36.

Pifer, G., 2000. Casting and splinting: prevention of complications. Top. Emerg. Med. 22 (3), 48–54.

Prior, M.A., Miles, S., 1999a. Casting: part 2. Nurs. Stand. 13 (29), 43–47.

Prior, M.A., Miles, S., 1999b. Casting: part 1. Nurs. Stand. 13 (28), 49–53.

RCN, 1999. Education and training in casting. Royal College of Nursing, London.

Schuren, J., 1998. Working with softcast: A manual on semi rigid immobilization, fourth ed. 3M Publication and IF Publication Service Monchengladbach, Germany.

Smith, J., 2004. A literature review of the care of babies and young children in hip spicas. J. Orthop. Nurs. 8, 83–90.

Sparks, L., Rush, M., Aubuchon, P., 2005. Meeting the developmental needs of a child in a body cast. J. Orthop. Nurs. 9, 35–38.

Stone, J., 2000. Foreword. In: Royal College of Nursing. (eds) A framework for casting standards. RCN, London.

Further reading

Dandy, D.J., Edwards, D.J., 1998. Essential orthopaedics and trauma, third ed. Churchill Livingstone, Edinburgh.

Jolleys, J.V., Caring for a child in a cast. Presented by orthopaedic products, 3M Healthcare, Bracknell.

Kelly, A., Miljesic, S., Mant, P., et al., 1996. Plaster checks by nurses: safe and efficient? Accid. Emerg. Nurs. 4 (2), 76–77.

McRae, R., Esser, M., 2002. Practical fracture management, fourth ed. Churchill Livingstone, Edinburgh.

Miles S and Members of the Royal College of Nursing and the Society of Orthopaedic Nursing, 2000. A practical guide to casting, second ed. BSN Medical, Hull.

Royal College of Nursing (RCN), 2000. A framework for casting standards. RCN, London.

Williamson, M.J., 1994. Paediatric forearm fracture. Orthop. Nurs. 13 (3), 65–68.

Chapter 20

Positioning, handling and exercises

Victoria Demery & Susan Rideout

CHAPTER CONTENTS

Introduction   211
   Learning outcomes   211
   Rationale   211
   Factors to note   212
   Guidelines   215

Pre-term babies   215

Acutely sick children   217
   Respiratory system   217
   Central nervous system   218
   Skin   218

Chronically/long-term sick babies   218
   The floppy child   218
   The neurologically impaired child   219
   Observations and complications   219
   Dos and Don'ts   220

INTRODUCTION

Correct positioning is an integral part of the care of sick children, or those with a physical disability, and can be used to enhance their speed of recovery, promote normal development and prevent deterioration in their condition (Turrill 1992, Short et al 1996). Competent handling is a crucial part of holistic care, as is the provision of appropriate opportunities for exercise, both active and passive (Jones 1999).

LEARNING OUTCOMES

By the end of this section you should be able to:

- Understand the benefits of correct positioning
- Assess the most appropriate positions and specific handling needs for children according to age, size, developmental level and condition
- Recognise the dangers of incorrect positioning
- Determine whether specialised advice and equipment is necessary
- Be aware of the need to assess the risk of moving and handling loads
- Be aware of the child's exercise requirements according to age, developmental level and condition.

RATIONALE

Any child with limited ability to move, whether because of age or condition, requires assistance to ensure appropriate and comfortable positions are achieved (Finnie 1997). This will maximise recovery and minimise deterioration. Some children have specific handling requirements, for example premature infants or those with certain conditions such as cerebral palsy. Others may require intervention by means of active, or passive, exercise.

FACTORS TO NOTE
Positioning

In order to practice good positioning, it is necessary to understand how it is used and the benefits it affords. Variations in position will allow the child to be comfortable and ease the pressure exerted on any one area. Changing positions will help prevent the skin becoming sore or breaking down and the subsequent pain and limitation of movement which might result. Certain positions can be used to help facilitate play. Allowing the child to experience movement in a range of different positions encourages normal development (Bly 1994). Specific positioning may be an important part of training a child to feed by ensuring correct head-on-body alignment. Positioning can assist the child with respiratory difficulties to drain secretions or reduce the work of breathing (Hough 1984, Badr et al 2002, Harcombe 2004). Positioning can have an influence on an infant's ability to lose heat and on the speed of gastric emptying (Hallsworth 1995). Children who have limited ability in movement need regular alterations to their positions in order to prevent the formation of muscle contractures and deformities (Dubowitz 1969, Goldspink et al 2002). It has also been shown that children with abnormal movement patterns and involuntary movements can have their problems reduced by correct positioning (Finnie 1997).

Healthy infants
The Department of Health (2007) advises that babies should be placed on their backs to sleep from the beginning to reduce the risk of sudden infant death syndrome. The 'Back to Sleep' campaign has been avidly supported across the globe since the 1990s, in an effort to reduce the incidence of sudden infant death (Efe et al 2007, Waltemyer 2008). The risk is further reduced by ensuring that they are positioned on their backs. The Department of Health (2007) also suggests that babies should be positioned with their feet close to the foot of the bed so that they cannot slide down under the covers.

Recent evidence has advised that all babies should be encouraged to have 'tummy time' when awake and being observed (Department of Health 2007). The prone position will reduce the risk of positional occipital plagiocephaly, i.e. cranial moulding/flattening of the head, and will provide an opportunity for the baby to develop shoulder girdle strength (AAP 2000, Persing et al 2003).

Moving and handling
It is important to understand the potential risks associated with incorrect positioning and poor posture to both the child and the carer. The risks of musculoskeletal problems to which all who work with children are exposed should be recognised, whether they come from continual lifting, stooping or working at an awkward level (Alexander 1997). Musculoskeletal injuries can be any injury which affects the musculoskeletal system but the most frequently seen injury resulting in work absence in the UK is back pain (Dolan & Adams 2005). Furthermore, it is estimated that four out of every five adults (80%) will experience back pain at some stage in their life (Maniadakis and Gray 2000). It is estimated that back pain along with stress is the biggest cause of sickness absence in the NHS, with a staggering 40% of this leave being attributed to back pain (HSE 2008). The prevalence of musculoskeletal injuries is further compounded by a lack of risk assessment being undertaken (CSP) in 2005 (cited in Glover et al 2005). The consequences of losing experienced professionals is obvious but the broader picture shows a huge financial burden on the healthcare sector to care and treat these injured individuals. It is estimated that every year, the healthcare sector spends on average £1.6 billion treating individuals with back-related pain, many of whom are injured healthcare professionals (Maniadakis & Gray 2000). In particular, a study carried out by The Chartered Society of Physiotherapy (CSP) in 2005 estimated that 67.5% of physiotherapists reported career prevalence of work-related musculoskeletal injuries (CSP, 2005).

Although much of the moving and handling literature focuses on preventing injury to the carer, it is imperative that the patient does not sustain an injury as the result of these activities; a commonly forgotten misconception. The incorrect handling of children can cause undue distress to the child and if handled with controversial handling techniques, can cause discomfort and injury to the child. Over time, experts in the field of moving and handling have advised against the use of uncomfortable and high risk handling techniques, because of the risk of sustaining an injury to the handlers (Ruszala 2005). As more evidence is presented, these controversial techniques are updated. It is the responsibility of any healthcare professional working with patients to ensure that their practice reflects this evidence-based practice as stated in the professional Codes of Conducts. These controversial techniques include, but are not limited to, the orthodox lift, the through-arm lift, the Australian lift, the front assisted transfer (also known as the bear hug and clinging ivy), and the drag lift (Ruszala 2005). Although the use of patient handling belts and handling slings have been very popular in the past, these handling aids are not advisable within children's nursing due to the poor posture and damage they can cause to both the child and the carer. It is worth noting that in some situations, physiotherapists and rehabilitation professionals will use both adapted front assisted transfers and handling belts to assist the handling of some children. These practitioners have received a greater depth of training in these practices compared with nursing practitioners and will use detailed risk assessments to reduce the risks associated with these practices. Indeed, Mutch (2004) suggests that the main difference between therapists and handlers is the observation method, in which handlers develop their specialist techniques compared with the specialist training the therapists receive. The Moving and Handling Advisor within each healthcare setting will be best placed to update and inform professionals on these techniques.

Healthcare Professionals must comply with the relevant legislation within this field of practice paying particular attention to the requirements of The Children's Act (HMSO 1989); The Human Rights Act (HMSO 1998); and the Disability Discrimination Act (HMSO 1995/2005) to ensure that any treatment encompasses the holistic needs of the child.

In order to reduce the risks associated with poor posture and handling techniques, it is imperative that appropriate risk assessments are conducted prior to carrying out any moving and handling activity. The Manual Handling Operations Regulations (as amended) (HMSO 1992), identify a specific approach to risk assessing a manual handling activity which can be applied to both animate and inanimate load handling. In summary, the employees' responsibilities are:

- To avoid the activity where there is risk of injury so far as is reasonably practicable
- To assess the risks in those operations that cannot be avoided
- To take action to reduce risks to the lowest level reasonably practicable
- To inform others of the actions taken to reduce these risks.

In order to undertake a risk assessment, there are many factors that must be taken into account. These can generally be classified into five categories as follows:

1. Task: frequency, duration, distance, posture (twisting, top heavy, kneeling etc), actions (push, pull, lift, lower, etc.)
2. Individual capability of the person carrying out the activity: fatigue, training, height, weight etc.
3. Load can be animate or inanimate. When considering the load as a child the following factors should be considered: the child's weight, age, muscle tone, compliance/comprehension, level of consciousness, medical condition, medical attachments, i.e. plasters/splints, drains, etc.
4. Environment: space, light, temperature, working at different levels, floor condition, etc.
5. Other factors: time, workload, uniform/footwear, personal protective equipment, etc.

Once these risks have been identified the employee must work to reduce these risks where reasonably practicable. This may include using handling equipment to assist with the activity.

When participating in moving and handling activities, healthcare professionals must ensure that they adhere to the legislative framework concerning paediatric care. In particular, consideration must be taken with regard to the informed consent process. Those healthcare professionals working in the paediatric setting must ensure that they act as advocates for the child or young person with whom they are working (CSP 2008).

There are a wide range of moving and handling aids currently available within the healthcare market. This equipment is designed, when used appropriately, to minimise the risk of injuries to both patient and carer, associated with handling patients. Each healthcare provider must carry out a detailed risk assessment to identify the most appropriate moving and handling aids to suit the needs of the client or patient group for which they care. It is important to ensure that there are adequate supplies of this equipment available to meet the needs of the patient group.

The most commonly used handling equipment include mobile and ceiling track hoists, low friction sheets, transfer boards, hand blocks and standing aids. There are many different types of hoist, all of which will facilitate a varying degree of movement for the patient. For example, there are hoists available which can facilitate safe walking with the more able patient and some hoists which will facilitate the patient to stand up supported. A walking hoist or standing hoist will require the individual patient to have an appropriate degree of ability and strength to facilitate these movements. However, the most commonly used hoists are generally used to move the dependent patient and do not require the patient to have any ability in order to facilitate their movement. Furthermore, this type of hoist will be able to move the patient in a prone position, a reclined position or a seated position depending on the type of hoist sling and hoist attachments used.

The patient sling can be professionally altered to meet the tailored needs of the patient, ensuring their safety throughout the hoisting activity. When considering children, additional safety belts and head supports are often featured on paediatric slings to maximise both comfort and safety for the child. Furthermore, slings designed for children are often colourful and incorporate features which will appeal to the younger patient; for example slings in the design of a popular children's cartoon character or specially designed fabric which will attract the younger child.

Orchard (2005) suggests that the key to successful and comfortable hoist transfers lies in the correct fitting of the sling, both in terms of size and type. The patient sling can be designed to meet the needs of individual patients and most popularly include features which facilitate patients to carry out tasks equivalent to toileting, bathing, walking and standing where the hoist can accommodate this. With such variety, it is imperative that a thorough risk assessment is carried out to ensure the correct selection of the sling is made for the various activities required by the patient. In addition, slings come in varying sizes, weight limits and fabrics and this needs to be taken into account when choosing the most appropriate sling for use.

Low friction sheets (more commonly known as slide sheets) are used to facilitate patients to move while in bed by reducing the friction between the slide sheets and allowing the top sheet to slide over the bottom sheet. Two main types exist in today's market; roller/cylinder sheets and flat sheets, which are required to be used in pairs. Both use the same principles to allow patients to move and turn while in a prone position. Low friction sheets can be used with a variety of dependency patients and are a valuable resource in both the hospital and community setting. It is worth noting, however, that low friction sheets should never be used with patients with a suspected or confirmed spinal or head injury due to the unpredictable movement associated with this equipment. A smaller version of the low friction roller sheet designed to lock in position in a single direction is invaluable with patients who slide down the seat of a chair and are very popular with younger children who cannot reach the floor with their feet when sitting down.

Transfer boards are available in a wide variety of shapes and sizes and are designed to facilitate safe assisted transfers for patients. Undoubtedly the most renowned transfer board is the PATslide which is commonly used for the transfer of the prone patient from one surface to another. Commonly available in the Emergency Department and Intensive Care settings, this transfer board can be used for the unconscious patient and is often used for transferring patients between beds/trolleys. More recently, the use of slide sheets with the transfer board has proved a very successful combination among the moving and handling community.

Smaller transfer boards are designed to assist patients to transfer between two surfaces in an upright sitting position by acting as a bridge between the two surfaces. These patients require adequate strength within their arms and upper body to facilitate their movement. Those patients who have weakness in their lower limbs can use a turn disc placed beneath their feet to allow their feet to follow the direction of their moving body. As with any moving and handling aid, a thorough risk assessment is required to ensure that the patient is both capable and safe to use with this type of transfer board. Although some patients will safely be proficient at using the transfer board independently, the majority of patients will require supervision and support to use this equipment. In particular, children are often anxious about using the transfer board initially but adapt very well to this equipment which facilitates much independence. The patient's handling plan and risk assessment will direct this. For some children, play specialists may be able to help in reducing this anxiety and facilitating compliance with this handling activity through structured play.

Moving and handling equipment is designed to meet the needs of the dependent patient to the semi-independent patient. It is therefore important that the most appropriate equipment is used to ensure that the needs of the patient are met without over-riding their own ability or independence. As with all patient activities, the patient should be encouraged and empowered to participate in the activity when they are able and it is appropriate to do so. As a patient progresses and becomes more independent it may be necessary to reduce the support offered by moving and handling aids to encourage their own independence. The healthcare professional must ensure that the risk assessment and subsequent treatment plan is reviewed and updated on a regular basis to reflect these changes in the patient's condition and ability (CSP 2008).

As with any piece of equipment, it is important that those using the equipment are trained in its correct use and are competent to use it safely. This training needs to take place with the involvement of specially trained advisors to ensure that the users receive the most appropriate advice on each piece of equipment and are aware of the requirements of the moving and handling aids.

It is important that all moving and handling aids are kept clean in accordance with the manufacturer's instructions and the recommendations of the infection prevention and control guidance applicable to each individual place of work. Disposable low friction sheets and slings can be obtained for use with the infectious patient. Likewise, all equipment should be well maintained and in good working order, and that appropriate measures are taken to ensure their safe use. All equipment is covered by the Provision and Use of Working Equipment Regulations (HMSO 1998) which details how equipment must be maintained and kept safe. Similarly, the Lifting Operations and Lifting Equipment Regulations (HMSO 1998) inform the user about maintenance and servicing requirements of all patient hoists and slings.

It is important to note that this is only a brief guide to risk assessment and that each employer will have its own local code of practice with which its employees have a duty to cooperate (RCN 1993). Furthermore, when considering patient handling, a patient handling plan identifying the various risks must be completed in line with the employer's guidelines to direct the type of equipment and technique used to assist the patient to move. In addition, when caring for children, the child and family must be consulted and involved in the handling plan and should be kept updated on the child's progress throughout their care in line with the philosophy of family centred care.

Exercise

Exercise is the practice or training of a movement (Larin 1998) and is a natural and essential part of development. It provides children with an outlet for energy (Montgomery et al 2003) and enables them to learn about themselves, their environment and others (Aarnion et al 2002).

GUIDELINES

Whenever possible, all carers should be aware of the specific positioning, handling and exercise needs of their child as detailed in the child's handling plan, and careful explanation should be given at all times to the family to maximise their input and support.

PRE-TERM BABIES

A full-term infant spends the last 4–6 weeks *in utero* in an increasingly compressed position. A pre-term infant does not experience this time in flexion and so when born, exhibits a floppy, extended posture. Babies who are born early, typically have low muscle tone and often require special life-supporting care. The above, together with immature development at birth, is likely to limit their ability to move against gravity and hence encourages them to lie in a flattened, frog-shaped posture (Fig. 20.1). Meanwhile, hypotonic neck muscles cause the head to rest flat on the side, resulting in narrow elongated head shape moulding. The aim of positioning must therefore be to:

- Stimulate active flexion of the trunk and limbs
- Encourage midline orientation

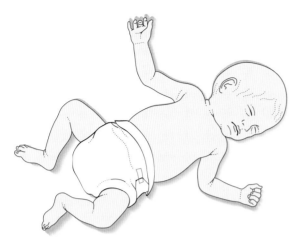

Figure 20.1 A typical frog-shaped posture adopted by a pre-term infant.

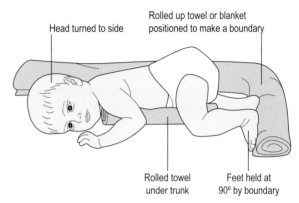

Figure 20.2 A baby positioned in prone.

- Minimise facial moulding and ensure full range of active head rotation
- Encourage a balance between extension and flexion
- Allow more symmetrical postures and enable postural stability
- Facilitate smooth antigravity limb movements (Updike et al 1986).

Pre-term babies should be cared for in a variety of positions mimicking normal development. However, some babies may be given specific positions by a physiotherapist because of 'particular concerns following a birth history indicating abnormal factors that are likely to cause handicap' (Sweeney & Gutiernez 2002).

When a baby is first admitted to a neonatal intensive care unit, the primary goal of care is to achieve physiological stability. Commonly, the prone position is best able to facilitate this, leading to improved oxygen saturation, heart rate and pulmonary resistance, and also helping to prevent gastric reflux and aspiration. Energy expenditure and heat loss are less in the prone position and babies are found to sleep better and startle and cry less.

When positioning a baby prone, Turrill (1992) suggests that the arms should be placed close to the body with the hands symmetrically brought up close to the mouth; the head then needs to be turned to one side. To discourage asymmetrical development, ensure that the head is not always turned to the same side. The legs should be encouraged to flex, with the knees brought up towards

the chest, raising the hips slightly. This position is best maintained by using a soft rolled blanket to make a boundary (Fig. 20.2).

There are times when sick, pre-term babies will be nursed in a supine position, for example to enable necessary equipment to be placed on the baby, for medical procedures or to make observation easier. This position does nothing to assist with the acquisition of a flexed posture, and so should be avoided whenever possible. To minimise the detrimental effects of this position the baby should be 'nested', i.e. given adequate support using small fabric rolls (Fig. 20.3) or carefully swaddled (Short et al 1996). This will help to achieve the following desired position while giving the baby security and comfort:

- Head in midline
- Shoulders protracted
- Hands to midline
- Hips abducted and flexed (supported in neutral)
- Knees flexed
- Feet 'neutral' (Hallsworth 1995).

From this position, the baby will be able to begin to develop head control, maintain a symmetrical

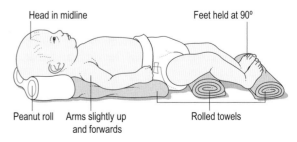

Figure 20.3 A baby positioned in supine.

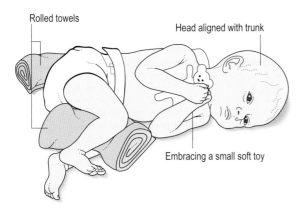

Figure 20.4 A baby positioned in side-lying.

posture, achieve normal flexor tone and establish visual skills (Sweeney & Gutiernez 2002). It will also encourage the baby to bring the hands together in the midline and to kick against gravity.

Side-lying is a valuable position that can be used to encourage flexion and symmetry in the pre-term infant. It is important to ensure that the trunk is held perpendicular to the cot surface by the use of a roll along the baby's back (not touching the back of the head, as the baby may be stimulated to push back into it). The legs should be flexed, and the upper leg supported in a neutral position by the use of a folded nappy or roll between the legs (Fig. 20.4). In this position, the head is already in the midline and the arms can be placed forwards and up towards the mouth. It is also suggested that a thin soft towel can be placed for the baby to hold between the arms to give a stimulus to flex towards (Turrill 1992).

Note that 'the baby's position can affect the parents' perceptions. A comfortable curled baby with hands touching face looks far more appealing than a flat, extended baby (Warren 1993).

When handling pre-term babies, it is important to consider certain principles:

- Handling of sick, pre-term babies should be kept to a minimum, as handling in any way will usually cause their condition to deteriorate, typically by making them hypoxic (Gagnon et al 1999).
- It is valuable to maintain positions of flexion during handling, either by lifting babies in a side-lying or prone position, with appropriate head support, or by swaddling them before they are lifted (Turrill 1992).

- Massage therapy has been found to be beneficial in terms of increased weight gain in certain medically stable pre-term infants (Maimous 2002, Deiter et al 2003) (see Ch. 5).

ACUTELY SICK CHILDREN

The positioning of an acutely sick child will often be a compromise in order to allow two or more body systems to be cared for simultaneously. However, it is important to understand the rationale for positioning for each of the different problems encountered.

RESPIRATORY SYSTEM

Drainage of secretions

The child is positioned to assist the drainage of secretions from specific areas of the lungs by means of gravity. The positions relate to the anatomy of the bronchial tree. A physiotherapist may choose to leave a child in a certain position, the relevance of which is indicated in Table 20.1. Babies should only be positioned head down following specific instructions by the physiotherapist, due to the high risk of reflux.

Improving gaseous exchange

Lung volume can be increased by helping a child to sit upright rather than slumped, or by positioning in side-lying when the abdominal contents will fall forwards away from the diaphragm (Kim et al 2004). Adequate gaseous exchange is dependent on adequate ventilation and adequate perfusion.

Table 20.1	Positions to aid postural lung drainage
AREA OF LUNG TO BE DRAINED	**POSSIBLE POSITIONS**
Right or left upper lobes	Sitting Supine lying – flat Three-quarters prone lying – flat
Right middle lobe	One-quarter left side-lying – head down 15°
Lingula	One-quarter right side-lying – head down 15°
Right or left lower lobes	Prone – head down 20° Supine – head down 20° Left or right side-lying – head down 20°

Inadequate ventilation can be caused by pneumonia, paralysed hemidiaphragm or pneumothorax. Inadequate perfusion can be caused by pulmonary vasoconstriction or pulmonary embolus. In unilateral disease (only one lung affected), gas exchange is optimum when the child is side-lying with the good lung uppermost and the child should therefore be positioned thus.

Reducing the work of breathing

When in respiratory distress, there are six relaxed positions a child could adopt: high side-lying; forward lean sitting; forward lean kneeling; relaxed sitting; forward lean standing; and relaxed standing (Davis 1983).

CENTRAL NERVOUS SYSTEM

Control of raised intracranial pressure

These children may be nursed in a head-up position with a 30° tilt, in order to reduce cerebral blood flow and with the head in midline, in order to prevent any compression of the cerebral vessels.

SKIN

The avoidance of breakdown of pressure areas demands frequent changes in position. Children who are at particular risk are those with reduced active movement, diminished sensation or poor circulation. Often a regular 30° turn is all that is necessary (see Ch. 23).

Following a burn, skin or joint contractures may develop. Collagen formation and contraction begin before the wound is healed and continue until the scars are fully mature. A child in pain will assume a position of comfort, generally a position of flexion (Sadowski 1992). Therapeutic positioning and exercises must be performed as soon as possible, and continued with regular monitoring throughout rehabilitation, to prevent the onset of contractures and subsequent disability. The use of splints and/ or pressure garments may be necessary.

CHRONICALLY/LONG-TERM SICK BABIES

Chronically sick babies often suffer from delayed development due to inadequate nutrition, recurrent illnesses and lack of stimulation. It is important to try to provide them with a position and environment from which they can get satisfaction in play with minimal effort. This should then increase their motivation to further explore their environment. Side-lying with a roll behind the back, to stop them falling back, helps to bring their hands together and position their head in midline, which is crucial in the development of coordination between the two sides of the body (Bly 1994). Sitting in a car seat, bouncy chair or tumble form chair enables them to see their surroundings and toys more easily, and will encourage them to try to reach out for them. Baby walkers are not recommended as they are considered dangerous and are thought to delay rather than facilitate walking (Siegal & Burton 1999, AAP 2001).

In addition, prolonged hospitalisation may interfere with parental bonding. The parents may be reluctant to be involved with the normal care of the child (cuddling, feeding, changing, playing, etc.). When medically stable, these babies should be exposed to as much handling and interaction during such activities as possible.

THE FLOPPY CHILD

A child may be floppy for many reasons, for example:
- Acute illness (infection, dehydration)
- Paralysis
- Neuromuscular diseases (muscular dystrophy, spinal muscular atrophy, neuropathies)
- Other disorders of the central nervous system (some types of cerebral palsy, Down syndrome)
- Metabolic disease.

When positioning these children, special consideration should be given to the prevention of deformities, which could eventually prove to be a greater disability than their weakness (Dubowitz 1969). They must, therefore, have regular changes of position throughout each day (sitting, prone, supine and side-lying) with an emphasis on providing enough support through the use of pillows, cushions or rolled towels to maintain a symmetrical posture. Floppy children, because of their inability to move against gravity, will find side-lying and sitting helpful positions to enable them to develop their skills.

In order to help prevent the development of contractures, active movement, coupled with passive movement of the joints through their full range, should be encouraged. Passive movements must only be carried out by an appropriately trained carer as the joints are very vulnerable to damage. Spinal braces or foot splints, where provided, must be worn.

When lifting a floppy child, remember that such children are likely to be unstable (owing to their lack of trunk control) and difficult to grasp (characteristically 'falling through' when lifted from under the arms). Special care should therefore be taken by the lifter to ensure that there is no accidental damage to the child's lax joints.

THE NEUROLOGICALLY IMPAIRED CHILD

Disorders of the central nervous system are the result of either abnormal development of the central nervous system itself or an insult to the brain or spinal cord, commonly affecting the sensorimotor activities of the child (Bedford & McKinlay 1993). The largest group with these problems will be children diagnosed as having cerebral palsy. The principles of positioning and handling for these children can be extended to other children with neurological impairment such as head injury, cerebrovascular accident, cerebral tumour or other acute insults including meningitis and encephalitis.

The main feature of this type of disorder is abnormal movement, which may be:

- Limited, stiff and in stereotyped patterns due to spasticity
- Floppy, feeling loose and with greater range than one would normally expect
- Athetoid – almost continuous and unwanted movement which the child cannot control
- Ataxic, jerky and uncoordinated.

Children with neurological impairment may have various combinations and distributions of any of these abnormal movements, and the first step towards effective handling and treatment calls for a full assessment of the child by a physiotherapist (Finnie 1997). Good positioning and handling are vital to help to:

- Reduce abnormal movements
- Break up and control stiffness
- Maintain the improved muscle synergies achieved through active treatment.

Poor positioning will potentially worsen these children's problems (Appleton & Baldwin 1998). A general guideline is to place and carry children in a different position from that which they assume naturally, but abnormally.

The extending child should not be left flat supine (Finnie 1997). In this position, the force of gravity pulls the body into an increasingly extended posture, making it more difficult for the child to move.

Side-lying, with the inclusion of semi-flexion at the neck, hips and knees, the legs separated by a towel or pillow and the arms placed forwards, is helpful. In addition, sitting in a chair may be useful. It can provide support to ensure a position with 90° hip and knee flexion, trunk and head alignment in the midline, and the shoulders prevented from being retracted. When carried, the child should first be moved into a more flexed and symmetrical position (e.g. sitting) and then held facing the lifter, with the legs apart and flexed at the hips and with the arms up and forwards on the lifter's shoulders.

In contrast, predominantly flexed children should be carried on their side or front in an extended position, with arms reaching up and legs held apart (Finnie 1994). It may also be appropriate for them to be positioned to sleep on their tummy, but it is important that they are fully assessed by a physiotherapist before this is attempted. The child should be monitored while in this position to ensure they have no problems (AAP 2000). A child who is strongly asymmetrical and usually holds the head turned to one side is helped most if the bed, or seating, is positioned so that all stimulation is from the opposite side (Finnie 1997).

Both athetoid and ataxic children need stability when they are being lifted or carried, and so handling should be steady and firm; the child usually responds well to generally flexed positions.

OBSERVATIONS AND COMPLICATIONS

Having positioned any child, always stand back and observe the child in the new position:

- Have you achieved what you were aiming for?
- Is the child comfortable?
- If you are having difficulty making the child comfortable, contact a physiotherapist for advice at the earliest opportunity.

COMMUNITY PERSPECTIVE

Prior to the discharge of a child who has a specific problem of mobility, it must be ensured that the parents are aware of any special procedures and that they have been taught how to carry them out. Moving and handling techniques should be explained, demonstrated and assessed.

Consideration should be given to the fact that one parent is likely to be on their own for the majority of the time and that the average home is not designed to cater for carrying older children from one room to another, or up and down stairs. These factors may pose a considerable risk to both carer and child. An assessment should be made of the home, involving other members of the multidisciplinary team as necessary, for example the occupational therapist to advise on bath aids, hoists and possible adaptation/extension of the home.

Part of the role of the CCN is to monitor the impact that constant moving and handling is having on the carers and to act accordingly. The families may have no-one else who can help and the CCN may need to organise respite care or press for a speedy implementation of adaptations and provision of equipment.

DOS AND DON'TS

- Do think before you start: 'What am I trying to achieve for the child?'
- Do keep the handling of acutely sick children to a minimum.
- Do remember to involve a physiotherapist.
- Do remember to assess any manual handling/lifting situation for risk.
- Do not put a baby to sleep on their front, unless advised by the medical staff or physiotherapist. The baby should be monitored closely during this time.
- Do not put a stiff extended child onto their back, unless advised by the physiotherapist or for medical reasons.

References

Aarnion, M., Winter, T., Kujala, V., et al., 2002. Association of health related behaviour, social relationships and health status with persistent physical activity and inactivity. A study of Finnish adolescent twins. Br. J. Sports Med. 36, 360–364.

Dolan, P., Adams, M.A., 2005. Biomechanics of low back pain. In: Smith, J. (Ed.), The guide to the handling of people. fifth ed. BackCare, Sheffield.

Alexander, P., 1997. Handling babies and young children. In: National Back Exchange (eds.), The guide to the handling of patients, fourth ed. National Back Pain Association/Royal College of Nursing, London.

AAP American Academy of Pediatrics, 2000. Task force on infant sleep position and sudden infant death syndrome. Changing concepts of sudden infant death syndrome: implications for infant sleeping position. Paediatrics 105 (3), 650–656.

AAP American Academy of Pediatrics, 2001. Committee on Injury and Poison Prevention. Injuries associated with infant walkers. Pediatrics 108 (3), 790–792.

Appleton, R.E., Baldwin, T. (Eds.), 1998. Management of brain-injured children. Oxford University Press, Oxford.

Badr, C., Elkins, M., Ellis, E.R., 2002. The effect of body position on maximal expiratory pressure and flow. Aust. J. Physiother. 48 (2), 95–102.

Bedford, S., McKinlay, I., 1993. Disorders of the central nervous system. In: Eckersley, P.M. (Ed.), Elements of paediatric physiotherapy. Longman, London, pp. 115–155.

Bly, L., 1994. Motor skills acquisition in the first year. Therapy Skill Builders, Tucson.

Childrens Act, 1989. HMSO, London.

CSP (2005). Work-related musculoskeletal disorders. CSP, London.

CSP Chartered Society of Physiotherapy, 2008. Guidance on manual handling for physiotherapy, third ed. London.

Davis, A.J., 1983. Medical chest physiotherapy. In: Downie, P.A. (Ed.), Cash's textbook of chest, heart and vascular disorders for physiotherapists. Faber and Faber, London, pp. 298–329.

Deiter, J.N., Field, T., Hernandez-Reif, M., et al., 2003. Stable preterm infants gain more weight and sleep less after five days of massage therapy. J. Pediatr. Psychol. 28 (6), 403–411.

DoH Department of Health, 2007. Reducing the risk of cot death. An easy guide. DH Publications, London.

Dubowitz, V., 1969. The floppy infant. Heinemann, London.

Efe, E., Sarvan, S., Kukulu, K., 2007. Sleep practices and environment and the risk of sudden infant death syndrome in Turkey. J. Spec. Pediatr. Nurs. 12 (4), 253–263.

Finnie, N.R., 1994. Handling the young cerebral palsied child at home. Butterworth-Heinemann, Oxford.

Finnie, N.R., 1997. Handling the young child with cerebral palsy at home., third ed. Butterworth-Heinemann, Oxford.

Gagnon, F.E., Leung, A., McNab, A.J., 1999. Variation in regional cerebral blood volume in neonates associated with nursery care events. Am. J. Perinatol. 16 (1), 7–11.

Glover, W., Sullivan, C., Hague, J., 2005. Work-related musculoskeletal disorders affecting members of the Chartered Society of Physiotherapy. London Online. Available: www.csp.org.uk/publications.

Goldspink, G., Williams, P., Simpson, H., 2002. Gene expression in response to muscle stretch. Clin. Orthop. Relat. Res. 1 (403), S146–S152.

Hallsworth, M., 1995. Positioning the preterm infant. Paediatr. Nurs. 7 (1), 18–20.

Harcombe, C.J., 2004. Nursing patients with ARDS in the prone position. Nurs. Stand. 18 (19), 33–39.

HSE Health and Safety Executive, 2008. Online. Available: www.hse.gov.uk/healthservices/msd/index.htm 21 September 2008.

HMSO, 1992. Manual handling operations regulations and guidance on regulations L23. HMSO, London.

HMSO, 1998. Human Rights Act. Elizabeth II, London.

HMSO, Statutory Instrument No. 2306. 1998. The Provision and Use of Work Equipment Regulations 1998. Stationery Office, London.

HMSO, Statutory Instrument No. 2307. 1998. The Lifting Operations and Lifting Equipment Regulations 1998. Stationery Office, London.

HMSO, 1995/2005. Disability Discrimination Act. Elizabeth II, London.

Hough, A., 1984. The effect of posture on lung function. Physiotherapy 70 (3), 101–104.

Jones, A., 1999. Teamwork is vital for spasticity. Ther. Wkly. May, 6.

Kim, H.Y., Lee, K.S., Kang, E.H., et al., 2004. Acute respiratory distress syndrome: computed tomography findings and their applications to mechanical ventilation therapy. J. Comput. Assist. Tomogr. 28 (5), 686–696.

Larin, H.M., 1998. Motor learning: a practical framework for paediatric physiotherapy. Physiother. Theory Pract. 14, 33–47.

Maimous, R.O., 2002. Infant massage as a component of developmental care. Past, present and future. Holist. Nurs. Pract. 17 (1), 1–7.

Maniadakis, A., Gray, A., 2000. The economic burden of back pain in the UK. Pain 84, 95–103.

Montgomery, C., Jackson, D., Kelly, L., et al., 2003. Intensity of physical activity and its relationship with energy expenditure in young children. Obes. Res. 11, 127.

Mutch, K., 2004. Changing manual-handling practice in a stroke rehabilitation unit. Prof. Nurse 19 (7), 374–378.

Orchard, S., 2005. Lying to sitting. In: Smith, J. (Ed.), The guide to the handling of people. fifth ed. BackCare, Sheffield.

Persing, J., James, H., Swanson, J., et al., 2003. Prevention and management of positional skull deformities in infants. Pediatrics 112 (1), 199–202.

Royal College of Nursing, 1993. Code of practice for the handling of patients. RCN, London.

Ruszala, S., 2005. Controversial techniques. In: Smith, J. (Ed.), The guide to the handling of people. fifth ed. BackCare, Sheffield.

Sadowski, D.A., 1992. Care of the child with burns. In: Hazinski, M. F. (Ed.), Nursing care of the critically ill child. Mosby, St Louis, pp. 875–927.

Short, M.A., Brooks-Brunn, J.A., Reeves, D.S., et al., 1996. The effects of swaddling versus standard positioning on neuromuscular development in very low birth weight infants. Neonatal Netw. 15, 2–31.

Siegal, A.C., Burton, R.V., 1999. Effects of baby walkers on motor and mental development in human infants. J. Dev. Behav. Pediatr. 20 (5), 355–361.

Smith, J. (Ed.), 2005. The guide to the handling of people. fifth ed. BackCare, Sheffield.

Sweeney, J., Gutiernez, T., 2002. Musculoskeletal implications of preterm positioning in the NICU. J. Perinat. Neonatal Nurs. 16 (1), 58–70.

Turrill, S., 1992. Supported positioning in intensive care. Paediatr. Nurs. 4 (4), 24–27.

Updike, C., Schmidt, R.E., Macke, C., et al., 1986. Positional support for premature infants. Am. J. Occup. Ther. 40 (10), 712–715.

Warren, I., 1993. How to place a baby. MIDIRS Midwifery Dig. 3 (4), 452–453.

Waltemyer, C.L., 2008. Educating parents about SIDS. Lippincotts Nurs. 4 (4), 22–26.

Chapter 21

Postoperative care

Jennifer McKenna

CHAPTER CONTENTS

Introduction   222
    Learning outcomes   222
    Rationale   222
    Factors to note   223

The immediate recovery period   223

The intermediate stage of dependency: return to the ward   224
    Hydration   224
    Pain   225
    Method   225

Discharge planning: return to normality   226
    Dos and don'ts   227

INTRODUCTION

Postoperative care commences as the child leaves the operating theatre and ends when discharged from the ward. However, in today's ever-changing national health service environment, hospital in-patient stays are reducing and more children are having surgery undertaken on a day-case basis. Consequently, postoperative care may continue into the home care setting and be supported in part by community children's nurses (Scottish Office 1994, O'Connor-Von 2000, Pfeil et al 2004).

LEARNING OUTCOMES

By the end of this section you should be able to:

- Understand the three stages of postoperative care
- Understand fundamental postoperative care
- Recognise the role of the child and family carer in the child's recovery
- Recognise the involvement of the multidisciplinary team.

RATIONALE

Care of the child in the postoperative phase is aimed at preventing complications and ensuring as quick a recovery from the operation and anaesthetic as possible. Postoperative care covers many different surgical specialities; however, the fundamental principles of care can be applied to any surgical procedure. The care of the child continues after discharge (Pfeil et al 2004) and often requires further nursing input while they are at home.

FACTORS TO NOTE

There are three stages of postoperative care:

1. The immediate recovery period
2. The intermediate stage of dependency
3. Returning to normality (Lyon & Best 1994, Andersen et al 2000, Discolo & Hirose 2002).

These three stages are not perhaps thought of consciously but are planned for from the moment the child is admitted. Surgery can be planned, emergency or day-case (see Ch. 22). A good preoperative preparation can make a difference to the child and their family postoperatively (Tazbir & Cronin 1999). If children are treated honestly, with realistic values and expectations, they can begin to accept the surgery and the consequences of it.

THE IMMEDIATE RECOVERY PERIOD

Immediate recovery from anaesthesia should be in a fully equipped recovery unit with a one-to-one ratio of nursing personnel trained in children's nursing (Association of Anaesthetists of Great Britain and Ireland 2002). Recovery units may be known by a different name in some areas, such as reception or post-anaesthetic care units (PACU). The recovery unit is usually situated near the operating theatres. This enables easy access to the patients by the surgical and anaesthetic staff should an emergency arise.

While the child has been in theatre and recovery, the bed/cot area should have been prepared for return to the ward. In some areas, the bed may have been transferred to the recovery unit perioperatively to minimise pain and distress for the child postoperatively. All beds must have a tilt facility and must be able to be raised up and down. (The tilt facility is important if children are experiencing postoperative shock or vomiting as it allows the child's head to be lowered or raised according to need.)

It is imperative that the bed space has access to working oxygen and suction. It may also be necessary for the child to be moved nearer the nursing station for closer observation. Neonates may need to be transferred in an incubator or Baby Therm and the same principles apply to them. Equipment that may be required postoperatively such as infusion pumps and monitoring equipment should be tested and ready when the child is transferred back to the ward. During the perioperative phase of nursing, the theatre nurse is responsible for the child while under anaesthetic and serves as the patient's advocate.

Once the theatre nurse has handed the child over to the recovery unit, immediate postoperative management is the responsibility of the anaesthetist involved in the surgery and the unit staff (Andersen et al 2000). Handover should incorporate the condition of the child while under anaesthetic, any problems which may have occurred and any analgesia which has been administered.

Serious complications can occur during the initial stage after surgery; hence the child receives short-term intensive care nursing while in the recovery unit. The duration of a child's stay in the unit depends on the type of surgery undertaken and the child's reaction to anaesthesia. If the child's condition indicates further intensive nursing intervention, the child will be transferred to the high-dependency unit (HDU) or the intensive care unit (ICU) (Tazbir & Cronin 1999, Andersen et al 2000). In the recovery unit the child is attached to a multifunctional monitor which tracks the following: heart rate, ECG, respiratory rate, oxygen saturation, non-invasive blood pressure and skin temperature. This kind of monitoring reduces disturbance to the child yet provides more detailed information for the nurse. Not all children will need all these facilities, as this depends on their condition and the type of surgery undertaken.

All vital signs, e.g. temperature, pulse, blood pressure, respirations and conscious level, are affected by surgery and the anaesthetic. On recovery from anaesthesia initially, the child will be supine with their head tilted; this ensures that the jaw is kept forward, positioning the tongue so that it does not obstruct the airway. Airway management is one of the most important areas of recovering a child from anaesthesia and should only be undertaken by appropriately trained staff. The airway requires support and this usually entails the administration of oxygen via a facemask and continuous monitoring of oxygen saturation. If the child has an airway *in situ*, the nurse waits for signs of returning consciousness before it is removed.

Anaesthesia-induced unconsciousness will mean normal reflexes are absent and respiration must be supported. During semi-consciousness the reflexes, e.g. breathing, coughing, swallowing and blinking, begin to return and finally the patient should be awake and orientated with the return of all normal reflexes. The airway is usually removed when the patient coughs it out or tries to remove it.

It should be stressed that monitoring is only an aid to continuous nursing observation. One of the most common surgical complications is haemorrhage, which can lead to shock. Any deterioration in condition is usually rapid and demands urgent attention. When shocked, the child will be pale, tachycardic and not responding as normal. In children, and especially neonates, it only takes a small amount of blood loss to make transfusion or rapid fluid replacement essential.

It is imperative that each bed/trolley space has working oxygen and suction, an emergency buzzer and easy access to the resuscitation trolley. The nurse should observe the colour of the child, and whether it is good for that particular patient. This type of information is often gained during the preoperative visit or from the ward's nursing documentation. Many children with special needs or those with cardiac/pulmonary problems can be pale or even cyanosed. Their oxygen saturations may also be lower than is normal. The promotion of safety and comfort is paramount and the use of cot sides is universal.

Although the child may feel alert and capable of moving, the remaining effects of the anaesthesia and sedation may mean that movements are uncoordinated. Special consideration should be given to children who have had spinal and epidural anaesthesia. Frequent assessment of the lower extremities should be made to determine the return of function. Temperature, colour and range of sensation and movement should be observed. In recovery, the relief of pain and encouragement to rest are also of high priority. The inclusion of parents in the recovery unit is a relatively new idea. The child has to be sufficiently recovered, e.g. fully conscious and maintaining their own airway, for the inclusion of the parent.

The presence of the parent affords reassurance and comfort and is effective in reducing postoperative distress and anxiety (Smith & Dearmum 2006). However, the presence of parents who are themselves visibly distressed, or anxious, can have an adverse effect on the child's emotional condition. It must also be stressed that not all hospitals allow a parent into the recovery unit, although this is becoming more common.

Before the child is transferred back to the ward certain criteria must be fulfilled:

- The child is conscious (but may be asleep)
- The protective reflexes have returned
- The child is maintaining their own airway and respirations are satisfactory
- The child's colour is good for that particular patient

- Postoperative observations have been stable
- The child is comfortable and pain is adequately controlled
- The child's temperature is above 36°C
- The child is clean and tidy.

THE INTERMEDIATE STAGE OF DEPENDENCY: RETURN TO THE WARD

Postoperative observations may include:

- Temperature, pulse, respirations, blood pressure, colour and conscious level of the child
- Observation and monitoring of the wound site
- Maintenance of intravenous infusion
- Monitoring of drains and urinary catheters.

These will be dependent upon the type of surgery that the child has undergone.

The frequency of routine postoperative observations may vary and is dependent on the child's condition (Andersen et al 2000). Observation of pulse and respirations is more frequent when intravenous opiate analgesia is in progress. One of the side-effects of opiates is respiratory depression, so the rate, depth and quality of respiration are monitored. Reduction in frequency of postoperative observation is based on the nurse's assessment of the child's condition.

Research has shown that the nurse often carries out more frequent observations than the patient's condition dictates, mistakenly believing that the regime had been prescribed by the hospital or by nursing policy (Botti & Hunt 1994).

HYDRATION

Normally, the reintroduction of oral fluids is left to the discretion of the nurse and is determined by the type of surgery undertaken. However, if the surgery requires that the child has no fluid, or dietary, intake for a long period of time, e.g. following bowel surgery, hydration needs will have to be met by intravenous means until the child can tolerate fluids orally (Andersen et al 2000). In this instance, a fluid balance chart is crucial to monitor all input and output. Output includes urine, vomit, wound leakage, gastric aspirate and stool. The nurse should also observe for signs of dehydration, e.g. decreased urine output, dark sunken eyes and dry mucous membranes.

The RCN (2005) recommends the reintroduction of fluids first when the child is fully awake and then diet if fluids are tolerated, but only if there are no medical, surgical or nursing contraindications. In day-case surgery, the RCN (2005) recommend that children should not be required to drink prior to discharge. However, in more complex surgery, it is common to wait until bowel sounds have returned, and fluids should be commenced as advised by the surgeons. Should it be anticipated that the child is going to be 'nil by mouth' for some time, a nasogastric tube will be inserted for the purpose of draining the stomach of bile and secretions. These losses are replaced millilitre for millilitre with intravenous fluid to prevent the child from becoming dehydrated.

Enteral feeding is usually started within 24 h of surgery unless contraindicated (Tazbir & Cronin 1999). For example, a child having undergone a fundoplication and/or gastrostomy may have to wait 48 h prior to commencing enteral feeds to allow primary healing. Parenteral nutrition may be administered to children who have been unwell for some time and have no expectation of being able to tolerate diet and fluids normally within a few days. Again, bowel surgery is a good example of this.

PAIN

Many hospitals have a pain management policy (see also Ch. 44) for children, which focuses on pain prevention and, where possible, children should be involved in assessing their own pain level. Pain assessment tools rely on the child's understanding of numbers, colours and drawings, so a selection of pain assessment tools is helpful in finding the right one to suit the child's level of understanding (Twycross 1995).

Parents play an important role in communicating with the child and, for those who cannot communicate verbally, pain management is something that should be discussed preoperatively.

As well as pharmacological pain relief, alternative methods include distraction, massage and snoezelen therapy. Snoezelen therapy works with all the senses, using aids such as soft music, optic fibre lights and tactile toys.

Pain is not just a consideration in the immediate postoperative period. The nurse has to prepare the child and family for potentially painful procedures such as removing drains and mobilisation. On these occasions, the play specialist can provide distraction therapy during the procedure. It is important, where possible, to carry out such procedures away from the bedside as the bed should be seen as a safe haven and a place of comfort. Privacy and dignity should be maintained at all times.

METHOD

1. Establish baseline information. Record temperature, pulse, respirations and blood pressure. Vital signs should be monitored and recorded regularly to detect any complications such as haemorrhage or compromise of the airway. They may also indicate that the child is experiencing pain. Assess consciousness level. Report any changes or concerns.

2. Observe the pallor of the skin. If oxygen is to be administered, ensure that the mask is correctly positioned and that the oxygen is delivered at the prescribed rate. Mouth care is essential to ensure patient comfort (see Ch. 9).

3. Check wound sites and drains. Monitor wound sites at regular intervals for signs of leakage and mark as necessary; change dressings or add additional padding as required. Report any excessive leakage. If drains are *in situ*, record output regularly and note the characteristics of the fluid, e.g. haemoserous fluid.

   Note: Aim to observe the wound site at the same time as these observations to reduce disturbance to the child.

4. Commence fluid balance chart. If an intravenous infusion is *in situ*, maintain it at the prescribed rate and record the amount infused hourly. Check the access point for signs of extravasation or phlebitis and report immediately. Reintroduce oral fluids as advised and increase intake as tolerated. All intake and output should be recorded. In the absence of oral fluid intake, ensure that adequate mouth care is provided.

5. Observe for signs of dehydration. Look for decreased urine output, poor skin turgor, dark sunken eyes, sunken fontanelle (in babies), dry mucous membranes and prolonged episodes of vomiting. Inform the medical staff of concerns. If an intravenous infusion is not in progress, it may be necessary to site one. Antiemetics may help to reduce nausea and vomiting and need to be prescribed and monitored as to their effectiveness.

6. Assess pain. Use a pain tool relevant to the child's age and development to assess the need

for analgesia. All analgesia should be given as prescribed and monitored for any adverse reactions and effectiveness. If intravenous analgesia is in progress, such as patient-controlled analgesia (PCA), maintain it at the prescribed rate and record pulse and respirations hourly, as some opiates may cause respiratory depression. Report any significant changes immediately. Liaise with the pain management team, if available, to regularly manage the child's pain safely and effectively.

7. Remember their reduced mobility. Observe and relieve pressure areas at regular intervals. Encourage the child to move by themselves where possible, but nursing staff should be there to assist. Changing position can also help to relieve any pain or discomfort the child may be experiencing. If appropriate, and if parents feel confident, babies and young children can be nursed on a knee or in a pushchair.

Encourage older children to cough and deep breathe. It may be necessary to involve the physiotherapist to relieve any chest problems and help with mobilisation. This type of involvement is usually for those who have had more major surgery, e.g. appendicectomy, nephrectomy. It is usual to mobilise as soon as the child's condition allows. Reduced mobility can also affect bowel movement. Monitor for signs of constipation and give aperients as prescribed if necessary. When diet and fluids have been re-established, encourage a good fluid intake and a diet which contains roughage. Depending on the type of surgery undertaken, for example following fundoplication, it may be advisable for the child to have smaller meals more frequently until normal dietary intake is re-established.

The family

Following the acute stage of surgical nursing care, the priority is to encourage a safe return to normality. It should be stressed to the parents and the family that the child still needs periods of rest. Sometimes this can be hard, especially when many paediatric wards and hospitals encourage an open visiting policy. Again it must be emphasised that not all wards will have this policy.

The paediatric nurse should always take account of the different ages of the children being cared for. Adolescents have specific needs and provision should be made to keep children of a similar age together where possible. Privacy and dignity should be maintained at all times.

DISCHARGE PLANNING: RETURN TO NORMALITY

The nurse should begin planning for discharge from the time of admission whenever possible. Usually, the initial assessment will identify potential problems, such as transport home and referrals to community nurses. Effective discharge planning can reduce any delay once the decision has been made to allow the patient home. Many areas have pre-printed discharge plans, which form part of the nursing documentation, and these often extend to printed discharge advice leaflets. The discharge plan should include any supplies that may be required, e.g. dressings, catheter bags, etc. Drugs required on discharge and specific instructions are important. Examples of such information are when the child should resume school and physical exercise. Information should also be given regarding pain relief, observation of the wound site and who to contact in an emergency.

Personal experience has shown that parents find it useful to have written instructions for reference, and contact numbers should be included for advice if they are having any problems.

If a child is a day-case, it may be appropriate to arrange for a district nurse, probably a paediatric community nurse, to visit the child the following day to perform a postoperative check and ensure that the parents are happy with their child's recovery. Again it should be noted that this is not always the case; local policy may dictate this practice.

COMMUNITY PERSPECTIVE

The role of the CCN in postoperative care can vary, particularly in reference to day surgery, from maintaining telephone contact with the family to check that all is well, to regular visiting to help with nursing care and monitor progress, ensuring that recovery is at the expected rate. This can be reassuring for parents, should any unforeseen problems occur. In some areas, this routine postoperative care may be undertaken by district nurses, who can refer cases to the CCNs if they feel this to be appropriate. It may be necessary to visit to change dressings or remove sutures.

DOS AND DON'TS

- Do encourage the parents to participate in their child's care.
- Do explain the planned care to the child and the family.
- Do explain the use of any equipment, e.g. infusion pumps, and also the purpose of any drains *in situ*.
- Do encourage the child to rest.
- Do explain discharge arrangements to the parents prior to discharge.

- Do outline the limitations, if any, when the child returns home, i.e. return to school and exercise.
- Do not allow the child to be discharged without arranging follow-up or community nurse input, if required.
- Do not forget that surgery is never routine for the child or the family.
- Do not assume that the parent or carer will want to participate in postoperative care. This should always be negotiated.
- Do not forget to give parents a contact number for advice should they have any problems.

References

Andersen, D., DeVoll-Zabrocki, A., Brown, C., et al., 2000. Intestinal transplantation in pediatric patients: a nursing challenge. Part 2: Intestinal transplantation and the immediate postoperative period. Gastroenterol. Nurs. 23 (5), 201–209.

Association of Anaesthetists of Great Britain and Ireland, 2002. Immediate post-anaesthetic recovery. AAGBI, London.

Botti, M.A., Hunt, J.O., 1994. The routine of post anaesthetic observations. Contemp. Nurse 3 (2), 52–57.

Discolo, C.M., Hirose, K., 2002. Pediatric cochlear implants. Am. J. Audiol. 11, 114–118.

Lyon, M.H., Best, B.J., 1994. Immediate postoperative recovery: management and care. Br. J. Nurs. 3 (17), 866–870.

O'Connor-Von, S., 2000. Preparing children for surgery – an integrative research review. AORN 71 (2), 334–343.

Pfeil, M., Mathur, A., Lind, J., 2004. Early discharge following uncomplicated appendicectomy in children. Paediatr. Nurs. 16 (7), 15–18.

RCN Royal College of Nursing, 2005. Clinical practice guideline: Perioperative fasting in adults and children. RCN, London.

Scottish Office, 1994. Caring for sick children: a study of hospital

services in Scotland. HMSO, Edinburgh.

Smith, J., Dearmum, A., 2006. Improving care for children requiring surgery and their families. Paediatr. Nurs. 18 (9), 30–33.

Tazbir, J.S., Cronin, D.C., 1999. Indications, evaluations and post operative care of combined liver-heart transplant recipients. AACN Clin. Issues 10 (2), 240–252.

Twycross, A., 1995. Children's nursing in Canada. Paediatr. Nurs. 7 (4), 8–10.

Chapter 22

Preoperative care

Jennifer McKenna

CHAPTER CONTENTS

Introduction 228
    Learning outcomes 228
    Rationale 228
    Factors to note 229
    Setting standards 230

Preoperative care 231
    General points 231
    Age-appropriate preparation 231
    Method 231
    Dos and don'ts 232

INTRODUCTION

Effective preparation of children who are to undergo anaesthesia and surgical intervention is an important factor in reducing the anxiety experienced by the child and their family during hospital admission (RCN 2004). Children provide a unique challenge in that the education and preparation that they require must not only meet their needs, but also the needs of their parents/primary carers (Kelly & Adkins 2003).

LEARNING OUTCOMES

By the end of this section you should be able to:
- Recognise the need for safe preparation for theatre
- Understand the role of the parent in the preoperative phase
- Identify the needs of different age groups and their level of understanding
- Recognise stressors affecting both parent and child
- Identify multidisciplinary involvement in preoperative care
- Assist in the safe preparation of a child for theatre
- Consider the importance of preparing for discharge within the preoperative period.

RATIONALE

Children, regardless of age, need to be appropriately prepared for theatre. This involves both physical and psychological aspects of care. Children who are familiar with their surroundings, and who are informed of events associated with surgical procedures, are more likely to cope with the overall experience (Newman & Scott 1990, O'Connor-Von 2000).

Parents who are fully informed and involved are confident and capable partners in the hospitalisation and recovery process of their child and on discharge (Darbyshire 2003). Children who are informed will have a reduction in anxiety related to the procedure and also to the hospital environment (LeRoy et al 2003).

FACTORS TO NOTE

Planned surgery

- Planned, or elective, surgery lends itself very well to good preparation prior to the day of surgery (O'Connor-Von 2000, Sexton & Redfearn 2003, Smith & Dearmum 2006, Bray & Sanders 2006). There is time to involve other disciplines who can make a contribution to the overall readiness of both the child and family for forthcoming surgery.
- Psychological preparation can begin at home well before the planned date of admission. There is a wide range of books and other visual aids available from libraries and bookshops, which offer the opportunity to talk through the need for hospitalisation and what to expect. Schools and nurseries will often facilitate role-play which involves dressing up and acting out the nurse/doctor roles. These are all recognised as ways of allaying the fears and anxieties of children and can help those parents who have little experience of hospitals themselves (LeRoy et al 2003). Preparation should include information on what will happen postoperatively including relevant information on wound care (Bray & Sanders 2006).
- The development of pre-admission programmes, such as Saturday morning clubs, facilitates interaction between hospital staff, children and parents and provides the opportunity to discuss pain control and the admission procedure. Efforts made at this stage of contact promote a feeling of well-being and aid in the speedy recovery of the child (LeRoy et al 2003, Sutherland 2003, Bray & Sanders 2006).
- On admission, there is the opportunity to involve play specialists and theatre staff. Thornes (1991), Hogg (1994) and Bray & Sanders

2006 highlight the value of play in hospital and this role has been further developed in paediatric areas. The benefit of the involvement of play specialists in overcoming operation anxiety, the use of photograph albums and visits made by recovery staff, all give a broader view of what the child will experience and the parents' role in the process (see Ch. 10).

Emergency surgery

- Unplanned surgery often means that there is little time for the psychological preparation of the parent or child. Some children go to theatre directly from the A&E department, and so there may be limited time for explanations or time for premedications. Sudden loss of contact with parents and siblings can cause additional stress to the child. The nurse should be aware of these factors and deal with them sensitively.
- When the child has been transferred to theatre, it is usual for the parents to be taken to the admitting ward to wait for the surgery to be completed. It is during this time that additional information and emotional/psychological support are given.
- When a child is transferred to the ward only a short time prior to surgery, emphasis is mainly on physical preparation, with medical staff completing tasks such as obtaining consent and examination of the child. There may be an opportunity for the parents to speak with the anaesthetist or surgeon, but this is not always possible. Fuller explanations of procedures and planned care usually take place while the child is in theatre and upon return to the ward.

Day-care surgery

- Day surgery has many advantages for both the child and family. Caring for Children in the Health Service is a consortium that was established by the Action for Sick Children charity. They have produced a number of reports concerning the preparation of children for surgery. Thornes (1991) on behalf of Caring for Children in the Health Service, explored the benefits of paediatric day care from an economic viewpoint, and from the child's needs with regard to avoiding the necessity for overnight admission. This was reinforced by the Audit Commission report, *Children First* (1993), which encouraged the development of such facilities.

- Morton and Raine (1994) defined some of the benefits as absence of parental separation, less disruption to the family and an increase in the amount of parental involvement. All of these should be supported by care being available in the community for children following attendance at a day-care facility.

- To shorten the admission time, it is preferable that routine preoperative investigations are completed during outpatient visits so that all necessary results are available on the day of admission. LeRoy et al (2003) suggest that younger children (age 3–5 years) should have the preparation as close to the day of surgery as possible, whereas older children (age 6–12 years) benefit more from earlier preparation, i.e. up to 1 week before.

- Written instructions for preoperative fasting should be given to the parents along with information about giving routine medications, e.g. inhalers. Parents should be encouraged to bring any medications with them on the day of admission.

- At some centres, children can travel to theatre on bicycles and in motorised cars which makes the journey much more acceptable and exciting. The wearing of their own clothes is becoming more widespread, but parents should be advised to bring a change of clothes as a precaution.

- Most areas now use topical anaesthetic creams such as EMLA or Ametop, and this can sometimes negate the need for oral premedications. The use of local anaesthesia (e.g. nerve blocks) during surgery was shown to reduce the complications of pain, nausea and vomiting. In addition, the children were awake more rapidly following anaesthesia, allowing diet and fluids to be accepted (Cohen et al 1990). This enables discharge to occur earlier, therefore minimising the stay in hospital.

- It should be stressed to the parents that there may be the possibility of an overnight stay if events change. This enables the family to make further arrangements if necessary.

- Arrangements should be made in advance for transport home (according to local policy), a discharge letter to be sent to the GP and, in some instances, a postoperative home visit.

Children with disabilities

- The preparation of children with disabilities may place more emphasis on the parents' or carers' involvement depending on the degree of disability. However, the basic principles of preoperative care still apply and the methods by which the children are prepared for theatre may need only slight adjustment. For example, the preparation of a child with visual impairment will be verbal rather than visual, but although photograph albums are of little use to the child, they may be helpful to the parent or carer, who in turn may help you to explain procedures in a language that the child can understand.

- Distraction therapy may be useful to reduce the anxiety of the child and involvement of play specialists is helpful in this instance (Honeyman 1994, Kelly & Adkins 2003) (see Ch. 10).

- For those children who cannot communicate verbally, one of the most important discussions which should take place prior to surgery, is that of pain control. The non-verbal signs used by the child to convey pain, or discomfort, are more readily known by the parent; similarly they usually know what comforts the child, such as rocking, stroking or talking. Richardson (1992) highlighted the fact that professionals sometimes underestimate the amount of pain experienced by children; it is therefore desirable to secure parental involvement in pain control when possible.

SETTING STANDARDS

The National Association for the Welfare of Children in Hospital (NAWCH, now known as Action for Sick Children) produced advice and 12 quality standards for children admitted as day cases in a report entitled *Just for the Day* (Thornes 1991). This covered the need for pre-admission programmes, literature available outlining parental responsibilities and a friendly environment. Some hospitals may have a designated area for children within an adult setting. (In these instances, great care must be taken to provide adequate facilities suitable for both children and their families.)

Hogg (1994) and the Audit Commission report, *Children First* (1993), made recommendations and set standards for children undergoing surgery. Hogg and Cooper (2004) updated the recommendations of Caring for Children in the Health

Service, but the underlying principles remained the same. These standards incorporate all aspects of the child's admission from decision to treat, preparation for theatre, anaesthetic room, recovery room, postoperative care and discharge. All standards reflect the need to provide appropriate child/family centered care.

PREOPERATIVE CARE

GENERAL POINTS

Parents within the anaesthetic room

Although policies for allowing parents into the anaesthetic room vary from hospital to hospital, Smith & Dearmum (2006) highly encourage parents' presence in the anaesthetic room. Adequate preparation of the parents as to their role in the anaesthetic room should remove one of the main reasons for their exclusion (Hall et al 1995). Where parents are excluded, the role of the named nurse or primary nurse has great importance in reducing separation anxiety (Gahan & Rogers 1993).

Parents, who do accompany their child to theatre, are the responsibility of the ward nurse who will ensure that the parent is not becoming distressed and will take them back to the ward once the child is asleep.

Toys and comforters

Any toys or comforters with the child will either be given to the parent or taken to the recovery room in readiness for the child being received from theatre.

Preparation

Whenever possible, the child should have every opportunity to be prepared for theatre by both professionals and parents. Their involvement may affect the level of cooperation the child is willing to give, and will lessen the amount of anxiety and stress felt by the child and family alike.

Preoperative fasting

It is now widely acknowledged that excessive fasting prior to surgery is inappropriate for children (Doswell et al 2002, Winslow et al 2002, Meurling 2004). As early as 1990, Schreiner et al (1990) showed that clear fluids up to 2 h before surgery for children of any age posed no additional risk of pulmonary aspiration during elective surgery. It is now accepted that children should not be fasted overnight prior to surgery/procedures and that a minimum fasting period of 2 h may be sufficient (Meurling 2004, RCN 2005). However, it is important for the nurse to be aware of hospital policy or protocol on fasting and, if unsure, to check with the appropriate anaesthetist.

AGE–APPROPRIATE PREPARATION

- Age-appropriate preparation is vital. Children have different attention spans and their ability to take in information and make sense of it may be limited. In these instances, it is more appropriate to direct most of the educational efforts towards the parents.

- Older age groups are looking for answers; knowledge gives them a sense of control and the ability to cooperate. They are more able to contribute to their own care by becoming involved in the planning and negotiating of preoperative care (Slote 2002). Explanations of the planned surgery and the sensations they will experience are appropriate (Stinson 1996).

- In the physical preparation, involve the parents as much as possible while giving them the opportunity to opt out of any part of the process with which they do not feel comfortable.

METHOD

1. Introduce yourself to the child and family as the nurse designated for the child's care.
2. Familiarise the child and family with the ward environment and the child's allocated bed.
3. Complete the admission procedure including baseline observations and current weight. Assist the medical staff with any preoperative investigations, e.g. haemoglobin levels, if necessary.
4. Encourage the child to bathe if not already done and remove any nail varnish. The fingertip colour is a good indication of the level of oxygenation in the bloodstream and is observed during the operative stage.
5. Remove any jewellery, or tape it if it cannot be removed, and either give it to the parents for

safekeeping or lock it in the hospital safe. (Jewellery can act as a conductor of electricity and may result in contact burns if not managed appropriately.)

6. Encourage the child to empty their bladder or put on a clean nappy prior to giving any premedication.

7. Make a note of any loose teeth and inform the anaesthetist. If a tooth is very loose, the anaesthetist may suggest that they remove it when the child is asleep to safeguard accidental ingestion or inhalation during the operation. Remove any dentures or plates.

8. If the child has long hair, tie it up using a non-metallic device.

9. Remove any prosthesis, hearing aids or spectacles. The latter two may be removed in the anaesthetic room at the last moment.

10. Some hospitals may allow children to wear their own clothes. If this is the case, ensure that they do not restrict access to the operation site; otherwise make sure that a suitable theatre gown is available for the child to wear. Small babies and neonates may also need to wear a hat as they lose most of their body heat through the scalp.

11. Check that the child has been fasted for a specified time.

12. Check that the child's name and hospital number are correct and legible on the wristband as sometimes these can become unclear after bathing.

13. Ensure that the premedication has been given by the prescribed route and at the prescribed time. If there are any queries relating to the premedication, check with the anaesthetist.

14. Check that the case notes, X-rays (if applicable) and nursing documentation are available, and that the consent form has been completed correctly.

15. Ensure that the operation site, if previously marked by the medical staff, is still clearly visible.

16. Complete the theatre checklist, as per local policy, and await confirmation that theatre is ready to receive the child. (The checklist should be completed immediately prior to the child going to theatre.)

17. Where the child's surgery has been delayed on the day of theatre, it is important to keep the family/parents informed. The anaesthetist must be contacted where the child is being maintained nil by mouth for an extended period as a result of delay, to avoid extensive fasting.

18. Accompany the child to theatre, having first checked the patient details with the theatre slip brought by the theatre porter. Some hospitals may check the details in theatre reception to confirm the identity of the child.

COMMUNITY PERSPECTIVE

Referral to the CCN team depends on the capacity and referral criteria of the team.

There are some cases where parents can be helped to organise specific equipment prior to admission, for example when a child is to have a hip spica plaster applied. It is always important to ensure that parents are well informed because any anxiety of the parent will be transmitted to the child. Preoperative therapeutic play can be undertaken in the home environment by community play specialists, where these are available (Shipton 1997). In this way, potentially traumatic situations can be defused by familiarising the child with medical equipment. Children with needle, or hospital, phobia may be referred prior to admission and, in the safe environment of the home, be helped to overcome their fears by various play techniques. In some centres, the play specialist can meet the children in the hospital on admission and continue to work with them. Children who are on the waiting list for a renal transplant can be prepared in advance in the home (Wilson 1992). This can be done by storytelling, playing with dolls and introducing medical equipment. In this way, children are helped to cope with some of their anxieties.

DOS AND DON'TS

- Do involve the parents in the preparation if they wish.
- Do be honest in answering the child's questions.
- Do remember that this is not routine to the family and be aware of their fears and anxieties.
- Do give clear and concise information.
- Do not assume that children who have had previous operations are not in need of support.
- Do not devolve total responsibility to parents to enforce fasting. Sometimes this can be misunderstood as meaning food only.

References

Audit Commission, 1993. Children first: a study of hospital services. HMSO, London.

Bray, L., Sanders, C., 2006. Preparing children and young people for stoma surgery. Paediatr. Nurs. 18 (4), 33–37.

Cohen, M., Cameron, C.B., Duncan, P.G., 1990. Pediatric anaesthesia morbidity and mortality in the perioperative period. Anaesth. Analg. 70, 160–167.

Darbyshire, P., 2003. Mothers' experiences of their child's recovery in hospital and at home: a qualitative investigation. J. Child Health Care 7 (4), 291–312.

Doswell, W.M., Jones, M., O'Donnell, J.M., 2002. One size may not fit all. Am. J. Nurs. 102 (6), 58, 61.

Gahan, B., Rogers, M., 1993. Recent advances in child health nursing. In: Glasper, A., Tucker, A. (Eds.), Advances in child health nursing. Scutari, London, pp. 91–105.

Hall, P.A., Payne, J.F., Stack, C.G., et al., 1995. Parents in the recovery room: survey of parental and staff attitudes: Comment. Br. Med. J. 310 (6983), 871.

Hogg, C., 1994. Setting standards for children undergoing surgery. Action for Sick Children, London.

Hogg, C., Cooper, C., 2004. Meeting the needs of young people undergoing surgery. Action for Sick Children, London.

Honeyman, L., 1994. Play for children with special needs. Paediatr. Nurs. 6 (3), 18–19.

Kelly, M.M., Adkins, L., 2003. Ingredients for a successful pediatric preoperative care process. AORN J. 77 (5), 1006–1011.

LeRoy, S., Elixson, E.M., O'Brein, P., et al., 2003. Recommendations for preparing children and adolescents for invasive cardiac procedures. Circulation 108, 2550–2564.

Meurling, S., 2004. Paediatric aspects: no fasting in children? Scand. J. Nutr. 48 (2), 83.

Morton, N.S., Raine, P.A.M., 1994. Paediatric day case surgery. Oxford Medical, Oxford.

Newman, J., Scott, G., 1990. Preoperative care. In: Paediatric nursing. Springhouse Clinical Rotation Guides, Springhouse, Philadelphia, pp. 219–224.

O'Connor-Von, S., 2000. Preparing children for surgery – an integrative research review. AORN J. 71 (2), 334–343.

RCN Royal College of Nursing, 2004. Sheet 3: Day surgery information. Children/young people in day surgery. RCN, London.

RCN Royal College of Nursing, 2005. Clinical practice guideline: Perioperative fasting in adults and children. RCN, London.

Richardson, J., 1992. Acute pain in childhood. Surg. Nurs. 22.

Sexton, K., Redfearn, M., 2003. Preadmission testing in a children's facility. AORN J. 78 (4), 604–617.

Schreiner, M.S., Treibwasser, A., Keon, T.P., et al., 1990. Ingestion of liquids compared with pre-operative fasting in paediatric outpatients. Anaesthesiology 72 (4), 593–597.

Shipton, H., 1997. Play at home. Cascade. Action for Sick Children, London, pp. 8–9.

Slote, R.J., 2002. Psychological aspects of caring for the adolescent undergoing spinal fusion for scoliosis. Orthop. Nurs. 21 (6), 19–30.

Smith, J., Dearmum, A., 2006. Improving care for children requiring surgery and their families. Paediatr. Nurs. 18 (9), 30–33.

Stinson, A., 1996. Cochlear implantations in children. AORN J. 64 (4), 561–571.

Sutherland, T., 2003. Comparison of hospital and home base preparation for cardiac surgery. Paediatr. Nurs. 15 (5), 13–16.

Thornes, R., 1991. Just for the day. Action for Sick Children, London.

Wilson, L., 1992. The home visiting programme. Paediatr. Nurs. (July), 10–11.

Winslow, E.H., Crenshaw, J.T., Warner, M.A., 2002. Best practice shouldn't be optional. Am. J. Nurs. 102 (6), 59, 63.

Chapter 23

Pressure area care

Louise Ford

CHAPTER CONTENTS

Introduction   234
   Learning outcomes   234
   Rationale   234
   Factors to note   235
   Risk factors to consider   235

Pressure sores   236

Prevention   237
   Developmental considerations   237

Education   237
   Equipment   237

Wound management   237
   Potential risks of inappropriate prevention and
   management of pressure sores   238
   Pressure risk and clinical governance   238
   Dos and don'ts   238

Conclusion   238

INTRODUCTION

Historically, scant attention has been given to the reporting of pressure sores in the child population (Tooher et al 2003). Waterlow's (1997) seminal study identified that children can develop pressure sores as a consequence of immobility, illness or hospitalisation, thus requiring the need for appropriate education, assessment and intervention. However, since then, the issue of research into the risk factors associated with the development of pressure sores has been scant but is now gaining momentum (Curley et al, 2003, Lane et al, 2004); although the majority of the evidence is based on studies undertaken with the adult and not the child population (Butler, 2006). More recently, however, Willock et al (2009) have developed and validated the Glamorgan Paediatric Pressure Area risk assessment scale, which is now being considered for introduction into many paediatric units across the UK.

LEARNING OUTCOMES

By the end of this section you should be able to:
● Understand the causes of pressure sores
● Explain the principles of pressure risk assessment
● Understand nursing care and pressure sore prevention
● Explain policy-driven changes to improve pressure risk assessment and management.

RATIONALE

Pressure sore risk assessment is now considered an essential element of care in adults as shown in the document *Essence of Care*; this focuses on quality of care and benchmarking to deliver evidence-based practice (DoH 2001). While this is a positive step forward, it does not specifically include the child population; there are essential elements of pressure sore risk assessment, care and management that can be applied in principle when caring for children and young people (Waterlow 1997, DoH 2001, NICE 2003a,b, Noonan et al 2006).

FACTORS TO NOTE

Historically, pressure ulcers in children were not seen as different to those in the adult population (Noonan et al 2006). Recent studies report pressure ulcer rates in the child population ranging from 4% to 13% (Willock et al 2000, McLane et al 2004). Pressure ulcers in the critically ill child have been reported to be 27% (Curley et al 2003).

While there are various pressure risk assessment scoring methods in use within clinical and community healthcare practice when caring for adults, until recently nothing existed for the assessment of infants and children with very little evidence available to inform and support the practice (Noonan et al 2006). Consideration needs to be given to the assessment of risk for infants and children and interventions used to maintain skin integrity that are evidence-based (Noonan et al 2006).

McGurk et al (2004) have developed two assessment tools for use with infants and acutely ill children. The neonatal scale measures and assesses skin integrity taking into account gestational age; the tool to measure skin integrity in children takes into account the needs of the acutely ill child.

Curley et al (2003) developed the Braden Q scale specifically for use in the child population: this has been modified further and validated for use with neonates (The Neonatal/Infant Braden Q (McLane et al 2004).

All formal assessments of risk should be documented and accessible for other professionals within the interprofessional team and also meet the requirements of good record-keeping and hospital/Trust policies (NMC 2009).

RISK FACTORS TO CONSIDER

Samaniego (2003) identified a higher incidence of pressure ulcers within specific risk groups of infants and children, e.g. children in plaster casts; in wheelchairs and wearing prostheses. In spite of these earlier studies, Butler (2006) maintains that there is still a paucity of information regarding the risk factors that are associated with pressure ulcer development in children (Butler 2006).

Butler (2006) identified factors which affect pressure sore risk as either extrinsic or intrinsic.

Extrinsic factors

- Pressure: compression on a local point, due to reduced or lack of mobility (Quigley & Curley 1996)
- Shearing: distortion of the skin beyond its ability to adapt, due to poor positioning
- Friction: the skin is in contact with the supporting surface, due to inappropriate manual handling techniques
- Moisture to the skin: delayed hygiene/elimination needs met.

Intrinsic factors

- Nutritional status: obesity or lack of body mass
- Oxygenation and tissue perfusion
- Dehydration: skin turgor.

Consideration of these factors provides identification of children who may be at risk of pressure sore development. Butler (2006) also recommends each child should be assessed with the participation and involvement of the family and should be evidence-based. The emphasis needs to be placed on accurate, consistent documentation that highlights the nature of the damage to tissues and the development and use of a skin care algorithm (Butler 2006, p 449). Although this presents a challenge when assessing the unwell child with an altered level of consciousness, an acute illness or complete immobility, a full and thorough assessment of pressure risks is essential (RCN 2001). It is important therefore to consider the following aspects in the assessment.

Body weight

Children who are underweight, overweight, or have excess weight due to fluid retention as a consequence of the side-effects of medications, may also experience difficulty in mobilising. Special consideration should be given to neonates who have less body mass, and therefore may experience increased risk over bony prominences and high localised pressure (e.g. the back of the head) (Willock et al 2000, Barnes 2004, McGurk et al 2004).

Elimination

The child who is experiencing continence problems is not only at risk of developing pressure sores but is also at increased risk of infection due to breakdown in skin integrity as a consequence of prolonged contact with urine and faecal matter (Zollo 1996). While infants may be considered as incontinent, it is prolonged contact with urine and/or faecal matter that will cause a break in skin integrity and not as a consequence of undue pressure (McLane et al 2004).

Skin integrity

Children with special needs may experience poor skin integrity due to reduced circulation, poor hydration and inactivity, and therefore have a tendency to have dry and fragile skin that excoriates easily. Conversely, these children may have a greasy or oily skin type, which may become sore and chaffed due to excessive perspiration. Children with thermal injuries are at particular risk of further skin breakdown due to excessive fluid loss (Bosworth-Bousfield 2002). Neonates are also vulnerable because their skin is very translucent and delicate (McGurk et al 2004).

Mobility

The body's natural response to prolonged pressure discomfort in any part of the body is to try to change position spontaneously. In the child with reduced mobility due, for example, to altered conscious levels, the child with special or complex needs; the child in traction or the severely thermally injured child, the increased risk of pressure sore development due to immobility is even greater (Samaniego 2003). It is therefore essential that a high quality of nursing care be provided to prevent pressure sores developing. Equally, the child who has been in theatre for a prolonged period or the ventilated child in intensive care is also at risk from breakdown in skin integrity (Barnes 2004, Noonan et al 2006).

Nutrition and hydration

These are vital aspects in reducing and assessing pressure area risk. Malnutrition increases the skin's vulnerability to pressure sore formation. It is essential that the child's dietary requirements are fully documented on admission and throughout the child's care. It is vital to liaise with other healthcare professionals such as the dietician to ensure that essential nutritional elements are provided, for example:

- Vitamin C – essential for collagen synthesis
- Vitamin E – to reduce tissue damage
- Protein – to encourage collagen synthesis and wound remodelling
- Zinc – if deficient, delays wound healing (McGurk et al 2004).

Accurate nutritional and fluid assessment by the nurse is fundamental, as other nutritional deficits such as failure to thrive and eating disorders can become more complex in the critically ill child. Therefore adequate fluids and nutrition are essential to reduce the risks of developing pressure ulcers and to help in the healing process (Butler 2006). If the infant or child is dehydrated, the skin can become dry, scaly and fragile and children that are oedematous can experience similar changes in skin integrity (Barnes 2004).

Medication

Some drug therapies cause skin to change, for example the use of long-term steroid therapy, anti-inflammatory and cytotoxic drugs. These pharmacological preparations can cause the skin to become fragile, dry and at increased risk of damage due to inhibition of the body's immune system. Some inotropes cause peripheral vasoconstriction. Sedation can also lead to altered consciousness, where the child is less likely to alter their position to relieve pressure (Barnes 2004).

PRESSURE SORES

Pressure sores can occur anywhere, depending on the cause, but typical sites for pressure sores in children will include any bony prominences, this is largely attributed to the fact that head and body sizes are disproportionate with the head being particularly at risk including the ears; other vulnerable areas include the sacrum, buttocks and heels (Butler 2006). Other risk factors in the acutely ill child include duration of intubation and the risks associated with the use of other medical equipment, such as tubing, leads or intravenous lines (Butler 2006).

Butler (2006) cites the work of Quigley and Curley (1996) and the Braden Q Scale as one to assessing children potentially at risk from pressure ulcers. For further details, read Butler (2006) and McGurk et al (2004).

PREVENTION

It is essential to carry out pressure risk assessment as part of the normal admission and in the ongoing assessment of the child while they are in hospital. The purpose of assessment is to identify areas of potential risk and implement interventions to reduce the chances of skin breakdown occurring.

Consideration of the child's environment is essential; lying on something hard such as monitor leads, intravenous lines or a toy even for a short period can initiate pressure sore development.

These interventions may be the subject of local policies and care pathways; however Cockett (2002) recognised that pressure sores can occur even when preventive aids are used.

DEVELOPMENTAL CONSIDERATIONS

- Age can affect the area of the body where pressure damage can occur: older children tend to develop sores at the sacrum/ coccyx with damage to the heels and occiput second (Willock et al 2000, Baldwin 2002)
- Skin damage in infants and children frequently occur on the occipital region, ears, sacrum and scapula (Amlung et al 2001)
- Regardless of age, most pressure ulcers are found to be partial thickness (Amlung et al 2001)
- Curley et al (2003) in a multisite PICU prospective cohort study reported a 27% incidence of pressure ulcers in the acutely ill child
- Assessment, identification and the correcting or avoiding of risk factors are the most important aspects of prevention and care (Curley et al 2003). For example, malnutrition and dehydration can be corrected through nutritional and fluid management; for the child experiencing continence difficulties, the nurse's

responsibility is to ensure effective hygiene care, which may include the management of continence.

EDUCATION

It is an essential component of pressure area risk assessment and management that parents and nursing staff are trained and competent in the use of pressure risk tools and equipment (Butler 2006). This can be achieved through liaison with other health professionals such as the tissue viability or wound management specialist nurses. It is also important to carry out pressure area care utilising evidence-based practice to improve standards of care (DoH 2001).

EQUIPMENT

Use of guidelines in conjunction with local policy will assist with pressure relief (RCN 2001). An in-depth assessment and accurate documentation of the child's needs is also vital (Butler 2006).

- Children deemed to be at low risk could use a standard mattress.
- For medium-risk cases, use of a pressure-relieving mattress or overlays is advisable, depending on local/trust policy. Other aids such as silicone gel or foam pads may be beneficial.
- Children at high risk of skin breakdown, e.g. children having prolonged surgery, should have access to a soft conforming theatre table along with the use of other appropriate pressure-relieving aids. Use of airwave inflation systems will help to reduce moisture and the use of a therapeutic mattress will help relieve pressure and help circulation (Butler 2006).
- For the child with total restrictions on mobility, e.g. the child with complex wound management needs or the thermally injured child, specialist equipment such as Clinitron air-fluidised therapy and low-flow therapy beds will assist in their nursing care.

WOUND MANAGEMENT

Wound management should follow accepted principles of wound care (see Ch. 37).

POTENTIAL RISKS OF INAPPROPRIATE PREVENTION AND MANAGEMENT OF PRESSURE SORES

- *To the child and family:* pain, scarring and disfigurement, low self-esteem, risk of further complications, septicaemia and death
- *To the nurse:* vulnerability to litigation for negligent practice; failure to fulfil obligations set out in the Code of Professional Conduct (NMC 2009); decreased job satisfaction
- *To the organisation:* cost of litigation cases; increased costs for inpatient care, due to prolonged bed occupancy. There is also a need to question the quality of service provision, which could have a negative impact upon the trust/hospital in question.

PRESSURE RISK AND CLINICAL GOVERNANCE

The prevention and management of pressure sores is a quality issue and therefore nurses have a responsibility to ensure that it forms part of the clinical governance agenda in their clinical area. Clinical governance in relation to pressure area care can be viewed under the following components:

- *Clinical risk management:* This is achieved through assessment, analysis and learning from actions seen and perceived
- *Clinical effectiveness:* Pressure risk assessment and management is monitored and evaluated as to the effectiveness of care. This includes evidence-based practice, clinical guidelines and clinical outcome measures (DoH 2001). Key aspects are education, information and critical appraisal
- *Clinical audit:* Ensures high standards of patient care, measuring current practice against standards of best practice; audit will then lead to improving clinical practice (McLane et al 2004, Groeneveld et al 2004).

COMMUNITY PERSPECTIVE

Children with a variety of conditions who are cared for at home may be at risk of developing pressure sores.

The responsibility of the CCN is to ensure that carers are aware of all potential problems. The CCN will need to educate the carers on pressure-relieving methods, such as positioning and turning, and on fluid and dietary requirements. Some families may require the loan of specialist equipment, the use of which will need to be demonstrated by the CCN. Some household equipment may need to be adapted to meet a specific need.

The CCN will need excellent knowledge of local resources in order to meet the needs of the family. Although some community nursing services have a good supply of equipment, the CCN may need to pursue and persist in order to obtain the optimum equipment for a particular child.

DOS AND DON'TS

- Do assess each child individually, taking into account potential/actual extrinsic and intrinsic factors.
- Do ensure all potential risks are documented accurately in the child's care record.
- Do utilise all available resources and literature to improve clinical practice and reduce potential risks of pressure development.
- Do not make assumptions that children do not get pressure sores.

CONCLUSION

It is essential that assessment of every child is thoroughly implemented, taking into account all known and potential risk factors. Accurate documentation of the child's skin integrity status is vital to assist with effective tissue viability management; it should also be noted that collaboration with other significant members of the multidisciplinary team should be encouraged to ensure that a seamless service of care is provided.

References

Amlung, S.R., Miller, W.L., Bosley, L.M., 2001. The 1999 National pressure ulcer prevalence survey: a benchmarking approach. Adv. Skin Wound Care 14, 297–301.

Baldwin, K.M., 2002. Incidence and prevalence of pressure ulcers in children. Adv. Skin Wound Care 15 (3), 121–124.

Barnes, S., 2004. The use of a pressure ulcer risk assessment tool for children. Nurs. Times. 100 (14), 56–58.

Bosworth-Bousfield, C., 2002. Burn trauma: management and nursing care, second ed. Whurr, London.

Butler, C.T., 2006. Pediatric skin care: guidelines for assessment, prevention, and treatment. Pediatr. Nurs. 32 (5), 443–450.

Cockett, A., 2002. A research review to identify the factors contributing to the development of pressure ulcers in paediatric patients. J. Tissue Viability 12 (1), 16–23.

Curley, M.A., Quigley, S.M., Lin, M., 2003. Pressure ulcers in pediatric intensive care: incidence and associated factors. Pediatr. Crit. Care Med. 4, 284–290.

DoH Department of Health, 2001. Essence of care. Patient focused benchmarking for healthcare practitioners. TSO, London.

Groeneveld, A., Anderson, M., Allen, S., et al., 2004. The prevalence of pressure ulcers in a tertiary care pediatric and adult hospital. J. Wound Ostomy Continence Nurs. 31 (3), 108–120.

McGurk, V., Holloway, B., Crutchley, A., et al., 2004. Skin integrity assessment in neonates and children. Paediatr. Nurs. 16 (3), 15–18.

McLane, K.M., Bookout, K., McCord, S., et al., 2004. The 2003 National Pediatric Pressure Ulcer and Skin Breakdown Prevalence Survey. J. Wound Ostomy Continence Nurs. 31 (4), 168–178.

NICE, 2003a. Pressure ulcer prevention. Clinical Guideline 7. National Institute for Clinical Excellence, London.

NICE, 2003b. The use of pressure relieving devices (beds, mattresses and overlays) for the prevention of pressure ulcers in primary and secondary care. National Institute for Clinical Excellence, London.

Noonan, C., Quigley, S., Curley, M.A., 2006. Skin integrity in hospitalised infants and children. A prevalence survey. J. Pediatr. Nurs. 21 (6), 445–453.

Nursing and Midwifery Council, 2009. Code of Professional Conduct. NMC, London.

Quigley, S.M., Curley, M.A., 1996. Skin integrity in the pediatric population: preventing and managing pressure ulcers. J. Soc. Pediatr. Nurs. 1 (1), 7–18.

Royal College of Nursing, 2001. Pressure ulcer risk assessment and prevention. RCN, London.

Samaniego, J.A., 2003. A sore spot in pediatrics: risk factors for pressure ulcers. Dermatol. Nurs. 16 (2), 153–159.

Tooher, R., Middleton, P., Babidge, W., 2003. Implementation of pressure ulcer guidelines: what constitutes a successful strategy? J. Wound Care 12 (10), 373–382.

Waterlow, J., 1997. Practical use of the Waterlow tool in the community. Br. J. Nurs. 2 (2), 283–286.

Willock, J., Baharastani, M.M., Anthony, D., 2009. The Development of the Glamorgan paediatric pressure ulcer risk assessment scale. Journal of Wound Care 18 (1), 17–21.

Willock, J., Hughes, J., Tickle, S., et al., 2000. Pressure sores in children: the acute hospital perspective. J. Tissue Viability 12 (2), 59–62.

Zollo, M.B., Schmidt, J.E., Gostisha, M.L., et al., 1996. Altered skin integrity in children admitted to a pediatric intensive care unit. J. Nurs. Care Qual. 11 (2), 62–67.

Further reading

Chambers, N., Jolly, A., 2002. Essence of care: making a difference. Nurs. Stand. 17 (11), 40–44.

NICE, 2001. Working together to prevent pressure ulcers: a guide for patients and carers. National Institute for Clinical Excellence, London.

Chapter 24

Radiography

Joanne Moore

CHAPTER CONTENTS

Introduction   240
   Learning outcomes   240
   Rationale   241
   Factors to note   241

General principles   242
   General environment   242
   Preparation of the child and parent/carer   242
   General care   243
   Sedation and general anaesthetics   244

Investigations   245
   Some common investigations   245
   Computed tomography (CT) imaging   246
   Ultrasound   246
   Magnetic resonance imaging (MRI)   246
   Nuclear medicine   247
   Interventional radiology   248
   Dos and don'ts   249

INTRODUCTION

This section is written to help nurses understand their role in preparing children for radiological investigation and assisting the radiologist/radiographer to perform radiological investigations on children. Some radiology departments may have a designated radiology nurse who is experienced in all aspects of the department and the procedures that are performed. When this facility is not available, the role will often fall on the ward nurse who accompanies the child to the radiology department. In some instances, even if there is a radiology department nurse available, it may be necessary for the nurse caring for the child to stay during the procedure to assist with holding, provide advice on the child's condition and utilise previously developed nurse–patient and parental rapport to gain optimal imaging. The role of the escort nurse will be primarily that of patient advocate but equally important will be the preparation of the child and carer, based on a thorough assessment of the child and knowledge of the examination required. The nurse may be involved in the preparation of equipment prior to the examination and will also be required to support the child and family. The nurse may also assist the radiographer in ensuring that the child remains in the correct position.

LEARNING OUTCOMES

By the end of this section you should be able to:
- Prepare a child and their family for X-ray examination
- Identify ways to minimise radiation

- Provide detailed explanation to child and family of what they will see, hear and feel throughout the radiological examination
- Observe and adhere to IRMER (TSO 2000) guidelines
- Explain the difference between ionising radiation and non-ionising radiation
- Assist in performing a radiological examination safely with or without sedation
- Describe the common types of radiological investigations.

RATIONALE

The need for an X-ray examination is usually for diagnostic purposes. The most common types of radiology modalities include plain film, ultrasound, computed tomography (CT), magnetic resonance imaging (MRI), interventional radiology/angiography and nuclear medicine. Interventional radiology is a rapidly growing subspecialty within radiology that is becoming increasingly popular and useful as both a diagnostic and treatment tool (Kaye 2000, Roebuck 2001). A child may also need to be supported during radiotherapy. If children are being treated in district general hospitals and require X-rays, in a department that mainly treats adults, the child's nurse will need to ensure that they are adequately prepared, taking into account the size and unfamiliarity of the equipment.

FACTORS TO NOTE

- All X-ray examinations must be requested either by a medical practitioner or by a nurse or other healthcare professional that has undergone the appropriate training and has been allowed by their trust/hospital to request certain radiology examinations. The benefits of radiological information that may aid in clinical diagnosis or treatment must be balanced against the potential hazards of the exposure to radiation (TSO 2000).
- The X-ray examination is clinically directed by the radiologist or trained physicist.
- The radiographer normally directs and is responsible for the examination.
- All X-rays hold a potential risk.
- It is important to remember that although the risk to the individual child is insignificant, it is general philosophy that the dose to the general

public from medical use of ionising radiation should be reduced.
- The dose to the child in diagnostic radiology is generally a very low or low dose. We are all exposed to background radiation on a daily basis and a child's chest X-ray is equivalent to 1 day of background radiation, therefore one could assume that a child undergoing a plain chest X-ray is 1 day older in radiation terms (Crawley 2002).
- The net gain should outweigh the risk; this is especially pertinent to children undergoing frequent X-ray examinations.
- Before any investigations are performed on any child, the principles laid down in the Ionising Radiation (Medical Exposure) Regulations 2000 must be adhered to (TSO 2000).
- Nurses should take responsibility and act as an advocate for the child, i.e. ensure there is no possibility of pregnancy in girls of child-bearing age.
- Nurses or mothers who are pregnant should not assist with X-ray examinations in order to protect the unborn child. It is the responsibility of the operator to determine whether or not the patient and/or their carers may be pregnant.
  It is sufficient to ask the accompanying adult if there is any chance they may be pregnant. Determining possible pregnancy in children undergoing tests requires diplomacy and sensitivity. If the child is competent to answer the question independently, you must determine whether they have started having regular periods. For patients with regular periods undergoing low-dose tests, e.g. plain chest film, who are sure their period is not overdue, you should proceed with the examination. Patients requiring high-dose procedures, e.g. barium enemas, CT of abdomen and pelvis, interventional procedures involving direct exposure of the abdomen and pelvis, and nuclear medicine tests with high fetal dose investigations, should be asked when their last period started. If it was within 10 days of the start of their last period, the test may proceed. If the test is requested more than 10 days since the start of their last period, it must be determined if there is any chance they may be pregnant. The answer to the pregnancy question should be documented on the radiology request form (TSO 2000). Staff that think they may be pregnant are asked not to accompany the child into the examination room,

and all young females are asked if they have started their menstrual cycle; if so, the steps outlined above are actioned, otherwise no further action is taken.

GENERAL PRINCIPLES

GENERAL ENVIRONMENT

Many radiology departments are largely adult focused, particularly in district general hospitals. It is important that consideration is given to the child in the environment of the X-ray department. The area should be child friendly with toys and games appropriate for different ages. Posters of current television favourites may be displayed. This helps to distract the child and may help in developing a relationship that will assist the radiographer. The *National Service Framework for Children* (DoH 2003) clearly states that children should be cared for in child-friendly hospitals and that hospitals should be safe and healthy places for children. Children should receive care based on their needs and the needs of their family. They should also be encouraged to participate in their care. Children should be encouraged to bring one of their favourite toys into the department with them so that they can be X-rayed together. Depending on the type of test being carried out, it may be possible for children to listen to their favourite CD or watch a video. These options should be discussed with the child prior to arriving at the radiology department and, if appropriate, the child can choose their entertainment or bring their own with them.

The X-ray room should be warm to avoid cooling of the child. Some clothing can be left in place, depending on the type of X-ray examination; if there is any doubt the nurse should check with the radiographer. It is advisable to remove any clothes with metal buttons or zippers beforehand. If it is anticipated that the procedure will be lengthy or if the patient is a neonate, a warming blanket should be placed on the bed. Children undergoing a MRI scan need to be checked more thoroughly by a trained person to ensure they have nothing on them that is incompatible with the MRI scanner. This includes any jewellery, body piercings, hair grips/slides, coins and medical implants. Anything metallic that can be removed should be, and any surgical implants should be thoroughly investigated prior to

the scan to ensure they are MRI compatible. Many MRI departments have a folder which lists devices and their compatibility.

The stability of the child's condition must be assessed before considering a move to the radiology department. The use of portable X-ray machines within intensive care units and isolation cubicles is common practice. Children whose access to the department is difficult or whose condition might be compromised, e.g. children in balanced traction or immune-suppressed children being reverse barrier nursed (nursed in protective isolation), should also be considered for a portable X-ray machine. Wall-mounted oxygen, suction and monitoring equipment should be available in every radiology room. Full resuscitation equipment for all ages of children must be present within the department.

PREPARATION OF THE CHILD AND PARENT/CARER

Preparation is one of the most important parts of any investigation in paediatric radiology. Parent participation is actively encouraged.

A full explanation of the procedure, equipment and process of events will help alleviate both the child's and the parent's anxiety. The provision of age-appropriate leaflets should be made available for the parent and child to take away with them to read at their leisure; this allows them the opportunity to think of any questions they may want answering prior to the planned procedure. A play specialist may also provide useful demonstrations using a favourite toy to show the child where they will be placed within the room and how close the X-ray equipment will come to them, but will not touch them. The explanation to the parents and the child should be provided before the child enters the investigation room. The language and depth of the explanation should be appropriate to the patient's age and understanding and will include any activity expected of the child, e.g. drinking the medication, holding their breath or micturating during the procedure. If the investigation requires the insertion of a cannula or catheterisation, the child and family will need to be given an indication of how and when this is likely to occur.

The child and parents need to know and understand that it is important for the child to remain still during the X-ray examination. If analgesia or sedation is to be used, this needs to be discussed with the parents as part of the preparation. There should also be a discussion on the most appropriate person to accompany the child to the department. This should be the person who is most able to comfort, calm, help restrain and offer reassurance to the child during the investigation.

An assessment of the child will be required as part of the admission process. If the child is an outpatient, an explanation of what will happen and reinforcement of the events during the procedure are necessary. The child should be weighed to enable the correct doses of drugs and radiopaque dye to be administered.

There needs to be communication between the nurse and radiologist to arrange the most suitable time for the procedure and to enable analgesia and sedation to be administered at the most appropriate time for it to be effective. Always check the name and date of birth of the child against the radiology request form prior to undertaking any investigation.

Preparation books

Books and leaflets written for children can help in explaining the type of equipment that will be used and the procedures involved. These will give a simple explanation of the process during the procedures and explain that the X-ray machines are large, can be mobile, i.e. move around the child, and that sometimes a tube above them may move towards them but it will never actually touch them during the procedure. The examination table on which the child is lying may also move at various times throughout the procedure. If a detailed explanation, including pictures, is given to the child and their parent/carer beforehand, it may help to alleviate unnecessary anxiety and make the equipment appear less frightening. Some departments may have an album with photographs of the various members of staff that the child and parents will meet and the various pieces of equipment they may encounter.

Play therapy

Some hospitals are fortunate in having a play therapy department. Play therapists are trained to help prepare the child for a variety of procedures, through play (see Ch. 10).

GENERAL CARE

Privacy

This is an important aspect of any procedure. All children should have their investigation in private and only people who are necessary for the investigation should remain in the X-ray room.

Protection

The nurse and/or parent must wear a lead apron and thyroid collar if assisting with the X-ray examination. Local protection for the child may be required, for example ovary/gonad pads. When X-rays are being taken on the ward using portable equipment, a safe zone should be established, ensuring that no unnecessary personnel are present in the area and that those who are required are wearing protective clothing. The nurse may be asked to help if the mother is pregnant and is unable to hold the child herself.

Positioning

The correct positioning of the child and the maintenance of the position during the X-ray examination is one of the most important aspects of the care. The radiographer will assist the nurse and/or parent in achieving the position that is required. The difficulty in positioning is greater with a child up to the age of 5 years (Gyll 1982) but does become easier as the child gets older. The radiographer may provide various adapted boxes or stools for the child to sit or lie on, to get the best picture/results first time.

It is the nurse's role to ensure that the child is not restrained against their will or for any great length of time and that appropriate explanation and reassurance are given. Where possible the nurse should anticipate and prevent the need for holding through giving the child information encouragement and distraction (RCN 2003).

In the case of a wheelchair-bound or physically handicapped child it is always advisable to ask the child's usual carer how to lift the child without harming yourself or the child. It may not be possible to obtain particular X-rays on some physically handicapped children because of their inability to move or maintain a particular position. The nurse should remember that they are the child's advocate on these occasions. Local lifting and handling policies must be adhered to.

Praise and reward

At the end of any X-ray examination, the child must be praised for their cooperation and, if appropriate, a bravery certificate, sticker or small present awarded.

SEDATION AND GENERAL ANAESTHETICS

As imaging technology advances, the need to keep children absolutely still during some X-ray procedures, especially interventional, MRI and CT scans, is increasing. It is highly unlikely that children under 5 years old or those with special needs will remain still while a MRI scan is being performed, as they may find the noise of the scan traumatic and feel very claustrophobic. Therefore the child may require intervention to help them tolerate the scan (Sury et al 2005). This may only be achieved by using either sedation or general anaesthesia. Local policy regarding fasting, preparation and monitoring during sedation and general anaesthesia must be adhered to. Invasive procedures require an appropriately trained nurse to remain with the patient, as any deterioration or distress may require intervention.

In very young babies, i.e. <6 weeks old, and/or those <5 kg, it is recommended that they be given their usual feed if this is not contraindicated, and then wrapping them snugly. Babies will often fall asleep as they usually would after their feed, thus avoiding the need for sedation. However while some babies are soothed by the constant noise of the scanner it appears that others are very distressed by it and are unable to tolerate the scan therefore a reduced dose of sedation may be administered.

If sedation is required, a doctor will prescribe it, the type and method of administration being adjusted according to the estimated length of the procedure. If children are attending as outpatients, sedation will normally be administered before they enter the examination room. If your radiology department does not have a day stay facility and, depending on local hospital policy, it is strongly recommended that a day bed be prearranged within the hospital so the child can recover fully before going home.

Children who have been given sedation should arrive in the department already asleep or drowsy. Monitoring of these children is the responsibility of the nurse present. A set of baseline observations should be taken pre-sedation, including pulse, respiration rate, oxygen saturation and colour.

During the investigation the child should be constantly monitored for colour, O_2 saturation, pulse and respiration. The child should be sent back to the ward after the investigation with a full set of observations and a complete handover should be given to the ward staff.

Some units have developed nurse-led sedation programmes which are finely tuned to meet the sedation requirements of their particular unit. Sury et al (1999) discovered that children require deep sedation to remain suitably still for successful completion of their MRI scan. This study showed that, with the appropriate training, a nurse-led sedation service can be safely used for MRI in children. They also found that sedating a child in the unit where the examination is to take place increases success of sedation, as opposed to transporting a drowsy child between departments. Great care must be exercised in adhering to the sedation policy of these units and ensuring that staff are appropriately trained.

A child with airway problems, raised intracranial pressure or difficult behavioural problems should be carefully reviewed prior to sedation. Sedation is not usually indicated under these circumstances and the child should receive a general anaesthetic. General anaesthesia is administered by an anaesthetist and anaesthetic nurse who will be responsible for all patient monitoring during and immediately after the procedure. The child should then be sufficiently recovered before returning to the ward (Sury et al 1999).

If the child requires a general anaesthetic, the ward nurse should accompany the patient with the parents into the anaesthetic area and check the patient's name, hospital number and date of birth with the anaesthetic nurse. A consent form should also be signed by the parents or carers prior to the investigation. In most anaesthetic areas one parent is usually allowed to stay until the child is asleep. Once asleep, the parent and ward nurse should leave the anaesthetic area unless the ward nurse is required to assist with the investigation.

Following the procedure and extubation, a recovery nurse should monitor the child until they are able to maintain their own airway and are rousable by speech. Once the child demonstrates they are able to maintain their own airway, they should be sent back to their ward or day stay unit until they have completely recovered and returned to their pre-anaesthetised state, before being discharged. Age-appropriate resuscitation equipment must be available in all areas where a child is sedated or given a general anaesthetic.

INVESTIGATIONS

The majority of radiological investigations require radiopaque dye to be administered, the method of administration usually involving an invasive procedure such as cannulation and sometimes catheterisation. These procedures should be carefully explained to the child and their parent prior to them arriving in the radiology department. Some children may have an allergic reaction to the contrast medium. Although the incidence of this is very rare, children or their carers should be questioned prior to administration to ensure they have not had any previous reaction to radiopaque dye or other iodine-based substance.

SOME COMMON INVESTIGATIONS

Plain X-rays

These are usually X-rays of the chest, skeleton or abdomen. The radiographer should explain exactly what is to happen, before the child is positioned. The aim is to keep the child still and correctly positioned, e.g. not rotated for a chest X-ray, so that only the minimal number of exposures are taken. They are non-invasive and should not give any discomfort to the child.

Micturating cystogram

A micturating cystogram is one of the most common investigations performed on children with any indication of pelvic, ureteric or bladder obstruction or malformation and urinary reflux.

Radiopaque dye is instilled into the bladder via a catheter. In most hospitals the catheter is inserted by the medical staff or radiologist but it may also be performed by the nurse if proficient in this practice. Some hospitals advocate the use of a local anaesthetic gel which is administered five minutes prior to catheterisation. The child is then encouraged to micturate and X-rays are taken. As the bladder contracts, malformations or abnormalities of the bladder or ureter may be demonstrated.

Barium study

Barium or contrast swallows, meals and follow-throughs are some of the most common upper gastrointestinal investigations performed in paediatric radiology. They are used to indicate the patency of the gastrointestinal tract and any abnormalities of anatomy or physiology within it. Barium swallow investigates the child's swallowing technique, the oropharynx, the oesophagus and the fundus of the stomach. According to the child's underlying condition, the choice of contrast medium will be at the discretion of the radiologist.

The child's age must be taken into account when selecting the vessel from which to drink the medium. A small baby can be given a bottle, but the hole in the teat has to be made slightly larger to allow the barium through. A toddler will normally take a drink from a beaker. It may be advisable to use the child's own beaker as the familiarity may encourage drinking the barium. Older children can use a straw or ordinary cup. Flavouring the barium is also advised. This can be achieved with either milk shake flavourings or powders.

A barium meal follows on from the barium swallow and follows the gastrointestinal tract into the stomach, the duodenum and jejunum. Barium meal and follow-through encompasses both of the above, but follows the entire intestinal tract to the terminal ileum and the ileocaecal junction.

A barium contrast enema is used to investigate the large bowel, its patency and any abnormalities. The contrast is administered by a rectal tube via the anus and rectum. In some sick children, the risks involved in contrast enemas are high and include perforation of the gut and respiratory distress in a child who is obstructed. The procedure should therefore not be undertaken lightly and must be under the direct supervision of a radiologist following a request from a surgical colleague. Oxygen, suction and full resuscitation equipment should be available.

Air enema

Intussusception is a commonly occurring condition in infants, characterised by the bowel backing up into itself. Air is instilled under pressure via a Foley tube placed in the rectum. It is important that a good seal is achieved and the pressure under which the air is instilled is increased gradually. Not all intussusceptions are fully reducible using this method and in some instances, reduction using air enema is contraindicated. If this is the case the child should be referred for surgical review (Bisset & Kirks 1988, Reijnen et al 1990).

COMPUTED TOMOGRAPHY (CT) IMAGING

A CT scan is a type of X-ray examination and refers to the way in which the equipment works.

X-rays, like radio waves, can pass through objects and be utilised to create a picture. During an X-ray examination, the beam of rays pass through the body, where it is absorbed to differing degrees by tissues such as bone, muscle and by organs. When the rays emerge on the other side of the body, they create a pattern of light and dark on a film, the image.

During a CT examination the child has to lie on a table which moves slowly through the CT scanner. The patient is rarely left alone in the room while the pictures are taken, parents/carers are encouraged to accompany them, however they must wear a lead apron and females must not be pregnant (see above).

The length of time of the CT scan varies, depending on the scan required. Generally CT scans take about 5–10 min duration. Often there is no patient preparation required prior to CT scanning, however, commonly CT of the abdomen requires oral contrast and intra-venous injection.

It is often necessary for the child to have an injection of a radiological contrast agent (sometimes referred to as a dye) into a vein via an intra-venous cannula, which may have been inserted on the ward. This contrast allows better visualisation of some organs. If an iodinated contrast agent is used this can make the child feel very warm when it is injected, but this feeling passes quickly and is quite normal. In some very rare cases a child may develop an allergic reaction to the contrast, and it is therefore imperative that any previous allergies are ascertained prior to the procedure. There are no long-term side-effects of this contrast as it passes quickly through the kidneys to the bladder.

While the pictures are being taken, the child may sometimes be asked to breathe in and hold their breath. This should be practised beforehand. Children find it difficult to keep still, which is why a good explanation beforehand is vital.

ULTRASOUND

This is a type of scan which takes place in the radiology department. It uses sound waves, not X-rays,

and is therefore safe. The sound waves pass through the body, giving back a signal and providing a black and white image which is produced on a television screen. This image is then interpreted by a radiographer or radiologist.

The preparation required will depend on the part of the body which is to be examined. When the pelvis is to be checked, it is useful if the bladder is full; however, this is not always practical in all age groups. A full bladder provides a 'window' to look through and see the other organs in the pelvis. The child lies on a couch and uncovers the part of the body which is to be examined. Gel is squirted onto the skin to give good contact between the machine and the skin. The transducer, which looks like a microphone, is then moved gently over the skin. The examination does not hurt at all; it tickles and the child may complain that the gel is cold. The child may be asked to breathe in and hold their breath while a clear picture is taken.

After the scan, the gel is wiped off and the child is free to go. As no X-rays are used, parents or nurses can accompany the child. The mother is often able to give the child a good explanation, as the procedure is similar to that used during pregnancy.

MAGNETIC RESONANCE IMAGING (MRI)

MRI is a way of looking inside the body without using X-rays. MRI can produce two- or three-dimensional images using a very large magnet, radio waves and a computer. The magnet is large enough to surround a patient, which is why it is sometimes referred to as a tunnel. There are no known harmful effects from exposure to a strong magnetic field, this allows children to have someone stay with them during their scan; however, expectant mothers are advised to remain outside the room.

Usually, there is no prior patient preparation required for an MRI scan, but no one is admitted to the MRI scanner without satisfactory completion of a detailed MRI safety questionnaire. Of particular concern are metallic implants or devices; MRI compatibility of such devices must be known before the patient is allowed to have a MRI scan. Cardiac pacemakers and external pacing wires are an absolute contraindication to MRI. Metallic objects are not allowed in the scanning room as they can cause serious injury to the patient or damage the scanner. This is because magnetic objects turn into dangerous projectiles when exposed to a very strong magnetic field.

Children do not have to undress as long as they are not wearing clothes with zips or other metal bits. They can come in pyjamas or zipperless jogging suits. The carer accompanying the child may leave gold or silver jewellery on but it needs to be removed from the child as it may heat up in the magnet and cause burns.

The child has to keep very still during the scan, as one movement can spoil all the images, unlike X-rays. This is because the images are built up from information collected during the whole of the scanning time. A child who is not able to keep still for about 30 min may have to be sedated. The child will be asked to lie on the table; they can be comforted and reassured and choose a video or music to play while they are being scanned. Before moving into the scanner, headphones should be placed over their ears so they can hear their chosen video or music clip and block out some of the noise made by the scanner. MRI scanning can be frightening for a young child who may therefore need sedation. Children over the age of 5 years may find it quite interesting. They can take a favourite toy in with them, as long as there is no metal in it.

Once the child is in the magnet, the machine starts to make a whirring and thumping noise which can get very loud and this continues for the whole of the scan. The child can talk to the radiographer while in the magnet. The child also has a bell to press should they wish the examination to stop. In practice, many children go to sleep and have to be woken up when the scan is finished.

Occasionally it is necessary to inject a small amount of contrast, which does not contain iodine, into the arm, allergic reactions are very rare with contrast agents used in MRI.

No special care is required following a scan, provided the child has not received sedation.

NUCLEAR MEDICINE

Nuclear medicine uses computers, detectors and radioactive pharmaceutical substances called radioisotopes to provide information about disease processes. The levels of radiation delivered in nuclear medicine studies are often less than, or comparable to, equivalent X-ray procedures, although they provide functional rather than anatomical images. The radiation risk received from nuclear medicine study is generally at a level considered negligible by the International Commission on Radiological Protection (ICRP 1977/1978). Nuclear medicine scans are

useful for detecting tumours, bony infection, irregular or insufficient blood flow to organs, blood cell disorders and inadequate function of organs such as thyroid and pulmonary function. The radioisotopes are usually injected into the bloodstream via an intravenous cannula, therefore children will need to be prepared for the insertion of a cannula prior to attending the nuclear medicine department for their scan. It is essential the person injecting the radiopharmaceutical has undergone special training so they are aware of what they are injecting and the precautions required to contain the radiopharmaceutical and dispose of waste matter appropriately. Local policy should be followed when doing so.

Some of the more common nuclear medicine scans are as follows.

Bone scans

Bone scanning detects radiation from a radioactive substance that, when injected into the body, collects in bone tissue. The substance accumulates in areas of high metabolic activity, and so the image shows 'bright spots' of high activity and 'dark spots' of low activity. Bone scanning is useful for detecting tumours and infection, which generally have high metabolic activity (Sharp et al 1998).

^{99m}Tc Dimercaptosuccinic acid (DMSA) and ^{99m}Tc diethylenetriamine–pentaacetic acid (DTPA)

There are a number of radiopharmaceuticals available for demonstrating renal function and imaging of the urinary tract. The most appropriate radiopharmaceutical is chosen for the examination and is dependent upon whether the examination is to look at the kidney and its function or the drainage characteristics of the urinary tract.

A DMSA and DTPA renal scan are most commonly used. The radioisotope or tracer is administered intravenously and is observed through a special gamma camera.

- DMSA is bound to plasma proteins and is cleared from the blood by uptake by the renal tubules. The proximal convoluted tubular tissue takes up DMSA, accumulating in the renal cortex. Because of the high specificity of the uptake in the renal cortex, DMSA is of use for the visualisation of the renal parenchyma. Therefore these scans are useful for assessing the size, shape and position of the kidneys and to demonstrate if renal dysfunction is occurring in both kidneys. DMSA scan also demonstrates scarring and narrowing of the renal cortex in pyelonephritis.

- DTPA is commonly used for renal transplant studies. When injected intravenously, it is distributed throughout the extracellular space. As it is excreted rapidly from the body by glomerulofiltration, it gives a good correlation with the standard measurements of glomerular filtration rate. DTPA is useful for both assessment of individual kidney function, and the study of renal function and drainage in obstructive uropathy (Sharp et al 1998).

INTERVENTIONAL RADIOLOGY

Interventional radiology is a medical specialty that uses image-guided, minimally invasive diagnostic and treatment techniques that are often an alternative to surgery. Interventional radiologists assist in diagnosis and treatment of diseases using small catheters or other devices guided by radiological imaging. Procedures performed by interventional radiologists are generally less costly and are less traumatic to the patient as they involve smaller incisions, less pain and shorter hospital stays.

Central venous access

As the demand for long-term central venous access increases, and with the recent publication of NICE guidelines (2002), many interventional radiology departments are now carrying out a large proportion of these procedures. These devices are increasingly used for the administration of antibiotics and chemotherapeutic drugs, for total parenteral nutrition, and for providing high-flow access for haemodialysis and plasmapheresis. Indwelling catheters also offer the ability to obtain frequent blood samples, which may be needed in some patients. Many children are reliant on lifelong central venous access for nutritional requirements and haemodialysis; repeated placement of such devices in these children proves challenging when traditional venous access sites are compromised by stenosis or occlusion of the central vessels. Placing central venous catheters in the interventional radiology department equipped with dedicated ultrasound and fluoroscopic machines allows the planned vascular access site to be evaluated prior to catheter placement. Ultrasonographic investigation of the neck

prior to the procedure may alert the operator to small collateral vessels instead of a single large jugular vein. This is important as it may be indicative of a stenosis or occlusion of the main vein. In many instances, one of the collateral veins can be accessed under direct ultrasonographic visualisation or the large brachiocephalic vein may be easily identified and punctured with ultrasound guidance. Therefore, by using fluoroscopic guidance, contrast material, guidewires and catheters, an interventional radiologist can usually bypass these thrombosed or stenosed vessels and access the central circulation, allowing placement of a catheter via vessels that could not otherwise be used.

Venous access under ultrasonographic and fluoroscopic guidance has the added advantage of significantly decreasing the rate of immediate complications such as inadvertent arterial puncture, pneumothorax and catheter tip malpositioning (Calvert et al 2002, NICE 2002, Silberzweig et al 2000).

Central venous line (CVL) insertion

This is a procedure that involves placement of a soft infusion catheter into a centrally located vein using vascular interventional techniques. The most commonly placed lines include:

- Peripherally inserted central venous catheter (PICC)
- Hickman lines (single and double lumens)
- Venous port device
- Temporary and permanent haemodialysis catheters.

Depending on the type of central venous access required, placement can be carried out under either local or general anaesthetic. For a PICC or other non-tunnelled central venous catheter, local anaesthetic with or without sedation is sufficient in the older child; however, for tunnelled catheter insertion such as a Hickman catheter which requires a large amount of compliance, a general anaesthetic is strongly recommended to ensure the procedure is carried out as safely and as pain free as practicable (Roebuck 2001, Calvert et al 2002) (see also Ch. 13).

A recent report from the National Institute for Clinical Excellence recommends ultrasound-guided placement of all central venous catheters into the internal jugular vein in adults and children in elective situations, and that ultrasound-guided placement should also be considered in emergency situations (NICE 2002).

Renal biopsy

Renal biopsy is undertaken to identify a specific disease process, determine extent of kidney damage, detect early transplant rejection and assess transplant failure (Roebuck 2001, Kessel & Robertson 2002). The kidney to be biopsied is visualised using ultrasound guidance, the intended biopsy tract is infiltrated with local anaesthetic and a thin needle is passed through the skin into the area of the kidney. Inside the needle is a sharp cutting edge that slices and removes small pieces of the kidney. In older children this procedure is successfully performed with sedation or demand-valve equimolar nitrous oxide (Entonox). If the child is young or not suitable for either sedation or Entonox, a general anaesthetic is recommended. As there is a small risk of postoperative bleeding, it is imperative that clotting results are obtained prior to the procedure and the operator is informed if the child is on medication that may interfere with clotting, for example children receiving aspirin for treatment of their underlying renal disease. Postoperative observations should include blood pressure monitoring for early detection of complications such as bleeding.

Angiography

Angiography is an X-ray examination of the arteries and veins to diagnose blockages and other blood vessel problems. Depending on the age and level of cooperation of the child, this procedure may be performed under local anaesthetic, sedation or general anaesthesia. The most common method for carrying out this procedure is with the child positioned supine; a small nick in the groin is made and the femoral artery is punctured. In small children, it is advisable to use ultrasound guidance to obtain femoral arterial access as their arteries are smaller and not as easily palpable as those in older children, making access more difficult (Roebuck 2001). Once arterial access is obtained, a guidewire is inserted and the access needle is exchanged for an arterial sheath; this allows the insertion of a guiding catheter which is advanced to the blood vessels of interest and an injection of contrast or dye gives the radiologist a clear picture of any abnormal vessels.

One of the most common reasons for angiography is to see if there is a blockage or narrowing in a blood vessel that may interfere with the normal flow of blood through the body. In many cases, the interventional radiologist can treat a blocked blood vessel without surgery at the same time as the angiogram is performed. Interventional radiologists treat blockages with techniques such as angioplasty where a balloon is guided to the site of narrowing and expanded to overcome narrowing; sometimes a small metal stent is inserted to aid in keeping the vessel open. Other conditions which may indicate an angiogram are arteriovenous malformations, trauma, vasculitis, renovascular hypertension and cerebral arteriovenous malformations (Roebuck 2001).

Postoperatively, bed rest is encouraged for at least 6 h or according to local hospital policy to minimise risk of bleeding from the puncture site. Circulation of the limb used for arterial access should also be assessed during routine postoperative observations.

DOS AND DON'TS

- Do ensure that the child and parents have received a full explanation of the procedure.
- Do maintain the child's privacy.
- Do remove jewellery or any metal fastenings.
- Do ensure resuscitation equipment is available for children of all ages.
- Do observe the child closely if any contrast medium containing iodine is used.
- Do ensure all radioactive material is disposed of correctly.
- Do ensure local radiation protection guidelines are available and adhered to by all staff members.
- Do not allow pregnant mothers/carers or nurses to be exposed to X-rays.

References

Bisset III, G.S., Kirks, D.R., 1988. Intussusception in infants and children: diagnosis and therapy. Radiology 168 (1), 141.

Calvert, N., Hind, D., McWilliams, R., et al., 2002. The effectiveness and cost effectiveness of ultrasound locating devices for central venous access. Anaesthesia 59 (11), 1116–1120.

Crawley, T., 2002. Ionising radiation safety: a handbook for nurses. York Publishing, York.

DoH Department of Health, 2003. National Service Framework for children. DoH, London.

Gyll, C., 1982. Investigations into and a comparative study of techniques for basic radiography in children's hospitals. Radiography 48 (573), 175–184.

ICRP, 1977/1978. Recommendations of the International Commission on Radiological Protection. ICRP Publication 26. Annals of the ICRP (1977) 1. No. 3; Annals of the ICRP (1978); 2: No. 3.

Kaye, R., 2000. Pediatric intervention: an update – Part II. J. Vasc. Interv. Radiol. 11, 807–822.

Kessel, D., Robertson, I., 2002. Interventional radiology – a survival guide. Churchill Livingstone, London.

NICE, 2002. Guidance on the use of ultrasound locating devices for placing central venous catheters. Clinical Guidance 49. National Institute for Clinical Excellence, London.

RCN, 2003. Restraining, holding still and containing children and young people. Guidance for nursing staff. RCN, London.

Reijnen, J.A., Festen, C., van Roosmalen, R.P., 1990. Intussusception: factors related to treatment. Arch. Dis. Child 65 (8), 871–873.

Roebuck, D.J., 2001. Paediatric interventional radiology. Imaging 13, 302–320.

Sharp, P.F., Gemmell, H.G., Smith, F.W., 1998. Practical nuclear medicine, second ed. Oxford University Press, New York.

Silberzweig, J., Sacks, D., Khorsandi, A.S., et al., 2000. Reporting standards for central venous access. J. Vasc. Interv. Radiol. 11, 391–400.

Sury, M.R., Harker, H., Begent, J., et al., 2005. The management of infants and children for painless imaging. Clin. Radiol. 60 (7), 731–741.

Sury, M.R., Hatch, D.J., Deeley, T., et al., 1999. Development of a nurse-led sedation service for paediatric magnetic resonance imaging. Lancet 353, 1667–1671.

TSO, 2000. Statutory Instrument No. 1059. The Ionising Radiation (Medical Exposure) Regulations 2000. The Stationery Office, London. Online. Available:www.opsi.gov.uk/si/si2000/20001059.htm.

Further reading

Chapman, S., Nakielny, R., 1988. A guide to radiological procedures, second ed. Baillière Tindall, London.

Kandarpa, K., Aruny, J., 2001. Handbook of interventional radiologic procedures, third ed. Lippincott, Williams and Wilkins, Philadelphia.

Milner, A.D., Hull, D., 1992. Hospital paediatrics, second ed. Churchill Livingstone, Edinburgh.

Chapter 25

Removal of drains and packs

Jennifer McKenna

CHAPTER CONTENTS

Introduction   251
   Learning outcomes   251
   Rationale   251
   Factors to note   252

Removal of drains and packs   253
   Equipment   253
   Method for removing wound drains   253
   Method for shortening a wound drain   254
   Method for removing a ribbon gauze pack   254
   Method for removing a foam pack   255
   Dos and don'ts   255

INTRODUCTION

Surgical wound drains and packs are primarily used to promote effective wound healing. Removing excess fluid from a wound will reduce the risk of infection and skin breakdown, while simultaneously easing wound pain through reducing swelling (McConnell 2001). While wound drains have an important function it is essential that nurses are familiar with the monitoring and removal of surgical drains in order to prevent complication and facilitate postoperative recovery (Walker 2007). Removal of the drain or pack at a time specified by medical and nursing assessment will help further promote wound healing by enabling earlier mobility, well-being and ultimately recovery.

LEARNING OUTCOMES

By the end of this section you should be able to:
- Be aware of the different types of wound drains and packs
- Be aware of their uses in wound healing
- Remove, or assist in the removal of, wound drains or packs, following observation
- Be aware of the initial follow-up care of the site.

RATIONALE

The aim of the drain or pack is to promote effective healing and therefore reduce the risk of complications. This in turn will lead to a quicker recovery and result in a shorter stay in hospital for the child.

FACTORS TO NOTE

Types of surgical wounds

- Clean wounds: where during surgery no infection is encountered and no organ is opened
- Clean contaminated wounds: where during surgery an organ has been opened with little content leakage
- Contaminated wounds: where during surgery an organ is opened and this is accompanied by extensive spillage of contents without pus. Also included in this category are fresh wounds occurring through trauma
- Dirty wounds: where during surgery pus or perforation in an organ is found. Also included in this category are old wounds caused by trauma. (i.e. >4 h old).

Types of healing

Wound healing is a complex process comprising four main phases: haemostasis, inflammation, proliferation and maturation. These phases occur concurrently, but the length of time taken in each phase can vary considerably. Factors which can affect the rate of wound healing include malnutrition (Clancy & McVicar 2002), poor wound care, inquisitive fingers and sleep disturbances. Normal healing occurs by either primary or secondary intention, both of which involve all four stages outlined above.

Primary intention

This occurs in wounds where there has been a clean cut, or incision, with little or no tissue loss. The edges can be brought together and held with sutures, tapes, etc. thus eliminating any space below the wound surface.

Secondary intention

This occurs when there has been substantial tissue loss and it is not possible to bring the edges together. These wounds heal from the base upwards by the formation of granulation tissue and wound contraction. Owing to the large amount of tissue involved, these wounds take considerably longer to heal (Zerbe et al 1996) (see also Ch. 37).

Types of packs

Packs are used to fill a resultant cavity when healing by secondary intention is the intended and preferred healing process. They include:

- Wicks: a variable length of ribbon gauze inserted into an open cavity after immersion in a suitable substance. Substances other than saline should be prescribed appropriately on the child's prescription sheet prior to use. An alternative to soaked ribbon gauze is an alginate-type dressing.
- Foam: a compound made from the mixing of a polymer and a base, which is poured into the cavity and expands to the contours of the wound, allowing for granulation, e.g. Cavi-Care.

Availability of dressings is subject to pharmacy guidelines and hospital constraints. Although the use of ribbon gauze (wicks) continues to be seen in practice, its benefit when compared to other dressing materials has been questioned (Pulman 2004). Pulman (2004) and Bale and Jones (2006) recommend the use of alginate dressings for cavity wounds, while Moore and Foster (2000) recommend an hydrofibre dressing. Moore and Foster (2000) identified that an alternative hydrofibre dressing facilitated an earlier discharge when compared to ribbon gauze. In Moore and Foster's (2000) study, although the cost of the dressing was more prohibitive, the overall net effect was more beneficial when considering earlier discharge and more effective use of hospital beds was seen as being advantageous. Watret and White (2001) do not recommend one particular dressing but do not encourage the use of ribbon gauze, and do recommend that each wound be assessed individually and the appropriate dressing used. They also encourage consultation with tissue viability nurses, especially for more complex wounds.

Types of wound drains

Drains are used when healing by primary intention is the intended healing process. The aims of drains are:

- To drain intra-abdominal collections of pus
- To drain any postoperative collections
- To re-route body fluids from a new suture line.

Types of drains include:

- Suction or sump drains: a vacuum is present to exert a low suction to remove any wound exudate from a cavity (Zerbe et al 1996, McConnell 1999), e.g. Redivac drain, Monovac drain, Shirley Sump drain
- Non-suction drains: these allow wound exudate to leave a cavity by a natural process, e.g. Penrose drain, Yates drain.

Note: The age and cooperation of the child should be taken into consideration by the surgeon when wound management is required.

All of these drains are removed when wound leakage has significantly reduced or stopped. Within adult patients, the use of closed suction wound drains has been questioned. Chandratreya et al (1998) identified that there was no difference in terms of mobilisation, postoperative infection and length of hospitalisation in adult orthopaedic patients who had a wound drain *in situ* when compared with those who did not have a wound drain. Purushotham et al (2002) concurred with this and indicated that using sutured wound flaps resulted in shorter hospital stays. However, no literature relating to children was identified to support these adult findings.

Analgesia

Effective analgesia and/or sedation must be taken into consideration and should be administered at least 30 min before the procedure is begun, to allow time for it to take effect. However, the recent introduction of Entonox as an acceptable form of analgesia for children gives an alternative and allows for effective pain control during difficult procedures (see Ch. 44). A study by Yiannakopoulos and Kanellopoulos (2004) in adults and adolescents suggested that the use of local anaesthetic significantly reduced the pain associated with drain removal and increased patient comfort during the post-removal period. However, this has not as yet become common practice in paediatrics.

Children are naturally inquisitive and may be more cooperative if they are able to participate in their own care. However, the nurse must continually assess the situation, and involvement by the play specialist can provide a useful distraction during procedures. Some ways in which the child can participate are by loosening or removing tape, holding tubing or counting down to the removal

of the drain. Not all children will be able to cooperate owing to their age or ability to understand; however, it is important to ensure that children are given information at a level that they are able to understand. In these instances, it is helpful to have support from the parents to assist in providing comfort and security whilst the removal of the drain or pack is being carried out.

REMOVAL OF DRAINS AND PACKS

EQUIPMENT

- Dressing pack
- Sterile stitch cutter or scissors
- Cleansing agent
- Selection of sterile dressings to cover or redress the wound
- Sterile forceps
- Gloves (non-sterile) and Sterile latex-free gloves, optional (these can be used in place of forceps)
- Wound swab (if required)
- Disposal bag.

Note: It is preferable to overestimate your required equipment rather than having to stop the procedure to obtain more (see also Ch. 37).

METHOD FOR REMOVING WOUND DRAINS

1. Explain the procedure to the child and parents/carers to facilitate understanding and cooperation.
2. Gather the required equipment and prepare your area for the procedure, i.e. the treatment room or bedside.
3. Wash and dry your hands.
4. If applicable, uncover the wound to obtain access to the drain site (wearing gloves if appropriate). At this point, if the drain is of a suction type, release the vacuum. Sometimes the drain can rest against tissue inside the wound; by releasing the vacuum, any remaining fluid can be drained. Wash and dry your hands. Apply non-sterile gloves.
5. Using aseptic technique (see Ch. 34), clean the wound if necessary to access sutures or clean away any exudate, which may be a source of infection.

6. Remove any sutures by holding the knot with sterile forceps and gently raising it from skin level; then cut the shortest end of the suture as close to the skin as possible. This prevents any part of the suture which has been exposed externally from passing through the tissue, reducing the risk of infection. This should allow the drain to be released.

   Note: Cut only one end of the suture.

7. Remove the drain slowly by holding the tubing close to the child and pulling gently, but firmly. If there is resistance, which does not yield with firm pulling, stop the procedure and seek advice.

8. Cover the drain site with a sterile dressing. This will minimise infection entering the drain site while it heals.

9. Dispose of soiled equipment safely and record the amount of drainage in the appropriate nursing documentation.

10. Regularly check the wound site for any excessive drainage or swelling which could indicate an internal collection of fluid, i.e. 2- to 4-hourly with routine observations.

11. Further wound management will be as per unit protocol.

METHOD FOR SHORTENING A WOUND DRAIN

1–2. As for removal of wound drain.

3. Wash and dry your hands. Apply non-sterile gloves. Remove wound dressing and expose drain. This is likely to be a tube type of drain, e.g. Penrose or corrugated latex. These drains usually have a sterile safety pin or suture to maintain their position outside the wound.

4. Wash and dry your hands again and apply non-sterile gloves. Clean the wound if necessary.

5. Remove the suture by raising the knot from skin level and cutting the shorter end as close to the skin as possible. When the suture has been removed, grasp the end of the drain and pull gently. It is usually sufficient to shorten the drain by 2–4 cm unless instructed otherwise by the medical staff. If unsure, seek advice. Shortening the drain will ensure that it does not remain in contact with any single structure for any length of time or impede the healing process. It also enables the drain to continue its

purpose throughout the depth of the wound. The excess tubing can be cut with sterile scissors.

6. Re-insert a new sterile safety pin just above wound level to prevent the drain slipping into it.

7. Re-dress the wound with an appropriate wound dressing. Copious amounts of drainage may be managed by placing a stoma bag over the drain site. This enables the bag to be emptied and prevents the frequent changing of dressings. This method of collection should be discussed with the child and parents/carers before implementation as they may not feel comfortable with using a stoma bag.

8. Dispose of soiled equipment and record the amount of drainage in the appropriate nursing documentation. This will aid further management of the drain.

METHOD FOR REMOVING A RIBBON GAUZE PACK

1–2. As for removal of drain. Confirm the length of ribbon gauze (wick) in situ by either checking the operation notes or consulting the medical staff.

3. Wash and dry your hands. Apply non-sterile gloves. Remove the outer dressing and assess the wound site.

4. Locate the end of the wick and gently ease it upwards out of the cavity. If there is any adherence, the wound and wick can be moistened with saline. Continue to ease the gauze from the cavity until no more is visible.

   Note: Some wounds are managed by shortening the wick gradually over a period of time.

5. Clean the wound as required.

6. Assess the wound bed for signs of healing and the possible need to insert a further wick. Consider the appropriateness of the dressing used and confer with the surgeon and tissue viability nurse if you think another dressing would be more appropriate. If a further wick is required, place an appropriate length in saline or a prescribed solution. (The wick is supplied as a tightly rolled coil in a sterile pack. Lengths are usually indicated on the packaging.)

7. Using two pairs of sterile forceps, one in each hand, grasp the wick with one pair while keeping it submerged in the solution, and locate the loose end. Take hold of the end with the other forceps. Gradually unravel the wick and re-roll onto the second forceps, ensuring that it is moistened throughout its length. The moistened wick can then be inserted into the wound from the base up. When the wound has been sufficiently packed, the wick can be cut with sterile scissors.
8. Dress the wound appropriately and dispose of soiled equipment.
9. Complete the nursing documentation and record the length of wick inserted.
10. If the wick has been removed, check the site for excessive leakage.
11. Further wound management will be as per local protocol.

METHOD FOR REMOVING A FOAM PACK

1–3. As for removal of ribbon gauze.
4. Grasp the edges of the pack with two pairs of sterile forceps and gently ease it from the wound cavity. Clean the wound if necessary.
5. Assess the wound healing to ascertain whether a further pack is required. If unsure, seek advice. If a pack is required, make up the foam preparation as per the manufacturer's instructions and pour it slowly into the cavity. Allow time for the expansion of the foam and, when it has solidified, cover the wound with an appropriate dressing. It may be necessary to secure the pack in position with tape, but this will depend upon the individual child and the location of the wound.
6. Dispose of soiled equipment and complete the nursing documentation.

COMMUNITY PERSPECTIVE

The removal of wound packs is frequently undertaken in the community, following conditions such as drainage of abscesses.

This procedure can be very frightening for the child and is potentially painful. The CCN must gain the trust of the child and family before undertaking the procedure and organise appropriate pain management (see Ch. 44). Analgesia should be timed to ensure maximum relief during the procedure. Older children may be able to use Entonox, but as this is self-administered, it is not suitable for the younger child. If the CCN feels that the pain cannot be adequately managed by drugs that can be given in the home, it may be necessary to request admission to hospital as a day case.

The CCN should be prepared to encounter less than adequate facilities for undertaking an aseptic non-touch technique in the home (see Ch. 34). It may be necessary to take additional equipment (sterile towels, plastic tray, hand-cleansing solutions).

DOS AND DON'TS

- Do be honest with the child when explaining procedures.
- Do involve and inform the parents/carers.
- Do ensure that the child's safety and privacy are maintained at all times.
- Do involve the play specialist if available.
- Do ensure that adequate analgesia has been given before commencing procedures.
- Do assess the wound and dressing to ensure appropriate dressing is replaced.
- Do not remove packs or drains without prior instruction.
- Do not assume that older children will cooperate or be brave.

References

Bale, S., Jones, V., 2006. Wound care nursing: A patient centred approach, second ed. Mosby, Edinburgh.

Chandratreya, A., Giannikas, K., Livesley, P., 1998. To drain or not to drain: literature versus practice. J. R. Coll. Surg. Edinb. 43, 404–406.

Clancy, J., McVicar, A., 2002. Physiology and anatomy: a homeostatic approach, second ed. Arnold, London.

McConnell, E.A., 1999. Clinical dos and don'ts: using a closed wound drainage system. Nursing 29 (6), 32.

McConnell, E.A., 2001. Clinical dos and don'ts: emptying a closed wound drainage device. Nursing 31 (7), 17.

Moore, P.J., Foster, L., 2000. Clinical cost benefits of two dressings in the management of surgical wounds. Br. J. Nurs. 9 (17), 1128–1132.

Pulman, K., 2004. Dressings in the management of open surgical wounds. Br. J. Perioper. Nurs. 14 (8), 354–360.

Purushotham, A.D., McLatchie, E., Young, D., et al., 2002. Randomized clinical trial of no wound drains and early discharge in the treatment of women with breast cancer. Br. J. Surg. 89 (3), 286–292.

Walker, J., 2007. Patient preparation for safe removal of surgical drains. Nurs. Stand. 21 (49), 39–41.

Watret, L., White, R., 2001. Surgical wound management: the role of dressings. Nurs. Stand. 15 (44), 59–69.

Yiannakopoulos, C.K., Kanellopoulos, A.D., 2004. Innoxious removal of suction drains. Orthopedics 27 (4), 412–414.

Zerbe, M., McArdle, A., Goldrick, B., 1996. Exposure risks related to the management of three wound drainage systems. Am. J. Infect. Control 24 (5), 346–352.

Chapter 26

Seizures

Louise Simmons

CHAPTER CONTENTS

Introduction   257
    Learning outcomes   257
    Rationale   257
    Factors to note   258

Seizures   259
    Types of epileptic seizures   259
    Guidelines   260
    Equipment   261
    Method   261
    Observations and complications   262
    Dos and don'ts   263

INTRODUCTION

Anyone can have an isolated seizure at some point in their life (NSE 2002a). They can happen for a variety of different reasons. Seizures are periods of sudden disturbance in neurological function that cause involuntary muscle activity, change in level of consciousness, or altered behavioural and sensory manifestations (Cameron et al 2005). Seizures can be frightening and disturbing to observe, both for the professional and the family. A number of dangers can occur during a seizure, i.e. apnoea, airway obstruction, aspiration and injury. The nurse's role is to provide a safe environment for the duration of the seizure and respond appropriately to the situation.

LEARNING OUTCOMES

By the end of this section you should be able to:

- State the main causes of seizures in children
- Describe how to nurse a child during a seizure
- State the possible complications of a seizure
- Show awareness of the different anticonvulsant medication that may be administered during a seizure.

RATIONALE

At least 20% of children admitted to hospital have a neurological problem, either as the sole or an associated complaint. Seizures are the most frequently observed neurological dysfunction in children (Slota 2006). Although seizures are the main characteristic of epilepsy, a chronic disorder with recurrent and unprovoked seizures, a single seizure event should not be classified as epilepsy. Seizures are a symptom of an underlying disease process and they can occur with a variety of conditions involving the central nervous system (CNS) (Wong 2007). Approximately 20% of children will experience a seizure in the first 5 years of life, often associated not with epilepsy, but with a febrile illness (Rudolf & Levene 1999). In children who have experienced a seizure associated with a febrile illness, about 15% of cases will have a further seizure within the same illness; 60% of these children are at risk of at least one more febrile seizure before they are 6 years old, with a further third of these at risk of three or more seizures (Crisp & Rainbow 2007). The risk is even higher if the onset is before the age of 1 year and if there is a positive family history (Lissauer & Clayden 2001). It is therefore important for the paediatric nurse to know how to care for a child during a seizure. Education of parents is also important as to the cause, and how to handle possible future seizures.

FACTORS TO NOTE

Neonatal seizures

The newborn period is the time of life with the highest risk of seizures and epilepsy. The newborn brain is more susceptible to a large number of cerebral and systemic insults. The immature brain is relatively 'excitable' and more likely to seize (Appleton & Gibbs 2004). Neonatal seizures can be difficult to recognise. Many babies in the neonatal period can have abnormal and involuntary movements that must be differentiated from seizures, i.e. jitteriness, startling or spontaneous clonus (Lissauer & Clayden 2001, Appleton & Gibbs 2004).

The features of neonatal seizures are different from those seen in the older infant or child. Most seizure activity in neonates may be subtle, tonic, clonic or myoclonic. The main causes of neonatal seizures are (Crisp & Rainbow 2007):

- Acute infections acquired pre- and postnatally, i.e. toxoplasmosis, meningitis, septicaemia, encephalitis and herpes simplex
- Metabolic and electrolyte disturbances, i.e. hypo/hypernatraemia, hypoglycaemia, hypocalcaemia, hypomagnesaemia, which can be due to inborn errors of metabolism or to a

single illness, i.e. dehydration due to diarrhoea, vomiting or poor feeding
- Birth trauma, i.e. intracranial bleed or post hypoxia: hypoxic-ischaemic encephalopathy.
- Structural brain lesions.

At presentation, all of these possibilities should be considered and various tests, i.e. full septic screen (blood count/culture, urine, lumbar puncture (LP), chest X-ray), computed tomography (CT) scan, magnetic resonance imaging (MRI) scan and electroencephalogram (EEG), should help confirm/eliminate the various causes.

Many of these causes are treatable and reversible with medications, i.e. antibiotics and electrolyte infusions/medications.

Infants and older children

Convulsions in the infant and older child can still be due to some of the causes seen in neonates.

- Infections, i.e. meningitis, encephalitis and septicaemia can be seen as well as urinary tract infections, otitis media and many viral infections, i.e. colds and coughs
- Metabolic and electrolyte imbalances can be seen with periods of fasting, i.e. hypoglycaemia or hypernatraemia with dehydration
- Head trauma can be seen as a result of either accidental (e.g. road traffic accident) or non-accidental injury (e.g. shaken baby syndrome, physical abuse).

Certain neurological conditions, such as febrile seizures, occur exclusively in childhood. It is also important to remember that most of the neuromuscular and neurodegenerative disorders present early in life.

Febrile convulsions are one of the most common neurological disorders in childhood, affecting about 3% of children. They usually occur between 6 months and 3 years but can go up to 6 years of age (Lissauer & Clayden 2001). They are generalised seizures and occur in children as a result of rapid temperature rise above 39°C (102°F). Up to 75% of all febrile seizures involve a generalised onset, tonic–clonic seizure that lasts <15 min with no post-ictal neurological deficit or sequelae (Appleton & Gibbs 2004).

The same investigations will be needed on presentation to establish the cause of the seizure. Following the full septic screen, CT scan, MRI scan and EEG as in the neonate, the course of treatment will be determined.

Status epilepticus

Status epilepticus is defined as a continuous tonic-clonic seizure lasting >30 min or a series of repeated seizures between which the child does not fully regain consciousness (Moules & Ramsey 2008). It is an emergency situation which is life-threatening and in which the child is at risk of permanent brain damage. It is important to support the child's vital functions, i.e. maintain a patent airway, adequate oxygenation and hydration. Monitor vital signs and assess neurologic level. NICE (2002) recommends the use of benzodiazepines such as rectal diazepam or buccal midazolam for pre-hospital treatment, which if there was no response, could be repeated. Treatment with intravenous anticonvulsant/sedative drugs (i.e. lorazepam) will possibly be required. Loading doses of phenytoin, or phenobarbital, may be necessary if seizures persist. McIntyre et al (2005) suggest that buccal midazolam is more effective than rectal diazepam and does not have the side-effects of respiratory depression. Clonazepam or thiopental may then be necessary, but these drugs will suppress not only the epileptiform activity but also normal brain function. As this includes the breathing centres, these children will most probably require mechanical ventilation in an intensive care unit.

Epilepsy

Epilepsy is the commonest chronic neurological condition in childhood (SIGN 2003). It means having a tendency to experience recurrent seizures that originate in the brain, which happen when ordinary brain activity is suddenly disrupted. As the brain is responsible for a wide range of functions, seizures associated with epilepsy can take on many forms and affect areas such as memory, sensation, personality, consciousness, mood and movement. Any of these functions may be temporarily disturbed during the course of a seizure (NSE 2002a). The diagnosis of epilepsy has important health, educational and social implications for both the child and family (SIGN 2003). These can include behavioural and emotional problems that are sometimes caused by embarrassment or frustration associated with their epilepsy. Having epilepsy can affect your independence by restricting your access to driving and some people and their families live in fear of the next seizure.

Children diagnosed with epilepsy will be commenced on regular anticonvulsant medication. The type of seizure will determine which medications will be prescribed. Approximately 70–75% of children with epilepsy can be controlled with a single anticonvulsant drug. The current 'recommended' first-line drugs are sodium valproate for generalised seizures and carbamazepine for partial seizures (RCPCH 2003). It often takes time to find the drug most suitable for optimum treatment and dose adjustment is ongoing as the child grows and develops.

Adolescents

Teenagers with epilepsy are frequently caught between paediatric and adult services with neither service being able to understand, or satisfy, their specific needs and concerns. Emotional and social development is also important during this period, as young people try and find their place in society. Many young people at this time are emotionally impressionable (Barnes 2003). Adolescents who have epilepsy may find that the onset of puberty and its accompanying hormonal changes can lead to further seizures. This may occur, even although they were previously well controlled on medication. This can be particularly distressing, especially if they had been free of seizures for some time. In addition to the distress of seizures recurring, the adolescent in particular may be extremely sensitive about involuntary loss of control of bladder and bowel which can occur with some seizures.

SEIZURES

TYPES OF EPILEPTIC SEIZURES

Generalised seizures

These seizures involve the whole of the brain and consciousness is lost. They will often occur with no warning and the child will have no memory of the event (NSE 2002b).

Tonic–clonic

Formerly known as 'grand mal', these are the most commonly recognised seizure. There is a loss of consciousness, muscles contract and the body becomes rigid which is the tonic phase. The clonic phase involves the muscles relaxing and then tightening rhythmically, causing uncontrollable jerks. Respiration is usually irregular and laboured, which leads to cyanosis. Saliva may accumulate in the mouth and there may be biting of the tongue. Incontinence may also occur (Lissauer & Clayden 2001).

Myoclonic

Classic features of this type of seizure are brief contractions of a muscle or group of muscles – abrupt jerking of one or more limbs (Wong 2007). If the whole body is involved, the jerkiness is usually bilateral, symmetrical and mostly flexor or extensor jerks. If mild, the head may drop but if more severe, the child may be thrown suddenly forwards or backwards. Myoclonic seizures are frequently associated with learning disability, or abnormal neurological physiology. Infantile spasms are a type of myoclonic seizure with a poor prognosis for the development of an affected infant.

Atonic

Also known as drop attacks, these seizures involve momentary loss of muscle tone, causing a sudden fall to the floor or drop of the head (Glasper & Richardson 2006).

Absences

Formerly known as 'petit mal', these seizures occur when consciousness is interrupted. They last for only a couple of seconds and often go unnoticed. There is an appearance of staring, blankness and vagueness. Occasionally, there is blinking or twitching of the eyelids or face. There may be involuntary movements, e.g. chewing, lip smacking, loss of postural tone, semi-purposeful movements and peculiar sensations. Amnesia is usual throughout the episode and usually lasts for 5–10 s. Awareness quickly returns and the person continues with the previous activity (Glasper & Richardson 2006).

Partial seizures

These seizures, also known as focal seizures, begin in, or involve, one hemisphere of the brain. Experiences during these seizures will vary, depending on which area of the brain is affected. Partial seizures are classified according to whether there is an impairment of consciousness.

Simple partial

Consciousness is not impaired during these seizures. Symptoms include: numbness, tingling or pins and needles. There is also sensory disturbances to both auditory (manifesting in humming, buzzing or hissing) and visual sensations (manifesting as flashes of light or colours) (Wong 2007). The seizure may be confined to a rhythmic twitching of the face, one limb or part of a limb. Pins and needles are often felt in a specific part of the body.

Complex partial

Many symptoms are similar to those of simple partial seizures. They differ in that consciousness is affected so there is limited or no memory of the event. Disturbance of sensation occurs and may affect auditory, olfactory (smell), gustatory (taste) or emotional senses. The child may manifest automatisms (involuntary movements that look purposeful), i.e. lip smacking, mumbling, making chewing movements, fumbling with clothes and being generally confused. Colour change, wetting and vomiting can occur. Following the fit, the person may remain confused for a prolonged period (Glasper & Richardson 2006).

Secondary generalisation

A partial seizure starts from a focus in one cortex of the brain but the electrical activity then spreads to both hemispheres simultaneously, producing a generalised seizure. If this spread is rapid then there may be an unawareness of the partial seizure onset.

GUIDELINES

Parental involvement is vital when a child has recurrent seizures. A large part of the nurse's role is to provide support and education. Encourage parents to express their fears and anxieties and answer their questions honestly. This may be to teach about managing their child's fever, as in the case of febrile seizure. In a child who has recurrent seizures, it is likely to be necessary to teach the family how to administer rectal anticonvulsants in an emergency. If epilepsy is diagnosed, then as with any chronic condition, it is important for the nurse to provide support as well as education in order to help the child and family adjust to the diagnosis and realities of living with a chronic disease. At the start of any treatment, parents (and where appropriate the child) should be informed about; the seizure type (and whenever possible the specific epilepsy), the aims and duration of treatment, the likely and unlikely side effects of the medication, the importance of compliance and the likely prognosis (Appleton & Gibbs 2004).

EQUIPMENT

Very little equipment is required to actually care for a child during a seizure. The unpredictable nature of seizures is such that it will most probably have to be gathered as the child is experiencing the seizure. When a child is known to be affected with recurrent seizures, it may be possible to have appropriate equipment available at all times. For example, if the child is known to have problems maintaining adequate oxygenation during a seizure, a resuscitator bag and mask should be kept to hand.

- Pillows/blankets
- Record of seizures chart
- Watch, with second hand, with which the length of seizure can be established.

The following will be needed if the child is unable to maintain adequate oxygenation:

- Oxygen supply: mask and tubing from wall oxygen points if the child is by, or on, their bed. Portable oxygen will be needed if the seizure occurs in the toilet or corridor
- Suction equipment: as above with the oxygen
- Resuscitator bag and mask which is age appropriate should be easily accessible if needed
- Prescription chart: if the patient has just presented in casualty during a seizure, then one must be immediately available.

The following may be needed if the seizure does not stop spontaneously after about 5 min:

- Rectal diazepam, paraldehyde or intravenous lorazepam; this will be dependent on the individual hospital/patient protocol or ease of intravenous access
- Filling quill – to enable rectal administration of paraldehyde
- Non-sterile latex-free gloves
- Lubricating jelly.

Buccal midazolam or lorazepam (administered between gums and lips slowly) may also be administered (again dependent on hospital protocols).

Rectal paraldehyde administration

Rectal paraldehyde may be extemporaneously prepared immediately prior to use, using equal parts paraldehyde and olive or sunflower oil. The solution is now available ready mixed, so it is important to ensure the prescribed dose reflects that, i.e. if the child is prescribed 3 ml of paraldehyde then the prescription will have to state 6 ml of the solution. Avoid contact with undiluted paraldehyde as it reacts with rubber and plastics. This reaction may make it difficult to depress the plunger of the syringe. A plastic syringe can be used if the administration is immediate.

METHOD

1. If the nurse realises that the seizure is about to occur and the child is standing or sitting, they should be lowered gently to the ground and put on their side if possible. If the infant is sitting, they should also be placed on the ground or in their cot on their side. Do not attempt to restrain them in anyway or try to put anything into their mouth. It is impossible to halt a seizure once it has begun (Wong 2007).
2. Call for help and remain calm. A child should not be left unattended while they are having a seizure and a second nurse may be required to fetch equipment/drugs.
3. Note the exact time that the seizure started.
4. Remove any objects in the immediate area on which the child may injure themselves. It may be necessary to pad a rigid surface temporarily with a pillow to prevent the child hitting their head or a limb.
5. If possible, ensure privacy – draw curtains, ask onlookers to move away.
6. During (and sometimes after) a seizure, the swallowing reflex is lost, salivation increases, and the tongue is hypotonic. This means that there is a risk of aspiration or airway occlusion. It is important to place the child on their side to help the drainage of secretions and the airway clear (Wong 2007).
7. Observe the child/infant for signs of cyanosis. Be prepared to administer oxygen if they become cyanosed. If they are in repeated

spasm for any length of time, it may be necessary to use a resuscitator bag to administer oxygen if they are unable to breathe effectively for themselves. Suction of the oral cavity (if safe to do so) may also be necessary (Wong 2007).

8. If relatives are present, try to reassure them about what is happening. It can help to reassure them that the child is unaware of what is happening during most types of seizure, even if it looks painful and distressing. Talk calmly and reassuringly to the child during and after the seizure. This will be of comfort at a frightening time.

9. Be aware of how long the seizure has been in progress. Generally a seizure is self-limiting, the child will recover spontaneously and require no emergency intervention (Moules & Ramsey 2008). Determine from the child's prescription sheet when action may need to be taken to administer anticonvulsant drugs. For example, a child is often prescribed rectal diazepam for a seizure lasting longer than 5 min. Each child will have different criteria of when to treat the seizures. Children who rarely seize will have quick action but in some cases of degenerative/intractable seizures, it may be after 20–30 min.

10. If necessary, administer rectal or intravenous anticonvulsant drugs as prescribed, in accordance with local drug policy and procedure, and note their effect.

11. Once the seizure has finished, ensure the child is in the recovery position to continue to prevent aspiration or a hypotonic tongue from blocking their airway.

12. If the child has been incontinent, they may need a change of clothing. An infant or young child may require a change of nappy.

13. If it was a febrile seizure, take measures to cool the child down. Assess their temperature and identify whether or not they require to be given an antipyretic such as paracetamol or ibuprofen. This may be given rectally if the child is assessed as being insufficiently awake to take it orally, i.e. unable to protect their own airway with a safe swallow, cough and gag reflex. Remove any excess clothing and ensure that the room is not hot and stuffy, but comfortable and well ventilated.

14. Record the seizure and describe it in detail (see below). Record the precise duration of the seizure and whether or not intervention was required, e.g. oxygen, assistance with breathing or administration of drugs.

OBSERVATIONS AND COMPLICATIONS

Observation is especially important when caring for a child having a seizure. It can be important both in aiding diagnosis and in helping to achieve effective control. Carefully observe and record all aspects of the seizure. It is important to obtain an eye witness account of the convulsion so that a 'video' image of the episode can be determined (Rudolf & Levene 1999). When did it start? Which part of the body was affected first (focal or generalized)? Was more than one area of the body affected at one time? What kind of movements occurred? Did the movements change? Was there more than one phase of the seizure? Did it start with spasm and then progress to jerkiness? Did the movements affect more than one part of the body as the seizure progressed? Has the child had seizures before? Did the child appear to have any prior warning of any kind? What was the child doing before the seizure occurred? Did they cry out? Can they describe any 'odd' sensations prior to the seizure? Observe the child carefully for signs of cyanosis. Be aware that if the child has had rectal diazepam or i.v. lorazepam, it may depress their respiratory drive, particularly in the infant (Crisp & Rainbow 2007).

There are three life-threatening risks of a seizure:

1. A complication of a seizure – aspiration, suffocation, injury (including burns), drowning
2. Status epilepticus (convulsive)
3. A related underlying condition – neurodegenerative disorder, severe cerebral palsy (Appleton & Gibbs 2004).

COMMUNITY PERSPECTIVE

One of the most frightening occurrences for parents is to witness their child having a seizure. Much reassurance is required and in some circumstances, discussion in their home environment with a CCN may help the parents to adapt to living with a child who has seizures.

The CCN will be able to support the family by allowing time for them to talk about their anxieties and to help educate them about the seizures and any treatment required, as well as monitoring the child's progress. The parents may feel guilt and humiliation and may be concerned that the seizures will affect their child's mental capacity and future.

The CCN will be able to:

- Assess how much information the family have understood prior to discharge. Parents may need help to supplement their understanding once the child has been discharged home.
- Reinforce the education given in hospital, stressing the importance of drug compliance and the potential complications from sudden drug withdrawal.
- Ensure the parents/carers have a seizure management plan clearly stating how long to wait before administering rectal diazepam or sublingual/buccal midazolam/lorazepam.
- Ensure parents are competent in administering rectal diazepam/sublingual/buccal midazolam or lorazepam which is now widely used to treat seizures even though it is not licensed for this use (RCPCH 2003).
- Ensure parents know when to seek medical help:
  - 10 min for the first seizure, or
  - 2 min longer than the usual length of seizure, or
  - When a second fit occurs without the child regaining consciousness.
- Discuss with the family the information that should be given to playgroup, nursery or school staff and any other adults who may take responsibility for caring for the child. The school staff will need to be taught how to administer rectal diazepam (Joint Epilepsy Council 2004) or buccal midazolam/lorazepam either by the CCN or

the school nurse. It will be necessary for the child to have an individual seizure management plan for use in school, stating the action to be taken if the child has a seizure and the policy for safe storage of medication in school.

- Ensure that parents are aware that their children can undertake sports, although appropriate precautions should be taken, i.e. they should not be allowed to swim alone but with a companion, use of protective helmet during skating and cycling, supervision when using hazardous machinery/equipment (Wong 2007).

Most importantly, the family should be encouraged to take a positive attitude and encourage the child to take part in normal activities.

DOS AND DON'TS

- Do position the child on their side if possible.
- Do observe carefully and thoroughly.
- Do be prepared to provide assistance with breathing.
- Do try to protect the child from injury.
- Do be prepared to administer rectal anticonvulsant drugs if the seizure does not stop spontaneously within 5 min.
- Do record all seizure activity.
- Do keep families updated.
- Do speak to the child and give reassurance.
- Do not attempt to restrain the child in any way.
- Do not attempt to put anything into the child's mouth; you may get your finger badly bitten and push their tongue backwards causing a blocked airway.

References

Appleton, R., Gibbs, J., 2004. Epilepsy in childhood and adolescence, third ed. Martin Dunitz, London.

Barnes, K., 2003. Paediatrics: A clinical guide for nurse practitioners. Butterworth-Heinemann, Oxford.

Cameron, P., Jelinek, G., Everitt, I. et al., 2005. Textbook of paediatric emergency medicine. Churchill Livingstone, London.

Crisp, S., Rainbow, J., 2007. Emergencies in paediatrics and neonatology. Oxford University Press, Oxford.

Glasper, A., Richardson, J. (Eds.), 2006. A textbook of children's and young people's nursing. Churchill Livingstone, London.

Joint Epilepsy Council, 2004. A guideline on training standards for the administration of rectal diazepam. JEC, Leeds.

Lissauer, T., Clayden, G., 2001. Illustrated textbook of paediatrics, second ed. Mosby, Edinburgh.

McIntyre, J., Robertson, S., Norris, E., et al., 2005. Safety and efficacy of buccal midazolam versus rectal diazepam for emergency treatment of seizures: a randomised controlled trial. Lancet 366 (9481), 182–183.

Moules, T., Ramsey, J., 2008. The textbook of children's and young people's nursing, second ed. Blackwell Publishing, Oxford.

NICE, 2002. Newer drugs for children with epilepsy. National Institute for Health and Clinical Excellence, London.

NSE National Society for Epilepsy, 2002a. Epilepsy: an introduction to epileptic seizures. Chalfont St Peter, Bucks.

NSE National Society for Epilepsy, 2002b. Epilepsy: information on seizures and status epilepticus. Chalfont St Peter, Bucks.

RCPCH, 2003. Medicines for children. Royal College of Paediatrics and Child Health, London.

Rudolf, M., Levene, M., 1999. Paediatrics and child health. Blackwell Science, Oxford.

SIGN, 2003. Diagnosis and management of epilepsies in children and young people. Scottish Intercollegiate Guidelines Network, Edinburgh, pp. 1–7.

Slota, M. (Ed.), 2006. Core Curriculum for pediatric critical care nursing. second ed. Saunders, London.

Wong, 2007. Wong's nursing care of infants and children, eighth ed. Mosby, St Louis.

Chapter 27

Stoma care

Stella Snell

CHAPTER CONTENTS

Introduction   265
   Learning outcomes   266
   Rationale   266
   Factors to note   266
   Guidelines   267

Changing a bag   267
   Equipment   267
   Method   269
   Observations and complications   270

On discharge   271
   Dos and don'ts   272

INTRODUCTION

The word 'stoma' comes from the Greek word for mouth or opening. Stoma formation in childhood is generally a temporary measure in the surgical correction of congenital abnormalities. Occasionally, a stoma may be permanent. This may be due to trauma, tumour or inflammatory bowel disease. Conditions that may require stoma formation include:

- Imperforate anus
- Hirschsprung's disease
- Necrotising enterocolitis
- Cloacal exstrophy
- Ulcerative colitis
- Familial polyposis coli
- Bladder tumour
- Crohn's disease
- Meconium ileus.

There are three main types of diverting/output stoma; these may be temporary or permanent and act as an outlet for elimination of body waste (Williams 2004).

1. Ileostomy: a portion of the ileum is brought out through the abdominal wall and is normally sited in the right iliac fossa
2. Colostomy: a portion of the colon is brought through the abdominal wall and is normally sited in the left iliac fossa. (In children, the transverse colon, descending colon or sigmoid may be used.)

3. Urinary diversion:
   a. Vesicostomy: the neck of the bladder is brought through the abdominal wall low down in the pelvis
   b. Ureterostomy: one or two of the ureters can be brought out to the abdominal wall, either side by side or at either side of the abdomen
   c. Ileal conduit: a small segment of the ileum is isolated to act as an outlet into which the ureters are implanted. This stoma can be sited in the left or right iliac fossa.

There are two main types of continent stoma (a non-refluxing catheterisable channel; Malone et al 1990), neither of which requires a pouch collection system.

1. *Antegrade continence enema (ACE)*: the appendix or portion of ileum is tunnelled out through the abdominal wall, usually in the right iliac fossa, to form a continent catheterisable channel which, when flushed with an enema such as bisacodyl or phosphate and diluted with saline, irrigates the colon. Faeces are passed via the anus.
2. *Mitrofanoff*: the appendix, a portion of ileum or ureter is used and channelled from the bladder through the abdominal wall. A Mitrofanoff can be sited in the left or right iliac fossa or through the umbilicus, forming a continent catheterisable channel to give access for intermittent bladder drainage.

A stoma nurse, if employed in a hospital where surgery is performed, should be involved in the care of all children requiring stoma surgery (DoH 2003). However, this may not be a specialist paediatric stoma nurse. If there is no stoma nurse within the hospital, attempts must be made to refer the child and family to a stoma nurse within the community.

Practice should be evidence-based and care should be given by appropriately trained staff. The National Service Framework for Children, Young People and Maternity Services (DoH 2004) is working towards ensuring that everyone receives the same standard of care, irrespective of where they live. This is still an ongoing process in 2009, with multi-agency working and care pathways being put in place.

LEARNING OUTCOMES

By the end of this section you should be able to:

- Identify and describe different types of stoma
- Be aware of any dietary implications following stoma formation
- Recognise potential problems with stomas
- Change a stoma appliance efficiently and effectively
- Be aware of how to dispose of used appliances
- Help maintain a healthy stoma and peristomal skin integrity
- Identify recurring or continuing problems with management of the stoma
- Describe how families obtain stoma appliances in the community.

RATIONALE

Children undergoing stoma surgery and their families will need to be taught how to care for a stoma and be aware of the implications of stoma surgery. Support is needed throughout what can at times be a traumatic experience. The specialist stoma nurse, play therapist and clinical psychologist should all be involved in the care of the child and their family.

FACTORS TO NOTE

Neonates and babies

- After surgery on the small intestine, a large number of babies will have a temporary intolerance to lactose (Shaw & Lawson 2007). Ileostomy output is normally loose; however, if lactose intolerance occurs, the effluent will be extremely loose/watery, greater in volume, and test positive to sugar, increasing the risk of dehydration and failure to thrive. Many will initially be fed by total parenteral nutrition (TPN). Enteral feeding is slowly introduced using a hydrolysed or amino acid formula such as Pregestimil (Mead-Johnson) or Neocate (SHS). These milks are easier to absorb as loss of intestinal length results in loss of surface area for absorption and loss of digestive enzymes (Shaw & Lawson 2007).
- If an infant is taking special formula milk, the parents should follow dietetic advice when weaning.
- It is usual for infants to take a milk-free diet until the ileostomy is closed.
- Babies with colostomies who take regular formula milks can have a normal weaning diet.
- Sodium depletion can be a common problem for babies and children with ileostomies.

The ileum is important in absorption of fluid and electrolytes. Losses can be high, especially in sodium (Shaw & Lawson 2007).

● Dehydration can occur very quickly: if the stools are very loose and an adequate oral intake cannot be taken, especially in the case of gastroenteritis, intravenous therapy will be needed (Shaw & Lawson 2007).

Children and adolescents

● Privacy should be maintained at all times.
● Children from 3 years onwards with ileostomies should be encouraged to take plenty of fluids in hot weather to avoid dehydration. As a guide, normal intake of fluid should be six to eight drinks per day of water or water-based drinks. This can be supplemented with isotonic drinks.
● Young people and their parents need to be aware of the problems that can be caused by some foods. Examples include:
    – Popcorn and dried foods, if eaten in large amounts, can swell in the gastrointestinal tract and cause small bowel obstruction.
    – Onions, fish, eggs and cheese can cause a more odorous stool.
    – Beans, greens, onions and fizzy drinks can cause increased flatus.
    However, it must be remembered that children need a healthy balanced diet and that nutrient and energy needs are high in relation to their body size compared with adults (FSA 2005).
● Children with urinary diversions may benefit from eating foods with a high vitamin C content, which helps to keep urine acid. By doing this and drinking plenty of fluids, especially in hot weather, urine is prevented from becoming concentrated. There is some evidence to suggest those prone to recurrent urinary tract infections may benefit from taking cranberry juice, but studies are few in the paediatric population (Kemper 2006). Cranberry also helps to reduce mucus production but is contraindicated if on anticoagulant therapy such as warfarin, as it may enhance its effect (CSM 2004). Diabetics must be aware to take the low sugar variety. Older children may wish to manage their colostomy by means other than a pouch, e.g. colostomy irrigation. This is done by the instillation of warmed water or saline through the stoma via a cone and irrigation equipment.

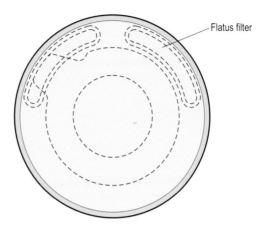

Figure 27.1 Stoma cap.

After evacuation of the bowel, a small stoma cap (Fig. 27.1) can then be used instead of a pouch. This system can be used to regulate the colostomy function; however, it is time consuming – up to 1 h – and may need performing daily (Williams 2004). A colostomy plug is again used to gain control over stoma function. This is a soft foam plug, gently inserted into the stoma, often used in association with irrigation (Williams 2004). A stoma nurse must first assess the patient, as not all patients are suitable for these procedures.

● Some children and parents may need extra psychological support in coming to terms with an altered body image. Preoperative planning with informed decision-making can prevent later negativity (Bray 2006). All families need support and information to help them cope with the illness (DoH 2003).

GUIDELINES

The carers of the child should be taught all aspects of stoma care prior to discharge into the community. Support and information should be given to help families plan for getting on with life after leaving hospital (DoH 2003).

CHANGING A BAG

EQUIPMENT

● Disposable gloves for hospital staff (parents may choose not to wear gloves as they would not normally do so when changing their child's nappy; however, they must be taught correct hand washing procedures to reduce infection). However, if a hospital acquired infection develops it would be prudent to advise the use of gloves for parents too

- Bowl of warm water
- Dry wipes
- Bag to dispose of used pouch and cleaning materials
- Scissors
- Template: a pattern of the stoma size, usually the adhesive release paper of the previously applied pouch
- Adhesive remover (silicone-based).

Before changing the pouch, make sure you have everything to hand. If the stoma is longstanding, the new pouch can be prepared beforehand.

Stoma pouches

There are many different pouches produced by a number of manufacturers. However, there are basically two designs: a one-piece pouch has an adhesive flange with a pouch bonded onto it (Fig. 27.2A); a two-piece pouch has an adhesive base plate or flange and a separate pouch that attaches to the flange (Fig. 27.2B). Some of these systems also now include a floating flange, which allows you to place your fingertips underneath the plastic ring on the base flange for support when attaching the bag. Pressure is not then exerted on the abdomen when securing a seal. Both types can be either closed, for formed stool (Fig. 27.3), or open-ended (drainable) for loose stool (Fig. 27.2), or with a tap for drainage of urine (Fig. 27.4). In the early postoperative period it is advisable to use a transparent drainable pouch. This ensures that the stoma can be observed easily and can be drained rather than changed frequently.

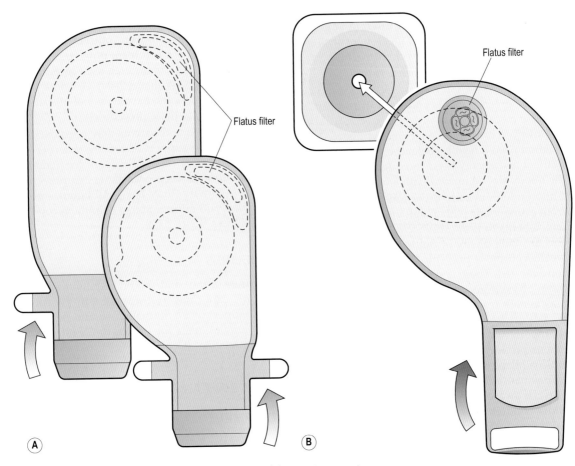

Figure 27.2 Drainable appliances. (A) One-piece pouch; (B) two-piece pouch.

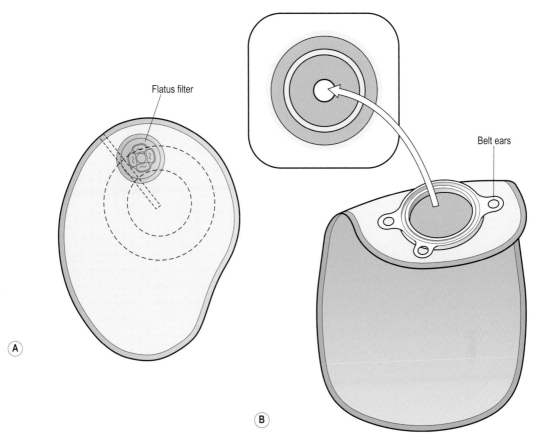

Figure 27.3 Closed appliances. (A) Closed one-piece pouch; (B) two-piece pouch.

METHOD

1. Position the child – babies lying down, older children lying or standing.
2. If a drainable or pouch with a tap is worn, empty contents before removing. In the immediate postoperative period, the stoma output may require measuring, therefore the pouch will be emptied into a measuring jug, the amount recorded on a chart, and then emptied into a toilet. Before discharge home, children and their carers will need to be taught how to empty the pouch directly into the toilet.
3. By using a silicone-based adhesive remover, the bag can be removed easily, causing little discomfort and without causing peristomal skin breakdown (Rudoni 2008). After application, gently peel away the flange from the top to the bottom with one hand, while supporting the skin with the other, re-applying

the remover as the bag is peeled downward. Place the used pouch into a disposal bag.

4. Clean the peristomal skin with warm water and dry wipe. If some residue of paste or pouch adhesive is left on the skin, remove this first with a dry wipe or adhesive remover. Do not use cotton wool or tissue as this can deposit strands that will stick to the stoma and surrounding skin which will cause problems with pouch adhesion. Once clean, dry the peristomal skin with a dry wipe. Prepare the new pouch if not already done. The aperture should be cut to fit snugly around the stoma with no peristomal skin exposed. Put on the new pouch. If a one-piece is being used, fold the adhesive in half, placing the pouch on the underside of the stoma first, then flip the adhesive over the stoma and secure all round. If a two-piece appliance is being used, secure the base plate and then attach the pouch.

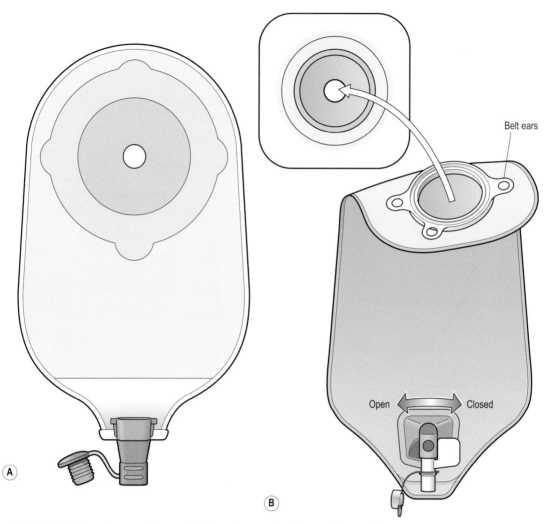

Figure 27.4 Drainable urostomy appliances. (A) One-piece pouch; (B) two-piece pouch.

5. If a drainable pouch is being used, ensure that the clip/integral closure is secured correctly at the bottom of the pouch. If a tap pouch is used, ensure that the tap is closed.

6. Used pouches should not be put down the toilet. Empty it into the toilet, then wrap in newspaper or place in a disposal bag designed for this purpose (most ostomy companies provide these free of charge along with dry wipes); it is then placed in a dustbin or clinical waste bin in hospital. Some local authorities view this as clinical waste. The stoma nurse or healthcare professional should advise you on local policies.

OBSERVATIONS AND COMPLICATIONS

- In the immediate postoperative period, the stoma should be observed to determine if there is a good blood supply. To aid easier observation of the stoma, a clear pouch should initially be applied, without a filter; medical staff will want to know when bowel sounds are returning – any wind passed will inflate the pouch.

- The normal colour of a healthy stoma is pink or red. Any signs of the stoma changing colour to a dusky purple must be reported to medical staff immediately as the blood supply to the stoma could be compromised, risking necrosis (Collett 2002). Observe also for haemorrhage around the stoma and/or into the pouch and excessive oedema.

- When first formed, the stoma will be oedematous due to handling of the bowel (Collett 2002), but over a period of approximately 6 weeks, the stoma will shrink in size. It is important to check the size before fitting a new pouch to ensure that no peristomal skin will be exposed. The size of the stoma can be checked by using a template.
- Check for any peristomal skin soreness; this can be caused by stoma effluent being in contact with the skin as a result of incorrect fitting of the pouch or the pouch adhesive not being cut accurately.
- Specific stoma barrier preparations are available to protect the skin around the stoma. They come in creams, pastes, powders, sprays, etc. All have instructions for use and these should be studied carefully. Remember that babies have sensitive skin and alcohol free based preparations should be used.
- Surface bleeding can happen if the cleaning routine is too vigorous, the stoma is knocked or the child scratches it. Unless the bleeding is prolonged it should cause no alarm. If the bleeding comes from inside the stoma it should be reported to a doctor.
- It is not uncommon in children for the stoma to prolapse. This is when the bowel intussuscepts (telescopes) out of the skin opening, becoming longer (Burch 2004). This may occur after a period of crying, coughing or strenuous exercise. Generally, the stoma will return to normal size at rest. If it does not and becomes tense or darker in colour, medical advice should be sought.
- The stoma may become retracted, this is when the stoma sinks below the level of the skin causing leakage of stool and poor bag adhesion. This can be remedied in some cases by using a pouch with a convex flange. If not, the stoma may need re-fashioning.
- Some children may experience rectal discharge. Usually it is only mucus which continues to be produced in the rectal stump. If the child cannot pass it into the toilet or nappy, or it becomes copious in amount, a gentle rectal washout may

be required, which should be carried out by an experienced practitioner.

- Children with stomas can get gastroenteritis like any other child. If a child's stoma output becomes loose or watery they should be encouraged to drink plenty of fluids and an electrolyte replacement drink. Dehydration can occur very quickly, especially in the child with an ileostomy.
- Any complaints of cramp from children with an ileostomy should be noted and urinary sodium levels checked. If below 20 mmol/L children should be encouraged to take more salty foods or an electrolyte replacement/isotonic drinks.
- Babies and toddlers with a persistent urinary sodium below 20 mmol/L should have prescribed oral sodium supplements.
- Children with urinary diversions can be susceptible to urinary infection due to a shortened urinary tract system (Burch 2004). If infection is suspected, a specimen of urine should be examined. It is important for a child with a urinary stoma to drink plenty of water or water-based fluid.

ON DISCHARGE

On discharge the family need to be given 1–2 weeks' supply of the type of pouch the child is using. Order numbers along with the manufacturer's name should be written down and given to the parents. This is to ensure that the GP knows which product to prescribe (DoH 2003). The supplies can be obtained either on prescription from the GP and taken to the pharmacy or by registering with a home delivery service (all companies now use one) who will:

- Deliver supplies to the home (usually within 48 h)
- Arrange prescription collection after receiving a telephone request from the parent
- Offer a flange cutting service once the stoma has settled and size remains constant
- Supply complimentary scented disposal bags and dry wipes
- Offer help when travelling abroad to arrange for supplies to be collected in country of destination.

However, they are unable to organise/deliver medication

- All children in full-time education are exempt from prescription charges
- The child may also be eligible for disability living allowance for personal care, the hospital social worker or stoma nurse will be able to advise on this
- The child should be referred to a stoma care nurse who covers their community area, as well as a children's community nurse and the health visitor (if appropriate), thus ensuring that the team give care in a holistic manner (Black 2000).

COMMUNITY PERSPECTIVE

It is good practice to refer babies and children with newly formed stomas to a CCN before discharge from hospital. The CCN, in conjunction with the stoma nurse or paediatric continence nurse specialist can support the family in adapting to coping with a stoma and the child's underlying condition. The CCN will liaise and coordinate care between other agencies such as health visitor, GP, referring hospital, and school nurse, as well as developing close links with education staff. Individualised child-specific training will need to be undertaken for school staff to enable them to carry out healthcare procedures. Comprehensive training with a teaching plan, and an individual healthcare plan must be drawn up. This may be from the school nurse, CCN, or paediatric continence nurse, with assessment of competence and an annual review (PromoCon 2006). For children with special needs, provision of their personal care needs must be included in the educational statement.

DOS AND DON'TS

- Do refer to a stoma care nurse any child for whom stoma surgery is planned or has taken place.
- Do refer to a children's community nurse prior to discharge.
- Do keep a template of the size of the stoma. This will make preparing new pouches easier. The template will need to be altered as the stoma shrinks postoperatively.
- Do not use cotton wool or tissue to clean the stoma. They deposit strands which can hinder pouch application.
- Do not cut the pouch adhesive bigger than the stoma as the peristomal skin will become sore.
- Do not cut the pouch adhesive smaller than the stoma as the pouch will leak. It may also restrict blood supply to the stoma.
- Do not use general barrier creams on sore peristomal skin; use only preparations specific for this use, otherwise the pouch may leak.

References

Black, P., 2000. Holistic stoma care. Baillière Tindall, Edinburgh.

Bray, L., 2006. Preparing children and young people for stoma surgery. Paediatr. Nurs. 18 (4), 33–37.

Burch, J., 2004. The management and care of people with stoma complications. Br. J. Nurs. 13 (6), 307–318.

Collett, K., 2002. Practical aspects of stoma management. Nurs. Stand. 17 (8), 45–55.

CSM Committee on Safety of Medicines, 2004. Enhanced effect of warfarin. Medicines and Healthcare Products Regulatory Agency, London.

DoH Department of Health, 2003. Essence of care: patient-focused benchmarks for clinical governance. NHS Modernisation Agency, DoH, London.

DoH Department of Health, 2004. National Service Framework for Children, Young People and Maternity Services. DoH, London.

FSA Food Standards Agency, 2005. Feeding your growing child. Food Standards Agency Publications, London.

Kemper, K., 2006. Cranberry therapy for children's urinary tract infections. Arch. Paediatr. Adolesc. Med. 160 (4), 451–452.

Malone, P.S., Ransley, P.G., Kiely, E.M., 1990. Preliminary report: the antegrade continence enema. Lancet 336, 1217–1218.

PromoCon, 2006. Managing bowel and bladder problems in schools and early years settings. PromoCon, Manchester.

Rudoni, C., 2008. A service evaluation of the use of silicone based adhesive remover. Br. J. Nurs. 17 (2), S4–S9.

Shaw, V., Lawson, M., 2007. Clinical paediatric dietetics, third ed. Blackwell Publishing, Oxford.

Williams, J., 2004. A stoma for incontinence. In: Norton, C., Chelvanayagam, S. (Eds.), Bowel continence nursing. Beaconsfield, Oxford, pp. 165–173.

Further reading

NHS Modernisation Agency, 2003. Good practice in paediatric continence services –

Benchmarking in Action. DoH, London.

Rogers, J., 2003. Successful inclusion of a child with a stoma in mainstream schooling. Br. J. Nurs. 12 (10), 590–599.

Support groups

Children's Continence Action Groups
Tel: 0161 214 5959
e-mail: promocon2001@disabledliving.co.uk

Contact a Family – offers advice, information and support for specific conditions and rare disorders

Tel: 020 7608 8700
Family Freephone Helpline: 0808 808 3555
website: www.cafamily.org.uk

National Advisory Service to Parents of Children with a Stoma (NASPCS)

Tel: 01560 322 024 – 24 hour answerphone
website: www.naspcs.co.uk

Royal Association for Disability and Rehabilitation (RADAR) Key Scheme (for access to disabled toilets)
Tel: 0207 250 3222
website: www.radar.org.uk

Chapter 28

Suctioning

Michaela Dixon

CHAPTER CONTENTS

Introduction   274
   Learning outcomes   274
   Rationale   274
   Factors to note   275

Resuscitation   275
   Equipment   275
   Indications   276
   Factors to note   276
   Method   276
   Technique   276
   Observations and complications   278
   Dos and don'ts   279

INTRODUCTION

Although suction is most often used in intensive care, theatres and emergency departments, it is essential for all healthcare workers to understand the principles and techniques, as it forms a vital component of resuscitation and of essential care for both the acutely ill child as well as the child with complex ongoing health needs. Suction may be performed by the nurse, physiotherapist, doctor or parent/caregiver. For this reason it is important that there are established evidence-based guidelines on an individual unit basis. There remains a dearth of child focused literature available and therefore practice is based upon adult studies with supporting evidence from within the child field where available.

LEARNING OUTCOMES

By the end of this section you should be able to:

- Understand the indications and contraindications for suctioning
- Demonstrate and understand the common techniques used for suctioning
- Understand the problems associated with suctioning.

RATIONALE

Normally, children and babies will keep their airway clear by coughing, sneezing, blowing their noses and by the protective mechanism of the gag reflex. Suction is an invasive procedure, and as such may be traumatic to both the child and family; it should therefore be used with care after thorough assessment, where less invasive interventions have been ineffective. The use of careful positioning can also help maintain a patent airway.

FACTORS TO NOTE

Infants and toddlers do not always have the necessary ability to clear their airway, due to immaturity of the respiratory system and its functions. Although the respiratory system of a child is essentially mature and fully functional by the age of 8 years, there is a group of children who will continue to have poor respiratory function due to underlying pathology at this age and when older. Infants are more susceptible to airway compromise when they have an upper or lower airway infection causing overproduction of mucus and secretions, due to the magnified effect of oedema on their airway when compared with the adult airway (APLS 2005). It can be helpful to give suction prior to a feed in infants to minimise the risk of the infant gagging and vomiting with suction immediately post-feed.

There are some childhood conditions which can cause overproduction of mucus, or a difficulty in combining swallowing and breathing. Examples include cystic fibrosis, tracheoesophageal fistulae prior to surgical repair, some laryngeal disorders and tracheostomy.

After some types of surgery, the child may bleed postoperatively, increasing the potential for airway compromise (e.g. after tonsillectomy). These children may require gentle suctioning to remove excessive secretions and prevent airway obstruction.

Some children may not have learnt the coordination skills required to keep their airways clear, whereas others may have lost their previously acquired skills due to illness and/or injury. These children may be unable to cough and clear the airway and so may require suction to prevent airway compromise.

RESUSCITATION

If the child has stopped breathing, first assess whether the airway is compromised and, if so, clear it, using suction, if the obstruction is thought to be secretion related. If there is a history of inhalation of foreign object, be very cautious about the use of suction – this may push the obstruction further down into the child's airway, increasing the degree of obstruction present.

EQUIPMENT

- Suction catheters:
  - For oro/nasopharyngeal suction: select size according to age of child, size of nostril or Guedel airway, amount and type of secretions, condition of mucosa. If suctioning orally, a larger size of catheter can be used. A smaller-sized Yankauer catheter can be very effective, but should be used with care, due to its more rigid structure. There is no particular formula for calculating suction catheter sizes for oro/nasopharyngeal suction – if you are uncertain then seek advice from a more senior member of staff.
  - For endotracheal tubes/tracheostomy tubes: the tube size of the suctioning catheter should be approximately twice the internal diameter of the endotracheal tube. Consequently, for a size 3.5 mm tube, use a size 6 or 7 Fg suction catheter. Using a larger suction catheter would completely occlude the internal diameter of the tube and as a consequence increase the detrimental effects of suction (see below). It is also important to know the length of the endotracheal/tracheostomy tube to ensure that you only suction to an appropriate depth
- Disposable gloves (non-powdered)
- Stethoscope
- Suction tubing
- Collection device, e.g. disposable bag and container, special suction specimen container
- Wall-piped suction or portable suction machine
- Tap water/clean container
- Sterile normal saline (endotracheal suction only); see discussion below
- Emergency equipment including oxygen and Ambu bag, with appropriately sized face mask, should be available.

All emergency equipment should be checked at the beginning of every shift in accordance with local unit policy.

INDICATIONS

If the child is able to clear their secretions independently, do not use suction. Physiotherapy techniques for clearing secretions should be considered, for example percussion and postural drainage and discussion with physiotherapists will assist in planning effective care.

- Suction should be considered if the child's respiration is compromised by excessive secretions; this can be assessed visually and through auscultation of the child's chest, using a stethoscope.
- If the child's oxygen saturation is low, i.e. <92% in a child without a cyanotic heart lesion, and the respiratory rate and effort high, then breathing may be obstructed and the child may need suction. The child's colour should also be assessed, in conjunction with heart rate and peripheral perfusion, as these may give an indication of inadequate respiratory function.

FACTORS TO NOTE

- Suction must never be carried out on a child in whom a diagnosis of epiglottitis is suspected. *This is a life-threatening condition –* seek urgent anaesthetic assistance and wait with the child until help has arrived in the department.
- Suction should only be undertaken following careful assessment, not as a matter of routine.
- Any child who requires suction to maintain airway patency should receive effective humidification to assist in loosening secretions.
- Laboratory analysis of nasopharyngeal (NPA) or endotracheal secretions will aid in the diagnosis of respiratory infections, e.g. respiratory syncytial virus (RSV[+ve]) bronchiolitis.

METHOD

Preparation

1. Assess the need for suction as described above.
2. Explain the procedure fully to the child and family to reduce anxiety levels.

3. Check all equipment is set up correctly and functioning before commencing.
4. Pre-set suction to appropriate pressure – as a guide the following pressures have been identified (Linton 2000, Pollard 2001):
   a. Neonates: 60–80 mmHg (8–10.6 kPa)
   b. Child: 80–100 mmHg (10.6–13.3 kPa)
   c. Adolescent/adult: maximum setting of 120 mmHg (16 kPa).

   When considering nasopharyngeal suctioning, ET suctioning and tracheostomy suctioning, the evidence has shown that there is no difference in the amount of secretions removed using 100 mmHg of suction pressure when compared with secretion removal using a higher suction pressure of 200 mmHg.

   There was, however, an increased risk of mucosal trauma when using higher suction pressures and most authors would recommend a maximum pressure of 120 mmHg (16 kPa) (Linton 2000).
5. Place the child in a comfortable, secure position; if necessary, ask for assistance.
6. If the child is receiving oxygen therapy, care must be taken to ensure that the supply is not interrupted to minimise the potential effects of hypoxia.
7. Put on gloves. The glove which is in contact with the suction catheter should be kept clean, and glove and catheter should be changed every time suction is performed. This will depend on local policy – some units will use one suction catheter per suction episode, whereas others will use one for each catheter pass. There is currently limited evidence to support decisions regarding frequency of use.
8. Positioning: If the child is conscious, the best position is lateral, to prevent inhalation of vomit, preferably on a parent's or carer's lap for comfort and reassurance. However, if the child is unconscious the procedure can occur in any position, either lateral or supine.

TECHNIQUE

There are two main techniques for suctioning, which will be considered separately:

- Oro- and nasopharyngeal suction
- Suctioning of an artificial airway, e.g. endotracheal tube/tracheostomy suction.

Oro- and nasopharyngeal suction

- Gently insert the suction catheter, not yet applying suction, upwards and backwards into the child's nostril or mouth:
  - If the child has a gag reflex, the child will cough.
  - If the child does not have a gag reflex, measure the catheter from nose or mouth to the suprasternal notch to estimate length (Fig. 28.1), then insert the catheter as above.
- Do not advance the catheter if early resistance is felt, instead withdraw the catheter and then reintroduce as above.
- Gently withdrawing the catheter, apply intermittent suction.
- Do not rotate the suction catheter as this will increase the risk of mucosal trauma.

Endotracheal suction

It is common practice in many units to instil small amounts of sterile saline (the volume of which is dependent on the size of the child) into the child's endotracheal or tracheostomy tube to assist with secretion removal during suctioning. It is important to note that this is a practice that is not evidence based and there is considerable debate in the published literature with most of the evidence being empirical in nature and inconsistent (Moore 2003, Celik & Kanan 2006, Kuriakose 2008).

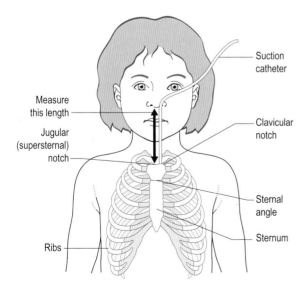

Figure 28.1 Measuring the suction catheter in a child with no gag reflex.

Most studies have involved small groups of adult patients and have examined other variables, e.g. hyperoxygenation prior to suctioning, in addition to the instillation of saline. Akgul and Akyolcu (2002) found a small but not statistically significant detrimental alteration in oxygen saturations and arterial blood gas levels after the instillation of saline for endotracheal tube suction. Other studies have looked at the volume of secretions removed with and without the use of saline and found no statistically significant benefit with the use of saline (Gray et al 1990, Raymond 1995). Other researchers have questioned the amount of saline that is not removed with suctioning and whether this has significant impact on the patient (Blackwood 1999). Much of the evidence is also rather old, appearing first in the 1970s and most recently in the 1990s.

It is suggested that, rather than routinely using saline to decrease the viscosity of secretions before suctioning of children with endotracheal tubes *in situ*, practitioners should concentrate on ensuring adequate airway heat and humidity, paying careful attention to the child's hydration status, and using mucolytic agents/nebulised saline as methods of maintaining the patency of the artificial airway (Blackwood 1999, Thompson 2000, Akgul & Akyolcu 2002).

Closed-system suctioning, designed so that the endotracheal tube does not need disconnection from the ventilator has been shown to be beneficial in reducing some of the adverse effects associated with suctioning, in particular hypoxia. These systems are normally only used in the intensive care setting and their use does not alter the responsibility of the practitioner in terms of assessment and preparation prior to carrying out suctioning.

It is recommended that the length of the catheter is pre-measured prior to starting the procedure to minimise the risk of mucosal trauma and to reduce the incidence of right upper lobe collapse in children (Boothroyd et al 1996, Pollard 2001).

Pre-oxygenation of the child should also be considered – this may be achieved by increasing the FiO_2 by 20% on the ventilator or by manually ventilating the child using an anaesthetic T-piece circuit (sometimes known as an Ayres T–piece circuit or a Mapleson Circuit). If you are unsure about either of these actions, seek advice from a more senior member of staff.

- Gently insert the catheter into the endotracheal tube, with no suction applied

- Insert the catheter to 0.5 cm beyond the end of the endotracheal tube only; see above regarding selecting appropriate tube size
- Apply suction and gently withdraw the catheter, interrupting the vacuum briefly every 1–2 s to reduce the potential for hypoxia. If secretions are particularly tenacious then vacuum may need to be continuous rather than intermittent to effect secretion clearance.

Tracheostomy suction

The technique is as for endotracheal suction, but with two important differences:

- Insert the catheter to the tip of the tracheostomy tube, not beyond it (see Ch. 30).
- Suctioning a tracheostomy tube should take less time as the tube is shorter in length than an endotracheal tube.

General

- Ensure that the catheter is withdrawn within 10 s in a child to reduce hypoxia (Pollard 2001)
- Ensure a minimum of 30 seconds must be allowed between each suction attempt; this may need to be increased if the child's saturations do not recover adequately within this timeframe
- Flush the suction tubing with tap water to clean it at the end of the procedure or between suction catheter passes if secretions are tenacious
- Ensure that the child is left in a comfortable position, has recovered from the procedure and their condition is stable (see below)
- Dispose of waste and change equipment as per local procedures.

OBSERVATIONS AND COMPLICATIONS

Observations

- Observe and record the child's colour, oxygen saturation, respiration rate and effort, and heart rate after the procedure to assess the child's response and recovery.
- Inspect and record the colour, viscosity and amount of secretions.

Possible complications

For further reading on complications, see Johnson (1999), Thompson (2000), Turner & Loan (2000), Moore (2003), Fiske (2004) and Coughlin (2005).

- Increased intracranial pressure, caused by raised blood pressure (see below)
- Hypoxia: during suction the child receives less oxygen than normal, especially if the procedure is prolonged and the child has pre-existing lung/cyanotic heart disease
- Laryngospasm caused by traumatic stimulation of the larynx
- Mucosal trauma from the same source
- Microatelectasis, related to trauma and negative pressure
- Pneumothorax: traumatic suction may perforate the lung
- Discomfort/pain: described by some children as 'gagging, suffocating'
- Overstimulation of secretions, often from too frequent suctioning
- Sepsis, due to poor infection control techniques and a child who may be more susceptible to infection
- Hypo/hypertension: caused by indirect vagal stimulation through hypoxaemia, as well as direct stimulation of the vagal nerve by the suction catheter
- Tachycardia/bradycardia, due to direct and indirect vagal stimulation and hypoxaemia.

COMMUNITY PERSPECTIVE

Some babies and children will be discharged home with ongoing care needs including the need for suction. There are an increasing number of children who require long-term home ventilation, have artificial airways (tracheostomies) *in situ* for airway protection, or who have complex medical conditions and are unable to maintain a patent airway independently. For many of these children, their parents/caregivers have primary responsibility for their day-to-day care, with support from a children's community nursing (CCN) team. It is vital that parents are, first of all, comfortable with the responsibility involved and, second, have received full training, prior to the child's discharge from the acute setting.

A partnership involving the child, their family and all health professionals involved is important to facilitate a smooth transition from hospital to home care. Consideration should be given to the following prior to discharge:

- Provision of both home and portable equipment in the event of mains failure

■ Availability and supply of disposables, e.g. suction catheters and gloves

■ Regular servicing of equipment and availability of loan equipment

■ Resources available in the event of equipment failure.

Most families are likely to need ongoing support from the CCN team, although the intensity of the input required will obviously vary according to the individual family. For some children, particularly those with complex needs, an 'open door' access agreement with the appropriate hospital/paediatric intensive care unit will be necessary.

DOS AND DON'TS

● Do check the emergency equipment at the beginning of every shift as per local policy.

● Do seek advice from a more senior member of staff if you are uncertain about carrying out suction on any child.

● Do wear gloves when carrying out this procedure.

● Do note the infant/child's colour and other vital signs and document these in the nursing records.

● Do not undertake suctioning as a matter of routine.

References

APLS Advanced Paediatric Life Support Group (APLS), 2005. Advanced paediatric life support: the practical approach, fourth ed. BMJ Publishing, London.

Akgul, S., Akyolcu, N., 2002. Effects of normal saline on endotracheal suctioning. J. Clin. Nurs. 11, 826–830.

Blackwood, B., 1999. Normal saline instillation with endotracheal suctioning: primum non nocere (first do no harm). J. Adv. Nurs. 29 (4), 928–934.

Boothroyd, A.E., Murthey, B.V., Darbyshire, A., et al., 1996. Endotracheal suctioning causes right upper lobe collapse in intubated children. Acta. Paediatr. 85, 1422–1425.

Celik, S.A., Kanan, N., 2006. A current conflict – use of isotonic sodium chloride on endotracheal suctioning in critically ill patients. Dimens. Crit. Care Nurs. 25 (1), 11–14.

Coughlin, A.M., 2005. Clearing the air about suctioning. Nursing made Incredibly Easy September/October, 59–63.

Fiske, E., 2004. Effective strategies to prepare infants and families for home tracheostomy care. Adv. Neonatal Care 4 (1), 42–53.

Gray, J.E., MacIntyre, N.R., Kronenberg, W.G., 1990. The effects of bolus normal-saline instillation in conjunction with endotracheal suctioning. Respir. Care 35 (8), 785–790.

Johnson, L., 1999. Factors known to raise intracranial pressure and the associated implications for nursing management. Nurs. Crit. Care 3, 117–120.

Kuriakose, A., 2008. Using the synergy model as best practice in endotracheal tube suctioning of critically ill patients. Dimens. Crit. Care Nurs. 27 (1), 10–15.

Linton, M., 2000. Endotracheal tube suctioning. In: Sinha, S.K.,

Donn, S.M. (Eds.), Manual of neonatal respiratory care. Futura, New York.

Moore, T., 2003. Suctioning techniques for the removal of respiratory secretions. Nurs. Stand. 18 (9), 47–53.

Pollard, C., 2001. Endotracheal suction in the infant with an artificial airway. Nurs. Crit. Care 6 (2), 76–82.

Raymond, S.J., 1995. Normal saline instillation before suctioning: helpful or harmful? A review of the literature. Am. J. Crit. Care 4, 267–271.

Thompson, L., 2000. Suctioning adults with an artificial airway, The Joanna Briggs Institute for Evidence Based Nursing and Midwifery Systematic Review No. 9.

Turner, B., Loan, L., 2000. Tracheobronchial trauma associated with airway management in neonates. AACN Clin. Issues 11 (2), 283–299.

Chapter 29

Temperature control

Toby Aslam Mohammed

CHAPTER CONTENTS

Introduction 280
    Learning outcomes 281
    Rationale 281
    Factors to note 281

Controlling temperature 281
    Equipment 281
    Guidelines 281
    Observations and complications 282
    Dos and don'ts 282

INTRODUCTION

Despite wide fluctuations in environmental temperature, through homeostatic mechanisms the human body can maintain the internal temperature at $37 \pm 1°C$. This internal temperature is referred to as the core temperature or set point. Thermoregulation involves complex physiological processes that aim to return the body temperature to the 'set point', and is controlled by the hypothalamus (Tortora & Grabowski 2005, RCN 2007, DTB 2008). The difference between the core temperature and that of the body surface can be as much as $0.5°C$ in normal circumstances (Casey 2000). Heat loss is increased by vasodilatation and sweating, while heat production and conservation are stimulated by shivering and vasoconstriction (DTB 2008). The balance between heat production and heat loss is controlled by a group of specialised neurones located in the anterior portion of the hypothalamus.

If the blood temperature rises, these neurones fire nerve impulses more rapidly; if the temperature decreases, the opposite occurs (Tortora & Grabowski 2005). These impulses are sent to other portions of the hypothalamus, which stimulate either a temperature increase or decrease. Thus these cells serve as an internal thermostat. An increase in body temperature is one of the most common symptoms of illness in children and may be caused either by an infection or by a head injury in which the temperature control centre of the hypothalamus has been affected.

LEARNING OUTCOMES

By the end of this section you should be able to:

- Identify the child at risk of pyrexia
- Initiate appropriate action to reduce or maintain a child's body temperature
- Understand the use of antipyretic medication and environmental interventions to reduce temperature in the fevered child
- Appreciate the problems of maintaining temperature in the term and pre-term neonate (see Ch. 15).

RATIONALE

The primary aim of reducing an ill child's temperature is to promote comfort by relieving the discomfort caused by the fever.

FACTORS TO NOTE

Research has indicated that fever has a therapeutic purpose (Holtzclaw 2003, DTB 2008). Fever is caused by the raising of the set point as a result of the initial infection (Purssell 2009). The raising of the set point is thought to be stimulated by the action of protein-like substances, produced by phagocytic white blood cells, on the cells of the hypothalamus. This action causes a release of prostaglandins, which resets the set point or core temperature at a higher level. The resetting of the core temperature may induce shivering and vasoconstriction to enable the body to reach the new temperature even if the body temperature is recorded at a higher than normal level. This will occur until the new set point has been reached (Tortora & Grabowski 2005). The rise in body temperature decreases the level of free serum iron required for bacterial/viral growth, as well as damaging the cell membranes of the microorganisms (O'Connor 2002).

Under normal conditions, body temperature fluctuates throughout the day. The temperature of a child is higher in the late afternoon and early evening. As children have a higher metabolic rate, they tend to have higher body temperatures.

An increase in temperature caused by bacterial, or viral, infection renders the child more prone to febrile seizure (see Ch. 26). The incidence of febrile seizures in children up to age 5 years is thought to be between 3% and 8% (Sadleir & Scheffer 2007). Reducing the temperature of a child may not affect the course of the child's illness, but may aid in the reduction of parental/carer anxiety (DTB 2008).

In the infant, overheating has been identified as a risk factor for sudden infant death syndrome (Lynch 2004). Infants and young children are highly susceptible to alterations and fluctuations in temperature. Their body temperature is altered not only by the environmental temperature, but also by crying, playing and emotional upset. Body proportions of infants and young children are different from those of the older child or adult, with the head of the infant or young child being larger in proportion to the rest of the body. Consequently, a greater amount of heat can be lost via the head (Wong 1997) (see Ch. 15).

Parental anxiety is increased in situations where their child has an increase in temperature. This often entails that they treat the temperature aggressively and use proprietary 'over the counter' preparations inappropriately. It is important that the children's nurse checks with the parents/carers what they have been giving for their temperature increase (DTB 2008, Purssell 2009).

Measurement of body temperature in children from age 4 weeks to 5 years can be achieved through the use of electronic thermometers, chemical dot thermometers or infra-red tympanic thermometers. For infants <4 weeks, an electronic thermometer applied to the axilla should be used (NICE 2007).

CONTROLLING TEMPERATURE

EQUIPMENT

- Thermometer
- Cotton sheets/blankets
- Cool fan
- Medicine cup/spoon for antipyretic medication.

GUIDELINES

The main reason for treating a fever is to relieve discomfort; however, it is widely recognised that clinical practitioners continue to believe that diminishing a child's temperature will alter the outcome of febrile illness (Holtzclaw 2003, NICE 2007). In fact, Casey (2000) recommends that elevations <38°C, in otherwise healthy children, probably should not be treated and left to run their course. However, within clinical practice, measures are routinely taken to reduce the temperature, including pharmacological and environmental intervention. It must be remembered for the reasons aforementioned that this practice does not alter the course of the illness, but relieves discomfort. The most effective intervention is the use of antipyretic medication (O'Connor 2002).

Pharmacological intervention

- The most effective way of reducing a child's temperature is to utilise an antipyretic medication to lower the set point (O'Connor 2002), although the use of such medication in children is controversial. Paracetamol and ibuprofen are both used in attempts to reduce temperature. Used separately or in combination both have been seen to reduce temperature, however the differences between these are clinically minimal (DTB 2008). Care should be taken when administering antipyretic drug therapy as non-steroidal antiinflammatory drugs, e.g. ibuprofen, can cause gastric irritation. For children who are dehydrated or have renal impairment, paracetamol should be used and ibuprofen avoided, as ibuprofen can exacerbate or cause renal impairment (RCN 2007, DTB 2008).
- There is a misconception among nurses and medical staff regarding the route of administration of paracetamol, with most thinking that rectal administration is a quicker way of reducing temperature (Chandler 2000, O'Connor 2002). The Royal College of Paediatrics and Child Health (1997) identified that rectal paracetamol was absorbed at a much slower rate than oral doses, with absorption being 90–120 min compared with 60 min, respectively.
- The antipyretic of choice will be given at the prescribed amount.

Environmental intervention

The use of environmental measures to reduce a child's temperature has been much debated within the literature (Harrison 1998, Blumenthal 2000). Environmental measures that can be taken following administration of an antipyretic to aid the comfort of the child include:

- Reducing the amount of clothing
- Using loose-fitting cotton clothing

- Reducing the amount of bedding; use sheets and blankets rather than quilts
- Reducing the room temperature by opening windows, using a cool fan (directed away from the child)
- Encouraging cool oral fluids.

Avoiding chilling is imperative, as this will cause the child to shiver and subsequently raise the set point.

OBSERVATIONS AND COMPLICATIONS

- Check the child's temperature (see Ch. 6) after an antipyretic has been given to assess its effect. This will normally be done around 30 min to 1 h after the dose. There is no need for continued frequent monitoring; however, a return to regular monitoring, e.g. 4-hourly, would help in the continued evaluation and assessment of the effect of the intervention.
- The child should be observed to ensure that they are gaining some comfort from the antipyretic, i.e. becoming more settled, reduced flushing.
- The child should be observed for seizure activity.

COMMUNITY PERSPECTIVE

Temperature taking by the CCN is usually only required for children who:

- Have malignant disease
- Are prone to febrile seizures
- Are particularly vulnerable to infection.

Routine temperature taking can heighten the parents' anxiety.

DOS AND DON'TS

- Do ensure that the child's temperature is monitored regularly (see Ch. 6).
- Do ensure that the parents are provided with information related to febrile seizures. This helps relieve anxiety.
- Do ensure that parents are provided with both verbal and written information on discharge.
- Do advise parents/carers on the appropriate use of proprietary, 'over the counter', medicines used for temperature reduction.
- Do not administer non-steroidal antiinflammatory drugs, e.g. ibuprofen, to

children with gastritis, as this may exacerbate further gastric upset and/or bleeding.

- Do not administer non-steroidal antiinflammatory drugs, e.g. ibuprofen, to children who have renal impairment or are dehydrated, as this may affect renal function.
- Do not use tepid sponging or cool moist compresses on the skin.

- Do not use environmental measures to reduce the temperature in the febrile child before the use of antipyretics. They may induce shivering, which will cause a further rise in the temperature.
- Do not use aspirin for fever in children under 12 years of age because of its identified correlation with Reye's syndrome (McGovern et al 2001).

References

Blumenthal, I., 2000. Fever and the practice nurse: measurement and treatment. Community Pract. 73 (3), 519–521.

Casey, G., 2000. Fever management in children. Nurs. Stand. 14 (40), 36–42.

Chandler, T., 2000. Paracetamol doses: practice variation. Paediatr. Nurs. 12 (4), 7–8.

DTB, 2008. When the child has a fever. Drug Ther. Bull. 46 (3), 17–21.

Harrison, M., 1998. Childhood fever: is practice scientific? J. Child Health 2 (3), 112–117.

Holtzclaw, B.J., 2003. Use of thermoregulatory principles in patient care: fever management. Cinahl Information Systems, Glendale.

Lynch, E., 2004. A bed of their own. Nurs. Stand. 18 (48), 18–19.

McGovern, M.C., Glasgow, J.F., Stuart, M.C., 2001. Reye's syndrome and aspirin: lest we forget. Br. Med. J. 322 (7302), 1591–1592.

NICE, 2007. Feverish illness in children. Clinical Guideline 47. Quick reference guide. NICE, London.

O'Connor, S., 2002. Antipyretics in the paediatric A&E setting: a review. Paediatr. Nurs. 14 (3), 33–35.

Purssell, E., 2009. Parental fever phobia and its evolutionary correlates. J. Clin. Nurs. 18 (2), 210–218.

RCN, 2007. Caring for children with fever. RCN, London.

Royal College of Paediatrics and Child Health, 1997. Prevention and control of pain in children: a manual for health care professionals. BMJ Publishing, London.

Sadleir, L.G., Scheffer, I.E., 2007. Febrile seizures. BMJ 334 (7588), 307–311.

Tortora, G.J., Grabowski, S.R., 2005. Principles of anatomy and physiology, eleventh ed. HarperCollins, New York.

Wong, D., 1997. Whaley and Wong's essentials of pediatric nursing, fifth ed. Mosby, St Louis.

Chapter 30

Tracheostomy care

Sue Fidment

CHAPTER CONTENTS

Introduction 284
    Learning outcomes 285
    Rationale 286
    Safety equipment 286
    Factors to note 286

Tracheostomy suction 289
    Rationale 289
    Equipment 289
    Method 290
    Observations 290

Cleaning the tracheostomy site 290
    Factors to note 290
    Equipment 290
    Method 291
    Observations 291

Changing the tracheostomy tube tape 291
    Equipment 291
    Method 291
    Observations 292

Changing a tracheostomy tube 292
    Equipment 292
    Method 292
    Observations 293
    Tips for day-to-day life 294
    Decannulation 297

Acknowledgements 297

INTRODUCTION

A tracheostomy is an artificial opening into the trachea via the neck (Fig. 30.1). It therefore provides an alternative route for effective respiration and for the removal of tracheobronchial secretions. A tracheostomy is required when circumstances make breathing impossible or difficult via the mouth and nose (Wilson 2005).

Indications for a tracheostomy (Wilson 2005, Trachsel & Hammer 2006) include:

- Congenital abnormalities, which may occlude or obstruct the airway such as: laryngeal papilloma, laryngeal haemangioma, laryngeal webbing, vocal cord paralysis, choanal atresia, subglottic stenosis, tracheo-oesophageal anomalies and micrognathia (underdevelopment of the mandible as in Pierre–Robin syndrome and Treacher–Collins syndrome)
- Trauma, which may occlude or obstruct the airway such as: subglottic stenosis (could be caused by prolonged or repeated intubations) and emergency situations, e.g. road traffic accidents and burn injuries to face and neck
- Facilitating long-term ventilation, for conditions such as: tracheomalacia, bronchopulmonary dysplasia, spinal muscular atrophy and polyneuritis (e.g. Guillain–Barré syndrome).
- Traumatic brain and spinal injury
- Face and neck tumours
- Foreign body may occlude the upper airway resulting in the need for an emergency tracheostomy

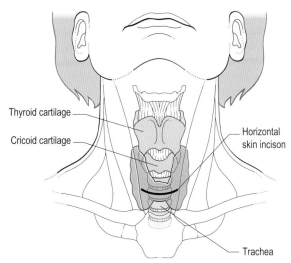

Figure 30.1 Landmarks of the neck and the incision site for tracheostomy.

Thyroid cartilage

Cricoid cartilage

Horizontal skin incison

Trachea

- Infections, which may cause acute swelling around the airway such as: acute epiglottitis or laryngo-tracheobronchitis (the introduction of the HIB vaccine has caused this category of patient to diminish significantly).

To be able to provide safe effective care, it is essential that children's nurses are aware of the signs and symptoms of respiratory distress and airway obstruction:

- Increased respiratory rate: at rest, tachypnoea can indicate that increased effort of breathing is needed, indicating further assessment is required (ALSG 2005)

- Stridor: a high-pitched sound produced by narrowing within the more rigid confines of the larynx or trachea. In laryngeal obstruction the stridor is inspiratory; in tracheal lesions it is usually both inspiratory and expiratory (Bull 2002)
- Stertor: the noise produced by obstruction in the throat, i.e. above the larynx; it is usually a low-pitched choking type of noise (Bull 2002)
- Recession and use of accessory muscles: intercostal, subcostal or sternal recession indicates increased effort of breathing (Fig. 30.2). Babies and younger children may use their diaphragm and abdominal muscles to aid respiration
- Pallor: due to hypoxia causes sweating and restlessness
- Nasal flaring: seen especially in infants with respiratory distress
- Tachycardia: due to hypoxia and anxiety
- Cyanosis: this is a late sign of respiratory distress (ALSG 2005)
- Exhaustion: a late and pre-terminal sign of hypoxia. The child makes less effort to breathe, stridor and recession become less pronounced and apnoea is not far off (Bull 2002, ALSG 2005).

LEARNING OUTCOMES

By the end of this section you should be able to:

- Identify the conditions which require the formation of a tracheostomy in children
- Discuss the nursing care required to maintain a patent airway in a child with a tracheostomy

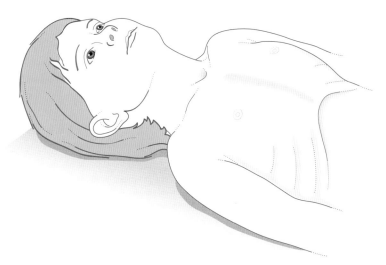

Figure 30.2 Sternal and intercostal recession.

- List the equipment required for safe, effective care
- Discuss the rationale of when different procedures are required
- Describe the skills that staff and the child's carers need to acquire (achieve competency in) to care for a child with a tracheostomy
- Discuss the multidisciplinary support required by the family prior and after the child's discharge.

RATIONALE

Children requiring a tracheostomy formation may initially be nursed on an intensive care unit or in a high dependency area. Another child with a tracheostomy, who's condition is more stable will be cared for on a children's ward or at home. The main safety concern when caring for a child with a tracheostomy is to maintain patency of the tube, ensuring a clear airway at all times. Suction via the tracheostomy is required to achieve this. The frequency of suction varies from child to child, and is dependent upon the age of the child and the viscosity and amount of secretions. The child may need humidification of inspired gases to help keep the secretions thin and easily removable, preventing inspissation (thickening and drying of secretions through evaporation) (DoH 2007). This can occur because the normal mechanisms of warming and humidifying air as it is breathed (i.e. passage through the nose) are bypassed while a tracheostomy is in place (Harkin & Russell 2001). If necessary, humidity can be administered, with a humidifying unit and tracheostomy mask or with a heat and moisture exchanger (e.g. Artificial/Swedish nose). Regardless of the method of humidification used, the equipment must be used according to the manufacturer's instructions and local policy.

Family support and training

Nurses and the multidisciplinary team need to support and empower the family of a child with a tracheostomy. To do this they must provide information, support and resources, to ensure that the family can learn and eventually provide care competently and safely for their child. Skills families require include suction, cleaning the stoma site, changing the tapes and changing the tracheostomy tube. Theoretical knowledge they require includes recognising changes in secretions, signs of infection or aspiration, signs of a mucus plug or blocked tracheostomy tube, and cardiopulmonary resuscitation (CPR).

To be able to achieve this, nursing staff who are to teach and support family training should be competent at teaching and assessing clinical skills to others. In addition they must have sound knowledge and understanding of the airway anatomy; predisposing factors which may lead to the formation of a tracheostomy; operative procedures; preparation of safety equipment; immediate post-operative care (including the treatment of potential complications); care of a child following decannulation; care of a humidifier; and discharge planning. Nurses should also advocate and facilitate the development of evidence based practice in regard to tracheostomy care.

SAFETY EQUIPMENT

The following pieces of equipment are required to be with the child with a tracheostomy at all times, both in hospital and at home. So that accidental displacement, or obstruction of the tracheostomy tube and suctioning can be dealt with immediately. See Figure 30.3 for emergency care of the child with a tracheostomy.

- Oxygen point (or oxygen cylinder), oxygen tubing and tracheostomy mask (not required in the community unless the child is oxygen dependent)
- Suction apparatus with tubing and a box of suction catheters of appropriate size; one catheter attached to the suction tubing
- Spare tracheostomy tube with tapes attached (same size as the child has *in situ*)
- Spare smaller tracheostomy tube with tapes attached (one size smaller)
- Disposable gloves (latex free, non sterile, non-powdered) and disposable aprons
- Water based lubricant
- Water (to rinse the suction tubing)
- Disposal bag for hazardous waste
- Spare tracheostomy tape
- Scissors.
- 10 mL syringe (only required if the child has a cuffed tracheostomy tube *in situ*).

FACTORS TO NOTE

- Hand washing and universal precautions are used (disposable gloves and disposable aprons are worn) when providing tracheostomy care. This is to prevent the spread or introduction of infection (DoH 2007). Parents may prefer not to wear gloves and apron, when caring for their child.

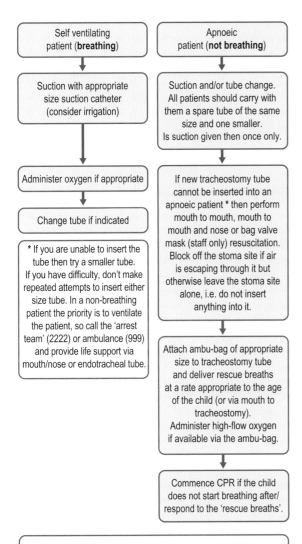

Self ventilating patient (**breathing**)	Apnoeic patient (**not breathing**)

Self ventilating patient (**breathing**) → Suction with appropriate size suction catheter (consider irrigation) → Administer oxygen if appropriate → Change tube if indicated

* If you are unable to insert the tube then try a smaller tube. If you have difficulty, don't make repeated attempts to insert either size tube. In a non-breathing patient the priority is to ventilate the patient, so call the 'arrest team' (2222) or ambulance (999) and provide life support via mouth/nose or endotracheal tube.

Apnoeic patient (**not breathing**) → Suction and/or tube change. All patients should carry with them a spare tube of the same size and one smaller. Is suction given then once only. → If new tracheostomy tube cannot be inserted into an apnoeic patient * then perform mouth to mouth, mouth to mouth and nose or bag valve mask (staff only) resuscitation. Block off the stoma site if air is escaping through it but otherwise leave the stoma site alone, i.e. do not insert anything into it. → Attach ambu-bag of appropriate size to tracheostomy tube and deliver rescue breaths at a rate appropriate to the age of the child (or via mouth to tracheostomy). Administer high-flow oxygen if available via the ambu-bag. → Commence CPR if the child does not start breathing after/respond to the 'rescue breaths'.

All parents/carers of children with tracheostomies should be taught Basic Life Support techniques after they are competent at changing the tracheostomy tube and prior to discharge. This training should be provided by the Resuscitation Training officers or an approved trainer. The ambu-bag will be provided on discharge.

Figure 30.3 Sheffield Children's Hospital emergency tracheostomy management flow chart (*with permission*).

- Latex-free gloves should be worn to reduce the incidence of latex allergy.
- Non-sterile gloves are used because tracheostomy care does not need to be performed as a sterile procedure. A clean 'non-touch' technique, i.e. thorough hand washing and not touching the part of the suction catheter that goes inside the tracheostomy, is sufficient.
- Irrigation (the instillation of a small amount of saline directly into the tracheostomy tube) prior

to suction may be performed to aid the removal of thick tenacious secretions. However, this is a potentially hazardous procedure and must be undertaken with care (Clarke 1995). Evidence consistently shows that such instillation is detrimental in adults, most often resulting in decreased oxygen saturation and distress to patients. More recent studies are again questioning the benefit of this practice (Akgul & Akyolcu 2002, Neil 2001), and alternative practices such as: effective humidity therapy, assessing the child's hydration status and the use of saline nebulisers are advocated as alternatives to thin secretions (O'Neal et al 2001, Klockare et al 2006). Therefore, irrigation should not be performed routinely and local policy should be followed (NHS QIS 2008).

- Tracheal dilators may cause trauma to the trachea. As a result of this these are rarely used in practice. However, some hospitals may still have them in the tray at the child's bedside for emergency purposes; therefore local policy should be followed.
- The ward resuscitation trolley should contain an appropriately sized Ambu bag for use in an emergency. The 15 mm connector fits directly onto almost all tracheostomy tubes. Ambu bags are given to parents in the community in some areas; therefore local policy should be followed.

Tracheostomy tube selection

The type of tracheostomy tube selected for a child is primarily the responsibility of the ENT surgeon and the respiratory team. Often the most important factor in determining the appropriate type of tube is the age of the child. There are many reasons why a child may need a tracheostomy, and manufacturers produce a wide range of models and sizes of tracheostomy tubes, therefore selection of an appropriate tube should be carried out on an individualised basis (Eber & Oberwaldner 2006).

Shiley tracheostomy tubes

These are plastic tubes with an introducer (Fig. 30.4). Sizes are measured by the internal diameter (ID) in millimeters (mm) 3.0, 3.5, 4.0 and 4.5 in the neonatal design and 3.0, 3.5, 4.0, 4.5, 5.0 and 5.5 in the paediatric design. Neonatal tubes have a different design of flange from the paediatric tubes; the angle of the curve also differs although the internal diameter is the same. The Shiley tracheostomy tube needs to be changed every 29 days, although they may be

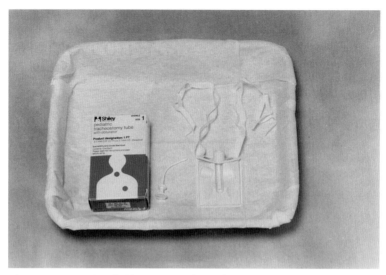

Figure 30.4 Shiley tracheostomy tubes: box (left); introducer (centre); spare tracheal tube with tapes attached (right).

changed more often depending on local practice and policies. Parents and other family members may be keen to do a weekly tube change in order to gain more practice and confidence. This type of tube is for single use only, and should be disposed of after removal (Wilson 2005).

Cuffed and fenestrated tubes

These are tracheostomy tubes only used in older children and adults, therefore their use in paediatric patients is less common. The cuff around the outer distal end of the tube is inflated with air which then sits below the larynx, and therefore makes it more secure and less likely to fall out (cuffed tubes are not indicated in younger children and neonates as the cuff causes pressure and damage to the tracheal wall). The cuff should be assessed several times a day with a manometer, to measure the pressure. Ensuring that the cuff is not over inflated and causing damaging pressure to the trachea wall, but also is inflated enough to be secure. A 10 mL syringe needs to kept with the emergency equipment to deflate/inflate the cuff in case of an emergency tube change.

Fenestrated tubes have a hole in the wall of the tube (therefore they allow the patient to breathe through and around the tube, aiding speech and secretion clearance). They also come with two types of inner tube for each outer tracheostomy tube; a fenestrated inner tube and non-fenestrated inner tube. When the non-fenestrated inner tube is in, the tracheostomy acts as normal, and routine suctioning can take place. When the fenestrated inner tube is inserted then both tubes have a hole, this can be used

for talking when the tracheostomy end is occluded (which forces air up through the larynx causing phonation). The fenestrated tube can also be used for assessing when the patient is ready for decannulation. The inner tubes need to changed regularly to clear the tracheostomy of secretions, the inner tubes can be cleaned with water/saline or mild detergent, dried and then reinserted.

Bivona tracheostomy tubes

This range of tubes comes in the same sizes (ID) as Shiley tubes. Bivona tubes are made of silicone and are soft and flexible to the shape of the trachea, and are therefore preferred by some units. They can also be custom made to the length required by the child. Bivona tubes are reusable following sterilisation.

Sheffield tracheostomy tube

This is a silver tube with an introducer, two inner tubes (one being a spare), a speaking tube and a blocker (Fig. 30.5). The inner tube can safely be removed and cleaned without disturbing the outer tube. Silver tubes may be used for children who require long-term airway management without ventilation. Due to advances in the manufacturing of disposable tracheostomy tubes and the extensive range of single use tracheostomy tubes available, means that silver tubes are rarely used now because of issues regarding vCJD and the re-sterilising of equipment. They must only be used for the same patient and thrown away after decannulation. If the child has a silver tracheostomy tube, an endotracheal tube connector will be needed to connect the Ambu bag to the tube in emergencies.

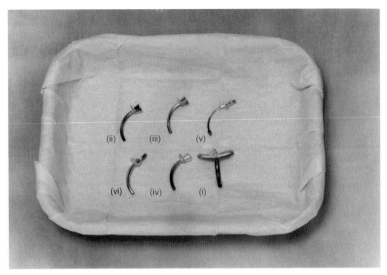

Figure 30.5 Sheffield tracheostomy tubes: (i) tracheostomy tube; (ii) and (iii) inner tubes; (iv) speaking tube; (v) introducer; (vi) blocker.

TRACHEOSTOMY SUCTION

RATIONALE

Suctioning of the tracheostomy tube prevents the build up of secretions, which may narrow the lumen of the tube and make it difficult for the child to breathe. Suctioning of the tube should be undertaken with care as, performed incorrectly, it can lead to complications such as; trauma, hypoxia, laryngospasm, bronchospasm and infection.

Factors to note

Each child's need for suction will vary and therefore should be individually assessed, a child who has a cold or newly formed tracheostomy will require more frequent suctioning (Wilson 2005). Often a child's condition will indicate when suctioning is required, e.g. coughing, audible or visible secretions and decreased oxygen saturations from mucous build up (Ireton 2007).

- Suction catheters: it is important to use the correct size of suction catheter (NHS QIS 2007). A catheter that is too small will not aspirate the secretions efficiently, and a catheter that is too large will block off too much of the airway during suction. As a rule, the size of the suction catheter (measured in French gauge, Fg) is twice the internal diameter of the tracheostomy tube, e.g. a 3.5 ID neonatal or paediatric tube will require a size 7 Fg catheter.

- There is still ambiguity around safe pressure required for effective suctioning for different age groups of children (Ireton 2007). It is important to apply only enough suction to remove secretions; suction that is too vigorous can damage the tracheal mucosa and cause atelectasis. Suction that is too gentle is inefficient at removing secretions and may mean that the procedure has to be repeated. Guidelines for adult suction pressures are recommended to be <120 mmHg when suctioning a tracheostomy (NHS QIS 2007). For children and neonates, recent guidelines recommend pressures of: 80–120 mmHg adolescents, 80–100 mmHg for children and 60–80 mmHg for neonates (Ireton 2007, NHS QIS 2008). Therefore local policies and guidelines should be followed. Some models of portable suction machines require a higher pressure to remove minimal secretions. The manufacturer's guidelines should be referred to before using such machines.

EQUIPMENT

- Suction equipment (either wall or portable)
- Appropriate size and type of suction catheters
- Disposable gloves and disposable aprons
- Disposal bag for clinical waste
- Bowl filled with tap water
- A pre-measured guide to measure the length of suction catheter, e.g. a piece of suction catheter that has been previously cut to the length required.

METHOD

1. To prevent trauma during the procedure, check that the suction equipment is set to give the correct pressure on applying the suction and that there is a suction catheter of the correct size attached to the suction tubing.

2. Allow the child to perform their own suction if this is usual. If not, explain the procedure.

3. To reduce the risk of infection, wash hands thoroughly and wear a disposable apron.

4. To minimise the risk of introducing infection, put on gloves and withdraw the suction catheter from the sleeve. Do not touch the part of the catheter that will be introduced into the tracheostomy.

5. To prevent damage to the tracheal mucosa, which can lead to trauma and respiratory infection, turn the suction equipment on, do not apply suction, check the length of suction catheter to be used against the pre-measured guide and gently introduce the catheter into the tracheostomy to this length. The length of the suction catheter should be equal to the length of the tracheostomy tube. Occasionally it may be necessary to perform deeper suction, past the end of the tracheostomy tube – this should only be performed by experienced staff using their clinical judgement, who are aware of possible effects/complications it may have on the child.

6. To minimise the risk of trauma, apply suction only when the catheter is gently withdrawn. Do not rotate or 'twizzle' the suction catheter while suctioning and withdrawing. Day (2000) states: 'It is not necessary to rotate the catheter in the fingers as withdrawal takes place if the preferred multiple eyelet catheters are being used'. Do not apply suction for more than 10 seconds at a time, as prolonged suction can damage mucous membranes and cause hypoxia (NHS QIS 2007). New paediatric guidelines recommend to apply suction for no more than 5 seconds in infants, and less than 10 seconds in children, as there is an increased risk of hypoxia and atelectasis in neonates (Ireton 2007). Therefore local guidelines should be followed.

7. Observe the suction catheter for amount, colour and consistency of secretions, then dispose of suction catheter and glove appropriately.

8. Allow the child to recover from the suctioning procedure, and assess their respiratory status.

9. Repeat the procedure if necessary, using both a fresh suction catheter and glove.

10. To prevent a build-up of secretions in the suction tube, rinse the tubing. Apply a fresh suction catheter to the tubing to ensure that suction can be rapidly applied when necessary.

11. Ensure that the child is comfortable and able to continue with the activity they were involved with prior to suction.

OBSERVATIONS

If the secretions are particularly copious, which often occurs routinely when a child first wakes up after sleeping, unusually tenacious (thick), green in colour, bloodstained or have changed in any way, record this information in the nursing documentation and liaise with medical staff (a specimen may be required for laboratory investigations). This ensures that any evidence of infection or other problems are detected as early as possible. If tenacious secretions persist, then humidified air (or oxygen depending on their oxygen saturation level) may be required until the secretions return to their usual consistency.

CLEANING THE TRACHEOSTOMY SITE

This is a socially clean technique, usually performed once or twice a day. Tracheostomy stoma care aims to keep the area clean and dry, reducing the risk of skin irritation and infection (Laws-Chapman et al 2000). It also allows you the chance to check for any redness or chaffing of the flange against the skin which, depending on the consultant's advice, may require treatment.

FACTORS TO NOTE

● Cotton wool must not be used to clean around the stoma, due to the risk of inhalation of fibres (NHS QIS 2007).
● A dressing is not generally required around the stoma, but if it is indicated, do not use a gauze (or similar type) dressing due to the risk of inhalation of loose fibres (NHS QIS 2007).

EQUIPMENT

● Sterile gallipot
● Cleaning implements, such as swabs or long-handled applicators as available and recommended locally

- Cool boiled water, a sachet of 0.9% saline or Saliwipes (impregnated sterile swabs with 0.9% sodium chloride) as per local policy
- Non-sterile gloves
- Bag/bin for disposal of clinical waste.

METHOD

1. Wash your hands; wear a disposable apron.
2. Explain the procedure to the child and parent.
3. Empty the normal saline or cooled boiled water into the gallipot/open Saliwipe pack.
4. Put on non-sterile gloves as per local policy.
5. Dip the swab or end of long handled applicator into the solution or using Saliwipe, wipe in one direction underneath the flange of the tracheostomy tube. Then dispose of the applicator or Saliwipe.
6. Using a clean applicator or Saliwipe, repeat the procedure as many times as necessary, i.e. until the area is clean.
7. Finally, dry under the flange with swabs or applicators.
8. Dispose of all used equipment appropriately.

OBSERVATIONS

Observe the appearance of stoma, document in the care plan, and report to medical staff:

- Any offensive smell which may indicate an infection
- Any bleeding which may indicate an excessive growth of new skin around the stoma (granulation) (Fig. 30.6).

CHANGING THE TRACHEOSTOMY TUBE TAPE

Securing the tracheostomy tube is vital to prevent it becoming dislodged or removed altogether (Docherty & Bench 2002). There are several different techniques for securing the tracheostomy tube, the method described below is one that allows one member of staff or one parent to perform the procedure safely. Tape changing is performed at least once a day, and more frequently if the tapes become wet or soiled.

EQUIPMENT

- Two equal lengths of tracheostomy (linen) tape
- Pair of clean scissors
- Blanket to wrap child in
- Neck roll (e.g. rolled-up towel).

METHOD

1. To minimise anxiety and gain cooperation, explain the procedure to the child and parent.
2. Wash your hands.
3. It may be easier to see the tracheostomy if the child's head is extended slightly. To do this, place a rolled-up pillowcase or towel under the child's shoulders.
4. If the child is young or a baby, it may be useful to wrap them up in a blanket to keep their arms secure.
5. Thread a piece of tape through the flange on each side of the tracheostomy tube.

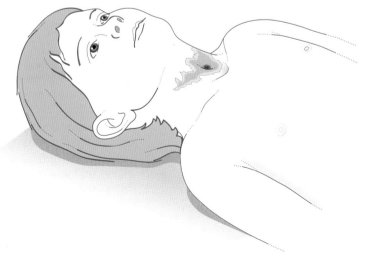

Figure 30.6 Excoriated skin with granulation.

6. To ensure that the tracheostomy tube does not fall out, *always* secure the new tapes by tying a reef knot (right over left and under, left over right and under) on one side of the neck before cutting the old tapes. Alternate the sides daily to prevent soreness. On young babies *never* fasten the tapes behind the neck, as this may become confused with the ties on a bib.

7. To ensure that the tapes are not too tight (which leads to sores) or too loose (which may allow the tube to fall out) check the tightness of the new tapes by inserting the tip of your little finger under the new tapes.

8. Carefully cut and remove the old tapes.

9. Remove the neck roll and ensure that the child is comfortable and able to continue with the activity that they were involved with prior to changing the tapes.

OBSERVATIONS

Observe, record and report immediately to medical staff any redness or excoriation around the child's neck.

Factors to note

- If the tracheostomy is new, the child's neck may be swollen, making it difficult to insert the clean tapes. This is made easier by wrapping a small amount of Sellotape around the end of the tracheostomy tape, like the ends of a shoelace (remove before securing).
- *Never* remove the old tapes before securing the new ones as the tracheostomy tube may fall out.
- The use of Velcro tapes on active children who are nursed on ward areas is not recommended. This is due to a lack of evidence regarding the security and safety of their use. However, children who have continuous supervision, i.e. on intensive care, may be suitable for Velcro tapes. Therefore, each child must be assessed individually, as to which tapes would be more suitable and safe (Wilson 2005).

CHANGING A TRACHEOSTOMY TUBE

It is advisable to change the tracheostomy tube routinely to prevent the gradual build up of secretions which can block the tube, rendering suction to be impossible and causing respiratory distress and requiring emergency tube change (Wilson

2005). Depending on the child and local policies a routine tube change may occur every couple of days or up to 28 days.

The first change of a tracheostomy tube is usually undertaken by the ENT consultant, senior registrars or competent nursing staff. However, in an emergency situation, a first tracheostomy tube change can be performed without the presence of specialist ENT staff, i.e. if the child is experiencing respiratory distress and suction has failed to clear the tube. Following the tube change, ENT medical staff must be informed. It is recommended that apart from in an emergency, a tube change should be avoided in newly formed tracheostomies for approximately 5 days to allow swelling to subside and the removal of the black stay sutures. If a new tube change needs to be performed as an emergency within the first 5 days, you can pull on these sutures to allow for traction on the opening in order to insert the tube (Bull 2002).

EQUIPMENT

- Water-based lubricant
- Sterile dressing towel
- Tracheostomy tube (appropriate size), tapes attached
- Tracheostomy tube one size smaller, tapes attached
- Scissors
- Hand towel or similar (used as a roll to extend the child's neck)
- Suction apparatus with the appropriate size of suction catheter connected
- Oxygen via a tracheostomy mask (may not be required in community setting)
- Non-sterile gloves and disposable apron.

METHOD

1. To ensure a safe procedure, prepare the correct equipment.
2. To minimise anxiety and gain cooperation, explain the procedure to the child and parent.
3. Wash your hands and put on non-sterile gloves and apron.
4. For tracheostomy tubes with inners, prior to starting the procedure ensure that the inner tube fits correctly inside the main tube, thus avoiding the need for a second tube change.
5. In order that the new tracheostomy tube can be secured immediately, insert the new tapes

into the flanges of the new tracheostomy tube prior to performing the tube change (Fig. 30.7).

6. To prevent trauma to the trachea, insert the introducer into the main tracheostomy tube and apply a small amount of water-based lubricant to the tip and place on the sterile towel.

7. To promote easy insertion of the tube, place a rolled towel under the child's head and ensure that the neck is extended and the child held securely.

8. Cut the old tapes, remove the old tube and immediately insert the new tube (Figs 30.8–30.12). *Immediately* remove the introducer as the airway is occluded while this is *in situ*. The child may cough following this procedure, so perform suction immediately and secure the tapes. If you are changing the tube in an emergency, after insertion, tie the tapes loosely before performing suction, then re-tie the tapes appropriately when the child's condition has improved.

9. Dispose of the used tracheostomy tube appropriately.

10. Observe the child carefully following the procedure for signs of respiratory distress. Oxygen therapy and suction may be required in an emergency or difficult tube change. Ask for a medical/surgical review if concerned.

OBSERVATIONS

Observe and report to medical staff any inflammation or excessive granulation around the site.

Factors to note

- If the tracheostomy tube is changed in an emergency situation (i.e. the tube has totally blocked), following this the child will need close monitoring, oxygen therapy and possibly require further suction until their condition stabilises.

- If the new tube is difficult to insert, i.e. the tracheostomy is newly formed, try a smaller size. Ensure that the appropriate ENT surgeon is informed immediately of the problem.

- For a routine tube change, plan to do this before a meal or feed, or at least 90 min after the last feed, to reduce the risk of inducing vomiting and aspiration (Tyco Healthcare 2004).

- To ensure the safety and well-being of the child, a person who is competent at caring for a child with a tracheostomy must accompany the child while away from the ward area, i.e. to X-ray, theatre, the playroom or schoolroom, etc.

- When the child is away from the ward area, they must have their safety equipment, and a suction unit (and portable oxygen if needed) with them at all times.

- If parents have received teaching on how to care for their child's tracheostomy and are deemed competent, they should be encouraged to take their child away from the ward unsupervised for short periods of time, if it is assessed safe to do so.

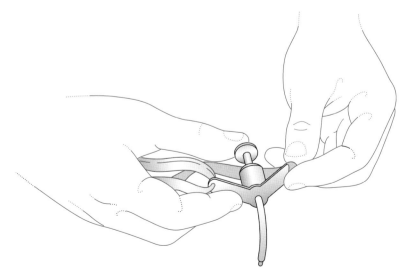

Figure 30.7 Tracheostomy tube is prepared for insertion: tapes are threaded and introducer is inserted.

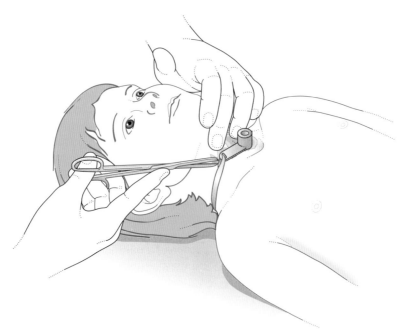

Figure 30.8 Existing tracheostomy tape is cut.

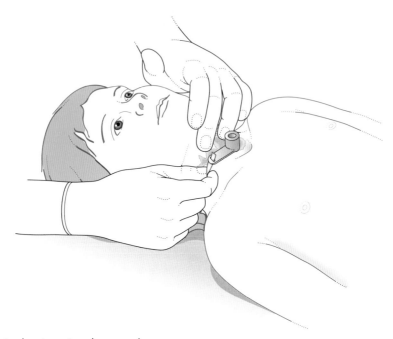

Figure 30.9 Existing tracheostomy tape is removed.

TIPS FOR DAY-TO-DAY LIFE

Multidisciplinary involvement in the child's care should include the speech and language therapist (SLT). The SLT team will advise on swallowing ability and communication. Speaking aids, such as a speaking valve can be used, to encourage vocalisation in children with tracheostomies.

● When bottle-feeding an infant, do not prop the bottle up or feed the child while they are lying down as liquid can enter the lungs via the

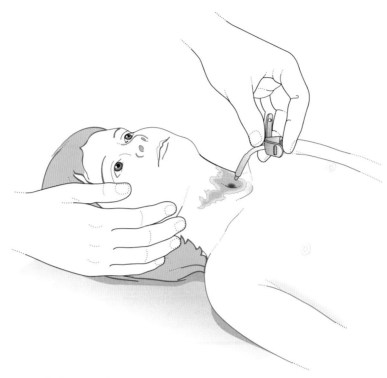

Figure 30.10 Tracheostomy tube is removed.

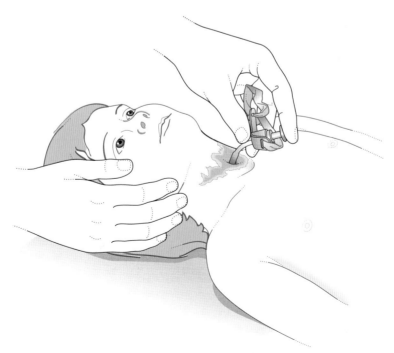

Figure 30.11 New tracheostomy tube is reinserted and introducer removed.

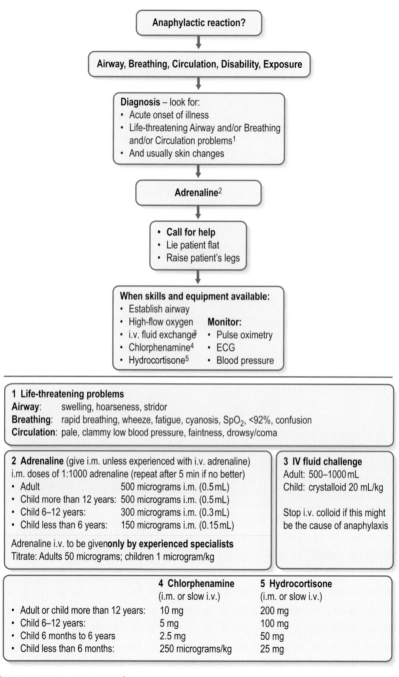

Figure 30.12 Tracheostomy tapes are secured.

tracheostomy tube. Hold the infant in a nearly upright position during feeding.

● Always prepare a shallow bath. Take care to prevent bath water from getting into the

tracheostomy tube because it goes directly into the lungs. For extra safety, attach an 'Artificial/Swedish nose' onto the tracheostomy, which will cover the end of the tube yet still allow active respiration.

- Do not use talcum powder on a child with a tracheostomy. The upper airway has been bypassed and this means that they lose the normal filtering mechanism of the nose and normal defences such as coughing (Griggs 1998). If talcum powder entered the tracheostomy it could cause the secretions to become thick and dry up, forming a plug, which could block the tracheostomy tube.
- Take care when placing children in car seats or bouncy chairs. You must make sure that they do not occlude the tracheostomy with their chin. If this is the case, the use of a thin neck roll placed over their shoulders should correct their position.
- If the child requires an inhaler, use an AeroChamber device, usually available from pharmacy. They work in exactly the same way as a volumatic device but connect neatly onto the tracheostomy tube.
- Likewise, if the child requires a nebuliser, use a standard nebuliser kit and replace the mask/mouthpiece with a tracheostomy mask (never connect the reservoir directly onto the tracheostomy tube as the vapour is unable to escape and will result in serious damage to the child's lungs).
- Should the child require oxygen therapy, there are several ways to achieve this. The use of oxygen via a Swedish nose is acceptable with a maximum flow rate of 2 L. Any dose higher than this would be required through a humidifying unit.

DECANNULATION

Decannulation is performed when the child no longer requires a tracheostomy, and will be able to maintain effective respiration via the nose and mouth. Prior to decannulation the child may have a bronchoscopy to assess the patency of the airway, and/or down sizing of the tracheostomy tube. When the child is assessed as ready for decannulation, the tracheostomy tube is occluded for 24 h, with close observation. If this is successful, then removal of the tracheostomy tube will take place and the stoma will be covered with an occlusive dressing. Careful observation of the child for signs of respiratory distress will be required for the first 24–48 h following decannulation (Carr 2007).

COMMUNITY PERSPECTIVE

It is essential that parents/carers of children with a tracheostomy have been fully trained in the necessary care and management of tracheostomies and assessed as competent in that care prior to planned discharge from hospital. The family and/or child will need to be able to take full responsibility for routine tracheostomy care. The specific details of tracheostomy care will depend on the child's individual needs, the type of tracheostomy device and the types of ancillary equipment being used. The CCN must be familiar with these variables before accepting a child for home care.

All children discharged home with a tracheostomy must have both a mains and a portable suction machine. A maintenance schedule must be agreed and cleaning instructions given. Responsibility for the supply of essential equipment such as tracheostomy tubes and suction catheters should be agreed before discharge.

Direct humidification, e.g. via an East Blower, should only be supported in the home at the direction of the referring paediatrician and then only if home conditions are appropriate and safe. Warm air delivered by a humidifier to a tracheostomy mask can be dangerous in the home environment as the child can suffer burns or scalds, or condensation can enter the tracheostomy tube. The hot humidifier containing boiling water is a danger to the child and others. The close supervision that is required if this equipment is to be used in the home may be impossible.

A sick child with a tracheostomy is likely to be extremely dependent and this can affect the freedom and mobility of the whole family. The CCN team, social care team and education (if appropriate), and local children's hospice (who will usually supplement statutory service provision) should be involved in the discharge planning. It is essential that a continuing care package is in place before discharge so that short breaks are provided in the home. It is very helpful for the child and family to have a weekend at home prior to the final discharge.

It is sensible to notify electrical and telephone companies in writing so that the home can be given priority for restoration of power in the event of a failure.

ACKNOWLEDGEMENTS

Thanks to the Tracheostomy Special Interest Group, and to Sarah Massey, Knowledge and Library Services Manager, Illingworth Library, at Sheffield Children's NHS Foundation Trust.

References

Akgul, S., Akyolcu, N., 2002. Effects of normal saline on endotracheal suctioning. Journal of Clinical Nursing. 11 (6), 826–830.

ALSG, 2005. Advanced paediatric life support – the practical approach, fourth ed. BMJ Publishing, London.

Bull, P.D., 2002. Diseases of the ear, nose and throat, ninth ed. Blackwell Science, Oxford.

Carr, M.M., 2007. Pediatric tracheotomy. Oper. Tech. Otolaryngol. 18, 127–133.

Clarke, L., 1995. A critical event in tracheostomy care. Br. J. Nurs. 4 (12), 676–681.

Day, T., 2000. Tracheal suctioning: when, why and how. Nurs. Times 96, 13–15.

Department of Health, 2007. High Impact Intervention No. 5 – Care bundle for ventilated patients (or tracheostomy where appropriate). Saving lives: reducing infection, delivering clean safe care. Online. Available: www.clean-safe-care. nhs.uk.

Docherty, B., Bench, S., 2002. Tracheostomy management for patients in general ward settings. Prof. Nurse 18 (2), 100–104.

Eber, E., Oberwaldner, B., 2006. Tracheostomy care in the hospital. Paediatr. Respir. Rev 7, 175–184.

Griggs, A., 1998. Tracheostomy: suctioning and humidification. Nurs. Stand. 13 (2), 49–56.

Harkin, H., Russell, C., 2001. Tracheostomy patient care. Nurs. Times 97 (25), 34–36.

Ireton, J., 2007. Tracheostomy suction: a protocol for practice. Paediatr. Nurs. 19 (10), 14–18.

Klockare, M., Dufva, A., Danielsson, A.M., et al., 2006. Comparison between direct humidification and nebulization of the respiratory tract at mechanical ventilation: distribution of saline solution studied by gamma camera. J. Clin. Nurs. 15 (3), 301–307.

Laws-Chapman, C., et al., 2000. Guidelines for the care of a patient with a tracheostomy tube. St Georges Healthcare NHS Trust and Sims Portex, Kent.

Neil, K., 2001. Normal saline instillation prior to endotracheal suction: a literature review. Nursing in Critical Care 6 (1), 34–39.

NHS QIS, 2007. Caring for the patient with a tracheostomy. Best Practice Statement. NHS Quality Improvement Scotland, Edinburgh.

NHS QIS, 2008. Children's Tracheostomy Project, Best Practice Statement (final draft). NHS Quality Improvement Scotland, Edinburgh.

O'Neal, P.V., et al., 2001. Level of dyspnoea experienced in mechanically ventilated adults with and without saline instillation prior to endotracheal suctioning. Intensive and Critical Care Nursing. 17 (6), 356–363.

Trachsel, D., Hammer, J., 2006. Indications for tracheostomy in children. Paediatr. Respir. Rev. 7, 162–168.

Tyco Healthcare, 2004. A parent's guide to paediatric tracheostomy home care, tracheostomy products. Tyco Healthcare Group Ltd, Basingstoke.

Wilson, M., 2005. Tracheostomy management. Paediatr. Nurs. 17 (3), 38–43.

Tracheostomy websites

Aaron's Tracheostomy Page: www. tracheostomy.com.

Breathing Easier, University of Chicago Children's Hospital: www.uchicagokidshospital.org/ specialities/pulmonary/patient-guides/breathing.

Care Card, Children's Mercy Hospital, Kansas: www. childrensmercy.org/content/ view.aspx?id=4362.

Stiftung NOAH Tracheostomy Care Guide: www.stiftungnoah.de/ downloads/ tracheostomy_care_guide_en.pdf.

The American Thoracic Society: www.thoracic.org.

Tracheostomy UK: www. tracheostomy-uk.com.

Tracheostomy, University of Michigan Health System: www. med.umich.edu/1libr/pa/ pa_tracheos_hhg.htm.

Support group

ACT – Action for Children with Tracheostomies
Lammas Cottage

Stathe
Bridgewater TA7 0JL
Tel/Fax: 01823 698398

Website: www.tracheostomy-uk.com
e-mail: support@actfortrachykids. com

Chapter 31

Traction

Kathy Gracey

CHAPTER CONTENTS

Introduction   299
   Learning outcomes   299
   Rationale   299
   Factors to note   300
   Equipment   300
   Guidelines   302

Application of traction   304
   Equipment   304
   Application of skin traction   304
   Nursing care of the child in traction   305
   Observations and complications   305
   Dos and don'ts   307

INTRODUCTION

Traction is a pulling force. In orthopaedics, traction therapy is used as a conservative intervention. It is used to reduce and maintain alignment of fractures, immobilise inflamed or injured joints, relieve pain, correct mild deformities and reduce muscle spasm. Skin traction was one of the first management techniques in orthopedics. Currently, skin traction is primarily used in managing trauma. Advantages include preventing further displacement of the fracture and maintaining or improving alignment so reduction of the fracture is easier when operated on (Anderson et al 1993, Harvey 1998, Needof et al 1993). In theory, this technique replicates the actions of the surgeon in reducing the fracture (Drapper & Scott 1998).

LEARNING OUTCOMES

By the end of this section you should be able to:

- Understand why traction is used
- Identify the different types of traction
- Recognise the methods of applying traction
- Care for a child on traction
- Recognise the common complications that may occur as a result of the use of traction.

RATIONALE

Traction, in all its many guises, is extensively used in orthopaedic practice, including paediatrics. Like many aspects of orthopaedic therapy, it does not remain constant and therefore requires a high degree of nursing input.

FACTORS TO NOTE

Effects of hospitalisation on the family

Traction is often indicated following trauma such as a road traffic accident. The parents often feel shocked, guilty or angry about the trauma and find the application of traction very stressful at an already difficult time. An emergency admission, however routine for nursing staff, or a planned admission, is a time of great stress for both the parents and child. It is essential that explanations of all that is happening and why are given to the child and parents. When appropriate, the child and parents should be encouraged to participate in care of the traction when they feel able to do so. It is important that they feel confident and happy with this and do not undertake it out of a sense of duty. Traction equipment can be daunting to a nurse unfamiliar in its use and may be very frightening to a parent. Traction is often used for prolonged periods of time. This can be disruptive to family life. Parents should feel welcomed onto the ward and be able to stay with their child if they wish, although this may be difficult if there are siblings at home.

EQUIPMENT

Traction equipment and terminology can be confusing and anxiety provoking to nurses who do not fully understand the components and how each attaches to the other. The type and method of traction used is indicated by the type and position of the fracture, the age of the child and the desired outcome. Other factors such as trauma, surgeon's preference and availability of equipment will also be considered. Nurses caring for patients on traction need a working knowledge of each of the various types of traction along with its rationale, correct set-up and maintenance. Folick et al (1994) recognise that there are many variations in practice, all of which fulfil the same purpose. What is essential is that a uniform approach is used once the traction is established. There are many types of traction and the names may vary from hospital to hospital. There may also be variations and alterations to accommodate individual needs.

Types of traction

Traction is either fixed or balanced:

- Fixed traction is achieved by exerting a pulling force on the point splinted between two fixed points
- Balanced traction exerts a pulling force on the part held between two mobile points, and works by using the patient's weight against the applied load.

Both skin and skeletal traction are used for children.

Skin traction

This is the first choice of treatment and involves applying adhesive strips of material to either side of the affected limb. The limb is then bandaged, taking care to leave the knee free. The skin traction kits include cords to allow a pull to be exerted on the strips, which is transmitted from the material and skin to the underlying tissues and bone. Only a moderate amount of pull can be exerted using weights and the bed end is then elevated.

Skeletal traction

This is used at the surgeon's preference if the alignment of the fracture is difficult to achieve and maintain and internal fixation is not possible. This involves the insertion of a sterile pin through an area of strong bone such as the femoral condyles, tibial tuberosity or calcaneum. This is performed under general anaesthetic using aseptic conditions. A metal stirrup is then attached to the pin ends and cord fastened to it. Weights are then attached to the stirrup and hang over a pulley; they are then left free hanging over the elevated bed end. Skeletal traction is also used following trauma, such as when the integrity of the skin is damaged and the application of skin traction would be difficult. Skeletal traction allows for easier access to wounds, dressings or any other injuries. It is now rarely used for children due to advances in orthopaedic surgical techniques in the management of complicated long bone fractures.

The following types of traction are most commonly used for children:

- Simple leg traction or Buck's extensions: used for pre- and postoperative positioning and immobilisation, best for inflammatory disorders such as irritable hip syndrome – this is either fixed or balanced, and is usually skin traction.
- Gallows or Bryant's traction: used in infants usually under 1 year of age for femoral fractures and preoperative positioning prior to hip surgery – this traction is always bilateral and is fixed (Fig. 31.1).
- Thomas splint traction: used for femoral fractures – this can be either skin or skeletal,

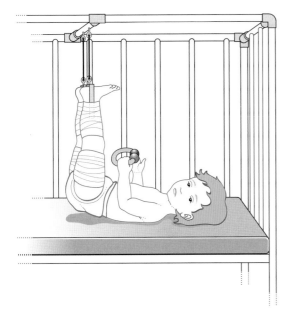

Figure 31.1 Gallows traction. This is fixed traction.

fixed or balanced. Now often used for femoral fractures splintage to allow swelling to subside prior to internal fixation of the fracture using the Nancy nailing system (Fig. 31.2).

- Slings and springs traction: often used for children with Perthes disease or other

hip conditions. Enables the child to have bed rest and the physiotherapist to teach and perform specific exercises of the hip and lower limbs.

The following forms of traction are now rarely used for children:

- Burns frame, Japanese frame or hoop traction: used in infants to correct congenital dislocation of the hip – fixed skin traction.
- Dunlop traction: used for contractures of the elbow and immobilisation of supracondylar fractures of the elbow – this can be skin or skeletal and is balanced (Fig. 31.3).
- 90–90 traction: used for displaced femoral fractures – balanced (Fig. 31.4).
- Pelvic traction: used for low back pain – fixed or balanced.
- Halter neck traction: used for torticollis, cervical injuries or disease processes – balanced (Fig. 31.5).
- Halo traction: used for cervical injuries – this is skeletal and fixed.
- Hamilton–Russell or modified Hamilton–Russell traction: used for immobilisation of fractured femur, postoperatively following hip surgery and for treatment of hip dislocation. It combines balanced traction with suspension – skin or skeletal (Fig. 31.6).

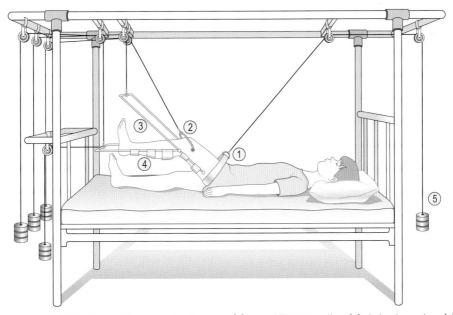

Figure 31.2 Thomas splint. The figure shows complex traction: (1) use of Thomas splint; (2) skeletal traction; (3) skin traction (below the knee); (4) Pearson knee piece; (5) counterbalance traction. This is balanced traction.

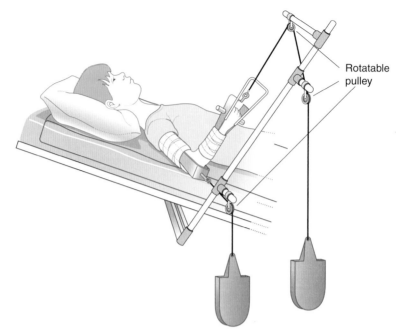

Figure 31.3 Dunlop traction. This is balanced traction.

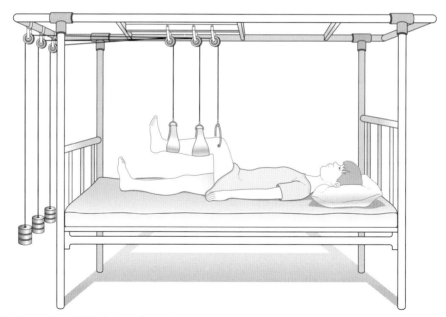

Figure 31.4 90–90 traction. This is balanced traction.

GUIDELINES

Developmental issues

Traction is used for all age groups from the new-born in gallows traction, to the adolescent on Thomas splint traction. It is an immobilising device and therefore restricts independence and the freedom to move. Consideration should be given to the environment and where these children are to be nursed.

Infants and young children should have their developmental needs met while in hospital. An

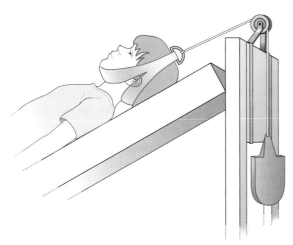

Figure 31.5 Halter neck traction. This is balanced traction.

open ward and the company of other children may provide a stimulating environment, but equal consideration must be given to parents who wish to be resident and will require a degree of privacy.

Young children often regress in their development, for example a child who is toilet trained may start to wet the bed. This can be upsetting for both the child and parent, but it is common and only temporary, so reassurance and support must be given.

Adolescents sometimes wish to be with their peer group, as they are often in for prolonged periods. However, some find it difficult to adjust to the loss of control over their environment and will prefer to be on their own.

All children and parents need to know what is expected of them; they need an explanation of the procedures and routine and they should be given choices (Houston 1996).

The multidisciplinary team

Children requiring traction have input from many members of the team during their stay in hospital.

Physiotherapists
Their role can be vital to the overall outcome of the traction. Their aim is to prevent complications of joint stiffness, muscle wasting and deformities by using exercises, which are taught and supervised. Early intervention is required to prevent complications arising and should be within 24 h of the application of traction.

Occupational therapists
If splints or slings are required as a result of complications such as foot drop or toe/finger deformities, the occupational therapist will assess the child's needs and organise the necessary equipment.

Play specialists
A child experiencing regressive behaviour may benefit from play therapy. Play specialists provide activities not only to prevent boredom but also to

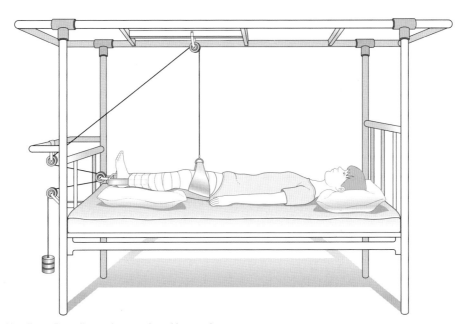

Figure 31.6 Hamilton–Russell traction – using skin traction.

support staff in carrying out painful procedures with the use of distraction therapy. Physiotherapy and exercise can often be disguised as play and can be quite imaginative and developmentally stimulating (see Ch. 10).

Ward-based schoolteacher

Traction is often a prolonged therapy and may cause long absences from school. Services for Children and Young People (DoH 1996) states: 'Your child has a right to receive suitable education while in hospital for a long time'. Liaison often takes place with the child's school to ensure continuity of education needs, and home education can be arranged if necessary.

Dietitian

The role of the dietitian is important as children on traction frequently have reduced appetite as a result of immobility and are subsequently more prone to constipation.

Parental participation

Once the traction has been established and is no longer daunting to the parents, they can often participate in their child's care. This is usually with the activities of daily living, but particular activities relating to the care of the traction, such as care of splints and greasing Thomas splint rings, can also be undertaken. Supervision of exercises as taught by the physiotherapists can be done by the parent and child together, although parents must be willing participants and must not feel that they have to undertake these roles.

When administering care, the nurse should be constantly thinking of ways to help the child care for themselves or assisting the nurse with the daily care of the traction system, e.g. helping to change bandages.

APPLICATION OF TRACTION

EQUIPMENT

For all skin traction

- Commercial skin traction kits, either adhesive or non-adhesive foam backed
- Bandages and securing tape
- Traction cord
- Traction beams and frames.

Other equipment that may be used for all traction

- Wooden blocks (for fixed traction, used to keep the heel off the bed)
- Weights and pulleys (for balanced traction)
- Balkan beams on four-poster frame
- Splints, e.g. Thomas splint
- Slings, e.g. foot and knee or halter neck
- Padding – gauze or cotton wool
- Monkey poles
- Polymer gel pads to prevent sore heels.

Equipment used specifically for skeletal traction

- Skeletal pins, e.g. Steinmann or Denham
- Stirrups, e.g. Bohler
- Knee piece, e.g. Pearson.

APPLICATION OF SKIN TRACTION

A full nursing assessment needs to have been completed prior to the application of traction to obtain baseline information upon which all plans of care are based (see Ch. 6).

1. Prepare the child and parent for the procedure with careful explanation of the plan of care.
2. Ensure that the child has had adequate analgesia prior to the procedure. Application of traction can be stressful and sedation may be required in addition to analgesia. Entonox (50% nitrous oxide and 50% oxygen) provides excellent pain relief for procedural pain (Pickup & Pagdin 2000). If manipulation of the fracture is required, a general anaesthetic will be given.
3. Maintain privacy.
4. Clean the skin prior to the application of traction.
5. Leave the ankle free. This allows for movement of the joint and prevents stiffness.
6. Bony prominences, especially of the malleoli and head of fibula, should be left free from pressure. Padding may be applied to these areas.
7. Strapping must be firm but not tight or constricting (Pritchard & David 1990) and must be applied wrinkle-free to prevent sores developing.
8. Two people are required to apply traction safely, one to do the application and one to support the affected limb.

9. If weights are to be used, pulleys and cord cut to the appropriate length will be required. The medical staff should indicate the amount of weight to be used. Too much can result in the child being pulled down the bed, and not enough will be ineffectual in providing any form of traction. When using weights, the bed end should be slightly elevated to provide some counter balance.

NURSING CARE OF THE CHILD IN TRACTION

Having applied the traction, the nursing care is then based on the care of the immobilised child, with additional factors implied by the traction.

Pain and discomfort

Once traction has been applied, the child is usually more comfortable. Pain needs to be assessed and analgesia given. One of the most common causes of discomfort is muscle spasm; this is resolved with antispasmodics but does settle after a short time on traction.

Positioning

Traction often demands the patient to be nursed in an unnatural position, such as lying flat, head down (e.g. gallows traction). This often affects the usual activities of daily living in the early stages but children quickly adapt.

Skin care

The skin on the injured limb needs to be checked at least daily. It is important to look for signs of allergic reaction to traction kits and adhesive tapes. Following trauma, damaged skin must be monitored and dressings applied as directed and necessary. Skin care also extends to washing and pressure area care as the child is immobile. Frequent change in position if possible, or relief of pressure on bony prominences such as sacrum, elbows and heels, is extremely important. Often the child will naturally move position and the use of a high-specification mattress, along with the use of a pressure-reducing device such as polymer gel pads, will reduce the risk of pressure sore development (Silverwood 2004).

When skeletal traction is in use, care of the pin sites is essential. The aim is to prevent infection which, if undetected or untreated, can develop into osteomyelitis. There may be variations in the care of pin sites; usually the dressings applied in theatre are left intact for the first 48 h, then a regime of daily cleaning with normal saline is established. The sites are then left exposed. Observe for redness and swelling or the presence of any exudate and report any changes to the medical staff.

Elimination

Changes in the child's usual bowel and bladder activities are common. Constipation frequently occurs owing to decreased gastrointestinal motility. A high-fibre diet and increased fluid intake can help. Bowel movements should be monitored. Urinary tract infections can also be an initial problem owing to awkward positioning and fear of using bedpans. Bed wetting due to regression in younger children is common.

Eating and drinking

This can be difficult because of the position of the patient, and reduced appetite can be expected. Frequent small meals should be encouraged and these can be in the form of milky drinks, or milk shakes, to promote high calcium intake. Fluid balance should be recorded.

Small children on gallows traction should always have their meal times supervised to prevent the dangers of choking.

OBSERVATIONS AND COMPLICATIONS

Trauma and constriction of a limb due to traction can cause disturbance to the circulatory system, the muscles and the nerve supply.

Neurovascular observations including colour, movement, sensation, pulse and pain should be recorded half-hourly for the first 4 h and then hourly for the first 24 h following the injury and at least 12 h following application of the traction. The orthopaedic team must be contacted immediately should any alterations in neurovascular observations occur.

The circulatory system

Circulatory problems are indicated by the change in colour of the injured limb, usually to a pale or blue colour, temperature change from warm to cool and the absence of a distal limb pulse.

The muscles

Damage to muscles can occur after injury or surgery to a limb. Muscle damage is known as acute compartment syndrome or Volkmann's ischaemic contracture. Early detection of damage to the muscle is critical as muscle, once infarcted, can never recover.

The signs and symptoms are:

- *Pain*: often disproportionate to the injury
- *Pallor*: a mottled, bluish or pale colour
- *Paraesthesia*: tingling or altered sensation
- *Paralysis*: inability to move the limb
- *Pulselessness*: absence of a distal pulse (Danby & Edwards 2003).

These are known as the five Ps. Not all symptoms are present at the same time. As with changes in the circulatory system, any change must be reported immediately.

Observation and monitoring of the above are undertaken for at least 24–48 h at a frequency of half- to 1-hourly intervals according to the child's condition.

Joints

Joint stiffness can result from bad positioning and inactivity. Passive and active exercise taught by the physiotherapist can prevent this. Excessive traction force or overdistraction (>2.5 cm (1 inch) of buttock off the mattress), especially in gallows traction, must be avoided as this can cause damage to infants' hips.

Nerves

Nerve damage is indicated by numbness, pins and needles or altered sensation. Prolonged nerve damage can cause foot drop.

Osteomyelitis

Infection of the bone is a potential but serious hazard of skeletal traction. Observation for signs of infection around pin sites and regular cleansing are necessary.

COMMUNITY PERSPECTIVE

In some areas, orthopaedic surgeons are in favour of children with femoral fractures or congenital hip dislocation being nursed at home on traction for part of the treatment (Clayton 1997, Orr et al 1994). A child nursed on gallows traction or with a Thomas splint can be considered for home traction.

Prior to discharge

The child should be well established on traction and fractures should be stable. Pain should be well controlled with oral analgesia.

Parents/carers must understand the principles of the traction, be familiar with the equipment and be able to recognise any problems. The suitability of the home to accommodate the equipment must be assessed by the CCN. This includes measuring the doorways to ensure that frames will go through and that there is sufficient room to negotiate round corners. A ground floor room will be most suitable as the child will feel more included in family life. It has to be accepted that some homes will be unsuitable for this type of home care and the family's hopes should not be raised unrealistically.

Parents need to be aware of whom to call in an emergency. If the CCN is able to provide 24-hour cover, this is not a problem. If this facility is not available, it may be necessary to involve ward staff (Clayton 1997) or have a re-admission policy organised which would need to include the ambulance service. The family should have access to a telephone. Liaison with the ambulance service will be necessary prior to discharge to prevent problems. Parents should be aware of the dates of their outpatient appointments and transport should be arranged.

Equipment to be supplied by the hospital

- Traction frame either specially adapted (Clayton 1997) or a hospital bed
- Weights and pulleys
- Supply of traction extension kits, cord, bandages and securing tape
- Tincture benzoin compound
- Pressure-relieving device may be necessary (see Ch. 23)
- Bedpan and urinal if required
- Incontinence aids if appropriate
- Hairwashing aids.

Following discharge

Initially, there should be daily visits by the CCN to check traction and pressure areas and ensure that the family are coping.

Strategies for relieving boredom can be suggested to the family. Work can be sent from school for the school-aged child. A home tutor may be arranged via the school education department.

All children will benefit from the involvement of a community play specialist if available.

Before the child returns to hospital for removal of the traction, the family will need information and reassurance concerning the child's mobility following the removal. They may also require information concerning physiotherapy. Children can be cared for with home traction most successfully, but there will need to be commitment from both family and professionals.

DOS AND DON'TS

- Do check the condition of equipment before assembly.
- Do size the patient correctly for traction to ensure comfort and maximum therapeutic outcome.
- Do ensure that traction pull is maintained at all times.
- Do check visible skin daily for signs of irritation or blistering.
- Do ensure that traction cords run in a straight line to aid smooth running in the pulleys.
- Do not allow traction cord to become knotted and frayed.
- Do not allow weights to rest on the floor – they must be free hanging.
- Do not bandage over the knee when the leg is in traction – the knee should be visible.

References

Anderson, G.H., Harper, W.M., Connolly, C.D., et al., 1993. Preoperative skin traction for fractures of the proximal femur. J. Bone Joint Surg. 75 (B), 794–796.

Clayton, M., 1997. Traction at home: the Doncaster approach. Paediatr. Nurs. 9 (2), 21–23.

Danby, D.J., Edwards, D.J., 2003. Essential orthopaedics and trauma, fourth ed. Churchill Livingstone, London.

DoH Department of Health, 1996. Services for children and young people. HMSO, London.

Drapper, P., Scott, F., 1998. Using traction. Nurs. Times 94 (12), 31–32.

Folick, M.A., Carina-Garcia, G., Birmingham, J.J., 1994. Traction: assessment and management. Mosby, London.

Houston, M.S., 1996. Care of the school-aged child in 90/90 traction. Orthop. Nurs. 15 (2), 57–64.

Needof, M., Radford, P., Langstaff, R., 1993. Preoperative traction for hip fractures in the elderly: a clinical trial. Injury 24 (5), 317–318.

Orr, D.J., Simpson, H.D., John, P.J., et al., 1994. Home traction in the management of femoral fractures in children. J. R. Coll. Surg. Edinb. 39 (5), 329–331.

Pickup, S., Pagdin, J., 2000. Procedural pain: Entonox can help. Paediatr. Nurs. 12 (10), 33–36.

Pritchard, A.P., David, J.A., 1990. The Royal Marsden manual of clinical procedures, second ed. Harper and Row, London.

Silverwood, B., 2004. Prevention of sore heels – evidence and outcomes. Paediatr. Nurs. 16 (4), 14–18.

Further reading

Apley, A.P., Solomon, L., 2003. Concise system of orthopaedics and fractures, third ed. Arnold, London.

Benson, M.K.D., Fixsen, J.A., MacNicol, M.F., et al. (Eds.), 2002. Children's orthopaedics and fractures. second ed. Churchill Livingstone, London, pp. 464–477.

Lee-Smith, J., Santy, J., Davis, P., et al., 2001. Pin site management. Toward a consensus: part 1. J. Orthop. Nurs. 5 (1), 37–42.

McGlone, R.G., Howes, M.C., Joshi, M., 2004. The Lancaster experience of 2.0 to 2.5 mg/kg intramuscular ketamine for paediatric sedation: 501 cases and analysis. Emerg. Med. J. 21, 290–295.

Nicol, D., 1995. Understanding the principles of traction. Nurs. Stand. 9 (46), 25–28.

RCN, 2002. Society of Orthopaedic and Trauma Nursing: traction working party 2002, traction update. Journal of Orthopaedic Nursing 6, 230–235.

RCN, 2003. Pinsite Care Project. Focus for research in orthopaedics group. RCN, London. Online. Available: www.man.ac.uk/rcn/ukwide/frogpinsite.htm.

Sponsella, P.D., Stevens, H.M., 1996. Handbook of paediatric orthopaedics. Little Brown, Boston.

Chapter **32**

Urine testing and urinary catheterisation

Jacqueline Winter

CHAPTER CONTENTS

Introduction   309
   Learning outcomes   309
   Rationale   309
   Factors to note   309

Urine testing   310
   Factors to note   310
   Equipment   310
   Method   311
   Observations and complications   311
   Dos and don'ts   311

Urethral catheterisation   311
   Factors to note   311
   Equipment   313
   Method   313
   Observations and complications   314
   Dos and don'ts   314

Catheter care   314
   Factors to note   314
   Equipment   315
   Method   315
   Observations and complications   315
   Dos and don'ts   315

Catheter removal   316
   Equipment   316
   Method   316

Bladder irrigation   316
   Factors to note   316
   Equipment   316
   Method   316

   Observations and complications   317
   Dos and don'ts   317

Suprapubic aspiration   317
   Factors to note   317
   Equipment   317
   Method   318
   Observations and complications   318
   Dos and don'ts   318

INTRODUCTION

Development of the urinary and renal systems starts around the third week of fetal development and continues until the fetus reaches a gestational age of 34 weeks (Tortora & Grabowski 2003). At 34 weeks' gestation, the urinary system is fully formed and the kidneys have their composite number of 1 million nephrons per kidney; however, these nephrons are immature and continue developing until around 12–18 months (Terrill 2002, Tortora & Grabowski 2003). The glomerulus of the fetal kidney will filter approximately 0.5 mL/min of filtrate prior to 34 weeks' gestation, increasing thereafter in a linear fashion with age to approximately 120 mL/min achieved during adolescence (Terrill 2002). In a healthy child, the volume and acidity of the urine and the concentration of solutes will vary according to the child's own metabolism. During pathological conditions, the composition of urine can change dramatically. An analysis of the chemical composition, the volume and the physical properties of the urine can tell us much about the metabolism of the child and the internal body environment (Poole 2002, Tortora & Grabowski 2003).

LEARNING OUTCOMES

By the end of this section you should be able to:
- Identify the normal constituents of urine
- Correctly use urine-testing equipment and recognise abnormal constituents in urine
- Prepare a child and parents for urethral catheterisation
- Select the appropriate size and type of urethral catheter
- Safely insert a urethral catheter, minimising trauma and distress
- Perform appropriate catheter care
- Understand the need for suprapubic aspiration of urine
- Provide comfort and support to child and parents during suprapubic aspiration understand the use of bladder irrigation
- Recognise the need for bladder irrigation
- Safely execute bladder irrigation.

RATIONALE

The examination of urine is the oldest clinical laboratory test. Performed either in the laboratory, or at ward level, urinalysis is one of the commonest clinical tests ordered and it can determine whether a child is dehydrated and/or infected, or has a renal or metabolic disorder (Liao & Churchill 2001, Poole 2002).

FACTORS TO NOTE

- Daily urinary output will vary with oral fluid intake, environmental temperature and the child's activity (Marshall 1995).
- Urine volume can also be influenced by blood pressure, diet, temperature and general health (Tortora & Grabowski 2003).
- Urinalysis is frequently performed both within the hospital and in the community.
- Urine is normally transparent and amber in colour with a variable odour.
- pH demonstrates the acidity or alkalinity of urine and consequently the pH of bodily fluids. Normal pH for urine is 4.0–8.0 (Fillingham & Douglas 2004). For accurate assessment pH measurement should be performed on fresh urine.
- Specific gravity is the concentration of urine and demonstrates hydration levels. Normal specific gravity should be between 1.003 and 1.030 (Simerville et al 2005).
- Traces of protein (> 200 mg/day), normally albumin and globulin, can be present, but are not detectable using strip reagent tests. This is normal and is insignificant (Marshall 1995, Cook 1996). Additionally, transient proteinuria may be seen in as many as 75% of febrile patients with little clinical significance (Liao & Churchill 2001).
- Minute traces of ketones and urobilinogen are normal in the urine; however, these are undetectable using strip reagent tests (Cook 1996). The diagnostic use of urobilinogen in urine is limited (Liao & Churchill 2001).
- A positive nitrate test indicates the presence of a significant number of bacteria in the urine (Poole 1999). The test is most sensitive when urine has been incubated in the bladder for approximately 4 h. Bayer multi-stix are commonly used.

- Leucocyte esterase is an enzyme present within white cells; therefore a positive test for leucocytes confirms the presence of white cells in an inflammatory response. This is quite possibly a UTI but it is not definitive as it is a generalised white cell inflammatory response (Simerville et al 2005). The presence of leucocytes and nitrites together are more reliable as a result indicative of UTI.
- A urine sample can be obtained from an infant, or child, in a number of ways including midstream specimen for children who are toilet trained and have urethral sphincter control. For those who are not toilet trained, a specimen can be obtained by clean-catch urine or obtaining the specimen using a sterile bag or absorbent pad (Ramage et al 1999, Farrell et al 2002, Poole 2002).
  - Midstream specimens are the method of choice in cooperative children who are toilet trained. This method ensures that the bacteria of the periurethral area do not contaminate the specimen by omitting to collect the first urine (Poole 2002).
  - Clean-catch technique has been identified as being an efficient method for collecting a sterile urine specimen (Ramage et al 1999). However, the method can be time consuming and technically difficult.
  - Bag specimens are obtained from attaching an adhesive sterile bag to the infant. Although an easy technique, there is a greater risk of bacterial contamination (Al-Orifi et al 2002).
  - Urine collection pads, launched in 1994, have been introduced widely within the NHS. This method is cheap and technically easy to use in infants; however, concern has been raised regarding the filtering effect of the pad fibres and reported high contamination rates (Farrell et al 2002, Poole 2002).
  - Suprapubic aspiration may be performed in emergency situations and will be addressed later in this section.
- The method used for urine sampling may be determined by the type of test that is being undertaken and may be considered as sterile or not sterile, e.g. a specimen for bacteriological analysis will mean that there should be minimal contamination and would be regarded as a sterile specimen, whereas one required for biochemical

analysis would not require a sterile specimen. In practice, however, bacteriological and biochemical tests are frequently done concurrently and therefore a sterile specimen would be obtained.

URINE TESTING

Urinalysis with reagent strips is a common routine examination seen both in the community and in hospital. It plays an important role in the diagnosis and screening of several diseases (Armstrong 2004). Urinalysis can also be used to monitor the progress of disease and in monitoring the efficacy of treatment. The reagent strips contain impregnated reagent areas and can test for one or more constituents when the reagent area comes into contact with the urine. Urinalysis with reagent strips is a cheap, reliable and simple non-invasive method of detecting and monitoring disease (Armstrong 2004).

The following practice guide refers to the testing of urine, using reagent strips, within the hospital or community setting.

FACTORS TO NOTE

- Urine examination can yield valuable information on the early signs of disease (Poole 2002, Armstrong 2004).
- Careful and accurate use of reagent strips for urine testing can prove to be cost-effective as this may help to reduce the number of sterile specimens that are analysed within the laboratory (Armstrong 2004). Reagent strips are also used within the laboratory setting. The use of an automated urine chemistry analyser has been shown to improve accuracy of urine testing (Rowell 1998).
- If urine is not to be tested within 1 h of being obtained, the specimen can be stored in a refrigerator until such time as it can be tested, when the specimen should be allowed to return to room temperature (Cook 1996).

EQUIPMENT

- Reagent strips
- Manufacturer's instruction for use
- Manufacturer's colour chart
- Urine container
- Stopwatch/watch with second hand

- Recording chart
- Non-sterile latex-free gloves
- Automated analyse (if available).

METHOD

1. Explain to both the child and parent the reason for the test and how the specimen is to be collected.
2. Obtain a sample of urine in a suitable container, which should be clean, dry and free from contaminants (Poole 2002).
3. Check the expiry date on the bottle of test strips; ensure that the test strips are not damp.
4. Read the instructions carefully.
5. Wearing non-sterile gloves, dip the reagent strip into the fresh urine specimen, ensuring that all reagent areas are covered. Remove immediately and tap the edge of the strip on the side of the urine container to remove excess urine.
6. Closely observe the reagent strip areas and compare with the manufacturer's colour charts at the stated times. If using an automated analyser, follow the manufacturer's instructions.
7. Record the findings on an appropriate recording chart and report any abnormalities.
8. Replace the cap on the container tightly and store as per manufacturer's instructions.

OBSERVATIONS AND COMPLICATIONS

- Preferably use a fresh urine sample.
- Urine which has been stored in the refrigerator should be returned to room temperature before testing.
- Check that the reagent strips are dry and have not exceeded their expiry dates.
- Ensure accurate timing by using a stopwatch or a watch with a second-hand. Inaccurate timing will give false results.
- Check the reagent area with the manufacturer's colour chart at the appropriate time.
- Always replace the lid of the bottle immediately after use, ensuring that it is tightly closed.

DOS AND DON'TS

- Do ensure that the reagent areas are fully covered with urine

- Do ensure accurate timing prior to comparing with the colour chart
- Do record results on the appropriate chart
- Do send a specimen of urine to the bacteriology laboratory if the specimen is foul smelling, cloudy, dark red/brown in colour. This may indicate infection.
- Do not use damp reagent strips.
- Do not cut the strips as this may alter their effectiveness.
- Do not check more than one urine specimen at a time.

URETHRAL CATHETERISATION

Urethral catheterisation is the insertion of a drainage tube into the bladder using aseptic technique for the purpose of evacuating or instilling fluid (NHS QIS 2004). Catheterisation has physical, mental and social implications beyond the drainage of urine. The promotion of best nursing practice in catheter care is integral to enhancing good patient care (Robinson 2001). Catheterisation can be intermittent or indwelling. Intermittent catheterisation is the preferred method for catheterisation when an indwelling catheter is not required (Niël-Weise & van den Broek 2005).

The following practice guide is focused on the catheterisation of the acutely ill child or the child requiring investigation. Adaptations to the practice may be made for intermittent catheterisation of the chronically ill child or the child with long-term urinary problems, as indicated below.

FACTORS TO NOTE

- The use of an indwelling urethral catheter is a safe and effective strategy to maintain bladder and renal health and contributes to improved outcomes (Griffiths & Fernandez 2005).
- Urethral catheterisation may be performed for acute urinary retention, characterised by a sudden inability to micturate or a failure to void 12 h after surgery, in addition to a palpable bladder (Choong & Emberton 2000). It is likely to be a result of a surgical procedure, drug related event or the use of spinal anaesthesia (Cropper et al 2003). Acute retention can also be secondary to constipation, spinal injury or urethral outflow obstruction. Past operative

urine monitoring – children who are critically unwell following injury, trauma or emergency surgery are likely to have a urethral catheter inserted to monitor fluid balance and assess specific gravity (to monitor hydration levels) (Willock & Jewkes 2000). Urinary catheters are also used to act as stents to the operated site, e.g. reimplantation of ureter and hypospadias repair. Urinary drainage allows wound healing, minimising infection, pain and discomfort. More complex surgery involved the positioning of urinary catheters which can remain *in situ* for several weeks, e.g. bladder augmentation and Mitrofanoff, where the bladder requires complete drainage during the healing process and the child often has both urethral and suprapubic catheter insertion to minimise post operative risk of bladder perforation. Catheterisation is also required for investigations, e.g. urodynamics and micturating cystogram.

- Intermittent catheterisation is the act of passing a catheter into the bladder in order to drain the urine and removing it immediately when the drainage has ceased (Getliffe & Dolman 2003). In children with spina bifida or spinal injury, intermittent catheterisation is used as a longer term form of bladder management for incomplete bladder emptying (Clanet & Brassat 2000, Getliffe & Dolman 2003). This is performed at home by parents and/or the child and is a clean procedure rather than aseptic. Where nursing staff perform the procedure, whether in the community or hospital setting, then the procedure should be aseptic to reduce the risk of infection (NHS QIS 2004).

- For intermittent catheterisation the genital area may be cleansed with soap and water and dried thoroughly.

- The use of anaesthetic lubricant is indicated in both boys and girls to protect the urethra from trauma. Increasingly, anaesthetic gels are being used for lubrication; this serves to make the procedure as pain free as possible and can reduce the incidence of infection due to such preparations being in sterile, ready to use packs (Gentry & Cope 2005).

- The advent of sterile, disposable, single use catheters has made intermittent catheterisation a safe procedure. Coated, low friction catheters are currently the market leaders. These catheters have a hydrophilic coating with very low friction when wet. Traumatisation of the urethral mucous membrane during catheterisation is thus minimised and these catheters are associated with a lower risk of haematuria, bacteriuria and urethral strictures than non-coated catheters (Hedlund et al 2001; Vapnek et al 2003; Stensballe et al 2005).

- Urinary catheters are deemed medical devices and health professionals have a responsibility to understand the consequences of using them, as outlined by the Medicines and Healthcare Products Regulatory Agency (MHRA 2001).

- Male and female members of staff who have been appropriately trained can catheterise male and female children. Patients have a right to be catheterised by someone of their own sex (Robinson 2004).

- The choice of catheter is important and based not only on the child's urethral size but also the reasons for use and whether or not the catheter is to be indwelling (Table 32.1) (EPIC 2001,

Table 32.1   Selecting an appropriate size-for-age urethral catheter

AGE OF CHILD	SIZE OF CATHETER	RATIONALE
New-born to 1 year	6–8 French Foley catheter	Small French Foley catheters are preferred for long-term drainage or where urinary debris is present. Catheters are manufactured using inert material, which reduces urethral discomfort
13 months to 13 years	6–8 French Foley catheter with 3 mL retention balloon	Preferred to feeding tube for prolonged drainage. Standard balloon sizes preferred over larger sizes, which increase bladder neck irritation and bladder spasm
13–18 years	8–14 French Foley catheter with 5 mL retention balloon	Smaller sizes promote comfort and adequate drainage

After Gray (1996).

Robinson 2001, 2004). Accurate assessment of the patient, along with evidence-based decision-making, record-keeping (time and date of insertion, type of catheter and any complications) should be made. Type and size of catheter are increasingly important aspects of care (Buckley 1999, EPIC 2001, NHS QIS 2004). Some clinical areas do not stock paediatric catheters and feeding tubes are sometimes used to catheterise children (Smith 2003). Inappropriate use of feeding tubes can result in knotting and harm to the patient (Faster et al 1992). Smith (2003) identifies this practice as persisting primarily as a result of suitable catheters not being available for their use. Smith urges that practitioners raise this with the manufacturers.

- There is little research evidence on the most appropriate catheter material for use in the paediatric patients (Smith 2003). Hydrogel coated and 100% silicone catheters are commonly used in practice (Bray & Sanders 2006). Latex-coated or latex catheters should not be used in patients who are at risk of latex allergy, this include children with chronic illness, especially those with neural tube defects and other urogenital abnormalities (Sapan et al 2002).

- Suprapubic catheterisation is increasingly being used as an alternative to urethral catheterisation (Addison & Mould 2000) and involves the insertion of a catheter directly into the bladder via an incision in the abdominal wall (Shah & Shah 1998). It is associated with many advantages including: no risk of urethral trauma, being more comfortable for wheelchair users and evidence of reduced infection. Initial suprapubic insertion in children is done under general anaesthetic (Robinson 2003). This may be used following bladder and ureteric surgery if there is a urethral problem (e.g. stricture) or if the child/family chooses this for long-term urinary management (Sanders 2001, NHS QIS 2004).

EQUIPMENT

- Sterile dressing pack
- Two pairs of sterile latex-free gloves
- Appropriate size of catheter
- Cleansing solution, e.g. sterile sodium chloride
- Lubrication anaesthetic gel
- Plastic apron

- Tape to secure
- Sterile water (for catheter balloon)
- Appropriate size of syringe for sterile water
- Urinary drainage bag.

METHOD

1. A careful explanation of the procedure and reasons for it being needed should be given to the child and parent.
2. The parent may be asked to comfort and support the child during the procedure.
3. The child may be sedated prior to catheter insertion. Sedation is prescribed by the medical staff.
4. Wash and dry your hands and put on a plastic apron.
5. Apply gloves and using sterile saline on gauze, clean the urethral meatus. There is no evidence to support cleansing the urethral meatus as a sterile procedure; it is recommended to use sterile saline on gauze (Bray & Sanders 2006).
6. Clean the trolley and lay out a sterile pack with equipment for catheterisation. Catheterisation is a sterile procedure and should be undertaken using a strict aseptic technique (NICE 2003).
7. Wash and dry your hands and put on sterile gloves.
8. Insert 2–3 mL (up to 10 mL for older children) of lidocaine local anaesthetic gel.
9. Allow 3–5 min for gel to have full effect.
10. Apply sterile lubrication to tip of catheter. Locate the urethral meatus and insert the catheter slowly. Continue inserting the catheter until urine drains.
11. When urine drains from the hub, insert the catheter at least a further 2 cm. This will prevent possible inflation of the balloon in the urethra and ensures correct placement (Bray & Sanders 2006).
12. Attach the syringe filled with sterile water to the channel hub on the catheter (sterile water prevents contaminations; saline must not be used as it can crystallise and cause harm to the patient on removal of the catheter).
13. The balloon should be slowly inflated with the recommended amount on the catheter. The guidance from the manufacturer is that the correct inflation must be adhered to, as over or

under inflation can cause uneven inflation causing the catheter tip to lie against the bladder wall resulting in irritation (Getliffe 2003).

14. If any resistance is felt during balloon inflation, stop the procedure and reposition the catheter. This prevents inflation of the balloon when not correctly in the bladder.
15. Attach a sterile drainage bag.
16. Gently pull back on catheter to ensure it is secure. This checks the location and prevents trauma.
17. Apply hydrocolloid dressing to the child's leg. This protects the skin against strong adhesive tapes.
18. Secure the catheter using appropriate tape. The catheter must be secure to prevent trauma.
19. Reassure the child and parent.
20. Document the make, type and batch number of the catheter used along with the water inserted and the time and place of catheter insertion.

OBSERVATIONS AND COMPLICATIONS

- An assistant to help with catheterisation is essential. Parents should *not* be used for this role.
- Assemble all equipment prior to going to the child and parent.
- Ensure that the anaesthetic gel has taken effect prior to inserting the catheter.
- Insert the catheter gently, using aseptic technique.
- Do not use excessive force to insert the catheter. Contact medical staff if any difficulty with insertion is experienced.
- Obtain a specimen of urine for bacteriology prior to attaching the drainage bag.
- Ensure that urine is flowing freely before insufflating the catheter balloon (if applicable) or securing the catheter (Belfield 1998).
- Ensure that there are no kinks in the tubing and that the drainage bag is properly positioned (see below).

DOS AND DON'TS

- Do ensure the catheter is secured in position.
- Do ensure that anaesthetic lubricant gel is used in both boys and girls.
- Do ensure that gloves are changed prior to insertion of the catheter.
- Do record the type/size of catheter and the amount of water in the balloon in the child's nursing documentation (Buckley 1999).
- Do ensure that a trusted chaperone is present to support a child who has been, or is suspected of having been, sexually abused.
- Do not use excessive amounts of lubricant jelly, as this may lead to infection (Willis 1995a).
- Do not use excessive force when advancing the catheter.
- Do not continue with the procedure if the child is extremely distressed.

CATHETER CARE

Urinary tract infections are one of the most commonly acquired hospital infections; the majority (80%) are associated with urinary catheters (Niël-Weise & van den Broek 2005, Parking & Keeley 2003). The risk of developing a catheter acquired infection increases with the period of catheterisation, with the highest risk factor associated with catheterisation lasting longer than 6 days, which increases the risk by seven-fold (Gentry & Cope 2005). Practice regarding catheterisation can often be ritualistic rather than evidence-based and it is important that nurses carrying out this procedure have received specific training and are competent practitioners.

FACTORS TO NOTE

- There are two main routes of bacterial infection in the catheterised child:
  - Periurethral: bacteria travelling between the urethral wall and the outside of the catheter
  - Intraluminal: bacteria travelling up the inside of the catheter lumen (Willis 1995b).
- Maintaining urethral meatus hygiene is of utmost importance in preventing periurethral infection. Maintaining meatal hygiene with soap and water is now thought to be sufficient (EPIC 2001). The use of antiseptic solutions is not recommended.
- Urinary pH has been recognised as being a contributory factor in catheter encrustation (Sanders 2001, Rigby 2004). An increase in urinary pH is thought to be the result

of bacterial infection, which causes an increase in bacterial colonisation of the catheter surface and subsequent encrustation (Getliffe 2002).

- Increasing fluid intake can aid in keeping indwelling catheters patent. The recommendations for children are 1500 mL/day over 5 years and up to 2000 mL for active teenagers (June Rodgers, director, PromoCon, Disabled Living, Manchester 2005, personal communication).

EQUIPMENT

- Catheter bag holder
- Alcohol wipes (for cleansing drainage port of catheter bag)
- Urine container
- Latex-free gloves and apron.

METHOD

1. Catheter care commences with the selection and insertion of the urethral catheter (see above).
2. Ensuring a closed system is important in reducing infection (NHS QIS 2004). However, all systems have points of entry for infection, normally at connection sites (Pomfret 2000).
3. Selection of drainage equipment is dictated by the reasons for catheterisation. Some drainage bags are designed for hourly or more frequent urinary volume measurement. Some are drainable, with others being totally closed.
4. Always ensure that the catheter drainage bag is kept below the level of the bladder. This ensures good drainage and prevents backflow of urine. Some bags may be fitted with a non-reflux valve; however, it is good practice to position the bag below bladder level to ensure that there is minimal chance of backflow.
5. Use an appropriate catheter bag hanger for suspending the bag. This should prevent contact of the bag with the floor (EPIC 2001).
6. When emptying the catheter bag, wear gloves and an apron. Clean the drainage tap with an alcohol wipe before and after emptying, and empty the urine into a clean container.
7. Urine drainage bags should be emptied frequently enough to maintain urine flow and

reflux (EPIC 2001). Drainage bags should not become more than two-thirds full before emptying (NHS QIS 2004).

8. Cleanse the urethral meatus with soap and water (Pomfret 2000). This can be performed during the child's normal bath-time routine (EPIC 2001).
9. Cleansing the urethra twice daily, morning and evening, is considered sufficient (Willis 1995b)
10. Cleanse:
    a. *For girls*: the labia majora, then the labia minora followed by the urethral meatus and down the catheter for approximately 3 cm. Dry the area.
    b. *For boys*: around the glans penis by retracting the foreskin, then cleanse from the urethral meatus down the catheter for approximately 3 cm. Dry and replace the foreskin over the glans penis. In young boys it is not desirable to retract the foreskin, as this may cause discomfort.
11. Always ensure that hands are washed before and after care.

OBSERVATIONS AND COMPLICATIONS

- Ensure that the catheter is secured with tape to the child's upper thigh. This will help prevent undue traction on the catheter.
- Use a catheter bag holder to ensure that the bag does not come into contact with the floor.
- Ensure that hands are washed before and after emptying the catheter bag. Gloves should also be worn.

DOS AND DON'TS

- Do involve parents.
- Do tape the catheter to the thigh to prevent undue traction.
- Do ensure that the urethral meatus is clear of debris.
- Do ensure that gloves are worn when cleaning the urethral meatus.
- Do keep the urine drainage bag below the level of the bladder.
- Do clean the drainage outlet before and after emptying.
- Do not allow the drainage bag to rest on the floor.
- Do not use a variety of different cleansing agents for cleansing the meatus.

CATHETER REMOVAL

As important as the insertion of the indwelling catheter, is the removal. Before catheter removal, the water in the catheter balloon has to be drained; the balloon will have expanded and stretched at inflation (Robinson 2003). At deflation, the balloon membrane collapses and deforms resulting in surface changes to the deflated balloon. These changes can form ridges and cuffing, all can cause discomfort to the patient on catheter removal and possible trauma of the urethra (Robinson 2003). Manual syringe aspiration is the most common method used to deflate catheter balloons.

EQUIPMENT

- Sterile pack
- Sterile saline
- 5–10 mL syringe
- Non-sterile gloves
- Plastic apron.

METHOD

1. A careful explanation of procedure and reasons for it being done should be given to the child and parent.
2. Prepare sterile equipment.
3. Wash and dry hands; put on sterile gloves.
4. Attach syringe to the inflation and deflation hub and gently draw back on syringe. The full quantity of original water may not be present. Osmosis causes the water in the balloon to decrease in volume over time.
5. When all the water has been withdrawn gently apply pressure to the catheter and pull in a smooth action away from the body.
6. If any resistance is felt reattach the syringe to the inflation and deflation hub and repeat the withdrawal technique.
7. When the catheter is removed, ensure that the child drinks adequate fluids and that pain relief is provided to aid the first passing of urine.

BLADDER IRRIGATION

Children with an indwelling urethral catheter may require bladder irrigation to relieve catheter blockage, the most common cause of which is encrustation of the catheter surface caused by mineral constituents of the urine (Winn 1996, Robinson 2004). In boys, following hypospadias repair, where a urethral catheter has been inserted to aid urinary drainage and/or act as a stent, blockage of the catheter may occur, necessitating bladder irrigation (Ellsworth et al 1999).

FACTORS TO NOTE

- Catheter blockage can be caused by bladder spasm, twisting of the tube or constipation (Simpson 2001). Each of these should be considered if a child's urinary catheter drainage diminished.
- Urine infection is known to increase the incidence of catheter blockage (Pomfret 2000).
- Urine infection produces alkaline urine, which encourages encrustations (Simpson 2001).
- Citric acid solutions may be used to dissolve crystals that have formed as a result of alkaline urine. Sodium chloride (0.9%) can be used to flush out bloody pus and mucus (NHS QIS 2004).
- Bladder washout does not prevent catheter-associated infection. Using antibiotic solutions for bladder instillations is not effective in treating catheter-associated infection.

EQUIPMENT

- Sterile dressing pack
- Sterile latex-free gloves
- Sterile solution for irrigation
- Syringe (catheter tipped if required)
- Drainage bag (if required)
- Sterile bowl for collecting returned fluid.

METHOD

1. Where possible, a closed system should be used, e.g. Urotainer system. However, it must be noted that performing a bladder irrigation will entail the opening of the closed system with the potential for introducing infection. Always follow the manufacturer's instructions when using these bladder irrigation solutions.
2. Explain to the child and parent the need for the bladder irrigation and what will happen.

3. This is an aseptic procedure and sterile equipment should be used.

4. Select an appropriate volume of bladder irrigation solution. The volume used will be dependent on the child's bladder capacity. Different volumes of solution in 'closed containers' are now available.

5. Wearing sterile gloves, clean the connection between the catheter and drainage bag (if used) with antiseptic solution, approximately 2.5 cm (1 inch) above and below the connection.

6. Disconnect the drainage bag from the catheter and attach the syringe/solution container.

7. Push the fluid into the catheter following the manufacturer's instructions. This will flush out the inside of the catheter.

8. Disconnect the syringe from the catheter and allow the fluid to drain into a sterile receptacle.

9. Repeat the procedure until the returned fluid flows freely.

10. Clean the insertion end of the catheter and attach a new drainage bag (if required).

11. Record the total amount of fluid used and returned.

OBSERVATIONS AND COMPLICATIONS

- Prepare equipment prior to collecting the child.
- Ensure that the solution has been warmed to room temperature prior to insertion.
- Ensure accurate recording of all fluid instilled and drained.
- Observe the returned fluid for clarity, blood or any particles.

DOS AND DON'TS

- Do ensure that the bladder irrigation fluid is at room temperature prior to insertion.
- Do use a closed system if available.
- Do record the volume of fluid instilled and returned.
- Do observe the returned fluid for clarity, blood and particles.
- Do not use excessive force to instil fluid.
- Do not apply negative pressure, using the syringe to drain the bladder.

SUPRAPUBIC ASPIRATION

Suprapubic aspiration of urine is performed by experienced medical staff to obtain a sterile specimen of urine for urinary investigation in infants and children <2 years old. This technique is used when the specimen is required urgently, dictated by the child's condition, normally when the child is unable to produce a specimen by the clean-catch technique. Suprapubic aspiration should be performed when the urinary bladder is known to contain urine; normally if the child has not passed urine for 1 h or the bladder is palpable above the symphysis pubis and is considered the best way to minimise bacterial contamination (Campbell & Glasper 1995, Jakobson & Esbjorner 1999).

FACTORS TO NOTE

- Suprapubic aspiration of urine is usually performed in young children who are not toilet trained, normally <2 years of age and who are very unwell – a specimen of urine being required to rule out urinary tract infection (Carter & Dearmum 1995).
- It is important that the child's bladder contains urine; therefore this procedure should only be performed if the child has not passed urine for at least 1 h.
- Although invasive, this method of specimen collection is the technique of choice in the sick febrile infant. The use of ultrasound assistance improves success rates in obtaining a urine sample (Ramage et al 1999).

EQUIPMENT

- Sterile dressing pack
- 70% alcohol
- Sterile latex-free gloves
- 5–10 mL syringe
- Size 20, 21 and 22 gauge needles
- Airstrip dressing
- Sterile urine container.

Cleanse around the glans penis by retracting the foreskin, then cleanse from the urethral meatus down the catheter for approximately 3 cm. Dry and replace the foreskin over the glans penis. In young boys, it is not desirable to retract the foreskin, as this may cause discomfort.

METHOD

1. Explain to the parent the need for the bladder aspiration.
2. The parent may wish to comfort the child during the procedure. This should be encouraged, however, the parents should not be coerced as they may find the aspiration distressing.
3. This is an aseptic procedure, therefore a sterile technique should be used.
4. The child should be in a supine position with legs in the frog-leg position and securely restrained to prevent undue movement.
5. The area above the child's symphysis pubis should be cleaned with 70% alcohol and allowed to dry.
6. A member of the medical staff will insert the needle into the bladder approximately 1 cm above the pubic bone at a 90° angle.
7. Urine is then aspirated from the bladder.
8. The needle is then withdrawn. Pressure should be applied to the insertion site for 1–2 min. A dry dressing, e.g. Airstrip, should be applied.

9. The urine should be put into an appropriate sterile urine container and sent for bacterial or biochemical analysis.

OBSERVATIONS AND COMPLICATIONS

- Ensure that the child is firmly held in the supine position during the procedure.
- Ensure that pressure is applied to the needle insertion site once the needle is removed. This helps to stem bleeding and leakage of urine.
- Advise parents that some fresh blood may be present in the urine for a short period following the procedure.
- Observe the child for signs of increasing abdominal pain, as bowel perforation during the procedure is possible.

DOS AND DON'TS

- Do ensure that the child is held firmly.
- Do observe the insertion site for signs of bleeding.
- Do observe nappies for haematuria.
- Do not perform the procedure if the child has voided urine within the previous hour.
- Do not coerce parents or carers into holding the child firmly.

References

Addison, R., Mould, L., 2000. Risk assessment in supra pubic catheterisation. Nurs. Stand. 14 (36), 43–46.

Al-Orifi, F., McGillivray, D., Tange, S., et al., 2002. Urine culture from bag specimens in young children: are the risks too high? J. Paediatr. 137 (2), 221–226.

Armstrong, K., 2004. Urinalysis. Pract. Nurse 27 (4), 25–30.

Belfield, P., 1998. Urinary catheters. Br. Med. J. 296 (6625), 836–837.

Bray, L., Sanders, C., 2006. Nursing management of paediatric urethral catheterisation. Nurs. Stand. 20 (24), 51–60.

Buckley, R., 1999. Keep it legal. Nurs. Times 95 (6), 75–166.

Campbell, S., Glasper, E.A. (Eds.), 1995. Whaley and Wong's children's nursing. Mosby, London.

Carter, B., Dearmum, A.K., 1995. Child health care nursing – concepts theory and practice. Blackwell Science, Oxford, UK.

Choong, S., Emberton, M., 2000. Acute urinary retention. Br. Int. J. Urol. 85 (2), 186–201.

Clanet, M.G., Brassat, D., 2000. The management of multiple sclerosis patients. Curr. Opin. Newrol. 13 (3), 263–270.

Cropper, J., Hutchison, L., Llewellyn, N., 2003. Post operative retention of urine in children. Paediatr. Nurs. 15 (7), 15–18.

Cook, R., 1996. Urinalysis: ensuring accurate urine testing. Nurs. Stand. 10 (46), 49–52.

Ellsworth, P., Cendron, M., Ritland, D., et al., 1999. Hydrospadias repair in the 90s. AORN J. 69 (1), 148–150 152–153, 155–156.

EPIC, 2001. Guidelines for preventing infections associated with the insertion and maintenance of short term indwelling urethral catheters in acute care. J. Hosp. Infect. 47 (Suppl), S239–S246.

Farrell, M., Devine, K., Lancaster, G., et al., 2002. A method comparison study to assess the reliability of urine collection pads as a means of obtaining urine specimens from non-toilet trained children for microbiological examination. J. Adv. Nurs. 37 (4), 387–393.

Fillingham, S., Douglas, J., 2004. Urological nursing. Ballière Tindall, London.

Foster, H., Ritchey, M., Bloom, D., 1992. Adventitious knots in urethral catheters: report of 5 cases. J. Urol. 148 (5), 1496–1498.

Gentry, H., Cope, S., 2005. Using silver to reduce catheter-associated urinary tract infections. Nurs. Stand. 19 (50), 51–54.

Getliffe, K., 2002. Managing recurrent urinary catheter encrustation. Br. J. Community Nurs. 7 (11), 574–580.

Getliffe, K., 2003. Catheters and catheterisation. In: Getliffe, K., Dolman, M. (Eds.), Promoting continence: a clinical and research source. Baillère Tindall, London.

Getliffe, K., Dolman, M. (Eds.), 2003. Promoting continence: a clinical and research source. Baillère Tindall, London.

Gray, M., 1996. Atraumatic urethral catheterisation of children. Pediatr. Nurs. 22 (4), 306–310.

Griffiths, R., Fernandez, R., 2005. Policies for the removal of short-term indwelling urethral catheters. Cochrane Database Syst. Rev. 1, CD004011.

Hedlund, H., Hjelmas, K., Jonsson, O., et al., 2001. Hydrophilic versus non-coated catheters for intermittent catheterisation. Scand. J. Urol. Nephrol. 35, 49–53.

Jakobson, B., Esbjorner, E., 1999. Minimum incidence and diagnostic rate of first urinary tract infection. Paediatrics 104 (2), 222–227.

Liao, J., Churchill, B., 2001. Paediatric urine testing. Pediatr. Clin. North Am. 48 (6), 1425–1440.

Marshall, W.J., 1995. Illustrated textbook of clinical chemistry, third ed. Lippincott Gower, London.

MHRA., 2001. Equipped to care: the safe use of medical devices in the 21st century. MHRA. London.

NICE., 2003. Infection control; prevention of healthcare – associated infection in Primary and community care. National Institute for Clinical Excellence, London.

Niël-Weise, B.S., van den Broek, P.J., 2005. Urinary catheter policies for short-term bladder drainage in adults. Cochrane Database Syst. Rev. 3, CD004203.

NHS, Q.I.S., 2004. Urinary catheterisation and catheter care. Best practice statement. NHS Quality Improvement Scotland, Edinburgh.

Parkin, J., Keeley, F.X., 2003. Indwelling catheter associated urinary tract infections. Br. J. Community Nurs. 8 (4), 166–170.

Pomfret, I., 1996. Catheters: design, selection and management. Br. J. Nurs. 5 (4), 245–251.

Pomfret, L., 2000. Catheter care in the community. Nurs. Stand. 14 (27), 46–51.

Poole, C., 1999. The use of urinary dipstix in children with high risk renal tracts. Br. J. Nurs. 8 (8), 512–516.

Poole, C., 2002. Diagnosis and management of urinary tract infection in children. Nurs. Stand. 16 (38), 47–55.

Ramage, I.J., Chapman, J.P., Hollman, A.S., 1999. Accuracy of clean-catch urine collection in infancy. J. Paediatr. 135 (6), 765–767.

Rigby, D., 2004. pH testing in catheter maintenance: the clinical debate. Br. J. Community Nurs. 9 (5), 189–194.

Robinson, J., 2001. Urethral catheter selection. Nurs. Stand. 15 (25), 39–42.

Robinson, J., 2003. Deflation of a Foley catheter balloon. Nurs. Stand. 17 (27), 33–38.

Robinson, J., 2004. A practical approach to catheter-associated problems. Nurs. Stand. 18 (31), 38–42.

Rowell, D.M., 1998. Evaluation of a urine chemistry analyser. Prof. Nurse 13 (8), 533–534.

Sapan, N., Nacarkucuk, E., Canitez, Y., Saglam, H., 2002. Evaluation of the need for routine pre-operative latex allergy tests in children. Pediatr. Int. 14 (2), 157–162.

Sanders, C., 2001. Suprapubic catheterisation risk management. Paediatr. Nurs. 13 (10), 14–18.

Shah, N., Shah, J., 1998. Percutaneous suprapubic catheterisation. Urol. News. 2 (5), 11–12.

Simerville, J.A., Maxted, W.C., Pahira, J.J., 2005. Urinalysis: a comprehensive review. Am. Fam. Physician 71 (6), 1153–1162.

Simpson, L., 2001. Indwelling urethral catheters. Nurs. Stand. 15 (46), 47–56.

Smith, L., 2003. Which Catheter? Criteria for selection of urinary catheters for children. Paediatr. Nurs. 15 (3), 14–18.

Stensballe, J., Looms, D., Nielsen, P.N., et al., 2005. Hydrophilic-coated catheters for intermittent catheterisation reduce urethral micro trauma: a prospective, randomised, participant-blinded, crossover study of three different types of catheters. Eur. Urol. 48, 978–983.

Terrill, B., 2002. Renal nursing: a guide to practice. Radcliffe Medical Press, Oxon.

Tortora, G.J., Grabowski, S.R., 2003. Principles of anatomy and physiology, tenth ed. Wiley, New York.

Vapnek, J.M., Maynard, F.M., Kim, J., 2003. A prospective randomised trial of the LoFric hydrophilic coated catheter versus conventional plastic catheter for clean intermittent catheterization. J. Urol. 169, 994–998.

Willis, J., 1995a. Intermittent catheters. Prof. Nurse 10 (8), 523–528.

Willis, J., 1995b. Catheters. Urinary tract infections. Nurs. Times 91 (35), 48–49.

Willock, J., Jewkes, F., 2000. Making sense of fluid balance in children. Paediatr. Nurs. 12 (7), 37–42.

Winn, C., 1996. Basing catheter care on research principles. Nurs. Stand. 10 (18), 38–40.

Chapter 33

Venepuncture and cannulation

Maureen Lilley

CHAPTER CONTENTS

Introduction   320
   Learning outcomes   320
   Rationale   321
   Factors to note   321

Venepuncture   322
   Equipment   322
   Method   322

Intravenous cannulation   323
   Equipment   323
   Method   323
   Observations and complications   324
   Care of *in situ* intravenous cannula   325
   Dos and don'ts   325

INTRODUCTION

Children may require blood sampling or the insertion of an intravenous cannula for many reasons, including the monitoring of the progress of a condition, the administration of medicine or the administration of fluids, blood or nutrition.

In the majority of circumstances, children's nurses are now undertaking venepuncture and cannulation as part of the holistic approach to patient care. Nurses undertaking extended practice must be appropriately trained and fit for purpose (RCN 2005, NMC 2008). However, nurses may also assist medical staff in this procedure by providing support to the child during the procedure.

LEARNING OUTCOMES

By the end of this section you should be able to:

- Demonstrate an awareness of the differences between arteries and veins
- Identify the common sites for venepuncture and intravenous cannulation
- Support the child during the procedure
- Choose the appropriate size of intravenous butterfly/cannula for the individual child (use the smallest gauge required for treatment)
- Safely perform venepuncture/intravenous cannulation if extending the scope of practice under supervision and as per local policy
- Apply the necessary precautions to prevent dislodgement of the needle/cannula
- Safely dispose of equipment used during the procedure.

RATIONALE

Obtaining access to the blood vessel of a child is a relatively common occurrence within paediatric practice. However, it should be borne in mind that obtaining a blood sample or insertion of an intravenous cannula is a traumatic and distressing event for the child and parents. The children's nurse plays an important role in performing this procedure with the necessary support and comfort to the child and/or parents but also provides expert assistance to any healthcare professional obtaining the blood sample or inserting the intravenous cannula. Firm support of the child will help to reduce the distress that they may be experiencing, bearing in mind the need to avoid excessive restraint (RCN 2003). More commonly, children's nurses, in a variety of settings, are extending their scope of professional practice to include such areas as venepuncture and intravenous cannulation.

Guidance from the Nursing and Midwifery Council (NMC) emphasises knowledge and skills as prerequisites for taking the responsibility for practice (NMC 2008).

FACTORS TO NOTE

- Intravenous access may be more difficult to obtain in young children owing to the size of their veins and the possibility of the veins being covered with subcutaneous fat, as well as because of their level of cooperation (Ingram & Lavery 2007).
- Both arteries and veins are composed of three layers or tunics and have a hollow core called the lumen (Tortora & Derrickson 2006).
- Arteries contain blood at higher pressure than within veins, with the blood moving within the artery in a pulsatile manner caused by the longitudinal arrangement of smooth muscle. Arterial blood is brighter in colour than venous blood.
- When an artery is punctured, the blood will leave in a pulsatile fashion. Greater quantities of blood can be lost from an artery; however, constriction of the walls of the artery helps to delay the escape of blood (Tortora & Derrickson 2006).
- Veins have less elastic tissue and smooth muscle than arteries; however, they contain more white fibrous tissue.

- Veins are distensible and adapt to changes in volume and pressure. Gentle squeezing of the area above a vein will cause the blood to pool within the vein and the vein to become palpable.
- Veins tend to be more superficial than arteries.
- The pressure of the blood within the vein is low and when the vein is punctured the blood will tend to flow out of the vein evenly.
- The venous anatomy differs in each individual child; hence a thorough assessment of all possible sites will help relieve distress by identifying the best site. Possible sites for intravenous cannulation and venepuncture are displayed in Figure 33.1. Care must be taken to avoid adjacent structures, e.g. arteries, nerves. The scalp vein should only be used as a last resort
- Accidental puncture of an artery may cause painful spasm and will result in prolonged bleeding.
- If the nerve is touched, severe pain may result.
- Venepuncture and intravenous cannulation are painful procedures. The use of local topical

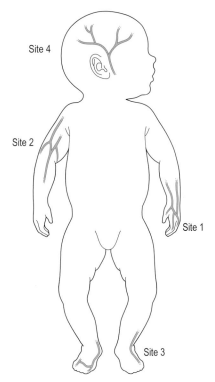

Figure 33.1 Common sites for venepuncture.

anaesthetic cream has been proven to reduce the pain of these procedures. EMLA (eutectic mixture of local anaesthetic) cream is one such cream that is universally used in children (Scales 2005, Tak & Bon 2006). In children < 6 months of age, the use of EMLA cream is contraindicated as the risk of methaemoglobinaemia is thought to be increased (RPS & BMA 2008) and therefore EMLA cream is only licensed in the UK for children aged ≥ 1 year. Tetracaine gel (Ametop) is another local anaesthetic and can be used in children/infants > 1 month old (Tak & Bon 2006, RPS & BMA 2008). Local topical anaesthetics should be applied as prescribed by medical practitioners or independent nurse prescribers.

- Methaemoglobinaemia is a condition wherein the haemoglobin of the blood has been altered to a form that cannot transport oxygen (Hockenberry & Wilson 2006).
- EMLA cream should be applied 1 h prior to the needle puncture; Ametop can be applied 30 min prior to procedure. A thick layer of cream/gel should be applied over the site and should be covered with an occlusive or semi-permeable dressing, e.g. Tegaderm (Scales 2005, Tak & Bon 2006).
- It is important to have a thorough examination of all sites to ensure that the best site is chosen. Distal sites should be used to preserve the proximal sites in case the initial attempts are unsuccessful (Hockenberry & Wilson 2006).
- Some hospitals/trusts employ phlebotomy technicians to perform venepuncture and cannulation. Healthcare assistants may also be trained to perform these tasks.
- Registered nurses should be fully conversant with the NMC Code of Standards of Conduct, Performance and Ethics (NMC 2008) if considering extending their scope of practice within this area.

VENEPUNCTURE

Venepuncture is the term used for the procedure of entering a vein with a needle, normally for the purposes of obtaining a blood sample for laboratory analysis.

EQUIPMENT

- Correct size of butterfly needle (smallest gauge required to obtain specimen)
- Tourniquet
- Gauze swabs or equivalent for spillage whilst sampling
- Syringe(s)
- Appropriate blood sampling bottle. This should be undertaken at the bedside after the sample is taken as this is the safest practice. Labels are not used
- Swabs of 2% chlorhexidine and 70% alcohol (DoH 2007)
- Non-sterile, latex-free gloves
- Cotton wool balls/gauze swabs
- Spot plasters.

METHOD

1. Explain the procedure to the child and parents prior to the venepuncture; obtain verbal consent.
2. Always examine all potential sites to ensure that the best vein is obtained. Ensure that this is explained to the child. Common sites used for venepuncture are the back of the hand, ante-cubital fossa and feet; however, the scalp may be used as a last resort (Fig. 33.1, site numbers 1–4).
3. Once sites have been identified, apply local topical anaesthetic, as prescribed, to the two most suitable sites for venepuncture and cover with a dressing.
4. Firmly hold the child's limb and provide tourniquet by gently squeezing the limb. Parents can support and hold the child, to reassure them, but should not be used to provide tourniquet. Always have someone to assist.
5. Wipe off the local topical anaesthetic.
6. Warming the child's limb will help the vein to dilate.
7. Palpate the vein to ascertain its calibre and direction. (Palpation – evaluate the vein by gently placing finger tips over the protruding vein.)
8. Wash hands prior to commencing the procedure.

9. The area should be cleaned with a 2% chlorhexidine and 70% alcohol swab (DoH 2007)

10. Allow it to dry.

11. Wearing non-sterile, latex-free gloves, insert the needle into the vein approximately 0.5–1 cm at a 30° angle.

12. Withdraw the appropriate amount of blood and instil into appropriate blood bottles. Paediatric vacuum systems are available for obtaining blood samples however may collapse small, fragile veins.

13. Once all samples have been obtained, release the tourniquet, place a cotton wool ball or gauze swab over the insertion site and withdraw the needle. Then apply pressure over the site for approximately 2–3 min.

14. Once bleeding has stopped, a dry dressing, e.g. Airstrip dressing, may be applied if the child does not have an allergy to this type of dressing.

15. Reassure the child and parents during the procedure and afterwards.

16. Dispose of waste and sharps as per local policy.

17. Most areas now give the child a bravery award following venepuncture. This may be a sticker, a badge or a certificate.

18. Document how much blood has been withdrawn (this is often relevant in neonates as well as when frequent blood sampling is required).

INTRAVENOUS CANNULATION

Peripheral intravenous cannulation is required when a child is to receive intravenous fluid therapy or intravenous medication. An intravenous cannula consists of a plastic catheter, which is inserted with the aid of a stylet or needle placed in the lumen of the catheter with the sharp point protruding from the end.

EQUIPMENT

- Correct size of intravenous cannula (smallest gauge required for treatment)
- Tourniquet
- Gauze swabs or soft paper for spillages whilst cannulating

- T-piece or equivalent, primed with heparin sodium (Hepsal) or 0.9% sodium chloride
- Tape to secure cannula: this should be a sterile transparent dressing (DoH 2007) for intravenous use, e.g. i.v. 3000
- Bandage
- Splint for limb/cover for cannula site (if sited in scalp)
- Swabs soaked in 2% chlorhexidine in 70% alcohol
- Latex-free gloves
- Hepsal to flush inserted cannula
- Intravenous administration set if fluids required
- Fluids or drugs as per drug prescription sheet
- Appropriate drug prescription sheet (as per hospital policy)
- Syringes if blood sampling
- Appropriate blood-sampling bottles correctly labelled at the patient's bedside after the blood sample has been obtained.

METHOD

1. Examine potential cannulation sites thoroughly. Apply local topical anaesthetic as prescribed.

2. As a last resort, the scalp vein can be used, however consent should be obtained from the parents for the shaving of the section of head.

3. Select the appropriate size of intravenous cannula (smallest gauge required to facilitate treatment).

4. Cut tape to desired length.

5. Gently hold/support the child in a supine position if possible, bearing in mind the need to avoid excessive restraint (RCN 2003). Ensure an assistant is available. Parents can assist in supporting their child and providing reassurance during the cannulation, if they feel able to do so.

6. Wipe off topical anaesthetic and clean the site with a 2% chlorhexidine and 70% alcohol-impregnated swab. Allow to dry (30 s).

7. Apply tourniquet to aid identification of the best vein for cannulation, enure some one is available to assist.

8. Insert the cannula at a 15–30° angle, advance the catheter and withdraw the stylet needle. A flash-back of blood should be seen before advancing the catheter.
9. Securely tape the cannula in place (Fig. 33.2).
10. Flush the cannula as per local policy to maintain patency.
11. Immobilise the limb using a suitable splint, which immobilises the joint close to the site of insertion, hence preventing excessive movement (Fig. 33.3).

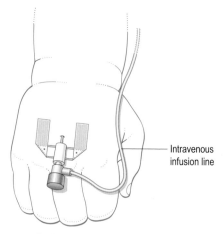

Figure 33.2 Taping of an intravenous cannula to secure its position.

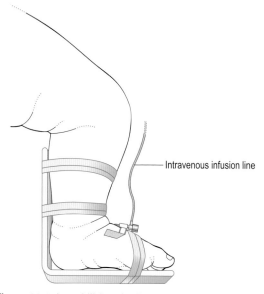

Figure 33.3 Immobilising the limb using a suitable splint.

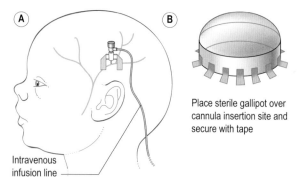

Place sterile gallipot over cannula insertion site and secure with tape

Intravenous infusion line

Figure 33.4 (A,B) Protecting the scalp cannula.

12. Protect a scalp cannula using a gallipot (Fig. 33.4).
13. Attach an intravenous fluid administration set to the cannula if it is to be used for intravenous therapy.
14. Apply a sterile device (either a white bung or ideally a needle-free system especially) if the cannula is to be used for intravenous medication.
15. Dispose of waste and sharps as per local policy.
16. Document date, time, size of cannula and where cannula sited in the patients health records.

OBSERVATIONS AND COMPLICATIONS

- Ensure that blood flows freely and that there is no swelling at the insertion site.
- Blood spurting into the syringe may indicate puncture of an artery. If this occurs, remove the needle and apply firm pressure for 5 min.
- Extreme pain may indicate nerve involvement.
- If either of the two aforementioned complications arises, immediately remove the needle, allow the child to rest and then try again.
- Failure to ensure a free flow of blood may result in haemolysis and an inaccurate biochemical result.
- Using a needle that is too small may lead to haemolysis.
- Intravenous cannulae should be secured with tape or dressings; however, approximately 1–2 cm above and below the insertion site should be clearly visible to allow for close observation.

- Splints should be used on limbs with an intravenous cannula sited, the aim being to immobilise the limb and prevent the cannula from becoming dislodged. These again should be secured in place by surgical tape and bandaged. Approximately 1–2 cm above and below the insertion site should be clearly visible to allow for close observation.
- Poor application of pressure following removal of the needle may result in bruising and swelling around the site.

CARE OF *IN SITU* INTRAVENOUS CANNULA

On a daily basis:

- Check patency of cannula by flushing as per local policy
- Check cannula is secured and remains in position
- Check site for redness, swelling, inflammation and pain as per local policy
- Record all checks in patient documentation.

The cannula should be changed on a weekly basis. High Impact Interventions (DoH 2007) states that cannula should be re-sited every 72 h, however, in children this may be extended but the reasons why needs to be documented.

COMMUNITY PERSPECTIVE

Children's community nurses (CCNs) trained in the techniques of venepuncture and cannulation may be able to save families out-patient visits by undertaking these procedures in the home and the procedure becomes less of an issue for the child. However, in practice, the necessity for the procedure may arise so infrequently that the CCN may need to consider whether they are having sufficient practice to retain the necessary skills.

Some areas may use Ametop, which is an alternative to EMLA and can be used on full-term babies from the age of 1 month. The CCN may carry sharps bins, although children having care requiring regular use of sharps may keep these in the home. Local collection for disposal can be arranged.

DOS AND DON'TS

- Do involve parents in the support of their child.
- Do ascertain the child's previous experience of venepuncture/cannulation.
- Do ensure that all possible sites for use are thoroughly examined.
- Do palpate the vessel to identify its position.
- Do ensure that local topical anaesthetic (EMLA or Ametop) is used, if the child wishes, to help prevent pain.
- Do ensure that the child has had an explanation of the procedure and obtain verbal consent.
- Do use the play therapist/leader if available to help with explanation and assist with distraction.
- Do ensure that the child is firmly yet gently supported. An experienced assistant will help ensure a successful procedure.
- Do apply sterile tape or sterile dressing to secure intravenous cannulae. The dressings should keep the site dry and prevent contamination. Dressings with a high water permeability should be used (Hockenberry & Wilson 2006).
- Do not coerce parents into being present. Some parents may not wish to be present or may feel anxious and scared, which will heighten the child's anxiety.
- Do not ask the parents to restrain their child. They should be providing support and reassurance. However, some parents may wish to help restrain their child.
- Do not tell the child that it will not hurt.
- Do not use EMLA cream on children <1 year old.
- Do not use fragile, inflamed or fibrosed veins.
- Do not use sites that may interfere with a child's normal activity, e.g. do not use the right hand of a right-handed child; avoid the feet of an active toddler if possible.
- Do not use wooden tongue depressors as splints.
- Do not use non-sterile tape to cover the insertion site of an intravenous cannula as this may contaminate the site. (This does not usually happen in practice where either Transpore or zinc oxide tape is used most commonly.)
- Do not use adult vacuum systems for venepuncture, as these are often not suitable and may cause the vein to collapse.

References

Royal Pharmaceutical Society of Great Britain and British Medical Association, 2008. British National Formulary, fifty sixth ed. Pharmaceutical Press, London.

DoH, 2007. High impact intervention. 2. Peripheral intravenous care bundle. Department of Health, London.

Hockenberry, M.J., Wilson, D., 2006. Wong's nursing care of infants and children, eighth ed. Mosby, St Louis.

Ingram, P., Lavery, I., 2007. Peripheral intravenous cannulation: safe insertion and removal technique. Nurs. Stand. 22 (1), 44–48.

Nursing and Midwifery Council, 2008. The Code: Standards of conduct, performance and ethics for nurses and midwifes. NMC, London.

RCN, 2003. Restraining, holding still and containing children and young people: guidance for nursing staff. RCN, London.

RCN, 2005. Competencies: an education and training framework for capillary blood sampling and venepuncture in children and young people. RCN, London.

Scales, K., 2005. Vascular access: a guide to peripheral venous cannulation. Nurs. Stand. 19 (49), 48–52.

Tak, J.H., Bon, W.H., 2006. Pain- and distress-reducing interventions for venepuncture in children. Child Care Health Dev. 32 (3), 257–268.

Tortora, G.J., Derrickson, B., 2006. Principles of anatomy and physiology, eleventh ed. Wiley, New York.

Further reading

Collins, M., Phillips, S., Dougherty, L., 2006. A structured learning programme for venepuncture and cannulation. Nurs. Stand. 20 (26), 34–40.

Fitzsimmons, R., 2001. Intravenous cannulation. Paediatr. Nurs. 13 (3), 21–23.

Glasper, A., Aylott, A., Prudhoe, G., 2007. Fundamental aspects of children's and young people's nursing procedures. MA Healthcare Ltd, London.

Lavery, I., Ingram, P., 2006. Prevention of infection in peripheral intravenous devises. Nurs. Stand. 20 (49), 49–56.

Moules, T., Ramsay, J., 2008. The textbook of children's and young people's nursing, second ed. Blackwell Publishing, Oxford.

SECTION 4

Infection control and prevention

SECTION CONTENTS

34. Aseptic non-touch technique   329

35. Isolation nursing   337

36. Specimen collection   344

37. Wound care   354

Chapter 34

Aseptic non-touch technique

Stephen Rowley, Simon Clare

CHAPTER CONTENTS

Introduction   329
   Learning outcomes   329
   Rationale   330
   Factors to note   330

Evidence: important components of ANTT   331
   Hand washing   331
   Gloves: should they be worn and what
   type?   332
   Environmental/air contamination   332
   Aseptic fields   332
   Risk assessment and equipment   333
   Observations and complications   334
   Dos and don'ts   335

INTRODUCTION

Every year it is estimated that as many as 5000 patients die unnecessarily in the UK as a direct result of healthcare associated infection (HCAI), and as many as 15 000 may die as an indirect result of infections they acquired from healthcare settings (National Audit Office 2000). Many of these infections are due to poor aseptic technique. Aseptic non-touch technique (ANTT) is an evidence-based aseptic technique, based on a theoretical framework and growing evidence base (Fig. 34.1). The principles of ANTT are applicable to all clinical procedures, such as wound dressing, catheterisation and intravenous (i.v.) therapy. Intravenous therapies are particularly important, as they are among the most commonly performed aseptic procedures in hospitals today and often provide the most direct infection risk to the patient. The principals of ANTT are increasingly acknowledged as the basis of good aseptic practice and as part of Department of Health (DoH) guidance for the prevention of HCAI (DoH epic2 2007).

LEARNING OUTCOMES

By the end of this section you should be able to:

- Understand the principles of achieving asepsis
- Apply the principles of the non-touch technique to any particular aseptic procedure
- Understand why it is important to use the correct and thus achievable terminology when referring to aseptic techniques.

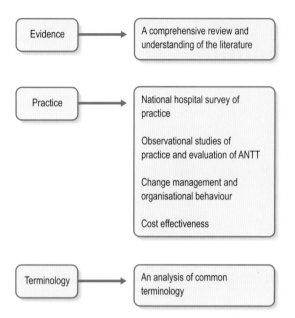

Figure 34.1 Theoretical framework (Rowley 2001).

RATIONALE

What is ANTT?

ANTT is based upon a series of peer reviewed clinical practice guidelines for the most common aseptic procedures. There are two main components to ANTT: the evidence underpinning the techniques used in the guideline and the processes involved in ensuring staff actually comply with it. This chapter is primarily concerned with the former. The latter, standard implementation process, is however very important to those concerned with implementing ANTT into clinical teams, and involves standardised assessment, audit, education and training. By following this approach, aseptic practice can be more easily standardised. Standardised practice is key, as it facilitates quality assurance and smoother skills acquisition. In addition, and significantly, ANTT becomes instantly recognisable to other staff and patients; which, in turn helps maintain compliance as well as providing greater reassurance to patients and families. ANTT dispenses with much of the mythology of the aseptic technique and provides straightforward clear guidance that has been tested in the clinical setting.

Why does ANTT work?

The easy-to-follow clinical guideline approach helps provide a simple and effective tool which signposts best practice, helping to establish safe, standardised aseptic technique.

First, staff are taught to identify and protect the key parts of any procedure, perform effective hand washing, institute a non-touch technique, wear only appropriate and necessary protective equipment (COSHH 2002), and use the most applicable infective precautions; implementing these actions in a logical order. Second, by introducing ANTT as an audit cycle using quality resources, staff are trained and retrained on an ongoing basis. In typical ward-based teams, these two approaches combined with patient involvement have the added value of creating a degree of peer pressure, which further helps promote standardised practice.

Terms used

Infective precautions
Equipment used to help maintain asepsis, e.g. gloves, aseptic towels, aprons, etc.

Key parts/key sites
Those parts or sites that if contaminated by infectious material increase the risk of infection.

In i.v. therapy, key parts are usually parts of equipment that come into direct or indirect contact with the liquid infusion.

Aseptic non-touch technique (ANTT)
An aseptic technique that helps to prevent direct and indirect contamination of key parts and key sites, by a non-touch method and by other appropriate infective precautions (Rowley 2001).

FACTORS TO NOTE

Correct use of terminology

Other terms, such as 'sterile' and 'clean technique', are often used inaccurately and can confuse practitioners (Box 34.1).

Equity in intravenous care

In intravenous therapy, ANTT should be used for both central and peripheral line care (see Ch. 41).

Healthy, sick and handicapped children

The definition or principles of the aseptic non-touch technique are not dependent on the diagnosis of the child. The principles of ANTT should

---

BOX 34.1 **Terminology should accurately reflect practice**

Sterile techniques – are not achievable

The word sterile means 'free from microorganisms' (Weller 1993). Therefore, due to the natural multitude of microorganisms in the atmosphere it is not possible to achieve a true sterile technique for procedures in typical ward/home environments.

Aseptic techniques – are achievable

For infections to occur in the bloodstream (in i.v. therapy) or local sites (in wound care, etc.), key parts or sites must be contaminated by a sufficient number of virulent, pathogenic organisms (Hendrick 1988). Therefore, a technique that prevents this level of contamination is safe. Such a technique is most accurately termed an 'aseptic technique', as the word asepsis means 'freedom from infection or infectious (pathogenic) material' (Weller 1993).

Non-touch techniques – are paramount

Pathogenic organisms cannot always be removed by effective hand washing (Church 1986). Additionally, hand washing is not always effective (Mallett & Dougherty 2000). Therefore, a non-touch technique is perhaps the single most important component in achieving asepsis.

---

always remain constant, although the infective precautions may change depending on the type of procedure and the technical difficulty involved in maintaining asepsis. According to Jones (1987), an ideal aseptic technique for intravenous catheter care is one that is safe and effective, yet requires a minimal amount of time and equipment. Choosing appropriate infective precautions for any particular procedure is achieved by an effective assessment of 'risk'. If the nurse considers that asepsis of key parts/sites cannot be maintained by a non-touch method, further steps must be taken to minimise the risk of contamination. This might entail the use of extra precautions such as forceps or sterile gloves.

A review of the literature indicated that aseptic techniques have evolved more from anecdotal evidence and ritualistic practice than from empirical research. In addition, the principles of aseptic technique require reappraising in nursing practice (Lund & Caruso 1993). These two factors underpin the theoretical framework of ANTT and emphasise the need for its simple, pragmatic and robust research base.

EVIDENCE: IMPORTANT COMPONENTS OF ANTT

HAND WASHING

Hand washing is the most important and central component of ANTT (NPSA website: www.npsa. nhs.uk). On each square centimetre of the skin, there may be as many as 3 million bacteria (Gould 1991a) and new research suggests that as many as 182 species of bacteria are present on the skin (Gao 2007). Some are normal or resident skin flora and some are transient organisms that can be carried on the skin for weeks or months (Gould 1991a). Studies have demonstrated the ability of pathogenic organisms to survive and breed on the hands of healthcare workers (Adams & Marrie 1982, Bauer et al 1990). Effective hand washing can significantly decrease bacterial counts (Leonard 1986, Rossoff et al 1995, Pittet et al 1999, 2000, Girou et al 2002, Lucet et al 2002). Effective hand hygiene and washing is as important both before and after glove use when bacterial counts will have rapidly risen (increased) in the warm humid environment created under gloves (Larson 1989, Gould 1991a, Pittet et al 1999, Pratt 2007, CDC 2002). Stringer et al (1991) found that failure to wash hands after the removal of gloves was one of the most common breakdowns in universal precautions. Further information on hand washing can be found in Chapter 4.

Hand cleansing has been identified as the single most significant procedure in preventing cross-infection (Maki et al 1973, Thomlinson 1990, Gould 1991a, Girou et al 2002, Cochrane 2003); however, paradoxically, despite these widely known facts, healthcare workers continue to exhibit poor compliance with effective hand cleansing practices (Thomlinson 1990, Gallagher 1999, Pittet et al 1999). The reasons for this remain complex and multifaceted including:

- Environmental factors such as heavy workload (Gould 1991a, Gallagher 1999, Pittet et al 2000)
- Inadequate hand washing facilities (Gould 1991a, 1994, Gallagher 1999, Pittet et al 2000, Girou et al 2002, Cochrane 2003)
- Lack of knowledge regarding infection control.

Practice issues such as failing to wash hands before and after wearing gloves (Stringer et al

1991, Pittet et al 2000) or use of poor hand-washing techniques have also been identified (Mallett & Dougherty 2000). In terms of improving compliance, the use of bedside alcohol hand-rubs has been shown to be effective (Rossoff et al 1995, Gallagher 1999, Pittet et al 2000, Lucet et al 2002, DoH 2005) and is more successful in decreasing bacterial counts than conventional soap and water (Pittet et al 1999, Girou et al 2002).

ANTT recommends a combination of effective hand washing with soap and water (Ayliffe et al 1978) to be used interchangeably with alcohol hand-rub during aseptic non-touch technique procedures. Hand cleansing before and after glove use is another important recommendation. It is possible for hands to be washed effectively this way in just 20–40 s (ICNA 2002) (see Ch. 4).

GLOVES: SHOULD THEY BE WORN AND WHAT TYPE?

Choosing between sterile, non-sterile or no gloves at all is often debated in aseptic techniques. In the absence of empirical research, sterile gloves seem to have been advocated simply on a 'better safe than sorry' basis. The aseptic non-touch technique recommends the use of non-sterile gloves for nearly all aseptic procedures. The rationale for this is based on the following:

- There is no substantial evidence demonstrating that any particular type of glove reduces the incidence of i.v.-related infection.
- Even sterile gloves cannot always be considered 100% sterile, due to a small but significant micropermeability (DeGroot-Kosolcharoen & Jones 1989).
- Key parts/sites should *never* be touched either by gloved or non-gloved hands, thus reducing the necessity for sterile gloves.
- Gloves should be worn in order to protect the healthcare worker from hazardous substances (drugs and body fluids) and to comply with COSHH regulations (1988, 2002). The wearing of gloves for all procedures involving potential exposure to body fluids such as blood and urine was recommended by the Expert Advisory Group on AIDS (HMSO 1990), and the Centers for Disease Control (1988).
- Ojajarvi (1990) established that colonisation of skin by transient bacteria is the likely outcome

when skin is repeatedly moist or damaged. Shredded skin caused by such damage can transmit bacteria via the contact route (Gould 1991b). Practitioners often have moist and damaged hands due to frequent washing and drying. Gloves may serve as a barrier to prevent de-scaling of bacteria onto key parts and sites.

- It has been reported that excessive precautions contribute to a false sense of security and thus a reduction in sensible precautions (Lund & Caruso 1993). This is supported by observations of staff who thought it was acceptable to touch key parts when wearing sterile gloves (Rowley 1996).
- A study conducted by Anderton and Aidoo (1991) revealed no contamination in any enteral feed samples gathered from systems assembled while wearing non-sterile gloves, indicating that non-sterile gloves could reasonably be considered aseptic.

ENVIRONMENTAL/AIR CONTAMINATION

Due to air-borne microorganisms, a flawless sterile technique is not possible in healthcare and home settings. Air-borne infections in hospital account for only 10% of all endemic infections (Eickhoff 1994). Therefore, the potential for harmful contamination of key parts and sites by air is insignificant compared with contamination by direct contact. It is possible to reduce the potential for environmental infection by taking 'sensible measures', i.e. not practising aseptic procedures at the bedside immediately after activities like bed-making and wound dressing – when the level of air-borne bacteria is at its highest.

ASEPTIC FIELDS

The nurse must decide what kind of aseptic field is required to maintain the asepsis of equipment and key parts. The need for sterile towels, dressing packs, etc. for all procedures is overly extravagant. For the majority of aseptic procedures, asepsis of only one or two small key parts/sites needs to be maintained. This can be achieved simply and effectively by a non-touch method and ad hoc aseptic fields (e.g. using the inside of equipment packaging).

In i.v. therapy, a large plastic or disposable tray is ideal. Such trays should be aseptic, large enough to provide an organised working space, be flat and have high sides in order to en-house sharps safely and to protect the nurse and child from spillages. Re-use of this equipment between patients is acceptable with appropriate cleaning as guided by local policy.

Preparation of the child

For any ANTT procedure it is essential that the child and their carer have the procedure fully explained. This explanation may take place at the child's bed or in the preparation room prior to the procedure taking place in a language that is suitable for the child's age. Involving the play therapist as considered necessary will help in the preparation of this practice.

RISK ASSESSMENT AND EQUIPMENT

It is impossible to provide a definitive list of equipment for all aseptic procedures. It is, however, possible to break down any aseptic procedure into five broad stages (Fig. 34.2), which require either a specific action, or a choice of

infective precautions. It can be seen that components 1, 4 and 5 are compulsory for all procedures. However, for some procedures, the nurse must make choices regarding the use of gloves and an aseptic field. These will differ depending on how difficult each procedure is, i.e. the degree of risk involved. Risk assessment is simple. The practitioner should simply ask whether it is possible to perform the procedure without contaminating key parts. Most aseptic procedures can be completed without touching any equipment that will be in direct contact with the patient. In ANTT, such equipment items are called key parts. An example of a key part in i.v. therapy is parts of equipment that will come into contact with the liquid infusate such as the syringe end, the needle used for drawing up the liquid, the inside of the syringe and so on. Key parts should also be properly accessed as per current best practice guidelines for medical device cleaning and in conjunction with the manufacturer's instructions for use, e.g. an infusion port that requires cleaning before the connection of a key part to infuse a solution (NICE 2003, Kaler and Chinn 2007). If it is not possible to complete the procedure without touching key parts due to the complexity, the length or the type of procedure, then more

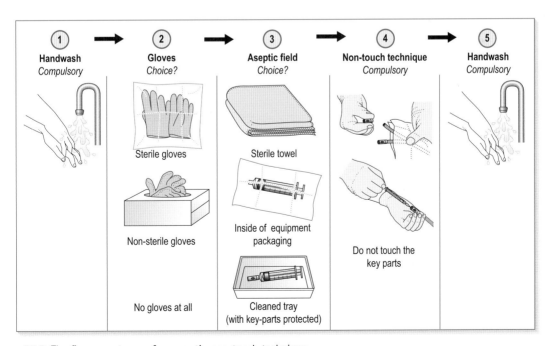

Figure 34.2 The five core stages of an aseptic non-touch technique.

BOX 34.2 The core stages of ANTT – a practice example

Aim: To prepare and administer an intravenous drug into a peripheral cannula
Setting: A typical hospital preparation room or the child's bedside

Method	Notes
Enter the prep room or be at the bedside with clean hands, i.e. just washed	Hand washing at key points during the procedure helps to break potential 'chains' of cross-infection
Clean your aseptic field according to local policy – making it 'aseptic', e.g. a good-sized plastic tray with sides (alternatively, a procedure trolley may be cleaned to create an 'aseptic' area, or a sterile disposable tray may be used)	A good-sized aseptic field will help you protect the key parts; a tray is also nicely portable Paper trays cannot be made aseptic by cleaning facilities available in a ward area
While the tray dries, gather all the equipment you need and lay around the aseptic field	You need to get all these 'dirty' activities done before you clean your hands again
Clean your hands with alcogel or soap and water	Hand asepsis can be compromised during the preparation stage
Put on non-sterile gloves	Gloves are used here in accordance with COSHH regulations, i.e. to protect the nurse from repeated drug exposure
Prepare drugs and equipment using a non-touch technique	Maintains asepsis
Do not touch any key parts but *do* touch non-key parts with confidence	Touching non-key parts with confidence will help the user develop good, safe handling skills
Remove gloves and wash hands	
When ready, go straight to the patient without delay and check patient's identification bracelet	Helps ensure the right patient gets the right drug
Prepare the patient, and gain free access to the i.v. site:	
Clearly explain the procedure to the child and involve the child's carer in this reassurance/consenting process	
Prepare the site (remove bandage, etc.)	
Ensure the i.v. site shows no signs of infection or trauma. In the event of complications, seek help and document in the nursing notes	
Put on a pair of non-sterile gloves	
Clean all key parts (in this case, the cannula port) and wait for it to dry (30 s)	A key part is not aseptic until dry
Administer drugs according to policy and prescription chart	
Dispose of all sharps and used products safely	
Clean tray or aseptic field	
Remove gloves and wash hands	
Document as appropriate	

---

infective precautions will become necessary, including the use of sterile gloves (Box 34.2). It should be noted, however, that such procedures in i.v. therapy are rare and sterile gloves should never be worn as a shortcut to asepsis.

OBSERVATIONS AND COMPLICATIONS

If key parts/sites are inadvertently contaminated, remedy the situation by cleaning with appropriate agents or by changing equipment.

COMMUNITY PERSPECTIVE

The principles remain the same within the home environment.

CCNs need to be aware that hand washing facilities may be inadequate in some homes and they will therefore need to carry appropriate hand-cleansing equipment and disposable towels.

A simple way to form an aseptic field is to clean a plastic tray with an alcohol solution immediately prior to the procedure.

In cases where families perform aseptic procedures, the CCN will need to ensure that they understand the rationale for, and methods of achieving, aseptic non-touch techniques as part of maintaining a safe environment. It is important that the procedure is clearly explained to the child and the carer. In some instances, it may be appropriate for the CCN to arrange for disposal of clinical waste, according to local policies.

DOS AND DON'TS

- Do explain the procedure fully to the child and the carer.
- Do touch non-key parts with confidence – this will make the procedure easier.
- Do concentrate on the key parts and key sites. As long as they are not touched/contaminated by you or anything else, you are practising safely.
- Do take time to develop your own handling technique. As long as it meets the principles of the aseptic non-touch technique, you are practising safely and efficiently.
- Do clean away from the wound in wound care. Only uncontaminated gauze, forceps, gloves, etc. should make direct contact with the wound.
- Do remember the importance of hand cleansing.
- Do not use unnecessary infective precautions, as this only wastes time and resources.
- Do not confuse your practice. For example, don't try to keep one hand 'clean' and the other 'dirty', as this will only make things more difficult.

References

Adams, B.G., Marrie, T.J., 1982. Hand carriage of aerobic gram-negative rods by health care personnel. J. Hyg. 89 (1), 23–31.

Anderton, A., Aidoo, K.E., 1991. The effect of handling procedures on microbial contamination of enteral feeds – a comparison of the use of sterile vs non-sterile gloves. J. Hosp. Infect. 17, 297–301.

Ayliffe, G.A.J., Babb, J.R., Quoraishi, A.H., 1978. A test for hygienic hand disinfection. J. Clin. Pathol. 31, 923.

Bauer, T.M., Ofner, E., Just, H.M., et al., 1990. An epidemiological study assessing the relative importance of airborne and direct contact transmission of microorganisms in a medical intensive care unit. J. Hosp. Infect. 15 (4), 301–309.

Centers for Disease Control and Prevention, 1988. Nosocomial infection surveillance. MMWR CDC Surveill. Summ. 35 (1), 17SS–29SS.

Centers for Disease Control and Prevention 2002 Guidelines for hand hygiene in health-care settings, 2002. Recommendations of the Healthcare Infection Control Practices Advisory Committee and the HICPAC/SHEA/APIC/IDSA Hand Hygiene Task Force. MMWR 51 (16), 1–45.

Church, J., 1986. Spread of infection: direct contact. Nursing 3 (4), 136–137.

Cochrane, J., 2003. Infection control audit of hand hygiene facilities. Nurs. Stand. 15 (17), 33–38.

COSHH, 1988. Control of substances hazardous to health [original]. HMSO, London.

COSHH, 2002. Control of substances hazardous to health. HMSO, London.

Degroot-Kosolcharoen, J., Jones, J.M., 1989. Permeability of latex and vinyl gloves to water and blood. Am. J. Infect. Control 17 (4), 196–201.

Department of Health, 2005. Saving lives: a delivery programme to reduce healthcare associated infection including MRSA. DoH, London.

Department of Health, 2007. Epic 2: National evidence-based guidelines for preventing healthcare-associated infections in NHS hospitals in England. NRIC, DoH, London.

Eickhoff, T.C., 1994. Airborne nosocomial infection: a contemporary perspective. Infect. Control Hosp. Epidemiol. 15 (10), 663–672.

Gallagher, R., 1999. This is the way we wash our hands. Nurs. Times 95 (10), 62–65.

Gao, Z., Tseng, C., Pei, Z., et al., 2007. Molecular analysis of human forearm superficial skin bacterial biota. Proc. Natl. Acad. Sci. 104 (8), 2927–2932.

Girou, E., Loyeau, S., Legrand, P., et al., 2002. Efficacy of handrubbing with alcohol based solution versus standard hand washing with antiseptic soap: randomised clinical trial. Br. Med. J. 325, 362–364.

Gould, D., 1991a. Nurses' hands as vectors of hospital-acquired infection: a review. J. Adv. Nurs. 16, 1216–1225.

Gould, D., 1991b. Skin bacteria: what is normal? Nurs. Stand. 18 (5), 25–28.

Gould, D., 1994. Infection control. Making sense of hand hygiene. Nurs. Times 90 (30), 63–64.

Hendrick, E., 1988. Infectious waste management: will science prevail? Infect. Control Hosp. Epidemiol. 9, 488–490.

HMSO, 1990. Guidance for clinical health care workers. Protection against infection with HIV and hepatitis viruses. Recommendations of the Expert Advisory Group on AIDS. HMSO, London.

ICNA, 2002. Hand decontamination guidelines. Infection Control Nurse Association/Regent Medical, London.

Jones, P.M., 1987. Indwelling central venous catheter related infections and two different procedures of catheter care. Cancer Nurs. 10 (3), 123–130.

Kaler, W., Chinn, R., 2007. Successful disinfection of needleless access ports: a matter of time and friction. JAVA 12 (3), 140–142.

Larson, E., 1989. Handwashing: it's essential – even when you use gloves. Am. J. Nurs. 89 (11), 934–939.

Leonard, M., 1986. Handling infection. J. Infect. Control Nurs. 82, 81–84.

Lucet, J.C., Rigaud, M.P., Mentre, F., et al., 2002. Hand contamination before and after different hand hygiene techniques: a randomised clinical trial. J. Hosp. Infect. 50, 276–280.

Lund, C., Caruso, R., 1993. Nursing perspectives: aseptic techniques in wound care. Dermatol. Nurs. 5 (3), 215–216.

Maki, D.G., Goldman, D.A., Rhama, F.S., 1973. Infection control in IV therapy. Ann. Intern. Ther. 79, 869–880.

Mallett, J., Dougherty, L., 2000. The Royal Marsden Hospital manual of clinical nursing procedures, fifth ed. Blackwell Science, Oxford.

National Audit Office, 2000. The challenge of hospital acquired infection. NAO, London.

National Patient Safety Agency (NPSA), 2000. Hand washing. Online. Available: www.npsa.nhs.uk.

NICE, 2003. Infection control: prevention for healthcare-associated infection in primary and community care (clinical guidelines 2) 234. NICE, London.

Ojajarvi, J., 1990. Effectiveness of hand washing and disinfection methods in removing transient bacteria after patient nursing. J. Hyg. 85, 193–203.

Pittet, D., Dharan, S., Touveneau, S., et al., 1999. Bacterial contamination of the hands of hospital staff during routine patient care. Arch. Intern. Med. 195, 821–826.

Pittet, D., Hugonnet, S., Harbarth, S., et al., 2000. Effectiveness of a hospital-wide programme to improve compliance with hand hygiene. Lancet 356, 1307–1312.

Pratt, R.J., Pellowe, C.M., Wilson, J. A., et al., 2007. Epic2: National evidence-based guidelines for preventing healthcare-associated infections in NHS hospitals in England. J. Hosp. Infect. 65S, S1–S64.

Rossoff, L.J., Borenstein, M., Isenberg, H.D., 1995. Is hand washing really needed in an intensive care unit? Crit. Care Med. 23 (7), 1211–1216.

Rowley, S., 1996. A safe and efficient handling technique for IV therapy: aseptic non-touch-technique. (Unpublished).

Rowley, S., 2001. Aseptic non-touch technique. Infection Control Supplement. Nurs. Times 97 (7).

Stringer, B., Smith, J.A., Scharf, S., et al., 1991. A study of the use of gloves in a large teaching hospital. Am. J. Infect. Control 18 (5), 233–236.

Thomlinson, D., 1990. Time to dispense with the rituals. Changing infection control practice. Prof. Nurse 5 (8), 421–425.

Weller, B. (Ed.), 1993. Encyclopaedic dictionary of nursing and health care. Baillière Tindall, London.

Chapter 35

Isolation nursing

Rachel Sales

CHAPTER CONTENTS

Introduction 337
    Learning outcomes 337
    Factors to note 338

Developmental and family considerations 338
    General principles 338
    Equipment 339
    Hand hygiene 339
    Personal protective equipment (PPE) 340
    Specimen collection 340
    Clinical waste 340
    Linen/laundry 340
    Environmental cleaning
    and decontamination 341
    Documentation and planning of care 341
    Dos and don'ts 342

INTRODUCTION

Microorganisms, as discussed in Chapter 4, can cause a variety of infections within children. Adherence to basic hygiene principles, standard precautions, wearing appropriate personal protective clothing, a clean environment and segregation of the child where necessary, will minimise the risk of cross-infection or colonisation by pathogenic organisms, by interrupting the chain of transmission (Curtis 2008).

Wilson (2006) describes four factors that influence the necessity for isolation precautions:

1. Ease of transmission
2. Route of transmission
3. Epidemiological significance, e.g. antibiotic resistance
4. Presence of susceptible individuals.

The isolation of a child in hospital will be either to protect them from infection (*protective isolation*, e.g. if they are immunosuppressed) or to protect other patients from infection (*source isolation*, e.g. diarrhoeal illness).

The principal objective of isolating nursing is to minimise the risk of transmission of microorganisms. Wilson (2006) specifically reminds us that it is *the microorganism that is being isolated rather than the patient.*

LEARNING OUTCOMES

By the end of this section you should be able to:

- Understand the principles of isolation nursing
- Know the importance of compliance to universal precautions

- Understand the need for additional transmission precautions
- Understand the effects that isolation nursing can have on the child and family and be able to:
  - prevent the spread of infection while caring for the child and family
  - plan safe individualised care for the child and family
  - alleviate any anxiety or stress felt by the child and/or family while the child is nursed apart from others.

FACTORS TO NOTE

Microorganisms cause a variety of infections and the incubation period and mode of transmission will vary according to the site of the infection and the micro-organism involved. Global and local epidemiological patterns of infection should be taken into account, e.g. *Clostridium difficile* and multi drug resistant organisms (MDROs), such as methicillin-resistant *Staphylococcus aureus* (MRSA), *vancomycin-resistant enterococcus* (VRE), and aminoglycoside-resistant Gram-negative bacteria such as *Klebsiella* (Curtis 2008, Pittet et al 2008, Purssell 2003, Smyth et al 2008).

DEVELOPMENTAL AND FAMILY CONSIDERATIONS

Isolation can be stressful for patients and relatives (Gammon 1999, Davies & Rees 2000, Rees et al 2000). Careful explanations must be given to the child and parents as to why there is a need for segregation from others. The child needs to be made aware that the isolation is not a form of punishment for anything they have done wrong. Details of the mode of transmission, the need for protective clothing and appropriate precautions to take should also be given. Consideration of the cultural and social implications some infectious diseases may have for the individual and family, such as tuberculosis, measles or human immunodeficiency virus (HIV), must be taken into account (Helman 2000). Rees et al's (2000) study reinforces the importance of addressing the emotional, communication and information needs for patients in isolation.

GENERAL PRINCIPLES

The isolation of any patient should be undertaken in a systematic way following risk assessment in compliance with local policy.

- Does the patient require isolation in a single room (such as protective isolation) or has an outbreak occurred which needs cohort isolation (nursing children together who have the same infection) such as a diarrhoeal illness or respiratory syncytial virus (RSV).
- Consider the environmental need for special high-efficiency particulate air filters (HEPA) for the child who is or may become severely immunosuppressed and needs protection from opportunistic infections.
- The area should be uncluttered and thoroughly cleaned at least daily, in accordance with local policy and national standards.
- Special attention should be paid to the child's toys, as these can be a source of infection (Avila-Aguero et al 2004). While in isolation, the child should have their own toys and not be sharing toys with other children or patients. All available toys need to be washable.
- Communal toilets should be avoided where the risk of transmitting the infection is increased, such as when the child has diarrhoea or vomiting.
- If en suite toilet facilities are available, they must be flushed after use, cleaned when visibly soiled and cleaned at least daily. Disposable toilet seats are not necessary.
- In the home setting, maintain standards of hygiene and cleanliness. Do not use communal washing/bathing equipment such as towels, flannels or toothbrushes as these can be a source of cross-contamination.
- Assess the need for a single room or for cohortion and how best to implement the appropriate transmission precautions. Consider whether the likely organism is transmitted via the air-borne, droplet or contact route and whether the door of the room should be open or closed.
- Respect the child and family's need for privacy by providing curtains/blinds for the bed area and knocking on the door before entry.
- Consider the precautions to be taken when visiting other departments such as the operating theatre or X-ray department. It may be advisable to place the child last on the operating list or to go to the X-ray department when the least number of children are there, such as at the end of the day.
- It is important that all children who are segregated from others receive the same care

and time allocation as others, such as play therapy and hospital schooling.

- If there is a history of communicable disease in the family (e.g. chickenpox or blood-borne viruses) or signs of infection such as diarrhoea and vomiting, rash, cough or pyrexia, initiate appropriate microbiological investigation (see Ch. 36) and precautions as soon as possible.

- Check the need for prophylactic antibiotics for the family with diseases such as *Neisseria meningitidis* – meningococcal disease (Fraser et al 2006). Check whether relevant exposure of healthcare workers to the disease warrants prophylaxis. Healthcare workers should seek advice from the occupational health department or infection control team.

- Discuss with the infection control team whether the infection is a disease notifiable (to local authority proper officers) under the Public Health (Infectious Diseases) Regulations 1988 (TSO 1988).

EQUIPMENT

- A notice on the door of the cubicle or area to indicate to staff and visitors:
  - The need for separation and the risk of cross-infection
  - The need to discuss entry to the area and visiting arrangements where individuals are non-immune to the infection, e.g. chickenpox
  - The necessity to comply with hand washing and the wearing of protective clothing
- Hand washing equipment: disposable hand towels, liquid soap or antiseptic solution, alcoholic hand-rub; basins should have lever-operated mixer taps or automated controls
- Personal protective equipment (PPE) and protective clothing, such as disposable gloves, plastic aprons, facial protection (mask, goggles, visor) as per local policy
- Foot-operated pedal bin with appropriately coloured, labelled disposable clinical waste bag with ties
- Sharps bin, if necessary
- Individual examination equipment, such as a stethoscope, auriscope with earpieces, tape measure, tongue depressors, ophthalmoscope, patella hammer, sphygmomanometer with

disposable or washable cuff, disposable thermometer

- Suction and oxygen equipment; easy access to resuscitation equipment
- Scales (if required)
- Scissors (blunt tipped)
- Pens, ruler, chart holder, calculator
- Disposable equipment according to the needs of the child such as suction catheters, sticky tape, sterile packs, syringes and disposable hypodermic needles, equipment for intravascular cannulation
- A clock with a second hand should be easily visible
- Equipment for summoning attention such as a call bell or intercommunication system
- Non-communal play equipment, television, radio and reading material, according to the needs of the child
- If last offices are to be performed, consider the requirements for protective body bags (see Ch. 7).

HAND HYGIENE

Hand washing is widely acknowledged to be the single most important activity for reducing the spread of disease (Bloomfield 2007, Curtis 2008, NICE 2003, Picheansathian 2004, RCN 2005). The need for and frequency of hand washing should be determined by actions and not routines.

Hands must be washed and thoroughly dried:

- When dirty
- Before entry to the cubicle or cohorting area
- Before and after caring for the child
- Before aseptic procedures
- Before handling food
- After dirty tasks such as toileting
- After removal of protective clothing including gloves
- After handling specimens
- On exit of the single room or cohorting area.

Hand washing facilities with appropriate liquid soap, antiseptic solution, alcohol handrub and disposable paper towels must be available inside the room, immediately outside it or in the cohorting area. Nurses also need to empower the child, family and visitors with the knowledge for safe hand washing and disinfection (Ward 2003).

PERSONAL PROTECTIVE EQUIPMENT (PPE)

Have available inside and outside the room or cohorting area, disposable gloves, aprons and facial protection (visors, goggles and masks as per local policy). Assess the risk of procedures which may contaminate the healthcare worker. If there is a risk of aerosols (fine sprays) or splattering of body fluid into the face or mucosal surfaces, facial protection must be worn. Additional protective clothing may be required if there is extensive bleeding or explosive diarrhoea or vomiting and the risk of contamination to the healthcare worker and the environment is high.

- Non-latex and/or powder-free gloves should be available for healthcare workers who are allergic to latex or starch powder
- The need for parents, siblings or visitors to wear protective clothing should be assessed individually and discussed with the child and parents.

Infection control guidance (NHS 2007) describes the order for putting on PPE as apron, mask, eye/face protection, gloves. To remove PPE they suggest the order: gloves, apron, eye/face protection, mask.

SPECIMEN COLLECTION

All specimens must be regarded as potentially infectious. Plan the need for appropriate specimens to be taken in consultation with the medical staff before explaining to the child and family. This aids better continuity of care and reduces the likelihood of unnecessary and repeated specimens. Document the date and time that specimens are taken.

- Wear protective clothing such as gloves when obtaining or handling specimens and remember to wash your hands before and after collection
- Ensure that containers are adequately sealed and not leaking. Do not contaminate the outside of the container
- Ensure that all specimens and laboratory forms are correctly labelled, safely packed and dispatched to the appropriate laboratory as per local policy as soon as possible
- Do not store specimens in food or drug refrigerators.

If disposable potties, bedpans or urinals are used, they must be covered during transportation to the dirty utility area and placed in a well-maintained macerator for disposal. The supporting frame should be washed in hot water and detergent and dried before storage.

In the home setting, faeces from nappies or colostomy bags should be put down the toilet and the nappy or bag wrapped in newspaper or biodegradable polythene and disposed of in the dustbin.

CLINICAL WASTE

The waste that is created during the care of a child in isolation may be contaminated and therefore requires safe disposal as per local policy. Ensure that waste is segregated at source, such as by the bedside, in accordance with nation and local policy (DoH 2006).

- Sharps bins may be a source of infection and should be removed and disposed of frequently, or when two-thirds full, and on discharge of the child.
- Use foot-operated pedal bins with lids for all clinical and non-clinical waste and laundry. Hands will become contaminated if used for opening lids.
- Follow local infection control policies for decontamination of the environment on discharge of the child.
- Ensure that the waste bins are cleaned regularly, and on discharge of the child, with hot water and detergent and dried to prevent the risk of cross-infection.
- Infected clinical waste, including sharps, generated in the home may be collected by special arrangement organised by the primary health care team.

LINEN/LAUNDRY

Under the Health and Safety at Work Act, health authorities have an obligation to prevent risk of infection to staff handling and laundering linen. Therefore, local policy for the safe handling of linen must be adhered to (DoH 2006, NHS Executive 1995).

Linen should be categorised as either used (soiled and foul) or infected and placed in an appropriately colour-coded container (see Ch. 4). Infected laundry should be placed immediately into a water-soluble bag or soluble stitched bag within an outer bag, secured with a tie and labelled as to its origin before it is removed from an area (NHS Executive 1995).

Well-maintained domestic washing machines on a hot wash cycle may be used to decontaminate laundry in the home setting. This includes infections such as those causing diarrhoeal illness and blood-borne viruses.

ENVIRONMENTAL CLEANING AND DECONTAMINATION

Cleaning and disinfection of high contact areas such as bedside tables and call bells, along with other surfaces will reduce the risk of cross-infection.

Curtains should be laundered frequently and changed if visibly dirty. If shedding of pathogenic organisms such as staphylococci is extensive, as on the skin scales of a child with eczema, then curtains should also be changed on discharge.

Mop heads should be laundered daily in a washing machine and stored dry. They should not be left soaking in disinfectants, as this increases the risk of contamination with organisms such as *Pseudomonas*. The same mop should not be used in other communal areas or kitchens because of the risk of cross-infection.

DOCUMENTATION AND PLANNING OF CARE

- Plan and document all care around the family and child, taking into consideration their cultural, spiritual, psychosocial and physical needs.
- Care should be individualised according to the risk of acquiring or spreading infection. Take into account the age of the child and their ability and understanding of the required isolation precautions.
- Assess the risk of infection to the child and staff and implement the wearing of appropriate PPE such as gloves, aprons, masks, visors or goggles. A careful explanation to the child and family must be given to avoid feelings of alienation. The wearing of protective clothing by family members will depend on the type of infection.
- Do discuss with parents and the child all precautions to be taken while the child is in

hospital. Ensure that there is a means of communication if the child is in a single room, e.g. a bell, two-way intercommunication apparatus or telephone. Include the need to extend precautions in the home, at school or nursery. Seek help from the infection control team if parents require further explanations.

- Assess the risk of infection to the family, siblings and other visitors. Consider the precautions they should take while visiting in hospital. For example, have the family members had chickenpox or are they incubating it? If they have had the disease they can visit, but if not, do they pose a risk to others on the ward? Should visiting be restricted?
- Assess, daily, the need for all the precautions.
- Report any changes or deterioration in the child's condition or any signs or symptoms of infection in the family.
- Inform the infection control team, primary healthcare team or transferring hospital/unit of any actual or potential infections. Report to the infection control nurse/doctor any suspicions of secondary cases such as other people with diarrhoea, rashes or chest infections.
- Obtain written information for parents and children about the infection and the need for restricted precautions.
- Medical/nursing notes should be kept safely outside the room where possible to avoid unnecessary entry to the isolation area.
- Consider the need for health education for the child and family and any wider social networks such as schools, or play groups (Cottingham 2004).
- If the child has an infection which could be transmitted through sexual contact, such as human immunodeficiency virus (HIV), then this should be discussed with the parents through the multidisciplinary healthcare team. Sex education, where necessary, should be given in accordance with government guidelines.
- Alleviate stress and anxiety felt by the child while separated from others through increased play activity, schooling, television/videos and, where necessary, plan visiting as appropriate. Consider the need for voluntary workers.

DOS AND DON'TS

- Do remember that hand washing is the single most important point in controlling cross-infection.
- Do keep all cuts and abrasions covered with a waterproof plaster. If inoculation of mucosal or non-intact skin contamination with blood or body fluids occurs, act immediately and report to your manager and the occupational health department as soon as possible.
- Dispose of laundry bags when two-thirds full.
- Do wear appropriate personal protective clothing.
- Do maintain confidentiality for both children and staff who have an infection or communicable disease.
- Do set an example as a role model for others to follow in basic hygiene principles.
- Do ensure that local infection control guidelines are easily available to both staff and parents.
- Do know how to contact the local infection control nurse/doctor for advice.
- Do not use laundry or waste bins with swing lids, as this may cause aerosols and increases the risk of hand contamination.
- Do not make the child and family feel responsible, guilty or alienated.

References

Avila-Aguero, M.L., German, G., Paris, M., et al., 2004. Toys in a pediatric hospital: are they a bacteria source? Am. J. Infect. Control 32 (5), 287–290.

Bloomfield, S.F., Aiello, E., Cookson, B., et al., 2007. The effectiveness of hand hygiene procedures in reducing the risks of infections in home and community settings including hand washing and alcohol-based hand sanitizers. Am. J. Infect. Control 35 (10), S27–S64.

Cottingham, A., 2004. Now wash your hands please. Paediatr. Nurs. 16 (8), 33–35.

Curtis, L.T., 2008. Prevention of hospital-acquired infections: review of non-pharmacological interventions. J. Hosp. Infect. 69, 204–219.

Davies, H., Rees, J., 2000. Psychological effects of isolation nursing (1): mood disturbance. Nurs. Stand. 14 (28), 35–38.

DoH Department of Health 2006 Health Technical Memorandum 07–01, 2000. Safe management of healthcare waste. Online. Available: www.dh.gov.uk Accessed 26 July 2008.

Fraser, A., Gafter-Gvili, A., Paul, M., et al., 2006. Antibiotics for preventing meningococcal infections. Cochrane Database Syst. Rev. 3, CD004785.

Gammon, J., 1999. The psychological consequences of source isolation: a review of the literature. J. Clin. Nurs. 8 (1), 13–21.

Helman, C., 2000. Culture, health and illness, fourth ed. Butterworth-Heinemann, Oxford.

NICE, 2003. Infection control. Prevention of healthcare-associated infection in primary and community care. No. 1: Standard principles. National Institute for Clinical Excellence, London.

NHS Executive, 1995. Health service guidelines: hospital laundry arrangements for used and infected linen. HSG (95)18. NHS Executive, London.

NHS, 2007. Pandemic flu. A summary of guidance for infection control in healthcare settings. Department of Health, London.

Picheansathian, W., 2004. A systematic review on the effectiveness of alcohol-based solutions for hand hygiene. Int. J. Nurs. Pract. 10, 3–9.

Pittet, D., Allegranzi, B., Storr, J., et al., 2008. Infection control as a major World Health Organization priority for developing countries. J. Hosp. Infect. 68, 285–292.

Purssell, E., 2003. Community-acquired MRSA in children. Paediatr. Nurs. 15 (2), 47–49.

RCN, 2005. Good practice in infection prevention and control. RCN, London.

Rees, J., Davies, H., Birchall, C., et al., 2000. Psychological effects of source isolation nursing (2): patient satisfaction. Nurs. Stand. 14 (29), 32–36.

Smyth, E.T., McIlvenny, G., Enstone, J.E., et al., 2008. Four country healthcare associated infection prevalence survey 2006: overview of the results. J. Hosp. Infect. 69, 230–248.

TSO, Statutory Instrument No. 1546. 1988. The Public Health (Infectious Diseases) Regulations 1988. The Stationery Office, London.

Ward, D., 2003. Improving patient hand hygiene. Nurs. Stand. 17 (35), 39–42.

Wilson, J., 2006. Infection control in clinical practice, third ed. Baillière Tindall, London.

Further reading

Centers for Disease Control and Prevention, 2007. Guideline for isolation precautions: preventing transmission of infectious agents in healthcare settings. Online. Available: www.cdc.gov/ncidod/dhqp/gl_isolation.html.

Hall, J., Roopnarine, S., Mclean, J., 2007. Introduction of an isolation policy in paediatric wards. Paediatr. Nurs. 19 (9), 14–17.

Chapter 36

Specimen collection

Christina Maddox, Beryl Pearson

CHAPTER CONTENTS

Introduction   344
    Learning outcomes   344
    Rationale   345
    Factors to note   345

Specimen collection   346
    Equipment   346
    Eye swab   346
    Nose swab   347
    Pernasal swab   347
    Sputum   347
    Throat swab   347
    Ear swab   347
    Wound swab   347
    Faeces   348
    Urine   348
    Vaginal swab   350
    Blood samples   350
    Analysis of antibiotic levels   351
    Vesicular fluid for electron microscopy   351
    Fungal samples of hair, nail and skin   351
    Gastric washings   351
    Biopsy material   352
    Cerebrospinal fluid   352

INTRODUCTION

Infectious microorganisms/biological agents can refer to the bacteria, viruses, fungi and internal parasites that create a hazard to human health; most harm through infection but they can also cause allergies or be toxic (ACDP 2003). Specimen collection is undertaken when laboratory investigation is required for the examination of tissue or body fluid, and as an aid to diagnosis. Specimen collection is a fundamental aspect of children's nursing practice that requires a diverse range of knowledge and skills. Specimens can be taken from a number of areas and the results used for screening, diagnosis, treatment and research. The validity of specimen test results is, however, dependent on using the correct collection technique and safe practice, to avoid contamination and cross-infection. Collecting specimens from children is further complicated by the child's ability to understand what is being asked of them and the parent's willingness and ability to assist. Nurses often have responsibility for both the collection and the safe transportation of samples to the laboratory.

LEARNING OUTCOMES

By the end of this section you should be able to:

- Acknowledge the physical and psychosocial implications to the child and family when collecting specimens
- Collect appropriate specimens and transport them safely to the laboratory

- Be aware of your responsibility and accountability in obtaining specimens, interpreting and communicating results in conjunction with medical staff and the family
- Understand the need to record the investigation
- Be aware of complications that may arise from specimen collection.

RATIONALE

Specimen collection is undertaken for the examination of tissue or body fluid. Most samples are sent to the laboratory but some tests are carried out on the ward, for example, blood glucose and urinalysis. Knowledge of correct procedural principles in collecting specimens is essential to effective child and family nursing.

FACTORS TO NOTE

- Always gain consent (NMC 2008, DoH 2001a,b) from the parents and the child by explaining the procedure clearly and appropriately and the reasons for taking the specimen. If specimens are obtained for research purposes, written consent should be obtained. The child and family have a right to refuse without any obligation (RCPCH & Hull 2000).
- Wherever possible, collect specimens before antimicrobial treatment begins as this may affect the results (Baillie 2001, Royal Liverpool & Broadgreen University Hospitals 2004). However, treatment must not be delayed in serious sepsis.
- The principles of specimen collection are the same, but local protocols may differ. To maintain safe practice the nurse should be familiar with these protocols. Requests for collection of any specimen should be made by a doctor – usually on a laboratory request form or sometimes in the medical notes.
- Perform a risk assessment before commencement of any procedure and decide if alternative or additional equipment is necessary. If you are in an unfamiliar environment, e.g. the home, it is important to make a risk assessment to ensure safe collection of the specimen (ACDP 2003, 2005).
- Pain assessment should be considered before specimen collection and, if required, pain relief should be administered prior to the procedure.

- Hands should be washed according to national protocol, before and after specimen collection. Gloves should be worn when collecting or handling all specimens to avoid cross-contamination of the specimen and the nurse (ICNA 1997, DoH 2003, Hilton & Baker 2003, Camm 2004).
- Contamination of the specimen must be avoided, as this may produce the need for a further sample with implications for the child. It may also cause misleading results and delay in appropriate treatment.
- When collecting the specimen, avoid infecting the child. For example, there is an increased risk of infection if an aseptic technique is not used when collecting a catheter urine specimen or during the collection of cerebrospinal fluid.
- For all specimen samples collected, examine the sample for abnormalities, e.g. colour, content, consistency and odour, and record observations. Record the acquisition of the specimen sample in the nursing documentation.
- All pathological specimens must be treated as potentially infectious and local written laboratory protocols should be followed for the safe handling and transportation of specimens (HSE 1999, 2005, Pratt et al 2007). Specimens for laboratory inspection should be collected in sterile containers with close-fitting lids to avoid contamination and spillage; however, this would only be necessary if examining for infection. For some urine and stool collections, where specimens are being examined for biochemical abnormalities, there would be no need for sterile containers. All specimen containers must be transported in a double-sided, self-sealing polythene bag, with one compartment containing the laboratory request form and the other the specimen.
- All specimens must be clearly labelled to identify their source (RCN 2005, Pratt et al 2007). A laboratory request form with the following information must accompany the specimen. This aids interpretation of results and reduces mistakes. Label with:
  - Patient's name, age, ward/department and hospital number
  - Type of specimen
  - How collected, e.g. pad urine, MSU, U-Bag
  - Date and time collected

- Diagnosis with history and relevant clinical signs and symptoms such as returning from abroad (specify country) with diarrhoea and vomiting, rash, pyrexia, catheters *in situ* or invasive devices used, or surgical details regarding postoperative wound infection
- Any antimicrobial drugs given
- Consultant's name and cost code
- Name of the doctor who ordered the investigation, as it may be necessary to telephone preliminary results and discuss treatment before the typed report is dispatched
- Biohazard label, if appropriate
- When collecting pus specimens, obtain as much material as possible, as this increases the chance of isolating microorganisms which may be difficult to grow or are minimal in number, e.g. in tuberculosis.
- Transport medium is used to preserve microorganisms during transportation. Charcoal medium, used for bacteria, neutralises toxic substances such as naturally occurring fatty acids found on the skin. Because many viruses do not survive well outside the body, a special viral transport medium is used.
- Specimens sent through the postal system must be packed and labelled according to Post Office guidelines. The specimen must be wrapped in a plastic bag, encased in absorbent material within another plastic bag, placed in a rigid cardboard container and firmly taped. A warning 'Pathological Sample' along with the sender's name and address must be visible on the outside (DoH 1998, HSE 1999).
- In children suspected of suffering from viral haemorrhagic fevers, such as Lassa fever, Marburg or Ebola virus, the infection control team must be consulted before any specimens are taken (ACDP 1997).
- Body fluid spillages should be soaked up with paper towels, after which disinfectant or hot soapy water should be used to clean any non-blood spillage (DoH 2004). For a blood spillage, sodium dichloroisocyanurate (NaDCC) or hypochlorite solution (10 000 ppm) should be sprinkled over and left for a few minutes before cleaning with hot soapy water (DoH 2004). Local protocols on cleaning bodily fluid spillage may differ (RCN 2005) but universal precautions should always be used and care must be taken, as release of chlorine fumes has occurred when chlorine-releasing agents were mixed with urine (DoH 1990, HSE 2002, 2005).
- For advice or further guidance on the collection of any specimen, contact the laboratory.

SPECIMEN COLLECTION

EQUIPMENT

Specific equipment is available in each clinical area for each particular procedure, and should be used. This will vary according to the specimen required but must include:

- Disposable gloves – sterile for blood cultures
- A protective tray
- A sterile container for the specimen
- Appropriate transport medium, if required
- Laboratory specimen form
- A polythene transportation bag
- Biohazard label, if required.

EYE SWAB

This procedure is carried out when infection is suspected. The procedure may be uncomfortable and the child should be prepared appropriately.

- Where possible ask the child to look upwards, then gently pull the lower lid down or gently part the eyelids
- Use a sterile cotton wool swab and gently roll the swab over the conjunctival sac inside the lower lid. Hold the swab parallel to the cornea to avoid injury if the child moves
- Place the swab in the transport medium
- For suspected *Chlamydia* infection:
  - Clean the eye first with sterile normal saline to obtain a clear view of the conjunctiva
  - Use a pernasal wire swab; part the eyelids and gently rub the conjunctival sac of the lower lid to obtain epithelial cells; identification of the organism is by fluorescent monoclonal antibodies
  - Wipe the swab over the marked area on the glass slide and allow to dry
  - Place the glass slide into a slide holder or Petri dish to protect the specimen.

NOSE SWAB

Nasal colonisation with *Staphylococcus aureus* increases the risk of staphylococcal infections at other sites of the body such as postoperative wounds and dialysis access sites. It is also associated with recurrent skin infections and nosocomial infections (HPA 2004).

- If the nose is dry, moisten the swab in sterile saline beforehand. This will also reduce discomfort for the child (Dougherty & Lister 2004)
- For viral investigation, moisten the swab in the viral transport medium prior to taking the swab
- Insert the swab into the anterior nares and direct it up into the tip of the nose and gently rotate. Both nares should be cultured using the same swab to obtain adequate material (Higgins 2008b)
- Plain sterile cotton wool swab. Sample the anterior nares by gently rotating the swab over the mucosal surface
- Place in transport medium
- The outside of the nostrils may be rubbed after the procedure to alleviate the unpleasant sensation of swabbing.

PERNASAL SWAB

This investigation is used specifically to diagnose whooping cough (*Bordetella pertussis*). When obtaining this specimen, the nurse must be proficient in the procedure and ensure that suction, oxygen and resuscitation equipment are easily available. The child should be held securely and observed carefully as the procedure may produce paroxysmal coughing and/or vomiting.

- Place the child in a good light to facilitate observation
- Use a special soft-wired sterile swab to minimise trauma to the nasal tissue
- Holding the child's head upwards, pass the swab along the floor of the nasal cavity to the posterior wall of the nasopharynx
- Gently rotate and withdraw the swab and place it in special transport medium or dispatch the swab in its container immediately to the laboratory to ensure maximum enhancement of growth of the organism.

SPUTUM

Supervised older children, given proper guidance, may be able to provide the specimen themselves.

Specimens from younger children and babies may be obtained using a mucus extractor or suction apparatus.

- Encourage the child to cough, especially after sleep, and expectorate into a container. Alternatively, nasopharyngeal/tracheal suction using a sputum trap can be undertaken
- Physiotherapy may help to facilitate expectoration
- Ensure that the material obtained is sputum and not saliva, and avoid collecting sputum specimens soon after the child had eaten as food particles may contaminate the specimen.

THROAT SWAB

- Place the child in a position with a good light source. This will ensure maximum visibility of the tonsillar bed
- Either depress the tongue with a spatula or ask the child to say 'aahh'. The procedure is likely to cause gagging and the tongue will move to the roof of the mouth and prevent accurate sampling
- Quickly, but gently, rub the swab over the tonsillar bed or area where there is exudate or a lesion
- Place the sample into transport medium.

EAR SWAB

- No antibiotics or other therapeutic agents should have been in the aural region for about 3 hours prior to sampling the area as this may inhibit the growth of organisms
- If there is purulent discharge, this should be sampled
- Place a sterile swab into the outer ear and gently rotate to collect the secretions
- Place the swab in transport medium
- For deeper ear swabbing, a speculum should be used. This procedure should be undertaken by experienced medical staff as damage to the eardrum may occur.

WOUND SWAB

A wound swab or a sample of wound exudate will help to identify the infection and determine the most effective treatment. Specimen collection from wounds often yields poor results because the swab dries out before it reaches the laboratory. This is a particular problem if the specimen is stored before it is examined. Wherever possible, pus or fluid should be aspirated, but if swabbing is the only practical method, two or three specimens will give more reliable results than a single sample (Gould 2001). Interpretation of results must be in conjunction with clinical signs. In the absence of clinical signs of infection, wound swabs may not provide any useful information (Hampton 2004).

- Obtain the specimen prior to any dressing or cleaning procedure of the wound. This will maximise the material obtained and prevent killing of the organism by the use of antiseptics.
- Use a sterile swab; gently rotate it on the area to collect exudate from the wound and place into transport medium. Where there is ample pus, collect as much as possible in a sterile syringe or sterile container and send to the laboratory.
- For detection of *Mycobacterium tuberculosis* a calcium alginate swab can be used. The swab gradually dissolves, maximising the isolation of the organism as its numbers are usually small.

FAECES

- A faecal specimen is more suitable than a rectal swab
- A specimen can be obtained from a nappy, clean potty or pulp bedpan liner
- Using a scoop, place faecal material into a container until it is approximately one-third full (Higgins 2008a)
- Some investigations require the fresh stool to be taken to the laboratory for analysis immediately (Royal Liverpool & Broadgreen Hospitals 2004). Check with the laboratory prior to specimen collection
- Where diarrhoea is present, a small piece of non-absorbent material lining the nappy can be used to prevent material soaking into the nappy
- Examine the sample for consistency, odour or blood and record observations to monitor changes
- If segments of tapeworm are seen, send them to the laboratory. Tapeworm segments can vary from the size of rice grains to a ribbon shape, 2.5 cm (1 inch) long
- For the identification of *Enterobius vermicularis* (threadworm/pinworm), material should be

obtained first thing in the morning on awakening by using a Sellotape slide. Place the sticky side of a strip of Sellotape over the anal region to obtain the material and stick the Sellotape smoothly onto a glass slide. The eggs of the worm can then be identified under the microscope. Threadworms lay their eggs on the perianal skin at night and therefore they will not be seen in a faecal specimen.

- Where amoebic dysentery is suspected, the specimen of stool must be freshly dispatched to the laboratory. The parasite causing amoebic dysentery exists in a free-living motile form and in the form of non-motile cysts. Both forms are characteristic in their fresh state but difficult to identify when dead.

URINE

Bedside urine testing for the presence of blood, protein, ketones and other analytes is usually undertaken with reagent strips, the results of which are indicative of further laboratory investigation (Deville et al 2004, Higgins 2008c). Urine samples should be dispatched to the laboratory as soon as possible, or after no more than 2 hours if kept at room temperature or up to 24 hours if kept at 4°C, to avoid multiplication of organisms and misleading results (Griffiths 1995, Higgins 1995a).

Some laboratories request the specimen to be put into a sterile specimen bottle containing boric acid which inhibits multiplication of most bacteria. However, the growth of some bacteria such as *Enterococcus faecalis* is inhibited by boric acid and therefore it is not always used.

Where laboratory access is limited or rapid testing is required, a commercial dip slide, which consists of a plastic tongue coated with suitable culture medium, can be dipped into the urine immediately after collection, a colour change noted and results obtained in 2 min. It tests for leucocyte esterase and nitrites, two indicators of infection. However, these are not 100% accurate and some organisms such as enterococci do not produce nitrites. Enterococci may therefore be missed where there is a real possibility of infection, such as in children with complex renal problems (Griffiths & Woodward 1993). It is also possible that, as the production of nitrites takes at least 4 hours, a young, non-toileting child's urine may be negative to nitrites on urinalysis but positive with later culture (Poole 2002).

Urine collection from disposable nappies for microscopy, culture and biochemical analysis has been described (Ahmed et al 1991). According to Poole (2002), this procedure is extremely difficult with modern nappies, due to the level of absorbency, and should be used with caution.

Normal social hygiene such as washing the genitalia with soap and water and drying thoroughly is considered sufficient to minimise contamination from the skin prior to collection of the specimen. Assess the clinical and psychosocial needs of the child as to whether cleaning the genitalia is necessary. The nurse must be sensitive to the cultural issues surrounding touching intimate parts of the body. With sufficient procedural knowledge the child's parents may be able to assist in urine collection.

Midstream specimen

The rationale of a midstream collection is that the first urine, which contains most of the contaminating bacteria from the periurethral area, is omitted, thereby reducing the contamination rate (Higgins 2008c). This is the most reliable non-invasive urine specimen collection method but may not be possible in the very young or uncooperative child. In the female, encourage separation of the labia to prevent perianal contamination while passing urine. In the male, encourage retraction of the prepuce, if appropriate.

- The first part of the urine stream is passed into the toilet to exclude meatal contamination
- The middle part of the urine stream is collected into a clean container
- The remaining urine is passed into the toilet
- Pour the urine into a sterile container
- For viral investigation pour the urine into viral transport medium.

Clean–catch, pad or bag specimen

The use of urine pads for collection of urine samples for microbiological analysis was introduced in the mid-1990s and has gained popularity, given that the child's comfort is enhanced and that it is possible to extract an appropriate amount of urine without difficulty (MacFarlane et al 2005). Given its ease of use, it is possible for parents to collect specimens. However, caution has been raised with regard to the filtering effect of the pad fibres and the high contamination rates of up to 68% (Poole 2002).

Bag samples are equally unhelpful (Al-Orifi et al 2000), whereas clean-catch samples are least likely to need repeating, with several studies reporting low contamination rates for the clean-catch method (MacFarlane et al 1999, Ramage et al 1999, Poole 2002, Whiting et al 2006).

1. Select the correct size of sterile urine bag to avoid leakage or contamination with faeces.
2. Remove the protective seal:
   a. For the female, place the bag over the vulva, starting from the perineum and working upwards, sticking the bag to the skin.
   b. For the male, place the bag over the penis.
3. Observe the bag frequently until urine is passed, to avoid leakage.
4. Remove the bag and pour the urine into a sterile container.
5. For viral investigation pour the urine into viral transport medium.
6. Wash the genitalia after the procedure to prevent soreness of the skin (see comments on clinical, psychosocial and cultural issues, above).

Catheter specimen

This is collected from the self-sealing bung of the urinary drainage tubing in a child who is already catheterised. Do not disconnect the closed drainage system, as infection may be introduced, nor take the sample from the urinary drainage bag, as the specimen may be contaminated.

- Using an aseptic technique, clean the bung with an alcohol swab and allow to dry.
- Using a sterile syringe and needle, insert the needle into the bung at an angle of 45°. This will minimise penetration of the wall of the tubing and subsequent needlestick injury.
- Gently withdraw the urine into the syringe.
- Remove the needle and syringe, wipe the area with the alcohol swab and allow to dry. The rubber bung will self-seal.
- Place the urine in a sterile container.
- Discard the needle and syringe into a sharps container.

Obtaining urine from a Mitrofanoff stoma

The specimen should be obtained by a nurse who is familiar with the Mitrofanoff operation and the specific anatomy of the area on the child.

- The specimen should ideally be taken in conjunction with normal bladder emptying.
- A new sterile catheter of the child's normal catheter size should be used.
- Clean the stoma with soap and water and dry.
- Gently insert the lubricated sterile catheter into the stoma and collect the urine into a sterile container. A water-soluble lubricant should be used.
- Ensure that the bladder is completely empty before withdrawing the catheter.
- Wipe the area dry with a tissue.

VAGINAL SWAB

The taking of this specimen in children should be avoided where possible because of its invasive nature. Also, because of potential legal implications (why the procedure is necessary), it is usually carried out by an appropriately trained health professional or police surgeon.

- In the case of suspected or actual sexual abuse, do not clean the area. Identification of semen or sexually transmitted diseases may be required for evidence.
- Expose the vaginal area and part the labia.
- Gently insert a cotton wool swab into the outer entrance of the vagina. Care must be taken not to tear the hymen, if intact.
- Place the swab into transport medium.
- For suspected *Chlamydia* infection:
  - Obtain special transport medium
  - Use a pernasal swab and gently rotate the swab in the vaginal orifice
  - Place in transport medium.

BLOOD SAMPLES

Venepuncture or capillary blood sampling may be performed by a nurse who is trained in the procedure (DoH 2007). As there are many haematological (Higgins 1995b, 1997), biochemical (Higgins 1996), immunological and microbiological blood tests, the nurse should check local protocols as to the appropriate laboratory containers required for specific tests and the amount of blood required. Protective clothing, such as gloves, aprons and facial protection as appropriate should be used along with an aseptic technique (Jackson 1997, Campbell et al 1999) (see also Chs 4, 33 and 34).

Blood culture

Isolation of a causative organism is enhanced by careful collection of the blood, using a sterile technique to avoid skin contamination (Higgins 1995c, Campbell et al 1999). Sterile gloves should be used. The specimen should preferably be taken during pyrexial episodes, as the organism may be present in greater numbers. The following procedure is based on the Department of Health (2007) taking blood culture best practice guidelines.

- Use blood culture bottles according to local policy.
- Always make a fresh stab. Existing peripheral lines/cannulae must not be used.
- The skin must be decontaminated with an alcohol-based antiseptic agent such as 2% chlorhexidine in 70% isopropyl alcohol, and allowed to dry.
- *Do not* palpate the site again once it has been disinfected.
- After withdrawing the blood, insert the blood into the container with a new sterile needle as there is a risk of contamination of skin organisms on the needle used to withdraw the blood. The top of the culture bottle should be cleaned with 2% chlorhexidine in 70% isopropyl alcohol and allowed to dry before inserting the blood specimen.
- Place as much blood as possible (up to 3–5 mL) in the bottles.
- Inoculation of the blood into the blood culture bottles should be performed first, before inserting blood into other bottles, as many of these other bottles are not sterile and accidental contamination may occur.
- In children in whom line sepsis is suspected, blood for culture may be taken from a peripheral vein stab and also from the appropriate intravascular lines to enable identification of colonisation of the line. In cases of suspected bacterial endocarditis, more than one blood culture (three where possible) should be taken to ensure isolation of organisms which may be low in number.
- Blood culture bottles should be placed into an incubator at 37°C to enhance growth of the organism.

ANALYSIS OF ANTIBIOTIC LEVELS

The relationship between drug dose, drug concentration in biological fluid and the individual child's metabolic process must be understood for interpreting results. The results may be affected by the route of administration, the age of the child and the disease process, such as liver and renal disease. Analysis involves testing levels in blood serum in direct relationship to drug administration.

- For intravenous antibiotic bolus administration, the first blood sample (trough) is taken just before the dose is given. The second sample (peak) is taken 30–60 min after the dose is given. The time may vary according to local policy and the drug given.
- Record on the laboratory form the drug, the dose and the mode of administration; the time the drug is given and whether the sample is a peak or trough level.
- Levels of antibiotics given other than intravenously must be discussed locally with the microbiologist because interpretation of the results will differ for drugs given by other routes.
- Blood for antibiotic assay must not be taken through the same catheter which has been used to give the antibiotic at any time. Antibiotics bind to plastic and the drug may release intermittently, giving false results. The same principle applies for some other drugs such as glucose.

VESICULAR FLUID FOR ELECTRON MICROSCOPY

Explain to the child that the procedure is usually pain-free, as the needle only penetrates the vesicle not the skin.

Virus particles can be seen under electron microscopy and, combined with the clinical presentation, may aid rapid diagnosis. The vesicular fluid should also be cultured in order to confirm the clinical diagnosis such as varicella-zoster (chickenpox or shingles) or herpes simplex.

- Obtain a glass slide with a marked area for the specimen, a slide holder, sterile syringe and needle, sterile swab and viral transport medium.
- Pierce the top of the vesicle with a sterile needle and, if there is sufficient fluid, draw up the exudate into a syringe. Keep the needle flush to the skin to prevent accidental stabbing if the

child moves. Remove the needle and seal the end of the syringe with a sterile cap. Dispose of the needle in a sharps bin.
- If there is minimal fluid, place the marked area of the glass slide over the vesicular fluid to allow the fluid to attach to the slide. Let it dry.
- Place the syringe in a safe container or place the glass slide in a slide holder.
- Dip the sterile swab into the transport medium, then rotate it gently over the vesicle fluid on the skin. Place the swab into the transport medium.
- Place a sterile dressing over the vesicle until dry.

FUNGAL SAMPLES OF HAIR, NAIL AND SKIN

Special containers may be obtained locally from the microbiology department.

- Samples of infected hair should be removed by plucking the hair with forceps or gloves. The root of the hair is infected, not the shaft.
- Samples of the whole thickness of the nail or deep scrapings should be obtained (Smoker 1999).
- The skin should be cleaned with an alcohol swab. Epidermal scales scraped from the active edge of a lesion or the roof of any vesicle should be obtained.

GASTRIC WASHINGS

Swallowed sputum containing tubercle bacilli may be obtained through gastric washings. Children generally do not produce sufficient sputum, therefore gastric washings are obtained for laboratory analysis to aid diagnosis of pulmonary *Mycobacterium tuberculosis*. If alcohol-acid-fast bacilli are seen under the microscope, further tests are performed to aid the provisional diagnosis. Culture of the organism may take between 6 and 12 weeks to confirm diagnosis. Three consecutive early-morning specimens should be obtained. There are usually only small numbers of organisms present, so as much material as possible should be obtained. As alcohol–acid-fast bacilli are often found in tap water, sterile water must be used.

- Fast the child for at least 6 hours overnight
- Pass a nasogastric tube (see Ch. 40)
- Aspirate the stomach contents and place in a sterile container

- Instil at least 30 mL of sterile water down the tube to obtain as much stomach content as possible
- Aspirate the contents and place in the same container
- Remove the tube, if appropriate.

BIOPSY MATERIAL

Specimens such as skin, muscle, kidney, liver, jejunal tissue or brain biopsies are generally obtained by medical staff under either general or local anaesthetic according to the site. A sterile technique is required for all these procedures. All biopsy specimens must be discussed with the relevant laboratory personnel in order that the most appropriate specimen and laboratory tests are undertaken to aid diagnosis; selection of tests may be necessary if the specimen is small. *Note*: a fixative such as formalin is not used for microbiological investigation.

CEREBROSPINAL FLUID

Cerebrospinal fluid (CSF) is commonly obtained via a lumbar puncture performed by medical staff (see Ch. 16). A sterile technique is required as there is a risk of introducing infection, or causing meningitis. Specimens of CSF should be dispatched to the laboratory immediately. Do not store the specimen in a refrigerator, as this causes the cells to lyse and deteriorate rapidly, thus giving rise to false results.

COMMUNITY PERSPECTIVE

The types of specimen that can be taken in the home are limited. These may include routine specimens of:
- Blood, urine and stools
- Swabs from wounds, skin, throat, eyes, etc.

Consideration must be given to the transportation of such specimens to the laboratory. It would not be appropriate for specimens to be carried around in a hot car for several hours, so visits will need to be planned. It is worth considering the use of a cool bag. Some specimens, e.g. stool and urine samples, can be taken to the GP's surgery, from where they are collected and taken to the local hospital. This may help the family and the CCN by diminishing the need for hospital visits.

References

Advisory Committee on Dangerous Pathogens, 1997. Management and control of viral haemorrhagic fevers. HMSO, London.

Advisory Committee on Dangerous Pathogens, 2003. Infection at work: controlling the risks. A guide for employers and the self employed on identifying, assessing and controlling the risks of infection in the workplace. TSO, London.

Advisory Committee on Dangerous Pathogens, 2005. Biological agents: managing the risks in laboratories and healthcare premises. TSO, London.

Ahmed, T., Vickers, D., Campbell, S., et al., 1991. Urine collection from disposable nappies. Lancet 338, 674–676.

Al-Orifi, F., McGillivray, D., Tange, S., et al., 2000. Urine culture from bag specimens in young children: are the risks too high? J. Pediatr. 137 (2), 221–226.

Baillie, L., 2001. Developing practical nursing skills. Arnold, London.

Camm, J., 2004. What does it take to ensure effective hand decontamination by nurses? Prof. Nurse 19 (12), 26–28.

Campbell, H., Carrington, M., Limber, C., 1999. A practical guide to venepuncture and management of complications. Br. J. Nurs. 8 (7), 426–431.

Department of Health, 1990. Spills of urine: potential risk of misuse of chlorine-releasing disinfecting agents. Safety Action Bulletin SAB (90)41, DoH, London.

Department of Health, 1998. Guidance for clinical healthcare workers: protection against infection with blood-borne viruses. Recommendations of the Expert Advisory Group on AIDS and the Advisory Group on Hepatitis. DoH, Wetherby.

Department of Health, 2001a. Reference guide to consent for examination or treatment. DoH, London.

Department of Health, 2001b. Seeking consent: working with children. DoH, London.

Department of Health, 2003. Winning ways: working together to reduce healthcare associated infection in England. Report from the Chief Medical Officer. DoH, London.

Department of Health, 2004. The NHS healthcare cleaning manual. DoH, London.

Department of Health, 2007. Taking blood cultures. A summary of best practice. DoH, London.

Dougherty, L., Lister, S., 2004. The Royal Marsden manual of clinical nursing procedures, sixth ed. Blackwell, London.

Deville, W., Yzermans, J.C., van Duijn, N.P., et al., 2004. The urine dipstick test to rule out infections. A meta-analysis of the accuracy. BMC Urol. 4, 4.

Gould, D., 2001. Clean surgical wounds: prevention of infection. Nurs. Stand. 15 (49), 45–56.

Griffiths, C., 1995. Microbiological examination in urinary tract infection. Nurs. Times 91 (11), 33–35.

Griffiths, D.M., Woodward, M.N., 1993. Use of dipsticks for routine analysis of urine from children with acute abdominal pain. Br. Med. J. 306, 1512–1513.

Hampton, S., 2004. Wound colonization explained. Nurse2Nurse 4 (4), 34–36.

Health and Safety Executive, 1999. Safe Transport of Dangerous Goods Act 1999. TSO, London.

Health and Safety Executive 2002 The control of substances hazardous to health regulations (COSHH), 1999. Code of practice. TSO, London.

Health and Safety Executive, 2005. A brief guide to the regulations. What so we need to know about the Control of Substances Hazardous to Health Regulations 2002 (COSHH). TSO, London.

Health Protection Agency, 2004. Online. Available: www.hpa. org.uk.

Higgins, C., 1995a. Microbiological examination of urine in urinary tract infection. Nurs. Times 91 (11), 33–35.

Higgins, C., 1995b. Full blood count (RBC, Hb, PCV, MCV, MCH and reticulocytes). Nurs. Times 91 (7), 38–40.

Higgins, C., 1995c. Microbiological examination of blood for septicaemia. Nurs. Times 91 (16), 34–35.

Higgins, C., 1996. Laboratory measurement of sodium and potassium. Nurs. Times 92 (12), 40–42.

Higgins, C., 1997. Erythrocyte sedimentation test as an aid to diagnosis. Nurs. Times 93 (6), 60–61.

Higgins, D., 2008a. Specimen Collection Part 3 collecting a stool specimen. Nurs. Times 104 (19), 22–23.

Higgins, D., 2008b. Specimen Collection Part 4 obtaining a nose swab. Nurs. Times 104 (20), 26–27.

Higgins, D., 2008c. Specimen Collection. Obtaining a midstream specimen of urine 104 (17), 26–27.

Hilton, S., Baker, F., 2003. Transmission of infection. Prof. Nurse 18 (9), Card insert 2.

Infection Control Nurses Association, 1997. Guidelines for hand hygiene. ICNA, Edinburgh.

Jackson, A., 1997. Performing peripheral intravenous cannulation. Prof. Nurse 13 (1), 21–25.

MacFarlane, P., Houghton, C., Hughes, C., 1999. Pad urine collection for early childhood urinary-tract infection. Lancet 354 (9178), 571.

Nursing and Midwifery Council, 2008. The Code. Standards of conduct, performance and ethics for nurses and midwives. NMC, London.

Poole, C., 2002. Diagnosis and management of urinary tract infection in children. Nurs. Stand. 16 (38), 47–55.

Pratt, R., Pellowe, C., Wilson, J., et al., 2007. Epic 2: National evidence-based guidelines for preventing healthcare associated infections in NHS hospitals in England. J. Hosp. Infect. 65S, S1–S64.

Ramage, I., Chapman, J., Hollman, A., et al., 1999. Accuracy of clean catch urine collection in infancy. J. Pediatr. 135 (6), 765–767.

Royal College of Nursing, 2005. Good practice in infection prevention and control. Guidance for nursing staff. RCN, London.

Royal College of Paediatrics and Child Health, Hull, D., 2000. Guidelines for the ethical conduct of medical research involving children. Arch. Dis. Child 82 (2), 177–182.

Royal Liverpool and Broadgreen University hospitals 2004 joint pathology services, 2000. Online. Available: www.rlbuht.nhs.uk/ jps/mibspcol.htm.

Smoker, A., 1999. Fungal infections. Nurs. Stand. 13 (17), 48–56; 13 (19):43–47.

MacFarlane, P., Ellis, R., Hughes, C., et al., 2005. Urine collection pads: are samples reliable for urine chemistry and microscopy? Pediatr. Nephrol. 20, 170–179.

Whiting, P., Westwood, M., Bojke, L., et al., 2006. Clinical effectiveness and cost-effectiveness of tests for the diagnosis and investigation of urinary tract infection in children: a systematic review and economic model. Health Technol. Assess. 10 (36), ii–iv x–xiii, 1–154.

Chapter 37

Wound care

Angela Deliah Rodgers

CHAPTER CONTENTS

Introduction   354
    Learning outcomes   355
    Rationale   355
    What is healing?   355

Phases of wound healing   355
    Factors affecting healing   356

Wound assessment   357
    Guidelines when undertaking wound care   358
    Equipment   361
    Method   364
    Dos and don'ts   364

INTRODUCTION

A wound can be defined as 'a cut or break in continuity of any tissue caused by injury or operation' (Weller 2000) and, as with adults, wounds in children can occur for a variety of reasons. In general, wounds can be classified in two categories: acute and chronic. Acute wounds include injuries caused by trauma, e.g. road traffic accidents, scalds, bites, lacerations, burns, and those caused by surgical intervention. Chronic wounds in children include congenital abnormalities (ulcerated haemangiomas), underlying medical conditions (epidermolysis bullosa, EB), pressure ulcers and lesions caused by acute medical conditions (meningococcal septicaemia). It is important to remember that any wound can become chronic if the healing process is interrupted, e.g. by infection, and gets 'stuck' in either the inflammatory or proliferative phase of healing (Sibbald et al 2000).

Although children have the same physiological response to injury as adults, they can regenerate the cells required for the wound-healing process more rapidly, resulting in faster wound closure (Tendra Academy 2004).

The nurse's role in paediatric wound care, therefore, begins with an understanding of the wound healing process and the factors which may affect healing. This understanding is paramount in making an accurate assessment of any child with a wound, as the subsequent treatment plan will be heavily dependent on the outcome of that assessment. The nurse, in collaboration with the multidisciplinary team, must be able to choose the appropriate wound management strategies for the child and their family. A fundamental part of this process is recognising the need for holistic, individualised, family-centred care.

LEARNING OUTCOMES

By the end of this section you should be able to:

- Understand the physiological processes involved in healing
- Describe the factors that can delay wound healing
- Describe each phase of wound healing and the associated wound tissue type
- Understand the need for holistic wound assessment
- Use a paediatric wound assessment chart
- Understand the theory behind wound bed preparation and the TIME framework
- Consider wound healing within the context of other childhood disorders
- Understand how wound dressings work and what role they play in wound bed preparation and wound management
- Recognise the role of the multidisciplinary team in the assessment and management of paediatric wounds
- Understand the importance of family-centred care in the management of paediatric wounds.

RATIONALE

Children's nurses learn to develop holistic nursing skills and this is no different in the field of wound management. The goals for holistic wound management in children are to control pain, reduce emotional discomfort and minimise the risk of scarring (Bale & Jones 2006). Many factors can delay and complicate healing: poor tissue perfusion and oxygenation, poor nutritional status, infection, underlying medical conditions and extremes of age (Bryant 1992). The principal objectives of wound care are, first, to restore the function of injured tissue and second, to do no damage during that process of restoration (Box 37.1).

WHAT IS HEALING?

Wounds heal in two different ways: by primary or by secondary intention. Healing by primary intention indicates a process in which the wound edges are

---

BOX 37.1 Aims of wound care

- Create the optimum environment for the natural healing processes to take place
- Promote moist wound healing
- Protect from trauma and cooling
- Remove devitalised tissue and excess exudate
- Prevent infection
- Promote dignity, comfort and well-being
- Restore the function of injured tissue
- Maintain the function of the skin
- Cost-effective

---

closed as soon as possible using sutures, staples, steri-strips or glue. As there is no tissue loss, healing is rapid and usually occurs within 24–48 h. When wounds are closed in this way, granulation tissue is not visible and scar formation is minimal (Collier 1996). Surgical wounds without complications heal in this way. Healing by secondary intention occurs when there is tissue loss into the dermis and deeper layers of the skin. The wound edges are not opposed and tissue gradually regenerates from the bottom of the wound to fill the defect. This type of wound requires skilful and holistic assessment (Russell 2002a).

Healing occurs more rapidly in children than in adults for the following reasons:

- Formation of granulation tissue is faster
- Production of collagen and elastin is faster
- Quantity of fibroblasts in the wound is greater (Tendra Academy 2004).

PHASES OF WOUND HEALING

An understanding of the physiological process of wound healing is vital in making an accurate assessment of any wound; subsequent treatment will depend on the outcome of the assessment. There are three phases of wound healing:

1. The inflammatory phase
2. The proliferative phase
3. The maturative phase.

Inflammatory phase

When tissue is damaged, blood vessels are also damaged and the clotting process is started. Damaged cells release histamine causing vasodilatation and increased permeability of the blood vessels, delivering neutrophils and monocytes to the area (Collier 1996). This inflammatory response, therefore, results in all of the signs and symptoms of inflammation:

- Pain
- Heat
- Swelling
- Erythema (redness)
- Exudate production.

This is a normal and natural response and does not indicate infection. The exudate produced by the inflammatory response contains factors which actively promote healing. Its greatest importance is that it contains antibodies, leucocytes and macrophages. These collectively keep bacterial invasion and infection under control. Providing there is no infection, further injury or invasion, the inflammation gradually subsides and the exudate drains back into the circulation.

The main function of this phase is to keep the wound bed free from bacteria or other contaminants so that the optimal environment for tissue regeneration can be achieved (Collier 2003).

Proliferative phase

The main cells involved in this phase are macrophages and fibroblasts. Macrophages influence the healing process in several ways: they clear the wound of devitalised and unwanted material, release enzymes which break down necrotic tissue and are responsible for producing the cells which regulate new tissue formation (Kingsley 2002).

Fibroblasts are responsible for the production of the delicate collagen matrix laid down in the wound at this time. The matrix acts as a frame on which new capillary loops 'grow' into the wound bed. This process is known as angiogenesis. The formation of the capillary loops in the wound bed gives it a red appearance; this is known as granulation tissue. The new capillary loops are numerous and very fragile and therefore are easily damaged (Kingsley 2002).

Maturative phase

Once the wound bed is filled with granulation tissue, re-epithelialisation begins. Epithelial cells divide and begin to migrate over newly granulating tissue. A moist wound healing environment has been shown to accelerate the rate of epithelialisation and dermal repair (Winter 1962, Field & Kerstein

1994, Miller 2000, Bryan 2004). Collagen fibres, which have been randomly laid down during the proliferative phase, are also reorganised into tighter positions and over time, scarring is reduced. The scar will also change from dusky red to white in appearance due to the progressive decrease in the vascularity of the tissue (Bryan 2004, Miller 2000).

FACTORS AFFECTING HEALING

Conditions or factors that may compromise wound healing should be considered when undertaking wound assessment.

Nutrition

Adequate intake of fats, proteins and carbohydrates are required for optimal wound healing (Meghan & Barbul 2006). Encouragement must be given to the child to maintain an adequate oral intake while acknowledging cultural needs and avoiding unfamiliar foods (DoH 2003, Young 2006). Encouraging small amounts regularly may be preferable to having three large meals daily. Simple snacks such as yoghurts, cheese, and fruit can be offered at regular intervals throughout the day.

- Children who are deficient in nutrients as a result of illness, or disease, are susceptible to impaired healing:
  - Vitamin C deficiency inhibits formation of collagen fibres and capillary development
  - Protein deficiency reduces the supply of amino acids for tissue repair
  - Zinc deficiency impairs epithelialisation
- Children with special needs may have difficulty eating, drinking and swallowing; skilled assistance is therefore needed to ensure adequate intake of nutrition
- The assistance of the dietitian is also useful to ensure nutritional requirements are being met (Shepherd 2003).

Disease or pathology

- Diabetes mellitus: hyperglycaemia impairs phagocytosis, which is the engulfing and destruction of bacteria, foreign bodies and necrotic tissue by phagocytes. It also inhibits collagen synthesis and impairs circulation and capillary growth.

- Anaemia: healing is likely to be impaired through the reduction in oxygen transportation (Casey 2000).
- Compromised immunological status, such as in children with a malignancy, HIV/AIDS or an immunodeficiency disorder: healing in these conditions is delayed because of reduced efficiency of the immune system. Secondary to this is a decreased resistance to infection, which in turn will delay healing.
- Impaired circulation, as seen in some children with cardiac disorders, reduces the supply of nutrients to the wound area, and inhibits the inflammatory response and removal of debris from the wound.

Medication

- Cytotoxic drugs and radiotherapy interfere with cell proliferation during the process of healing.
- Radiation inhibits fibroblastic activity and capillary formation; it may also cause necrosis.
- Prolonged steroid therapy delays healing during the inflammatory and proliferative phases (Bale & Jones 2006). It impairs phagocytosis, inhibits fibroblast proliferation, depresses formation of granulation tissue and inhibits wound contraction.

Other causes

- Pain and stress can affect the immune system and thus interfere with wound healing.
- Foreign bodies inhibit wound closure and prolong the inflammatory response.
- Infection prolongs the inflammatory response and increases tissue destruction.
- Mechanical friction damages or destroys granulation tissue.

WOUND ASSESSMENT

The importance of holistic assessment and early identification of any factors which could delay the natural healing response is essential for a successful patient outcome (Bale 2000). The practitioner must have the required information regarding the child and the wound prior to undertaking any wound care practice. The children's nurse, in consultation with other members of the multidisciplinary team, must make an informed decision on what approach is the most appropriate for a particular child and their family.

It is helpful to consider the following factors when assessing a wound:

- Cause of the wound – remove where possible (e.g. pressure)
- Site of the wound – this will have an impact on product choice
- Clinical condition of the patient – this will impact on healing rates
- Size of the wound.

After assessing these factors, the nurse must then assess the wound itself. Wounds that heal following the normal process can be managed by applying the aims of wound care (Box 37.1) and dressing requirements for children (Box 37.2). As the assessment process is so subjective, a standardised approach to wound assessment is advisable (Russell 2002b). The theory of wound bed preparation and the TIME framework (see below) can be applied to chronic wound care to facilitate the practitioner in developing a wound management plan by enabling them to identify and remove barriers to healing (Dowsett & Newton 2005).

T – tissue non-viable

It is necessary to remove all non-viable tissue from the wound bed as this can prevent wound closure and create a focus for infection (Ayello et al 2004, Schultz et al 2003)

BOX 37.2 Dressing requirements for children
▪ Comfortable
▪ Conformable
▪ Non-adherent
▪ Pain-free on application
▪ Pain-free on removal
▪ Easy to apply
▪ Hypoallergenic
▪ Waterproof
▪ Non-restrictive
▪ Non-bulky
▪ Manufactured in small sizes
▪ Skin-friendly adhesives
▪ Able to withstand children's activities: crawling, climbing, running, cycling
▪ Reasonable wear time.

Table 37.1   Methods of debridement

METHOD	DESCRIPTION	ADVANTAGES	DISADVANTAGES
Autolytic	Slough is liquefied with the use of hydrocolloid or hydrogel products	Minimal pain/trauma for child/family Cost-effective	Multiple applications may be required Consider alternative methods if no evidence of debridement
Surgical/Sharp	Removal of non-viable tissue with blade/scissors by a skilled surgeon/clinician	Fast and effective Also reduce bacterial burden	In children, a general anaesthetic is usually required Pain, bleeding, possible nerve/tendon damage Not suitable for poorly perfused or immunocompromised child or child on anticoagulants
Enzymatic	Topical application of exogenous enzymes	Can be used for patients Not suitable for surgical/sharp debridement	Daily/twice daily application required May sting on application Possible sensitivity to enzyme/carrying agent
Mechanical	Wet to dry dressings Hydrosurgery Whirlpool Irrigation	Fast/effective (hydrosurgery)	Pain, damage to newly formed tissue, drive bacteria deeper into tissue
Biological (maggot therapy)	Maggots of the *Lucilia sericata* fly secrete enzymes which break down non-viable tissue without harming healthy tissue	Fast/effective if used in sufficient numbers Also reduce bacterial burden	Child/family acceptance Excoriation of surrounding skin if not well protected Not suitable for hard eschar

Non-viable tissue can be removed by debridement. There are five methods of debridement available (see Table 37.1). Debridement is an ongoing process and more than one method may be required.

I – infection and/or inflammation

Contamination or colonisation of chronic wounds is considered to be normal, however if the wound becomes critically colonised or infected, the bacterial burden on the wound has to be reduced (Ayello et al 2004).

A critically colonised or infected wound is characterised by a host response, i.e. fever, warmth oedema, swelling, pain, erythema and purulent discharge (Schultz et al 2003).

An antimicrobial topical preparation or dressing along with antibiotics to treat systemic infection may be required and the frequency of dressing changes may need to be increased.

M – moisture imbalance

Excess amounts of exudate can cause maceration of the skin surrounding the wound which in turn can lead to dessication of the tissue and an increase in wound size. It can also lead to an increased risk of infection as the exudate can provide a medium for the growth of bacteria

If the wound is too dry, this can inhibit the migration of epithelial cells over the wound surface and delay wound closure.

E – edge of the wound non-advancing or non-migrating

If wound closure is not achieved, there may be a problem with the wound in relation to the T, I or M and/or the factors that may affect healing.

This is a useful tool in helping the nurse prioritise the various aspects of the wound itself by treating the dominant factor first (T, I or M) and is also an aid for product selection. An effective wound assessment should therefore consider the components identified above and document all findings accurately after each dressing change in the wound assessment chart or nursing notes. An example of a wound assessment chart is presented in Figure 37.1.

GUIDELINES WHEN UNDERTAKING WOUND CARE

Local policies and guidelines may be in place to help the nurse when undertaking wound care. An example of Best Practice Guidelines is presented in Box 37.3.

Ⓐ Paediatric Wound Assessment Chart

Name: . . . .

Unit No: . . . . DoB: . . . . Consultant: . . . .

Date of initial assessment: . . . .

Does drug therapy at present include any of the following:

	YES	NO
Steroids	☐	☐
Chemotherapy	☐	☐
Insulin	☐	☐
Antibiotics	☐	☐
Inotropes	☐	☐

Draw site of wounds:

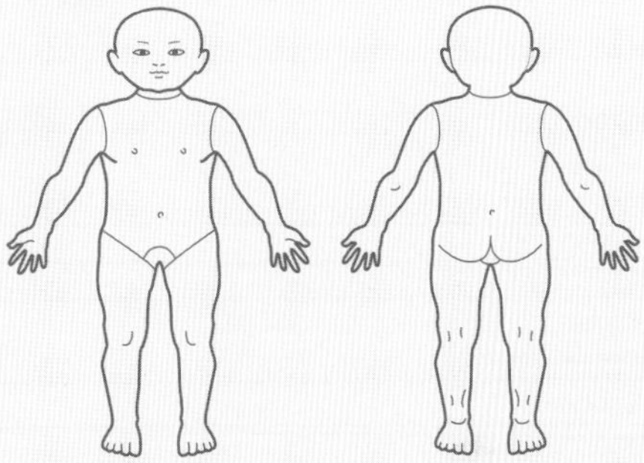

Front   Back

Cause of wound: . . . .

Now include wound care in nursing care plan

Initial wound assessment:

| NB | There may be more than one type of tissue in wound |

✓

Pink	☐
Red	☐
Yellow	☐
Black	☐
Dark red and raised	☐

Describe:
· Wound appearance . . . .
· Wound size . . . .
· Type of exudate (if any) . . . .
· Condition of surrounding skin . . . .

If wound is a PRESSURE SORE please plan to use a pressure relieving surface and document in care plan

Nutritional status: If poor contact Dietitian   Dietitian contacted: YES ☐   NO ☐

☐ Good   ☐ Satisfactory   ☐ Poor

Figure 37.1 (A,B) Paediatric wound assessment charts.

(Continued)

Wound cleansing

The purpose of wound cleansing is to remove dressing debris or wound debris (necrotic tissue, sloughy tissue), both of which can act as a focus for infection (Bale & Jones 2006). This procedure should only be performed when there is an indication that it will either benefit the healing process or prevent infection (Blunt 2001). It follows, therefore, that routine wound cleansing is not advised and may indeed be detrimental to the

(B)   Paediatric Wound Assessment Chart

Name .... Hosp No............... DoB............. Consultant ....

	Date	Date	Date
Analgesia used	YES ☐ NO ☐	YES ☐ NO ☐	YES ☐ NO ☐
Wound appearance and size (cm)			
Colour of wound bed:	Pink ☐ Red ☐ Yellow ☐ Black ☐ Dark red ☐	Pink ☐ Red ☐ Yellow ☐ Black ☐ Dark red ☐	Pink ☐ Red ☐ Yellow ☐ Black ☐ Dark red ☐
Exudate and type			
Odour			
Swab taken NB After wound cleansing			
Photograph (✓)			
Document treatment carried out			
Document dressing applied			
Reviewed by:	Dietitian / Tissue viability nurse / Medical staff	Dietitian / Tissue viability nurse / Medical staff	Dietitian / Tissue viability nurse / Medical staff
	Next dressing change / Signature and designation	Next dressing change / Signature and designation	Next dressing change / Signature and designation

Document wound care in care plan after each dressing change

Figure 37.1—Cont'd

wound healing process. Modern interactive dressings such as hydrocolloids and hydrogels can be used to soften and hydrate necrotic tissue before cleansing. This makes the process less traumatic when removing dead tissue. The use of this type of product has implications for practice and suggests daily changes of dressing and cleaning of wounds should be discouraged where possible to allow the product to work to its fullest potential.

Irrigation

Cleansing by irrigation with warmed solutions (tap water, sterile water, normal saline) will prevent the shedding of fibres into the wound bed and is less traumatic for the child. This technique is now being advocated (Bale & Jones 2006). However, one of the difficulties of this method is in assessing the amount of pressure to be used when irrigating; it should be enough to dislodge debris without causing damage to the underlying tissues (Wayne 2009).

Cleansing by bathing and showering

Bathing and showering are appropriate methods for wound cleansing (Joanna Briggs Institute 2008), particularly for children. The use of bathing and showering in paediatrics is much less frightening and traumatic than other methods of wound cleansing and it can also be a playful experience. Many children prefer to remove their own dressings by soaking them off in the bath or shower.

BOX 37.3 Best Practice Guidelines for caring for patients with wounds

Statement

Wound assessment and treatment should be based on a basic understanding of tissue repair and factors affecting the healing process.

The named nurse is personally accountable for their practice and, in exercising professional accountability, may therefore enhance their skills by caring for a patient with a wound as per trust hospital guidelines. The named nurse should recognise when they are unable to deal with a wound due to lack of experience/knowledge and should contact the tissue viability nurse for advice.

Aim

- Wound management will be approached holistically and tailored to the needs of the child and family
- Wound assessment will be carried out prior to application of any wound management products
- Wound management products used will be appropriate for the stage of healing
- Accurate documentation will be undertaken at each dressing change
- The nurse will work in partnership with medical staff, seeking their cooperation when necessary to ensure patient needs are met in a safe and effective manner

Guidelines

- Nursing staff caring for patients with wounds should have a basic understanding of the stages of wound healing
- Nursing staff caring for patients with wounds should be aware of factors affecting healing

- Wound assessment should take place prior to application of any wound management product
- Progress will be documented on the wound assessment chart at each dressing change

Dressing procedure

- Ensure the patient has had adequate analgesia prior to the procedure
- Assemble all equipment required prior to the procedure to ensure wound exposure time is kept to a minimum
- Apply the principles of aseptic technique to reduce the risk of infection
- Clean the wound only if necessary using warmed normal saline or tap water and a 20 mL syringe
- *Do not* dry the wound
- Select an appropriate dressing product using the wound assessment flow chart and wound formulary
- Document assessment and treatment on the wound assessment chart and in the care plan
- Plan and document the wound review date
- If the wound is complex or slow to heal, contact the tissue viability nurse
- Contact other relevant members of the multidisciplinary team if required (e.g. medical staff, community nursing team, pharmacy)
- If dressing products are required for wound care at home, contact the Community Nursing Team and provide the patient with a 7-day supply of products.

In surgical wounds, once skin edges have sealed, bathing or showering is not likely to present any further risk (Briggs 1997). In hospitals, the issue of cross contamination must be considered; therefore careful measures for disinfection of the bath must be taken between children using it. It is also not recommended that the wound be cleansed in a power shower as this may cause trauma to the wound bed.

Wound dressings

Children are a challenging group where wound dressings are concerned. Box 37.3 illustrates the specific requirements of wound management products for the paediatric population. There are many and varied dressings available for the paediatric nurse to choose from; Table 37.2 contains examples of and information on some products suitable for use on children.

EQUIPMENT

- Trolley or appropriate clean surface
- Sterile dressing pack containing plastic tray, non-woven swabs, sterile towel
- Sterile latex-free gloves
- Plastic disposable apron
- Large disposable plastic bag for soiled disposables
- Appropriate dressing materials.

Table 37.2   Examples of and information on dressings suitable for use on children

CATEGORY OF PRODUCT	EXAMPLE OF PRODUCT	MODE OF ACTION	INDICATIONS FOR USE	CONTRAINDICATIONS FOR USE	SPECIAL CONSIDERATIONS	FREQUENCY OF DRESSING CHANGE
Non-adherent contact layer	Mepitel (Mölnlycke) NA Ultra (Systagenix) Urgotul (Urgo)	Protects fragile tissue Non-adherent over wound surface area and helps to maintain a moist environment	Clean granular wounds Epithelialising tissue Wounds with low-moderate exudate	Necrotic tissue (unless conservative management being applied) Suitable for most wound types as long as correct secondary dressing chosen to absorb exudate	Requires secondary dressing Can be used with topical applications, e.g. silver sulfadiazine (Flamazine)	May be left in place for up to 7 days *Note*: If wound heavily exudating, not advisable to leave dressing for 7 days; 2–5 days more realistic in paediatric arena
Hydro-colloid	DuoDERM, Granuflex (ConvaTec) Hydrocoll (Hartmann)	Mixture of sodium carboxymethyl-cellulose, pectin and adhesive polymers Occlusive therefore fulfils many of ideal dressing criteria Forms a gel which bathes the wound as it absorbs fluid	Superficial grazes, minor skin abrasions (extra thin versions only) Rehydrating dry, crusty wounds, e.g. pressure sores Necrotic tissue	Wounds with large amounts of exudate critically colonized or infected wounds	Products come in an extra-thin variety and small sizes, particularly appropriate for paediatric population Waterproof therefore child can bath/shower with dressing *in situ* No secondary dressing required	May be left in place for up to 7 days Dressing needs to be changed when gel 'bubbles' in centre of dressing
Hydrofibre	Aquacel, Aquacel Ag (ConvaTec)	Hydrocolloid fibres Converts to gel when in contact with exudate Locks bacteria in dressing facilitating reduction of bacterial burden at wound surface area Aquacel Ag is combined with silver to increase bacteriostatic effect	Wounds with moderate–high exudate levels Heavily colonised wounds	Dry wounds or those with low exudate levels	Needs a secondary dressing Foam dressings appropriate if large amount of exudate otherwise a thin hydrocolloid may be more appropriate	May be left in place for up to 5 days *Note*: If wound heavily exuding, not advisable to leave dressing for 5 days; 2–5 days more realistic in paediatric arena
Film dressings	Tegaderm (3M) i.v. 3000 (Smith & Nephew)	Semi-permeable therefore allows passage of varying amounts of moisture from the wound surface Covers and provides protective layer over shallow, non-exuding wounds	Used to secure i.v. cannulae (i.v. 3000) and for the application of topical local anaesthetics, e.g. EMLA cream As a secondary dressing with hydrogels (Tegaderm only) to maintain moisture at the wound surface	Wounds with high levels of exudate which gathers under the film	Potential for adhesive trauma on removal from skin Use a non-toxic medical remover or lateral stretch technique to remove Can be difficult to apply as dressing can stick to itself if backing removed incorrectly	May be left in place for up to 7 days If used as secondary dressing with hydrogel, 2–5 days more realistic in paediatric arena
	Cavilon non-sting barrier film (3M)	Non-sting protective transparent barrier film 'Coats' skin to act as protective barrier from adhesive tapes, urine, faeces Is not removed by washing	Protects fragile and excoriated skin Used as treatment for severe nappy rash Good for prevention of excoriation under nasogastric/	Sensitivity to film contents Needs at least 30–60 s drying time after application Take care not to apply	Non-sting property means pain-free application Comes in foam applicator or pump spray	Re-apply every 48–72 h

Alginate	Sorbsan (Aspen Medical) Kaltostat (ConvaTec)	Manufactured from seaweed Combination of mannuronic and guluronic acid Also contain varying concentrations of calcium Turns to gel when in contact with exudate	Wounds with moderate–high exudate levels Donor sites/haemangiomas (Kaltostat is also a haemostat)	Dry wounds or those with low exudate levels	Needs a secondary dressing which will cope with exudate levels; foam dressings appropriate Can be difficult to remove from cavities Have potential to adhere if exudate level not sufficient to make dressing gel	May be left in place for up to 5 days Note: If wound heavily exudating, not advisable to leave dressing for 5 days; 2–5 days more realistic in paediatric arena
Hydrogel	IntraSite gel, IntraSite conformable (Smith & Nephew) ActiForm-Cool (Activa Healthcare)	Carboxymethyl–cellulose gel Draws exudate into gel while donating fluid to the wound Promotes a moist healing environment	Dry, necrotic wounds Superficial grazes and excoriated skin	Wounds with large amounts of exudate Maceration to surrounding skin	Needs a secondary dressing; film dressings most appropriate Be careful not to use a secondary dressing which will absorb the gel (e.g. foam)	May be left in place for up to 5 days Note: Not always appropriate to leave dressing for this long; 1–3 days more realistic in paediatric arena
Foam dressings	Tielle (Systagenix) Allevyn & Allevyn gentle border (Smith & Nephew) Mepilex border (Molnlycke Healthcare) Poly-mem (Aspen Medical)	Absorb exudate into dressing, thus controlling level of moisture at the wound surface Insulates wound Depending on product chosen, can also protect epithelialising tissue, e.g. Tielle Lite	Depends on type of foam used Will absorb varying degrees of exudate Wounds with moderate–high exudate levels, e.g. Tielle, Tielle Plus, Allevyn Flat wounds and shallow cavities Foam conforms to shape of cavity Wounds with low exudate levels, e.g. Tielle Lite, Allevyn Thin	Necrotic tissue Suitable for most wound types as long as correct type of foam chosen after exudate assessment	Some foams require a secondary dressing If using adherent foam dressing, remove carefully as adhesive can damage sensitive skin Some adherent foam dressings can be removed painlessly using water others have silicone gel adhesives for atraumatic dressing removal e.g. Allevyn gentle border, Mepilex border	May be left in place for up to 5 days Note: If wound heavily exuding, not advisable to leave dressing for 5 days; 3 days more realistic in paediatric arena
Antimicrobial dressings	Acticoat (Smith & Nephew) Aquacel Ag (ConvaTec) Urgotul SSD (Urgo) Activon products (Advancis Medical)	Reduces bacterial burden and odour in wounds Some honey dressings will also facilitate autolytic debridement	Wounds which are critically colonised or locally infected Product chosen will depend on tissue type and exudate level of wound	Sensitivity to silver Serum silver levels amy require monitoring in prolonged/repeated use of silver dressings Renal impairment	Some antimicrobial products require a secondary dressing	May be left in place for up to 7 days Note: If wound heavily exudating, not advisable to leave dressing for 7 days; 1–5 days more realistic in paediatric arena Some honey products can cause pain on application please remove and irrigate the wound and select a different product

METHOD

Preparation of the child

1. Assess the child for the need for analgesia, which should be given at least half an hour prior to the dressing change.
2. Explain the procedure to the child in an age-appropriate manner and to the main caregivers. Ensure understanding and identify their role throughout the dressing change.
3. Use play and involve the play specialist if appropriate.
4. Allow enough time between information giving and performing the practice – too much time may cause the child to become anxious, too little may not allow the play specialist time to prepare the child adequately.
5. Introduce the use of distraction, where appropriate.
6. Ensure that all the potential equipment required is on the dressing trolley.
7. Positioning of the child will depend on the site or location of the wound. Choose a position that is most comfortable and reassuring for the child, ensuring that the wound is easily accessible. Infants or small children can lie or sit on an adult's lap, if the wound site permits. Ensure that the child is in a safe position throughout.
8. If wound cleansing is required, a bath or shower is a less traumatic method for the child and is an effective way to soak off dressings.
9. Ensure that the child is kept warm and dressing time is kept to a minimum, thus decreasing heat loss and discomfort for the child.
10. Ensure that a young child has their favourite cuddly toy, or comforter, with them throughout.

Wound care practice

1. Ensure adequate time is available to undertake the wound dressing.
2. Explain all the steps of the practice, in advance of them occurring, and throughout, to the child and parent if considered appropriate.
3. Ensure thorough hand washing prior to commencing the procedure.
4. Perform the dressing using a non-touch technique.

5. If appropriate, allow the child, as far as is possible, to remove the dressing gently, avoiding damage to new granulation or epithelial tissue (this may be undertaken in the shower/bath or with the use of a non-toxic medical adhesive remover).
6. If further cleansing is required (including after the bath or shower), irrigate using a syringe with a warmed solution (water, normal saline).
7. Assess the wound and surrounding skin.
8. The choice of dressing for the contact layer, which is the primary dressing, will depend on the type of tissue categorised and the level of exudate (Harding & Jones 1996).
9. The choice of secondary dressing will often depend on the contact layer (Harding & Jones 1996).
10. Assess pain at the wound site.
11. Secure the dressing using an appropriate method.
12. For children who have special needs, it may be difficult to carry out aseptic non-touch technique at dressing changes. With this group of children, it is even more important that their dressing is secured; to avoid the use of tape that can be easily removed may require some creative thinking.
13. Document the assessment and management by completing the wound assessment and treatment chart, and record information in the child's nursing notes.

COMMUNITY PERSPECTIVE

The principles when undertaking wound care in the community are the same as in hospital; however, the CCN may need to adapt to maintain safe practice in the home (see Ch. 34). Analgesia, if required, may be given prior to the CCN's visit, allowing time for the drug to work; alternatively, Entonox may be self-administered by the child during the procedure.

DOS AND DON'TS

- Do involve the child and family.
- Do ensure that the multidisciplinary team are involved.
- Do individualise the child's wound care.

- Do assess the wound systematically, using where possible an assessment tool.
- Do record wound assessment and wound care on the wound assessment chart and in the nursing notes.
- Do minimise wound care problems by introducing evidence-based care.
- Do consider the factors that may influence wound healing.
- Do use play and distraction when undertaking wound care practice.

- Do assess the child for the need for analgesia.
- Do complete the dressing change as quickly as practical.
- Do encourage bathing or showering as a wound cleansing option.
- Do not use cotton wool balls.
- Do not routinely cleanse the wound.
- Do not use force to remove a dressing.
- Do not use alcoholic solution of povidone-iodine (Betadine) on wounds.

References

Ayello, E.A., Dowsett, C., Schultz, G.S., et al., 2004. TIME heals all wounds. Nursing 34 (4), 36–42.

Bale, S., Harding, K., Leaper, D. (Eds.), 2000. An introduction to wounds. EMAP Healthcare, London.

Bale, S., Jones, V., 2006. Wound care nursing. A patient-centred approach, second ed. Elsevier, London.

Blunt, J., 2001. Wound cleansing: ritualistic or research-based practice? Nurs. Stand. 16 (1), 33–36.

Briggs, M., 1997. Principles of closed surgical wound care. J. Wound Care 6 (6), 288–292.

Bryan, J., 2004. Moist wound healing: a concept that changed our practice. J. Wound Care 13 (6), 227–228.

Bryant, R., 1992. Acute and chronic wounds: nursing management. Mosby, London.

Casey, G., 2000. Modern wound dressings. Nurs. Stand. 15 (5), 47–57.

Collier, M., 1996. The principles of optimum wound management. Nurs. Stand. 10 (43), 47–52.

Collier, M., 2003. Wound bed preparation: theory to practice. Nurs. Stand. 17 (36), 45–52.

Department of Health, 2003. Getting the right start: National service framework for children. Standard

for hospital services. HMSO, London.

Dowsett, C., Newton, H., 2005. Wound bed preparation: TIME in practice. Wounds UK 1 (3), 58–70.

Field, C., Kerstein, M., 1994. Overview of wound healing in a moist environment. Am. J. Surg. 167 (Suppl. 1a), 25–30.

Harding, K., Jones, V., 1996. Wound management: good practice guidelines. Macmillan Magazines, London.

Joanna Briggs Institute, 2008. Solutions, techniques and pressure in wound cleansing. Nurs. Stand. 22 (27), 35–39.

Kingsley, A., 2002. Wound healing and potential therapeutic options. Prof. Nurse 17 (9), 539–544.

Meghan, A., Barbul, A., 2006. Nutrition and wound healing. Plast. Reconstr. Surg. Curr. Conc. Wound Heal. 117 (75), S425–S485.

Miller, M., 2000. Moist wound healing. Essential wound healing. EMAP Healthcare, London.

Russell, L., 2002a. Ch. 1. White, R., Harding, K. (Eds.), Trends in wound care. Quay Books, London.

Russell, L., 2002b. Ch. 10. White, R., Harding, K. (Eds.), Trends in wound care. Quay Books, London.

Schultz, G.S., Sibbald, R.G., Falanga, V., et al., 2003. Wound bed preparation: A systematic

approach to wound management. Wound Repair Regen. 11 (2), S1–S28.

Shepherd, A., 2003. Nutrition for optimum wound healing. Nurs. Stand. 18 (6), 55–58.

Sibbald, R.G., Williamson, D., Orstead, H.L., et al., 2000. Preparing the wound bed-debridement, bacterial balance and moisture balance. Ostomy Wound Manage. 46 (11), 14–37.

Tendra Academy, 2004. Best practice statement: issues in paediatric wound care. Minimising trauma and pain. Mölnlycke Health Care, Dunstable, Bedfordshire.

Wayne, L.E., 2009. Assessment and management of wounds in children. In: Kelsey, J., McEwing, G. (Eds.), Clinical skills in child health practice. Churchill Livingstone/Elsevier, London, pp. 309–318.

Weller, B.F., 2000. Nurses dictionary, twenty third ed. Baillière Tindall, London.

Winter, G.D., 1962. Formation of the scab and the rate of epithelialization of superficial wounds in the young domestic pig. Nature 193, 293–294.

Young, T., 2006. Principles of paediatric wound management. In: White, R., Denyer, J. (Eds.), Paediatric skin and wound care. Wounds UK, Aberdeen, pp. 58–69.

Further reading

Casey, G., 2002. Wound repair: advanced dressing materials. Nurs. Stand. 17 (4), 49–53.

Dowsett, C., 2002. The role of the nurse in wound bed preparation. Nurs. Stand. 16 (44), 69–76.

European Wound Management Association, 2004. Position document: wound bed preparation in practice. MEP, London.

Flecher, J., 2003. The benefits of applying wound bed preparation into practice. J. Wound Care 12, 347–349.

Hampton, S., 2004. Wound colonisation explained. Nurse2Nurse 4 (4), 34.

Miller, M., Glover, D., 1999. Wound management: theory and practice. EMAP Healthcare, London.

Morgan, D., 2000. Formulary of wound management products: a guide for healthcare staff, eighth ed. Euromed Communications, Haslemere, Surrey.

Stephen-Haynes, J., Gibson, E., 2003. Anatomy and physiology: wound healing and wound assessment. Wound Care Soc. Educ. Booklet 1 (2) Huntingdon.

Watret, L., White, R., 2001. Surgical wound management: the role of dressings. Nurs. Stand. 15 (44), 59–69.

White, R., Denyer, J., 2006. Paediatric skin and wound care. Aberdeen, Wounds UK.

Willock, J., Maylor, M., 2004. Pressure ulcers in infants and children. Nurs. Stand. 24 (18), 56–62.

World Union of Wound Healing Societies, 2004. Principles of best practice: minimising pain at wound dressing-related procedures. A consensus document MEP, London.

Useful website

http://www.tissueviabilityonline.com/

SECTION **5**

Nutritional and fluid management

SECTION CONTENTS

38. Blood glucose estimation   369

39. Feeding 1: Breast and bottle   374

40. Feeding 2: Enteral feeding   388

41. Intravenous therapy   401

Chapter 38

Blood glucose estimation

Mark Denial

CHAPTER CONTENTS

Introduction   369
   Learning outcomes   370
   Rationale   370

Educating the child and carer   370
   Guidelines   370
   Equipment   370
   Method   370
   Factors to note during the procedure   372
   Observations and complications   372
   Dos and don'ts   372

INTRODUCTION

Blood glucose estimation may be needed for a number of medical reasons within both the acute setting and the community. Within the hospital, the nurse may need to check a child's blood glucose level if the child is undergoing treatment which may *potentially* cause a rise in the blood glucose level, e.g. during the use of steroids. If the child is susceptible to hypoglycaemia or is unconscious, the blood glucose level will also be taken. Neonates in particular may be prone to hypoglycaemia and consequently may require regular blood glucose monitoring when cared for within the neonatal unit (Baumeister et al 2001). The most common reason for the monitoring of blood glucose may be associated with the management of diabetes mellitus, which also involves the education of the child and their parent/guardian.

At both ward-based level and within the child's home, blood glucose monitoring is undertaken using blood glucose meters. There are many types of excellent glucose monitors in use within the National Health Service and the selection of the meter for home use should be based on the age of the child and the skills level of the parents (Page et al 2001). In practice, however, significant inaccuracies may arise from operator related errors. Therefore healthcare professionals should use departmental devices only (Bergenstal et al 2000). The following guidelines are related to one specific method of blood glucose estimation using the Accu-Chek Advantage blood glucose meter, but the principles are the same for the majority of meters.

LEARNING OUTCOMES

By the end of this section you should be able to:

- Identify when an estimate of blood glucose level is needed
- Appreciate the need to use a finger-pricking device to obtain a sample of blood
- Appreciate the need to use the sides of the fingers for obtaining a capillary blood sample
- Use the Accu-Chek Advantage blood glucose meter
- Interpret the result, record it and liaise with other healthcare professionals when appropriate.

RATIONALE

Monitoring of blood glucose can give vital information on the current physiological status of the acutely ill child and also inform us of the effectiveness of the treatment that the child is receiving (Fain 2004). While near patient testing (NPT) can lead to improved patient care, it is considered imperative that wherever NPT is operated, it must be monitored and supervised by qualified staff with the relevant education and training. This complies with the principles of clinical governance related to standards of patient care and the control of clinical risk (Institute of Biomedical Science 2007).

EDUCATING THE CHILD AND CARER

Whenever possible, the diabetes specialist nurse, the diabetes ward link nurse or a nurse who has undergone appropriate education/training will teach the child and parent how to monitor the blood glucose levels. Staff performing NPT must be aware of the microbiological hazards of reagents and the physical or electrical hazards of any equipment in use. This equipment must be authorised for use within the setting of its proposed use and must be stored/sited so as to avoid unauthorised use (Institute of Biomedical Science 2007). This may be necessary when a child is diagnosed with insulin-dependent diabetes mellitus, or for children who are receiving treatment, or have a condition which affects their blood glucose level and who therefore require ongoing measurement within the home. When children or carers are being taught a practical skill, they need to know the importance of the procedure and how to interpret the results.

It is vital to the well-being of the child and family that adequate education is provided, as studies have shown that failing to meet the needs of the family increases the stress they feel and therefore the parents are less able to support their child (SIGN 2001).

To provide an appropriate teaching programme, the nurse has to assess the child and the child's family separately before undertaking an education plan for blood glucose measurement. Even young children have the ability to learn, and be competent in blood glucose monitoring. Play has the potential to greatly inform early childhood practice and can be used effectively in the therapeutic needs of young individuals (Hawes 2007).

GUIDELINES

It is vital that the principles of performing a capillary blood glucose measurement are followed both within the acute setting and during patient and carer education. When using a blood glucose meter, the manufacturer's instructions should be adhered to.

EQUIPMENT

- Accu-Chek Advantage blood glucose meter (Fig. 38.1)
- Advantage 2 test strips
- Finger-pricking device for multiple patient use or single patient use
- Appropriate lancet for finger pricker
- Cotton wool/gauze
- Latex-free disposable gloves
- Sharps bin.

METHOD

1. Explain the procedure to the child (if appropriate) and the family. This will help to alleviate any anxiety they may have.
2. Prepare all the equipment as listed. This will encourage a smooth procedure.
3. Ensure the meter has been quality controlled. If not, carry out this procedure first following the manufacturer's instructions.
4. Check the expiry date of the test strips. Out-of-date strips will give inaccurate results because of contamination, but if the strips have been stored correctly, they will remain stable until the expiry date.

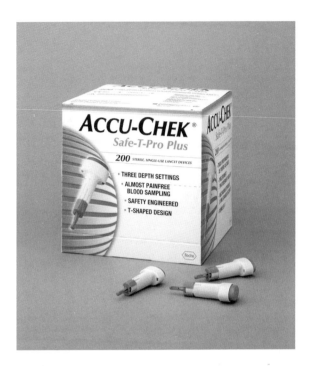

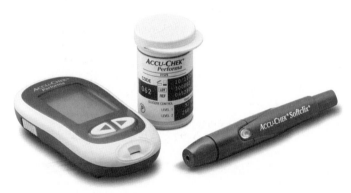

Figure 38.1 The Accu-Chek® Safe-T-Pro Plus device and the Accu-Chek® Performa blood glucose meter for use in primary care *(reproduced with permission of Roche Diagnostics Ltd).*

5. The person taking the blood sample should wash and dry their hands with soap and water to reduce the risk of cross-contamination.

6. Wash the child's hands with soap and warm water, remembering to rinse and dry thoroughly.

7. The nurse should wear gloves according to hospital policy.

8. Put the test strip into the meter and check the code on the screen with the code on the side of the box. If different, change the test strips and coding chip for new as per the manufacturer's instructions, as any results will be inaccurate.

9. Check that the length of the needle is appropriate for the child and prick the side of the finger, or heel, with either the child's own device or the one recommended by the hospital.

10. Milk the finger in a downward stroke until there is a reasonable hanging drop of blood. A drop of blood is needed to ensure full

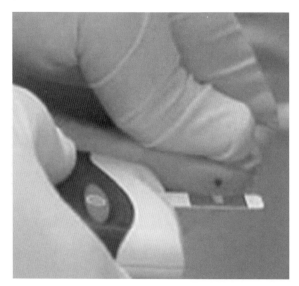

Figure 38.2 Obtaining a blood sample for checking.

- Washing hands and wearing gloves reduces the risk of cross-infection and removes any glucose from the skin.
- Warm water will also help promote blood flow to the fingers.
- A finger pricker should always be used because, owing to the measured depth of the device, it reduces the pain to the finger or heel.
- Heel pricks are needed in babies and young children to obtain a capillary sample.
- The sides of fingers should be used. Avoid using the pads of fingers as this reduces sensation. Young children use the pincer action for picking up objects and repeatedly pricking finger pads will cause more discomfort (Page et al 1999).
- If there is not enough blood, the meter will read 'ERROR'. You will need to re-check all of the above and re-test.

coverage (Fig. 38.2). *Note:* The manufacturer's instructions recommend using the *first* drop of blood acquired.

11. Move the blood glucose strip towards the drop of blood (strip will soak up blood). *Note:* Insufficient covering of the test strip will give an inaccurate result as will smearing or blotting the blood onto the pad.
12. When the strip takes up sufficient blood, the meter will beep. Count-down will then commence.
13. A second beep will be heard when the result is ready. If the meter reads 'Hi', the result is over 33.3 mmol/L; if the meter reads 'Lo', the result is under 0.6 mmol/L.
14. Record the result in a record book or on a ward/department recording sheet and report any abnormality to the medical staff if appropriate (refer to local guidelines for normal parameters).
15. Dispose of sharps immediately, according to local policy, to prevent needle stick injuries.

FACTORS TO NOTE DURING THE PROCEDURE

- Alcohol-based wipes should not be used as they will react with reagents in the strip and give a false reading.

OBSERVATIONS AND COMPLICATIONS

The normal range for blood glucose level should be 4–7 mmol/L (Page et al 1999). It is important to clarify with the medical staff at what point they should be informed if the blood test result falls outside of this range; depending on hospital policy, it may be necessary to send a blood sample for estimating true blood glucose level. This will also depend on the child's condition and treatment.

DOS AND DON'TS

- Do explain the procedure to the child and the family and the reason for the test.
- Do give the family adequate instruction and written instructions on the practice if they are to continue checking the glucose levels at home.
- Do explain the range that the blood glucose level should fall between, giving contact numbers for advice if the result is abnormal, if the family are to continue to monitor the blood glucose levels at home.
- Do ensure that the strips are stored at room temperature and the bottle is kept sealed at all times. Contamination is caused by moisture in the air and incorrect storage affects the readings.
- Do perform control tests on meters following the manufacturers' instructions. This should be

performed once a week if the child is cared for at home using a meter and as per local policy for meters in hospital.

- Do not change strips from one tube to another; all bottles have their own code number on the side of the bottle. This is especially important when using a blood glucose sensor for the

reading of the strip. There is also an expiry date on each bottle.

- Do not use Mediswabs, as they harden the skin and cause discomfort when the finger is pricked.
- Do not cut the strips, as this allows the chemicals to leak out and contaminate the rest of the strips.

References

Baumeister, F.A.M., Rolinski, B., Busch, R., et al., 2001. Glucose monitoring with long term subcutaneous microdialysis in neonates. Pediatrics 108 (5), 1187–1192.

Bergenstal, R., Pearson, J., Cembrowski, G.S., et al., 2000. Identifying variables associated with inaccurate self-monitoring of blood glucose: proposed guidelines to improve accuracy. Diabetes Educ. 26 (6), 981–989.

Fain, J.A., 2004. Helping your patient carefully weigh the available options so he can choose wisely. Nursing 34 (11), 48–51.

Hawes, D., 2007. In defense of child's play. PsycCRITIQUES-contemporary psychology: APA Review of Books 52 (19).

Institute of Biomedical Science, 2007. Point of care testing (near patient testing): guidance on the involvement of the clinical laboratory. Institute of Biomedical Science, London.

Page, N., Mackowiak, L., Bratt, K., 1999. Identifying and caring for the child with new onset Type 1 diabetes. J. Spec. Pediatr. Nurs. 4 (3), 128–130.

Page, N.E., Mackowiak, L., Bratt, K., 2001. Identifying and caring for the child with new onset type 1 diabetes. 'Ask the expert'. J. Soc. Pediatr. Nurs. 4 (3), 128–130.

SIGN, 2001. Scottish Intercollegiate Guidelines Network management of diabetes. National Clinical Guideline No. 55. SIGN, Edinburgh.

Further reading

Bannister, M., 1996. Promotion of diabetes self-care through play. Prof. Nurse 12 (2), 109–112.

International Society for Paediatric and Adolescent Diabetes, 2007.

Clinical practice consensus guidelines. Medical forum International, The Netherlands.

Selekman, J., Scofield, S., Swenson-Brousell, C., 1999. Diabetes update in the pediatric population. Pediatr. Nurs. 25 (6), 97–105.

Seley, J., 2000. Blood glucose testing. Am. J. Nurs. 100 (8), 24A–24G.

Chapter **39**

Feeding 1: Breast and bottle

Carolyn Patchell

CHAPTER CONTENTS

Introduction 374
  Learning outcomes 374
  Rationale 374
  Factors to note 375

Breastfeeding 375
  Breast milk 375
  Frequency and length of breastfeeds 376
  Equipment 376
  Method 376
  Observations and complications 378
  Expressing breast milk 379
  Dos and don'ts 380
  Eliminating 380

Artificial feeding 380
  Preparing artificial feeds 382
  Equipment 382
  Method 382
  Bottle-feeding an infant 382
  Observations and complications 384
  Dos and don'ts 384

Weaning 384

Toddler feeding 385
  Equipment 385
  Method 385
  Observations and complications 386
  Dos and don'ts 386

INTRODUCTION

A nutritionally balanced diet is essential to maximise a child's growth and promote normal development. Children are dependent upon adults to feed them safely and appropriately when young and, later, to teach them how and what to provide for themselves as they become independent.

LEARNING OUTCOMES

By the end of this section you should be able to:
- Explain how feeding impacts on a child's development
- Describe how to feed a baby and toddler
- List the benefits of breastfeeding
- Describe how to calculate a baby's feed requirements.

RATIONALE

Feeding supplies an infant with food and fluids to promote growth and to enhance recovery when ill. It also plays a vital role in development. A children's nurse must be fully aware of how, what and when to feed a child and be able to teach families, if necessary, how to feed their child.

Written guidance should be available on wards for families to support the advice they have been given. A number of publications are available from the Department of Health (DoH) and the Food Standards Agency (FSA), which give clear and easy to read guidance for families.

FACTORS TO NOTE

Assessment

The children's nurse should be familiar with how to assess the child's nutritional status. Being able to plot height and weight on a percentile chart and then interpret the results is an important skill. Children with abnormal nutritional status should be referred to a paediatric dietitian for assessment and advice. Local nutrition screening tools may be available to assist in this assessment, and if not advice should be sought from the dietetic department within the hospital.

Guidelines

Parental involvement in feeding is not just desirable, but essential. Feeding is one of the basic, vital life functions which parents undertake for their child and is an important part of the bonding process. Parents should always be included.

BREASTFEEDING

The ideal choice of feed for a healthy infant is breast milk. Breast milk is nutritionally the best feed for infants, and has been shown to promote optimum health, growth, development and immunity against illness (Heinig & Dewey 1996, 1997). There is significant evidence to support the existence of the significant advantages, both to the infant and the mother, of breastfeeding (British Paediatric Association Standing Committee on Nutrition 1994), which are summarised in Box 39.1. Despite the well-recognised advantages of breastfeeding, rates are low in the UK.

The *Infant Feeding Survey*, published in 2005 reported initial breastfeeding rates of 78% in England, a significant increase from the previous survey carried out in 2000. However, rates of breastfeeding reduced rapidly to only 22% of mothers exclusively breastfeeding their infant at 6 weeks of age; 8% at 4 months of age; and only a negligible number at 6 months of age. There is growing evidence of the lifetime benefits of exclusive breastfeeding and consequently, the World Health Organization (WHO 2003) recommend that all babies be exclusively breastfed until 6 months of age. This is supported by the UK government (DoH 2004).

A mother whose infant is sick should be given all the information to make a fully informed decision

---

> **BOX 39.1   Advantages of breastfeeding**
>
> **Advantages to the baby**
> **Reduced risk of developing:**
> - Gastrointestinal illness and gastroenteritis in particular
> - Middle ear infection
> - Respiratory system infection
> - Urinary tract infection
> - Insulin-dependent diabetes mellitus
> - Allergies, e.g. eczema.
>
> For the pre-term baby:
> - Optimum neurological development
> - Reduced risk of necrotising enterocolitis.
>
> **Advantages to the mother**
> **Reduced risk of:**
> - Premenopausal breast cancer
> - Some forms of ovarian cancer.
>
> **Social gains:**
> - Ready availability for feeding baby
> - Unique contact between mother and baby
> - May help mother to lose weight naturally.

---

about breastfeeding. The benefits of breastfeeding offer particular advantages to sick infants and many sick infants can breastfeed successfully. If the infant is too sick to feed at the breast, the mother can express her milk and it can be given to the infant via a nasogastric tube, cup and spoon or by bottle.

The reasons why a mother stops breastfeeding vary, but a recurrent issue is the lack of help and support to continue when difficulties are encountered (Hamlyn et al 2002). Social and cultural factors, e.g. early return to work, can also influence a mother's decision to cease breastfeeding. Lack of knowledgeable support can be a particular issue if the infant is admitted to a children's ward, especially straight from a maternity unit, as education about breastfeeding for children's nurses has been sketchy or non-existent in the past. The UNICEF Baby Friendly Initiative (1997) has supported specific guidance for good practice on paediatric units and these should be readily available for paediatric nurses on units where infants are admitted.

BREAST MILK

Breast milk is a unique fluid, which changes in nutritional composition over time from birth, to reflect the changing needs of a growing infant and also during an individual breastfeed. During the first 3 days after delivery, colostrum is produced, which is richer in electrolytes, protein and immuno-globulins and is lower in carbohydrate, fat and some vitamins than mature milk. The high levels of immunoglobulins found in colostrum confer the increased immunity seen in breastfed over formula-fed infants, and it is vital that infants, who are unable to feed directly from the breast in the first few days of life, receive this in an expressed form whenever possible. The first milk produced during a breastfeed is called foremilk. This milk is lower in fat and contains higher levels of maternal antibodies and immunoglobulins than the hindmilk which follows. Hindmilk is rich in fat and fat solu-ble vitamins and provides the bulk of calories in the feed. It is essential that infants receive a full breastfeed containing both foremilk and hindmilk for optimal growth.

FREQUENCY AND LENGTH OF BREASTFEEDS

Breastfeeding works on a supply and demand process, so the more the infant feeds the more milk is produced, and infant-led feeding is important for an adequate milk supply (Chadderton et al 1997). Many infants feed every 1–2h in the first few days after birth, and many will feed for long periods, sometimes up to 1 hour. As breastfeeding becomes established, the frequency of feeds reduces to an average of eight feeds over 24h (Hörnell et al 1999). If an infant continues to feed frequently and is unsettled after a feed, it is possible that the posi-tioning or attachment to the breast is poor and a breastfeeding specialist should review breast-feeding techniques. As breastfeeding is infant-led, the baby should come off the breast of their own accord. If they are still hungry, the second breast should be offered. The sucking pattern of the infant is rhythmical during breastfeeding and changes from quick short sucks to slow deep sucks with short pauses from time to time (Stables & Rankin 2005).

Correct positioning and attachment should be assessed if the mother is suffering from complications such as sore and cracked nipples or engorgement.

Mothers with insufficient milk supply should be encouraged to feed or express at night as maternal prolactin levels are highest at this time, and to feed at least every 3h throughout the day to promote increased supply.

EQUIPMENT

- The only 'equipment' necessary for breastfeeding will be a drink for the mother, close to hand.
- Breast pads or tissues may be required to clean any leakage from the breast from which the infant is not feeding.
- The mother must feel comfortable if she is to breastfeed well, so she may require a special chair or pillow in order to find her optimum position, and privacy, free from unnecessary interruptions.
- Nipple shields should be avoided as they can reduce the mother's milk supply, and also may exacerbate nipple problems such as fissures (Chadderton et al 1997).

METHOD

This method is based on Chadderton et al (1997).

1. Ensure that the mother is comfortable with a drink close at hand. The mother can either be sitting (Fig. 39.1) or lying down (Fig. 39.2).

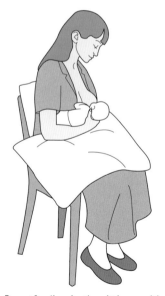

Figure 39.1 Breastfeeding in the sitting position.

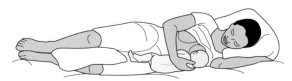

Figure 39.2 Breastfeeding in the lying position.

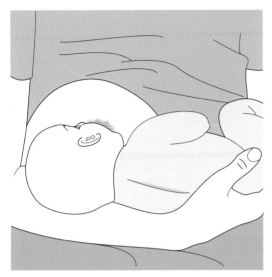

Figure 39.3 Position of the infant during a feed.

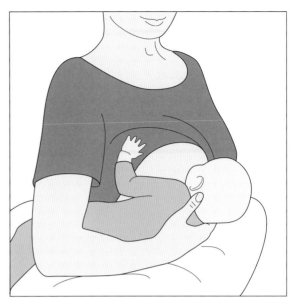

Figure 39.4 Supporting the baby during a feed.

2. If the baby is calm and relaxed, feeding is more likely to progress well.
3. Position the baby to lie comfortably, close to the mother with the baby's head and body in line and not twisted. The baby's head should be well supported, but free to move; do not hold the baby's head but support from the shoulders (Figs 39.3, 39.4). The baby's nose and mouth should be in line with the nipple.

4. Depending on its size and shape, the mother's breast may need support from her hand (Fig. 39.5). Place the mother's hand with fingers flat against her rib cage so that the breast is supported by the angle of thumb and forefinger. The breast can also be supported with the hand underneath and

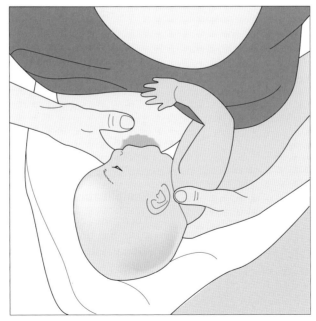

Figure 39.5 Supporting the breast during feeding (with approval from UNICEF UK Baby Friendly Initiative at: www. babyfriendly.org.uk).

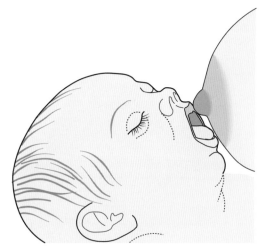

Figure 39.6 Infant rooting to the breast.

thumb lightly on top well back from the areola so that the mother can form her breast into a good shape for the baby to latch on to.

5. Allow the baby to root for the breast, letting tongue and lips touch the nipple (Fig. 39.6). Allowing the baby's head to tilt back slightly will encourage the baby to open the mouth wide. Then bring the baby back to the breast quickly, but smoothly, aiming the lower jaw at the base of the areola (Fig. 39.7). This brings the tongue over the lower lip to scoop up the areola, nipple and as much breast tissue as possible, ensuring that the tongue can reach the lactiferous ducts within the tissue behind the areola. The lactiferous ducts are small reservoirs of milk from which the milk is released.

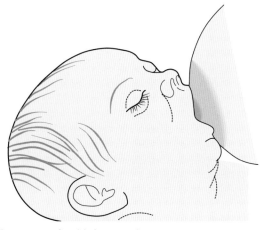

Figure 39.7 Good infant attachment.

6. Allow the baby to feed as long as desired from the first breast before moving on to the second, to ensure that both fore- and hindmilks are released. A baby should not have the feed stopped prematurely. While in hospital, any medical or nursing interventions should be timed around feeds and not be allowed to interrupt feeds.

OBSERVATIONS AND COMPLICATIONS

Observations (Chadderton et al 1997)

- Observe that the mother and baby are comfortable and relaxed. The baby should be close to the mother with the head and body straight, chin touching her breast (and in the young infant <6 months, with the bottom supported).
- Observe the baby's responses. Does the baby reach (root in the newborn) for the breast? Use the tongue to explore the breast? Stay attached? Are there signs of milk ejection (afterpains, milk leakage)?
- Is there evidence of emotional bonding (mother has a secure, confident hold, watches and touches her baby)? Does the baby watch her?
- Anatomy: Are the breasts soft and full? Are the nipples protractile? Is the skin healthy and breasts round during feeding?
- How does the baby suckle? Is the mouth wide, lower lip turned outward, tongue cupped around the breast? Are the cheeks round? Does the baby produce slow, deep sucks in bursts followed by short pauses? Can you see or hear the baby swallow?
- Note how long the baby feeds and record, if required.
- Observe for signs of possible difficulty (see below).

Complications/difficulties

There are no complications of breastfeeding as such, but there may be some difficulties in establishing effective breastfeeding. Examples are as follows:

- If the mother is tense and unrelaxed, give her time to talk through her worries and fears, and provide emotional and practical support. If the baby is uninterested at the start, try cuddling well into the breast, skin-to-skin between feeds.

This will help the baby become used to the smell, feel and appearance of the breast (Chadderton et al 1997). Do not give dummies, bottles or pacifiers which can confuse a baby trying to learn how to breastfeed (Shore 1998).

- If the mother's nipples become sore and/or cracked, this is usually due to poor positioning and attachment. Refer this complication to a breastfeeding specialist.
- Be aware that many drugs can be excreted in breast milk and therefore ingested by the baby (Hale 2004). Ask about any medication the mother is taking and check with the pharmacy about any possible contraindications.

EXPRESSING BREAST MILK

A mother may need to express her breast milk in order to:

- Help establish and maintain lactation
- Relieve her breasts if they are full or uncomfortable
- If her baby is unable to feed because of illness (e.g. too small or sick, or is being starved in preparation for an operation)
- If she is going to be away from her baby for more than an 1–2 hours, or going back to work
- Reduce engorgement.

There are three ways to express breast milk: (1) By hand (Fig. 39.8), (2) By hand pump (Fig. 39.9) and (3) By electric pump (Fig. 39.10).

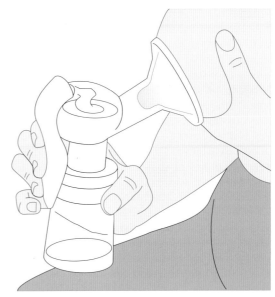

Figure 39.9 Using a hand pump (with approval from UNICEF UK Baby Friendly Initiative at: www.babyfriendly.org.uk).

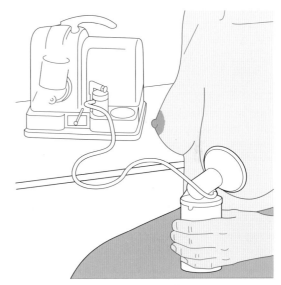

Figure 39.10 Using an electric pump (with approval from UNICEF UK Baby Friendly Initiative at: www.babyfriendly.org.uk).

Any equipment used for expressing milk must be sterilised before use and the mother's hands must be washed and carefully dried. In hospital, kits for electric breast pumps can be reused after autoclaving if recommended for multiple use by the manufacturer, e.g. Egnell breast pump kits. Nurses should familiarise themselves with the type of pump their department offers for mothers to use.

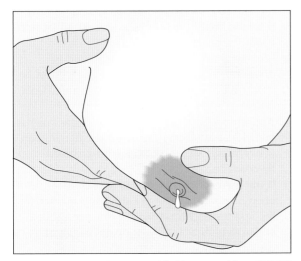

Figure 39.8 Expressing by hand (with approval from UNICEF UK Baby Friendly Initiative at: www.babyfriendly.org.uk).

If a mother is expressing milk to maintain a supply while her baby is unable to breastfeed, she should aim to express at least six to eight times in each 24 h, including once at night, and should ideally aim to express approximately the amount the baby would be taking if breastfeeding (i.e. 150–200 mL/kg). Some mothers are able to express large volumes of milk, but this should be discouraged in the long term as it may make establishment of breastfeeding difficult to achieve. The mother will be producing larger quantities of milk than the infant will take from the breast, leading to engorgement and possible difficulties with attachment.

Breast milk can be stored for up to 24 h in a refrigerator (which must maintain a temperature of 2–4°C), or up to 3 months in a freezer. However, from an infection control viewpoint, breast milk is a body fluid and therefore should be stored in a refrigerator or freezer containing nothing but breast milk, and an individual mother's bottles of expressed milk should be stored in a sealed box in that refrigerator. The expressed breast milk must be dated to avoid out-of-date milk being given, and the bottles should also be clearly labelled with the name and unit number of the mother and baby. Always refer to local policies and guidelines.

Breast milk that has previously been frozen should be thawed in a refrigerator, or by immersing the sealed bottle in cool water. This milk should be stored in a refrigerator and used within 24 h. Milk should not be defrosted in hot water or a microwave, and should never be refrozen. If not used, thawed milk must be thrown away.

Some hospitals recommend the pasteurisation of expressed breast milk. This process gently heats the milk and eradicates the majority of pathogenic organisms, which may have been introduced during the expressing process. Local policies and procedures should be followed for guidance.

DOS AND DON'TS

- Do provide encouragement, help and support to mothers who wish to breastfeed.
- Do ensure that a breastfeeding mother has access to a well-balanced diet and sufficient fluids.
- Do be aware of where to obtain expert help for the breastfeeding mother, if unable to provide it from available staff. Most maternity units and primary care trusts have breastfeeding advisors who are experts in their field.

- Do ensure that a breastfeeding mother has access to facilities to enable her to express milk when necessary.
- Do not give a breastfed baby a dummy or pacifier.
- Do not give a breastfed baby artificial milk, water or juice unless it is medically indicated, with fully informed parental choice and consent.
- Do not give a breastfed baby a bottle. If a breastfed baby has to be given anything by mouth, it should be fed using a cup, cup and spoon or nasogastric tube.

ELIMINATING

Breastfed babies should have a good urine output with frequent wet nappies. Their stool can vary but should be soft and yellow without being watery; frequency varies from every nappy to once a day, sometimes even less than this.

ARTIFICIAL FEEDING

Not all mothers will choose or be able to breastfeed their babies. Hull and Johnston (1993) list some contraindications to breastfeeding:

- Very premature infants may be unable to suck, and expressed breast milk can be given via nasogastric tube or cup and spoon.
- Infants with severe abnormalities of the mouth, e.g. severe cleft palate may be unable to feed from the breast but expressed breast milk can be given via nasogastric tube.
- Mothers who are HIV-positive should be discouraged from breastfeeding as HIV can be transmitted to the infant via breast milk (DoH 2004c).
- A mother who is severely malnourished or has poor renal function may find breastfeeding an unacceptable drain on her own nutritional reserves.
- Some medical conditions such as phenylketonuria require a strict special diet, and the infant may require either very controlled amounts of breast milk, or breastfeeding may be contraindicated.

A children's nurse must be able to undertake and advise on artificial methods of feeding and to

Table 39.1	Average fluid requirements of a healthy baby

AGE OF BABY	AVERAGE TOTAL FLUID REQUIREMENT IN 24 h IN mL/kg
Newborn	30
2 days	60
3 days	90
4 days	120
5 days	150
1 week to 8 months	150
9–12 months	120

calculate if a baby is taking appropriate amounts of feed to sustain expected growth and development.

Table 39.1 gives normal fluid requirements based on age. On the basis of these figures, a 3-month-old baby weighing 5.2 kg should receive: $5.2 \times 150 = 780$ mL in 24 h.

There may be exceptions to this calculation, such as a child who is failing to thrive whose fluid requirements may be increased to achieve weight gain, or a child who has fluid retention or is in renal failure who will require restricted fluids. In these circumstances, a paediatric dietitian or a paediatrician should devise a feeding plan.

It is a matter of parental choice as to which artificial feed their healthy baby is given. They may require guidance from healthcare staff as to the most suitable breast milk substitute, infant formula or follow-on milk to use and should be advised that cow's milk is not suitable as a feed for children under 12 months of age. Normal formula milks are made from modified cow's milk, containing cow's milk protein in the form of casein and whey. There are three basic types of formula milk (see Table 39.2).

Whey-dominant infant formulas have a whey to casein ratio similar to that found in human breast milk, and are the recommended artificial feeds for infants from birth.

All manufacturers produce second stage milks, marketed for hungrier babies. These have a higher casein to whey ratio and are more similar to cow's milk in their protein composition. Anecdotal evidence suggests that unsettled or hungry babies may be more settled on a casein dominant feed, however there is no scientific evidence to support this, and mothers should be advised that whey-dominant feeds are suitable for their infant until 12 months of age, and there is no clinical reason to change their infants formula from a whey-dominant one.

Follow-on milks have a higher iron, protein and vitamin content, and can be used from 6 months of age. They are particularly useful for infants whose weaning diet is suboptimal.

Many infant formula feeds are supplemented with long chain polyunsaturated fats (LCPs), prebiotics and nucleotides, to replicate the formulation of breast milk and to aid normal growth, development and protection from infection.

There are a large number of special formulas available for use in infants who require a special diet for medical purposes. A paediatric dietitian if available, or paediatrician, should advise on the use of these.

Vitamin supplements for women and children

The Department of Health advises that Healthy Start children's vitamins, containing vitamins A, C and D should be given to the following groups:

- Breastfed infants from 6 months of age, or from 1 month of age if there is concern over the adequacy of the mothers diet
- Formula-fed infants from 6 months of age if they are taking <500 mL formula feed daily

Table 39.2	Three basic types of formula milk		
FEED TYPE	EXAMPLES		INDICATIONS
Whey dominant feed	SMA Gold, Cow and Gate 1, Aptamil, Heinz Nurture Newborn		Recommended feed from birth. May be used to 12 months of age
Casein dominant feed	SMA White, Cow and Gate 2, Aptamil Extra Hungry, Heinz Nurture Hungry Baby		Can be used from birth, may be used to 12 months of age
Follow-on formula	SMA Progress, Cow and Gate 3, Aptamil Follow on, Heinz Nurture Growing Baby		Use from 6 months of age. Have higher levels of iron, some vitamins and protein than standard formula

- Children up to 5 years of age, particularly those with poor dietary intakes (NHS Healthy Start scheme).

Healthy Start women's vitamins, containing vitamins C, D and folic acid are recommended for all pregnant and breastfeeding women.

Both types of vitamin supplement are available free of charge from health centres for families on low incomes, and otherwise can be bought from health centres, pharmacies and should be available at NHS Trusts.

PREPARING ARTIFICIAL FEEDS

Larger children's units and children's hospitals will usually have a special feed unit or milk kitchen where infant feeds are made under clean conditions. If feeds are to be made on the wards, very careful attention must be paid to the risk of cross-infection. A separate area should be set aside for feed preparation, away from any other food, and basic food hygiene rules should apply. All staff who may be required to prepare or handle infant feeds or food, should have undertaken training in basic food handling.

Infant formula milk powders are not sterile, and the Department of Health have published recommendations on safe preparation (Food Standards Agency 2006). Staff should familiarise themselves with this guidance. Most normal infant formula feeds are available as sterile ready to use feeds, and these should be used wherever available.

EQUIPMENT

- Documentation listing type and quantity of feed to be made
- A washed and sterilised bottle with a fluid measure on the side
- A washed and sterilised manufacturer-supplied milk powder scoop
- Boiled water, cooled to no less than 70°C. Water should be boiled once and not artificially softened
- Formula feed powder of the same brand as the scoop; check that the feed powder is within its expiry date
- A washed and sterilised plastic knife with a straight-edged back
- A 70% isopropyl alcohol spray or impregnated swab
- Patient identification labels.

METHOD

1. Wash and dry hands thoroughly; put on a disposable plastic apron.
2. Ensure that the work surface is clean and dry; spray or wipe the surface with 70% isopropyl alcohol.
3. Water should be freshly boiled and should be cooled to no less than 70°C. Pour the required amount of boiled water into a bottle. The amount required is the total amount of feed per bottle. For example, if the infant requires 125 mL at each feed, put 125 mL of water in each bottle.
4. Using the correct brand of scoop for the type of milk powder being used, scoop up the milk powder. Do not pack the milk tightly into the scoop. Using the flat edge of the knife, level off the top of the powder with the top of the scoop. Add the powder to the water. One scoop of powder is added to each fluid ounce (30 mL) of water. Any less powder than this and the baby will be underfed; any more powder than this and the too-concentrated feed can lead to diarrhoea and even hypernatraemia.
5. Once all the powder has been added to the feed, put the lid on each bottle and shake well to mix the milk powder and water thoroughly.

Label the bottle with the baby's identification label, the type and the quantity of feed. Feeds should be made as required and not in advance of feeding.

BOTTLE-FEEDING AN INFANT
Equipment

- Plastic apron
- Freshly prepared bottle of milk of correct formula type and quantity
- Sterile teat
- Jug of hot water with sealable lid or bottle warmer to heat bottle
- Bib
- Comfortable chair with support for arm
- Sterilising unit containing 125 parts per million (ppm) of hypochlorite in solution
- Documentation to record feed given.

Method

1. Prior to feeding, ensure that the baby's nose is clean and also ensure that the baby has a clean, dry nappy. The baby is less likely to feed well with a nose blocked with mucus or when uncomfortable from a wet or soiled nappy.

2. Wash hands thoroughly and put on an apron (to prevent cross-infection).

3. If using a 'ready to feed' pre-prepared formula milk, first check the cap according to the manufacturer's instructions to ensure that the seal has not been broken.

4. Check that the expiry date of the feed has not passed and check again that the feed is of the correct make and the quantity to be given.

5. If the feed is to be heated, a bottle warmer should be used or, if one is not available, then a jug of water taken from the kettle may be used. The feed should be heated in the feed preparation area/ward kitchen and the warmed feed then taken to the infant to avoid any potential hazard from carrying a jug of very hot water through a ward area. If the feed is hot from recent preparation, it may need to be cooled in a jug of cold water to a feeding temperature of approximately 37.5°C to prevent scalding.

6. Test the temperature of the milk by squirting a small amount onto the skin on the underside of the forearm. Ideally the milk should be at approximately blood temperature (37°C), as breast milk would be, therefore it should feel just warm and not hot on contact with the skin.

7. Put the bib around the baby to protect clothing.

8. The baby should be held well supported for feeding, with the head above the stomach. This reduces the risk of accidental aspiration of stomach contents. A baby should never be bottle-fed while lying flat because of the increased risk of vomiting and aspiration of feed and vomit into the lungs.

9. Offer the bottle by placing it gently to the lips. Never force a bottle into a baby's mouth. If the baby is reluctant to accept the bottle, it may help to gently stroke the skin just to the side of the baby's mouth. This can stimulate the sucking reflex, as can stroking the baby gently under the chin.

10. Hold the bottle at a sufficiently steep angle to keep the teat filled with milk, to help prevent the baby sucking in too much air which can cause discomfort and vomiting (Hull & Johnston 1993). Most babies can take approximately half of the total amount of feed before requiring to be winded. Winding the baby helps to bring up any air swallowed during feeding (Hull & Johnston 1993), thereby promoting comfort and helping to reduce the incidence of vomiting after feeding.

11. Gently remove the bottle and sit the baby up, supporting the head if the baby is unable to do so. Gently rubbing the baby's back can help to bring up the wind. Some babies like to be put up onto the shoulder to be winded, but take care to protect the shoulder and back in case the baby regurgitates some milk with the wind. Regurgitating a small amount of milk with wind is normal and is known as posseting (Hull & Johnston 1993).

12. Remember that feeding is a time to promote physical contact, eye contact and verbal stimulation for the baby.

13. After the feed is completed, wind again and then make the baby comfortable. Ideally (and particularly if prone to vomiting), the baby should be allowed to sit up for 20–30 min after a feed to prevent aspiration and vomiting.

14. Record what feed was offered, how much feed was taken and note if there was any vomiting. If vomiting has occurred, describe the consistency and quantity.

15. Clear away. If the bottle and/or teat (if not a single-use teat) are to be used again, the bottle should be washed thoroughly in warm, soapy water then rinsed carefully. The teat should be washed thoroughly and salt may be rubbed inside it to remove all traces of milk. It should then be rinsed thoroughly to remove all salt. The clean bottle and teat are then submerged completely in the sterilising solution, ensuring that there are no air bubbles, and left in the sterilising unit for at least 30 min. The presence of any organic matter (e.g. milk, saliva) in a hypochlorite solution will destabilise it and render it incapable of sterilising. Hypochlorite solutions should be discarded every 24 h or if

there is evidence of contamination of the solution. It is not necessary to rinse the hypochlorite solution off the teat prior to offering it to the baby.

OBSERVATIONS AND COMPLICATIONS

Observations

Feeding is a good time to assess whether the baby is developing as expected for age. Be aware of how the baby is handling. Check that head control is appropriate for age. Is there any abnormal stiffness or floppiness or does the baby handle as would be expected of a child of that age? Observe the baby's face, expressions, eye movements, eye contact. Check that the baby is achieving developmental milestones, e.g. fixing and following by 4 weeks. Observe how the baby feeds, noting if there is a good, strong suck or if the baby is slow to feed and sleepy or unusually drowsy, or struggling to swallow. If there is vomiting, observe the physical nature of the vomiting and the vomit itself, e.g. is it effortless or projectile; is the vomit milky or bile-stained? Report any unusual findings.

Complications of bottle–feeding

As with any calculation, there is the risk of human error, resulting in too much or too little being given. Parents unaware of how much feed they should give their baby could overfeed, leading to excessive weight gain over a prolonged period, or underfeed, resulting in weight loss and dehydration. In addition, a child with medical problems such as congenital heart disease or renal disease may require fluid restriction and special attention may be needed to calculate the volume of feed to offer. Oral candida infection (thrush) is a common complication of bottle-feeding and is associated with poor or suboptimal sterilisation. In the pre-term neonate there is an increased risk of necrotising enterocolitis (NEC).

DOS AND DON'TS

- Do calculate the feed correctly.
- Do ensure that, if making up feeds, the correct brand of milk scoop is used for the correct type of milk powder.

- Do ensure that exactly one level scoop of milk powder is added to each fluid ounce (30 mL) of cooled, boiled water.
- Do ensure that the correct type of formula and amount of feed is given to the right baby.
- Do remember to test the temperature of a feed before it is given to a baby.
- Do not bottle-feed a baby who is lying flat.
- Do not reconstitute baby milk powder with water that has been boiled more than once.
- Do not re-heat bottle-feeds more than once, discard any unused feed.

WEANING

The Department of Health (DoH 2004) and The ESPGHAN Committee on Nutrition (Agostoni et al 2008) identify the following recommendations for weaning:

- Solid food should ideally not be introduced before the age of 6 months, and all infants should start solids by 26 weeks of age. At this age, breast and formula feeds provide insufficient nutrients, particularly iron for the growing infant and introduction of solids aids normal development. Infant-led feeding however is encouraged, and some infants are ready to start solid food before 6 months. The earliest time to start solids is 17 weeks of age, as earlier introduction of solids may lead to an increased prevalence of obesity and food allergies.
- The UK Infant Feeding Survey (2005) highlighted that 51% of infants in the UK are started on solids by 4 months of age. Early weaning predisposes infants to a greater risk of allergies and obesity.
- Suitable first weaning foods to be given by spoon are pureed fruit or vegetables, progressing onto a mixed diet in the first few weeks of weaning.
- Salt and sugar should not be added to weaning foods.
- First-stage foods should be smooth and runny in consistency and weaning foods should become increasingly thicker and contain small lumps by the age of 6 months. Infants should progress onto mashed and chopped foods by the age of 9–12 months.

- There is no evidence to support avoidance of potentially allergenic foods such as fish, eggs and wheat, unless this is medically indicated.
- Gluten-containing solids should not be introduced before 4 months of age or after 7 months of age.
- Diet should include adequate sources of iron, particularly for breastfed infants.
- Infants receiving a vegetarian diet should consume 500 mL breast or formula feed in addition to solids. A follow-on formula may be required to achieve adequate iron intake.
- Vegan diets are not recommended for infants and young children due to the risk of protein, energy, vitamin and mineral deficiencies.
- Breast or formula feeds should be given for the first year of life.
- Cow's milk can be introduced as a drink from 12 months of age.
- Drinking from a cup is to be encouraged from 6 months.
- If there is doubt that dietary iron is adequate, consider the continued use of iron-enriched follow-on milk.
- Discourage bottle-feeds from 12 months.
- Water should be the drink of choice when milk is not required.
- Prevent dental caries: promote healthy dentition by avoiding sugared or fizzy drinks and fruit juices. Give only at meal times via a cup, not a bottle or pacifier.

TODDLER FEEDING

Feeding is important for several areas of the toddler's development. Social, fine motor and perceptual development can be demonstrated, for example, by a 10-month-old boy attempting to grasp and manipulate the spoon with which he is being fed and his determination to try to feed himself (Bee 1997). While it can be frustrating for the child and carer to see him continually drop food just before he gets it to his mouth, it should not be discouraged. Neither should he be discouraged from handling food, as exploring texture teaches him about the surrounding world. However, it is important to distinguish between acceptable learning behaviour in comparison to what would constitute unacceptable social behaviour if it was

allowed to become established. Allowing the child to experience different textures of food aids the development of speech.

The normal toddler diet should contain a balance of foods providing protein, energy, vitamins and minerals. Salt and sugar should not be added, and the toddler should be offered a variety of foods, including finger foods to allow self-feeding. The food should be presented in an attractive way and served using appropriate cutlery, plates and bowls.

EQUIPMENT

- High chair
- Food of appropriate consistency according to age and level of development, e.g. finger foods and lumpy spoon feeds
- Bib
- Feeder beaker of water or diluted fruit juice; avoid fizzy drinks and sugary squashes
- Spoons for feeding. Give the toddler a spoon to encourage self-feeding but assistance will be required
- Use appropriate plates and bowls for age
- Documentation to record food given, if required.

METHOD

1. Wash the child's hands and utilise the opportunity to teach him about washing his own hands prior to meals.
2. Wash hands thoroughly and put on an apron (to prevent cross-infection).
3. Ensure that the toddler is strapped safely and securely into the high chair.
4. Allow him to hold a spoon of his own. He may accept help to put food onto his spoon.
5. Put a small amount of food onto the spoon. If he is managing well with his own spoon, let him carry on. Do not try to get him to take food from your spoon.
6. If he is having difficulty, intersperse his own efforts at feeding by placing your spoon just into the front of his mouth. Never force the spoon into his mouth.
7. Constantly encourage him and praise him when he manages to put food into his mouth himself and when he accepts food from you.

8. As children learn to manipulate their mouth and tongue muscles, inevitably some food gets spat out accidentally. However, it will become clear if there is a particular food which he does not like. He will try to spit it out and may well purse his lips and refuse to take another mouthful. Offer that particular food once more. If he still refuses or spits it out again, try another item of food from the plate instead.

9. Encourage him to feed himself finger foods, e.g. carrot, bread, fruit. This teaches him independence, different textures of food (not purée) and enables him to experience the achievement of feeding himself.

10. Offer him a drink from his feeder cup once or twice during the meal, at the end of the savoury course and at the end of the meal. The last drink of the meal would ideally be water to help rinse his mouth and prevent dental caries.

11. Allow him to feel his food if he so wishes, but discourage him from throwing his plate or utensils. Be firm and consistent in what behaviour is allowed and what is not tolerated.

12. At the end of his meal, clear away the remains and clean his face and hands.

OBSERVATIONS AND COMPLICATIONS

Observations

Observe how the toddler reacts to being fed. Does he help himself, or is he very passive? This can tell you something about his level of development.

Establish the toddler's likes and dislikes of different foods and textures. Relate your observations of how he feeds and what he does and does not like to the information given to you by his parents. Observe how he behaves when fed by his parents. Useful information about how he and his parents interact can be gained from observing them during a meal time.

Complications

There are few complications associated with feeding a toddler. There could be a risk of him choking on a piece of food, in which case he should be given emergency treatment for choking, following resuscitation guidelines. If the food he is given is too hot, there is a risk of him burning his mouth.

DOS AND DON'TS

- Do check the temperature of his food before feeding him.
- Do praise and encourage him when he succeeds in feeding himself.
- Do allow him to feed himself and help.
- Do let him touch and feel his food.
- Do be prepared for a messy meal time.
- Do not give him a lot to drink prior to a meal, as that would fill his stomach and make him less hungry.
- Do not ever force him to take food.

References

Agostoni, C., Decsi, T., Fewtrell, M., et al., ESPGHAN Committee on Nutrition, 2008. Complementary feeding: a commentary by the ESPGHAN Committee on Nutrition. J. Pediatr. Gastroenterol. Nutr. 46 (1), 99–110.

Bee, H., 1997. The developing child. eighth ed. Addison-Wesley, New York, pp. 128–129.

British Paediatric Association Standing Committee on Nutrition, 1994. Is breastfeeding beneficial in the UK? Arch. Dis. Child 71 (4), 376–380.

Chadderton, M., MacDonald, A., Munn, J., et al., 1997. A healthy start – infant feeding policy. South Birmingham Community Health Trust, Birmingham Children's Hospital NHS Trust, Birmingham.

Department of Health, 2004a. Birth to five: your complete guide to parenthood and the first five years of your child's life. DoH, London. Online. Available: www. dh.gov.uk.

Department of Health, 2004b. Breastfeeding. DoH, London. Online. Available: www.dh.gov.

uk/maternity/ maternalandinfantnutrition.

Department of Health, 2004c. HIV and infant feeding: guidance from the UK Chief Medical Officer's Expert Advisory Group on AIDS. Online. Available: www.dh.gov. uk/en/publications/ policyandguidance.

Department of Health, 2004d. Infant feeding recommendations. Online. Available: www.dh.gov. uk.

Food Standards Agency, 2006. Guidance on preparing infant formula. Online. Available: www.

food.gov.uk/news/newsarchive/2006/feb/infantformulastatementnov05.

Hale, T., 2004. Medications and mother's milk, eleventh ed. Pharmasoft Publishing, Amarillo, Texas.

Hamlyn, B., Brooker, S., Oleinkova, K., et al., 2002. Infant Feeding 2000. A survey conducted on behalf of the Department of Health, The Scottish Executive, The National Assembly of Wales and the Department of Health, Social Services and Public Safety in Northern Ireland. The Stationery Office, London.

NHS Healthy Start scheme, 2002. Online. Available: www.healthystart.nhs.uk.

Heinig, M.J., Dewey, K.G., 1996. Health advantages of breastfeeding for infants: a critical review. Nutr. Res. Rev. 9 (1), 89–110.

Heinig, M.J., Dewey, K.G., 1997. Health effects of breastfeeding for mothers: a critical review. Nutr. Res. Rev. 10 (1), 35–36.

Hörnell, A., Aarts, C., Kylberg, E., et al., 1999. Breastfeeding patterns in exclusively breast fed infants: a longitudinal prospective study in Uppsala, Sweden. Acta Paediatr. 88 (2), 203–211.

Hull, D., Johnston, D.I., 1993. Essential paediatrics. third ed. Churchill Livingstone, Edinburgh, pp. 75–89.

Infant Feeding Survey, 2005. Online. Available: www.dh.gov.uk/publications.

Shore, C., 1998. Good practice guidelines for breastfeeding in paediatric units. Paediatr. Nurs. 10 (1), 24–29.

Stables, D., Rankin, J., 2005. Physiology in childbearing with anatomy and related biosciences, second ed. Elsevier, Edinburgh.

UNICEF UK Baby Friendly Initiative, 1997. Breastfeeding guidance for paediatric units. UNICEF, London. Online. Available: www.babyfriendly.org.uk/paedunits.asp.

World Health Organization (WHO), 2003. Global strategy for infant and young child feeding. WHO, Geneva.

Further reading

Agnew, T., 1996. Battle of the breast in the classroom. Nurs. Times 92 (2), 15.

Baby Friendly website, 1996. Online. Available: www.babyfriendly.org.uk.

Coldicutt, P., 1994. Children's options. Nurs. Times 90 (13), 54–56.

Department of Health website, 1994. Online. Available: www.dh.gov.uk/publications.

Elia, I., 1994. Adoptive breastfeeding. Nurs. Stand. 8 (43), 20–21.

Food Standards Agency website, 1994. Online. Available: www.foodgov.uk/nutrition.

Henshel, D., Inch, S., 1996. Breastfeeding: a guide for midwives. Books for Midwives Press, Hale.

Payne, D., 1995. A lot of bottle. Nurs. Times 91 (17), 20–21.

Royal College of Midwives, 1991. Successful breastfeeding. Churchill Livingstone, Edinburgh.

Chapter 40

Feeding 2: Enteral feeding

Christopher Bunford

CHAPTER CONTENTS

Introduction   388
    Learning outcomes   388
    Rationale   388
    Factors to note   388
    Guidelines   392

Passing a nasogastric (NG) tube   392
    Equipment   392
    Method   392

Feeding via a nasogastric or gastrostomy
tube   395
    Equipment   395
    Method   396
    Observations and complications   397
    Dos and don'ts   399

INTRODUCTION

Enteral feeding is an artificial method of supplying the child with nutrition via a nasogastric tube or gastrostomy.

LEARNING OUTCOMES

By the end of this section you should be able to:

- Identify some typical situations in which a child may require enteral feeding
- Describe the techniques of providing enteral nutrition and hydration to the child who is unable to feed orally
- Understand the possible risks and side-effects associated with some feeding techniques.

RATIONALE

A children's nurse should be able to undertake enteral feeding, teach children and their families the different techniques and be aware of possible positive and negative effects of enteral feeding.

FACTORS TO NOTE

See also Factors to note in Feeding 1 (Ch. 39).

Hambridge et al (1995) give reasons why some children are unable to feed orally:

- The child has cancer and the treatment causes anorexia and vomiting
- The child is unable to take in sufficient nutrition for growth and development in an acute or

chronic illness, e.g. severe bronchiolitis, gross reflux, renal failure or liver disease, particularly when the child has increased calorific and nutrient requirements

- The child is unable to absorb the food, e.g. short bowel syndrome and severe, acute diarrhoea
- The premature infant may not yet have developed a swallowing reflex.

These children can be fed enterally via nasogastric (NG) tube or gastrostomy.

The multidisciplinary team is essential when a sick child has special dietary requirements:

- A children's dietitian and/or paediatrician may be required to prescribe a feed or extra calories (Maxijul) or additives, e.g. a thickening agent (Nestergel and Thixo D).
- A doctor may need to prescribe drugs, e.g. anti-reflux treatment, electrolyte supplements or intestinal motility regulators (domperidone, loperamide, ranitidine and omeprazole).
- Nutritional care nurse specialists may be available in some hospitals to help advise on practical aspects of feeding children.
- It is essential that a speech therapist conducts an assessment of the child's oral motor function if long-term NG feeding is required, and is a source of valuable advice with regard to the child's developmental needs associated with feeding (Langley 1994, NHS QIS 2007).
- Testing for acidity of gastric secretions to ensure correct positioning is essential to ensure safety. The pH of gastric secretions should be between 0–5 (NHS QIS 2007, Medical Devices Agency 2004, NPSA 2005).
- The use of pH indicator paper in neonates has been questioned by practitioners as their gastric secretions may not be sufficiently acidic to entail a change. Similarly, gastric acid pH response may be altered when infants/children are taking antacids. In these children, the pH reference range for testing with pH paper may be altered. Refer to local guidelines regarding type of pH paper and acceptable readings (Nutritional Care 2004, NPSA 2005). If there is any doubt that the tube may not be correctly positioned, it should not be used until its correct position in the stomach has been confirmed by senior nursing/medical staff.
- It used to be common practice to check the position of a NG tube by listening with a stethoscope for the sound of air injected into the stomach via the NG tube. Research has shown this to be an inaccurate and dangerous practice and should no longer be used (Hendry et al 1986, Metheny et al 1990, NPSA 2005).

Nasogastric tubes

There are two main types of NG tube commonly used. (1) Short-term tubes, which can be used for up to 7 days and (2) long-term tubes, which can last up to 30 days (refer to manufacturer's guidelines). The tubes are sized according to the width of their internal lumen; 6, 8 and very occasionally 10 French gauge (Fg) are most commonly used in children. If a thickening agent has been added to the child's feed, the small 6 Fg diameter tube may be too narrow to facilitate instillation of the feed. Tubes can come in various lengths which range from 50–85 cm in both short term and long term tubes. The length used will depend on how big the child is. The tube must be long enough to cover the length from the outer edge of the child's face, through the nasopharynx and down into the stomach (Fig. 40.1). Short-term tubes should be changed every 5–7 days and long-term tubes monthly, to prevent increased risk of bacterial contamination and the material of the tube being eroded by gastric secretions (Taylor & Goodison-McLaren 1992, Skipper et al 2003).

Gastrostomy tubes are made of silicone. There are three main types: skin-level 'button', percutaneous endoscopic tubes and surgically placed tubes. The skin around a gastrostomy site should be washed daily to prevent the skin around the site becoming sore (Coldicutt 1994). Frequency and timing of tube changes vary according to the device used and the child's condition.

The gastrostomy button is a device in which the exterior of the tube sits flush with the skin and, when not in use, resembles a button on the surface of the skin (Fig. 40.2). It is usually changed once every 3–6 months. However, in some areas, when the gastrostomy tract has been formed via a Stamm procedure (full surgical procedure), tubes are placed directly.

The percutaneous endoscopic tube (PEG) is a gastrostomy tube that is inserted through the skin into the stomach under endoscopic control, therefore avoiding the need for a full, laparoscopic surgical

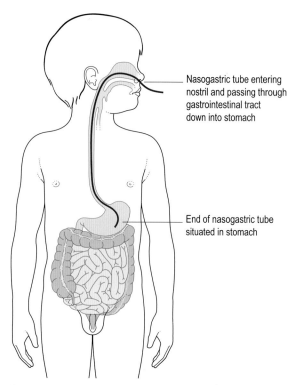

Nasogastric tube entering nostril and passing through gastrointestinal tract down into stomach

End of nasogastric tube situated in stomach

Figure 40.1 The length and position of a nasogastric tube *in situ*.

procedure (Booth 1991). It can stay *in situ* usually for up to 2 years.

A surgically placed tube is usually much shorter term in use and should only be changed by a surgeon or nurse who has received training in the procedure. If it becomes displaced in the first 2 weeks postoperatively, before the tract has properly formed, it must be re-inserted as a matter of urgency or the skin and tissues will close over. Gastrostomy tubes are most commonly sized between 9 and 15 Fg, although smaller or larger tubes may be used in small babies or older children (Bowling 2003).

Research–based practice relating to the risks of enteral feeding

Research has highlighted the risks of nasogastric feeding, in particular the risk of aspiration of feed because of misplaced tubes, blocked tubes, infection transmission and the excessive vacuum pressure caused by using smaller-volume syringes (Taylor & Goodison-McLaren 1992, Lord 1997, Anderton & Nivgough 1991, Skipper et al 2003).

Maintaining patency of nasogastric and gastrostomy tubes

NG and gastrostomy tubes must be flushed before and after a feed. During continuous feeding, or when not in use, NG tubes should be flushed regularly to maintain patency, e.g. every 4 h during the daytime (Lifshitz et al 1991, Paul et al 1993).

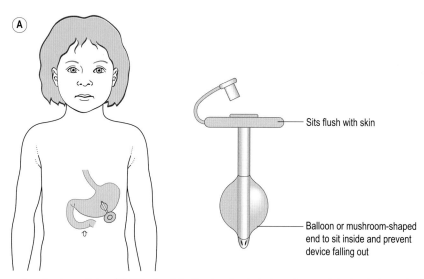

Sits flush with skin

Balloon or mushroom-shaped end to sit inside and prevent device falling out

Figure 40.2 Types of gastrostomy tube: (A) Skin-level 'button' or 'key' device; sits a coin's depth (2 mm) above the skin.

Continued

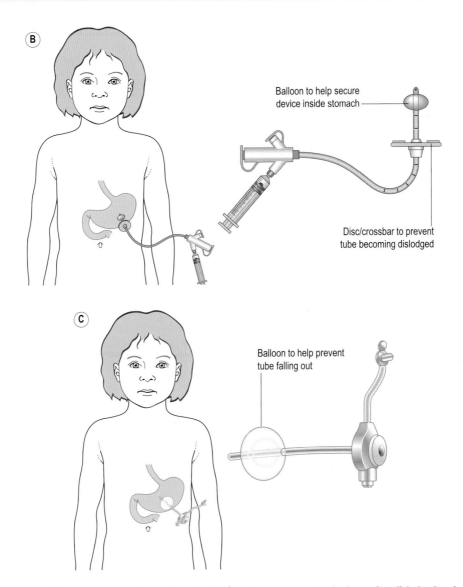

Figure 40.2—Cont'd (B) Percutaneous endoscopic tube; disc/crossbar to prevent tube becoming dislodged and migration of tube past stomach into duodenum. (C) Surgically placed tube, e.g. Foley catheter; held in place by suture depending on type of tube and surgeon's preference.

Preventing infection transmission via enteral feeding

Whenever an NG or gastrostomy tube is flushed, it should be done with cooled, boiled water, or Tap, depending on the age and condition of the child (Coldicutt 1994, Anderton 1995, Paul et al 1994, Skipper et al 2003). In addition, feeds should be prepared only on surfaces which have been cleaned thoroughly with soap and water, dried and then wiped with 70% isopropyl alcohol-impregnated wipes (Anderton & Nivgough 1991).

Any feed delivery systems should be single-use only, and feed containers (the visible external part of NG and gastrostomy tubes) should also be cleaned with alcohol-impregnated wipes prior to use (Paul et al 1994, Anderton 1995, Skipper et al 2003).

Size of enteral syringe used when administering feed/flush via nasogastric tube

A long-term tube is softer and more prone to damage. The smaller the syringe, the smaller is the bore (the hole in the middle) and the greater the pressure created when injecting with it; 1–5 mL syringes produce the highest pressure for a given force. Using a larger-sized syringe – 50 or 100 mL – reduces the pressure on the tube, thus minimising the risk of damage (Taylor & Goodison-McLaren 1992, Paul et al 1993, Sidey 1995).

GUIDELINES

Parents and older children should be encouraged to be involved with enteral feeding. This can include being involved in or even being trained to pass the NG or gastrostomy tube if they so wish. Involvement can help them to feel in control of the procedure and help their acceptance of the problem (Holden et al 1997).

PASSING A NASOGASTRIC (NG) TUBE

EQUIPMENT

- Plastic apron
- Disposable latex-free gloves
- Cooled, boiled water or sterile water for flushing tube
- Two sterile gallipots
- pH paper/strips capable of indicating an acid range of pH 0–5 (Metheney et al 1993)
- Two syringes – 5/10 mL for short-term NG tube or 50/60 mL for long-term NG tube (Lord 1997, Skipper et al 2003)
- 70% isopropyl alcohol-impregnated wipes
- Tape to secure the tube to the child's cheek (check that the child is not allergic to the tape)
- Scissors
- If the child has especially sensitive skin, you may need a hydrocolloid dressing such as extra-thin Granuflex to provide a protective layer between the child's skin and the adhesive tape holding the tube in place
- Dummy if the child uses it
- Drink of water if the child is older.

METHOD

Note: Generally, two people are needed to pass a NG tube; one to comfort and support the child and one to pass the tube.

1. Wherever possible, the child and family should have had psychological preparation to reduce the distress caused by the procedure (Holden et al 1997).
2. Wash hands thoroughly, dry them and put on a plastic apron to prevent cross-infection (Anderton 1995).
3. Clean the work surface/trolley on which equipment is to be placed as local policy, and wipe with alcohol (Anderton 1995). Allow alcohol to dry (it sterilises as it dries).
4. If using a hydrocolloid dressing, cut a piece and place it within easy reach. It should be wide enough to be at least three times the diameter of the NG tube and long enough to cover at least two-thirds of the child's cheek from the side of the nostril towards the ear (Fig. 40.3). Normally, a piece 1.5 × 5 cm would be adequate for most children except for a very tiny neonate who would need less.
5. Cut a piece of adhesive tape and place it in easy reach. It should be wide enough to cover the NG tube with overlap at each side sufficient to hold it securely in place, and long enough to secure at least 3 cm of tube. If a hydrocolloid dressing is used, the adhesive tape should not extend beyond the boundary of the hydrocolloid.
6. Draw up 2–5 mL of the water into one of the syringes. Place on one side, in easy reach.

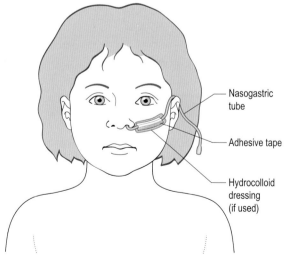

Figure 40.3 Size and position of tape securing nasogastric tube to cheek.

7. Put approximately 10 mL of water into a gallipot in easy reach.
8. Open up the second syringe and place it in easy reach.
9. Take a strip of pH paper/strip and place it in the second gallipot.
10. Wash hands thoroughly, dry them and put on disposable gloves to prevent bacterial contamination of the tube (Anderton 1995).
11. Take the NG tube out of its sterile packaging. Ensure that it is not damaged in any way. If the tube has a guide wire, check that the wire is not bent and is correctly inserted down the middle of the tube. Measure what length of tube is to be passed. With the fingers of your dominant hand, hold the distal end of the tube (the end which will sit in the stomach) by the child's nostril. Measure the first length of tubing from the nostril to the edge of the cheek, by the ear (Fig. 40.4A). Then, measure the second length of tubing from the edge of the ear down to the child's stomach and then two fingers below the xiphoid process (Fig. 40.4B). Mark this point on the tube by using a piece of surgical tape or a permanent marker pen (Nutritional Care 2004). Some tubes have black markings on the tubing at

10 cm intervals to give you a visual guide as to what length of tubing needs to be passed.
12. Ask the person assisting to position the child so that you can access the nostril. An older child should be encouraged to sit upright.
13. Maintain your hold on the proximal end of the tube (the end of which will remain on the exterior) at the end of the pre-measured length. Lubricate the distal end of the NG tube by dipping it in the gallipot containing water.
14. Gently pass the distal end of the tube into the child's nostril. Angle it slightly upwards and gently guide it over the back of the nose and into the nasopharynx.
15. Continue to pass the tube downwards. As it gets to the back of the throat, the child will gag. To ease the passage of the tube, encourage a baby to suck on a dummy and try to persuade an older child to have a sip of water. Advance the tube as the child swallows. This will help ease discomfort and reduce the risk of the tube passing into the trachea, as the epiglottis will cover the trachea when swallowing.
16. Continue to advance the tube. You may have to pause in order for the tube to pass through the cardiac sphincter into the stomach. When the place you have marked on the tube is at the opening of the child's nostril, the distal end should now be in the stomach.
17. Ask the person comforting the child, or the child personally, to place two fingers against the tube to prevent it slipping.
18. Check that the NG tube is in the correct position.
19. Connect a syringe 5/10 mL or 50/60 mL depending on type of tube and manufacturer's guidelines to the end of the NG tube and withdraw the plunger until fluid appears in the syringe – only a very small amount (0.5–1 mL) of fluid is required. Disconnect the syringe and close off the end of the tube.
20. Put the contents of the syringe onto the pH paper/strip and observe for an acid reaction (the aspirate must be in the pH range 0–5) indicating that the fluid originates from the stomach and the tube is correctly positioned.
    a. If no fluid was obtained, try changing the child's position and then aspirating the tube again. If still no fluid can be withdrawn and it is safe to do so, give the child a few millilitres (5 mL) of water, juice or milk orally and then aspirate the tube again.

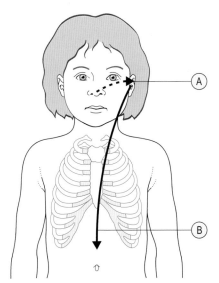

Figure 40.4 Measuring the length of nasogastric tube to be passed: (A) holding the tip of the tube, measure from nose to ear; (B) then measure from ear to stomach, aiming for two fingers below the xiphoid process.

b. If it is still not possible to be sure that the tube is correctly placed, it may need to be withdrawn a little, or passed further, in order to obtain acidic aspirate. In exceptional circumstances it may be necessary to obtain an X-ray picture to determine whether the tube is correctly positioned.

21. Having established that it is correctly placed, gently flush the tube with 2–5 mL of water to ensure that it is patent. Remove the guide wire if one has been used. Disconnect and close off the end of the tube.

22. Secure the tube to the child's cheek using the adhesive tape (and hydrocolloid if necessary).

Gastrostomy tubes

Changing a balloon gastrostomy device

The gastrostomy device should be changed every 3–6 months as recommended by the manufacturers. The device should only be changed by staff/carers who have had the appropriate training and experience.

Equipment

- New gastrostomy device (button or tube)
- 2 × 10 mL syringes
- Sterile water/cooled boiled water (to fill balloon)
- Small container
- Saline/cooled boiled water and swabs (or saliwipes)
- Water soluble lubricant (oil or petroleum jelly can damage the tube and therefore must not be used)
- pH paper (stored in an airtight container to prevent contamination)
- Gallipot (for testing the aspirate)
- Oral analgesia (prescribed if in hospital) and topical analgesia if required (prescribed)
- Sterile gloves
- Apron
- Rubbish bag.

Method/procedure

1. Seek consent and explain to the child what you are doing and position comfortably.
2. Wash and dry hands and prepare a clean surface.

3. Remove new device and place on clean surface.
4. Put on apron and gloves.
5. Check new balloon device by inserting 5 mL of water into balloon port, making sure there are no leaks and it inflates evenly, then remove water again.
6. Lubricate tip of device ready for use.
7. Remove old device by first attaching syringe and gently removing water from balloon, place a gauze swab under gastrostomy device and remove gently with slow steady pressure.
8. Clean and dry stoma site as shown with warm normal saline.
9. Gently guide new lubricated tube into the stoma.
10. If it is a button (skin level device) insert until device is flush with the skin.
11. If it is a Corflo or MIC tube, insert 3–4 cm into the stoma.
12. While holding the device in place, attach the syringe and fill the balloon with the recommended amount of water, and test for resistance (with Corflo/MIC tube, secure flange in place next to the skin).
13. Wipe away any excess lubricant and ensure the skin is dry.
14. Check the position of the gastrostomy using pH paper.
15. If unable to obtain aspirate, *do not use* and seek advice.
16. In order to detect migration, mark the tube at the insertion site. Ensure that the length of tube is documented in the patient's health records or equivalent, if at home.
17. Put used gloves, swabs, etc. into a rubbish bag.

Changing balloon water

Besides anchoring the tube inside the stomach, the balloon helps to prevent leakage. The water in the balloon should be changed on a weekly basis with the required amount of water.

Equipment

- Sterile water or cooled boiled water
- 2 × 10 mL syringes
- Non-sterile gloves (if worn).

Method

1. Equipment should be prepared on a clean surface.
2. Explain what you are doing to the child and reassure.
3. Wash hands before and after procedure and put on gloves (if worn).
4. Prepare a syringe with required amount of water to fill balloon.
5. Attach empty syringe to balloon port while holding gastrostomy device securely.
6. Remove as much water as possible from the balloon and discard syringe.
7. While still holding device securely, attach prepared syringe and re-inflate balloon with required amount of water.
8. Remove syringe and discard.

Confirming position of gastrostomy button

- Wash hands and put gloves on.
- Draw back on syringe and aspirate some stomach contents (small amount approx. 2 mL).
- Remove syringe and close tube.
- Test contents on suitable pH strips covering available areas with the abdominal secretions and check any changes against the appropriate pH chart. An acidic reaction is required.
- Always flush tube prior to feeding or medication with 5–10 mL of water.

What to do if ...

Tube falls out
The tube could fall out if the balloon holding the tube in place has not been checked on a regular basis or is faulty. Check with manufacturer's recommendations on frequency of testing the balloon and the amount of water to be placed.

Tube is pulled out
Tubes can also be pulled out accidentally or purposefully. If this occurs, replacing the tube quickly is essential, as some stomas can start to close within 1 h and have completely closed in 4 h. If the replacement tube cannot be placed, a smaller size French (Fg) gauge tube should be placed as a temporary measure until an appropriate tube can be placed that can be used for feeding purposes; the tract may need surgical dilatation. To prevent tubes from accidentally falling out, always ensure that tube is adequately secured.

Tubes need planned changes as per manufacturer's guidelines. Some tubes last up to 6 months.

Leakage
Leakage of feed/gastric contents around the gastrostomy tube on to the skin will cause skin redness, excoriation and breakdown. It is important to ensure the balloon is properly inflated, checking there is resistance when pulling gently on the tube and that the external fixator is secured

Infection
There is always a potential risk for gastrostomy sites to become infected. Signs that infection may be present are redness, excessive exudate, swelling and pain. A swab should be taken initially to identify if an organism is present and then an appropriate prescribed antibiotic should be commenced. Good hygiene should always be practiced regularly. If infection is suspected, keep the site as clean and dry as possible. There are a variety of creams, ointments and dressings that could potentially be used to treat infection, but these should always be assessed by a healthcare professional and prescribed.

Over granulation tissue
Over granulation tissue can occur as a result of the placement of a foreign device. It can become problematic, as it can be painful, bleeding may occur and it can be prone to infection. To reduce granulation tissue, the tubing should be secured to prevent excess movement, as this can potentially encourage further granulation tissue. There are a number of topical ointments and dressings available that have been beneficial in the reduction and complete removal of granulation tissue in some patients, e.g. Maxitrol eye ointment.

Silver nitrate (caustic sticks) should be used with caution and as a last resort and *must not* be used if any exudate is apparent, as this can potentially burn healthy surrounding skin. Always protect the surrounding skin with Vaseline if using silver nitrate.

FEEDING VIA A NASOGASTRIC OR GASTROSTOMY TUBE

EQUIPMENT

- Plastic apron
- Disposable latex-free gloves
- Cooled, boiled water or sterile water for flushing tube
- Two sterile gallipots

- pH paper/strips
- Two syringes: 5/10 mL for short-term NG tubes, or 50/60 mL for long-term NG tubes (see manufacturer's guidelines)
- 70% isopropyl alcohol-impregnated wipes
- Sterile feed – correct type and quantity at room temperature
- Bottle opener if required
- Documentation to record feed given.

For bolus feed

- Gravity feed delivery system with plunger if feed thickened or narrow bore (6 or 8 Fg)
- Separate clamp for gravity feed tube if roller clamp not integral to the system
- Dummy if appropriate (be aware that using a dummy may make establishing breastfeeding in the future more difficult)
- Toys related to feeding – plastic dishes, utensils, etc.

For continuous feed

- Enteral feeding pump with fully charged battery and lead to connect it to a mains electrical supply
- Continuous enteral feeding administration set. Labels to indicate when set changed.

METHOD

1. Clean the work surface/trolley, on which feed is to be prepared, with soap and water and wipe it with alcohol-impregnated wipes (Anderton 1995). Allow alcohol to dry (it sterilises as it dries).
2. Check that the expiry date of the feed has not passed.
3. Wash and dry the bottle opener and separate clamp if used. Clean bottle opener and clamp (if used) and top of feed container by wiping with alcohol-impregnated wipes to prevent cross-infection (Anderton 1995).
4. Open the feed administration system and put all equipment on the work surface.
5. Wash hands thoroughly and put on disposable latex gloves to prevent bacterial contamination of feed (Anderton 1995).

6. Reassure the child and parent; explain what you are about to do.
7. Ensure that the child is comfortable and is positioned with the head above the level of the stomach to prevent aspiration, preferably sitting or nursed at an angle of about 30° (Lifshitz et al 1991).
8. Draw up 5–10 mL of sterile water (for flushing tube) into the appropriate-sized syringe for the type of tube. Smaller volumes will be used in neonates or children on fluid restrictions.
9. Check that the NG/gastrostomy tube is in the correct position and patent (see steps 19–21 for checking the placement of a NG tube). A gastrostomy tube should be allowed to free drain a small amount of fluid onto pH paper/strip placed in a gallipot or a small amount of fluid can be withdrawn using a syringe.
10. Prime the feed administration system. Apply a clamp to the tubing, fill the barrel/bag/burette with feed and then fill the tubing by gradually releasing the clamp. If necessary, run excess feed into the second gallipot. When the tubing is primed and all air removed, apply the clamp again.

Then:

For bolus feeding

- Connect the feed administration set to the tube (Anderton 1995).
- Slowly release the clamp and raise the barrel of the feed system to allow feed to flow into the tube by gravity. The higher the tube is raised, the faster the flow rate. Administration of the feed should take the same length of time as it would take the child to have the same amount orally – usually 15–30 min.
  - If the feed is too thick, or the bore of the NG tube too narrow to allow feed to drip in by gravity, then the feed must be instilled using the plunger. Gently depress the plunger to deliver the feed at the same rate as if feeding by gravity. Never use excessive force; this will make the child vomit.
- Top-up the barrel with the remaining feed as it begins to empty. Do not allow it to empty as far as the tubing until the feed is complete (to prevent instilling air into the tube, leading to discomfort and wind).

- While the feed is being given, encourage the child to suck (on a dummy) so that sucking is associated with the sensation of feeding. The older child can be tube fed at the dinner table to encourage normal socialisation associated with feeding. Similarly, the older child should be encouraged to play with feeding utensils while being tube fed.
- When the feed is complete, remove the empty gravity feed system and close off the feeding tube before air can get into the tube.
- Gently flush the feeding tube with the remaining 2–5 mL of sterile water in the appropriate size of syringe. Cap off the feeding tube.
- Make the child comfortable and clear away equipment.
- A gravity feed set must be discarded and a new set used for each feed to reduce the risk of bacterial contamination (Enteral feeding-infection control guidelines, ICNA/Nutricia 2003).

For continuous feeding

- If the feed has preservatives and is sterile (e.g. a proprietary brand), the full amount of feed (up to 24 h worth) should be primed in the administration set to prevent the set being accessed frequently and therefore reduce the risk of bacterial contamination (Patchell et al 1998). If the feed does not have preservatives (e.g. it is made daily by a special feed kitchen), the set should be primed with enough feed for 4 h at a time (Skipper et al 2003).
- Plug in and switch on the enteral pump. Load the administration set into the pump.
- Set the pump to the correct rate (in mL/h) to deliver the desired quantity in the required time period. If it is important that a limited, specific, quantity of feed is to be delivered use the appropriate function on the pump and set a total volume for delivery.
- Connect the feed administration set to the tube.
- Set the pump to run. The nurse should check the pump hourly and document the amount of feed that the pump has administered.
- Aspirate the tube every 4 h to test that it remains correctly *in situ* in the stomach.
- The tube should be flushed with water every 4 h to ensure patency.

- If the set is to be topped up with feed 4-hourly, then a cleaned work surface/trolley should be used and apron and disposable gloves worn. The top of the feed container and the opening of the administration set are both wiped using alcohol wipes before feed is put into the system (Anderton 1995).
- Change the feed administration set every 24 h (Anderton 1995).

OBSERVATIONS AND COMPLICATIONS

Observations

- Check when the tube was last changed and is due to be changed.
- Check the skin around a gastrostomy site for any signs of soreness caused by leakage from the stoma.
- Always check the position of the tube before using it. Be aware that pH paper/strips will not indicate the recommended acid reaction if the child is on anti reflux treatment. An acid reaction of 0–5 using pH paper is the safest way to indicate an acidic aspirate, thus indicating that the tube is correctly placed (Metheney et al 1993, NHS QIS 2007, Medical Devices Agency 2004, NPSA 2005).
- While feeding, check that the child appears comfortable and is not showing signs of discomfort such as heaving or retching.
- Check the child's breathing and colour while administering the feed.

Complications

- Incorrect feed calculation could lead to too much or too little feed being given.
- The wrong feed or wrongly constituted feed could be given if not properly checked.
- The biggest risk of NG feeding is the tube being, or becoming, misplaced. This can cause feed to be delivered into the lungs, or feed to be aspirated. If at any time during a NG feed the child becomes blue or has difficulty breathing, the feed must be stopped immediately and the tube aspirated. The child may require suction.
- NG and gastrostomy tubes can also be misplaced in the wrong part of the gut. If either tube is in the small intestine rather than in the stomach, aspirate will be obtained, but will not

be acidic. In this case, the tube should be repositioned and re-checked for correct position before use.

- Vomiting can occur if the feed is given too fast.
- Tubes may become blocked, but excessive force should never be applied to try to unblock them as this could damage the tube and increase the risk of feed being instilled in the wrong place. If a tube remains blocked, it must be removed and a new one inserted if required.
- Rarely, a gastrostomy tube can migrate into the small intestine with the peristaltic action of the intestine. This can cause diarrhoea, vomiting and even intestinal obstruction and/or perforation, causing the child great discomfort and distress (Coldicutt 1994). Prevention is better than cure and the importance of correctly fitting and securing the tubes must be stressed.
- Bacterial contamination can lead to gastroenteritis.
- Prolonged absence of oral feeding can lead to developmental delay. Oral stimulation, sucking and swallowing can disappear and speech development can be affected (Evans Morris & Dunn Klein 1987, Taylor & Goodison-McLaren 1992). Manipulating food – chewing, swallowing, etc. – enables the child to learn the control of tongue and mouth muscles that is necessary to produce intelligible speech.

Without oral feeding, pleasant associations with oral stimulation such as gratification of hunger are lost and the child can become hypersensitive to touch and taste (Evans Morris & Dunn Klein 1987). This makes it increasingly difficult to reintroduce oral feeding after prolonged NG/gastrostomy feeding, when the only associations with oral feeding are unpleasant sensations, e.g. vomiting and suction (Langley 1994). This can then lead to problems with social development as the child may not learn appropriate social behaviour associated with meal times.

All these aspects of development must be considered and action taken to try to mitigate the negative side-effects in children who are unable to feed orally.

COMMUNITY PERSPECTIVE

Many children who require enteral feeding are cared for by their families at home. It is therefore imperative that the carers are aware of all aspects of this care, including potential problems; how to deal with problems and who to contact. Organisation of equipment is essential prior to discharge. This may include a feed pump and an ongoing supply of disposable equipment, nasogastric tubes, enteral syringes, feed bags, gastrostomy button extension tubes (NPSA compliant), pH paper, etc. It can be frustrating if a child's discharge from hospital is delayed because of lack of supplies. Parents also need to know who to contact for further supplies, whether this is a company supplying the entire package, a local chemist, a community dietitian or the CCN. They must also be aware of local policy regarding the servicing of feed pumps. In smaller homes, the sheer volume of supplies needing to be stored can be a problem.

The role of the CCN and/or commercial company nurse is to support the carers, ensuring that they are not only competent in the techniques required but are also happy to undertake them. Whereas enteral feeding is a routine procedure in hospital, it is a major commitment for families at home, both physically and emotionally. Concerns about altered body image may be problematic for parents, siblings and the child. The CCN will have the opportunity to recognise and address any concerns in the safe environment of the home and advise regarding referral for further psychological support if necessary.

Nasogastric feeding

Some parents are happy to undertake not only the technique of feeding but also replacing the tube. This is advantageous for carers and nursing staff, as tubes are frequently pulled out at the most inconvenient times, resulting either in parents having to travel back to hospital at short notice or community nurses having to reorganise their schedules to ensure that a child does not miss a feed. If the child is under the care of a children's hospice near to their home, they are usually able to facilitate the replacement of a nasogastric tube, thus avoiding going to hospital with potential long delays and parking costs.

Passing a nasogastric tube can be a frightening experience on the first few occasions and support for the carer at this time is vital. The opportunity to undertake the procedure in hospital prior to discharge is therefore most helpful and, on the first few occasions at home, the presence of a member of the CCN team is reassuring. There is the added advantage that the CCN can observe the carer's technique and check that they are confident and competent. Discussion can take place at this time on how to modify infection control measures, as the risk of cross-infection in the home is less, with the emphasis on hand washing techniques. The importance of including the tube-fed child at family meal times should not be overlooked. Parents should not be pressurised into taking on the responsibility of re-passing the nasogastric tube if they are reluctant. Often when they have gained confidence in managing feeds at home, they will feel ready to take on this skill. It is important to remember mouth care (see Ch. 9). Twice daily brushing of the teeth and the use of mouth washes (if appropriate) may improve the feel of the mouth as well as promoting good dental health. A useful tip to stop the skin on the cheeks becoming sore is to apply a strip of Stomahesive or Granuflex/DuoDERM to the cheek (see above), to which the tape is secured, rather than directly to the skin.

Gastrostomy feeding

Gastrostomy feeding is likely to be long term and, therefore, the child or the family will undertake the majority, if not all, of the care. The procedure should therefore fit in with the family's normal lifestyle and not dictate it. They should therefore be in a position to make decisions, in conjunction with medical, nursing and dietetic staff, relating to the type of device and the administration of the feed. In addition to the points related to nasogastric feeding, the family need to be aware of the following:

- The established stoma site which is free from infection should be cleaned in the bath or shower as part of the normal hygiene routine; care being taken to dry the area thoroughly.
- As part of this routine, the device must be turned daily. This helps form a healthy stoma and prevents the formation of adhesions (depends on make of tube).
- Treatment of over granulation of gastrostomy site:
  - Swab site for bacterial presence
  - Excessive moisture can be controlled by using an absorptive dressing
  - A steroid-based, antibiotic, antifungal cream may be prescribed for application to the gastrostomy site (Maxitrol is sometimes used)
  - Once a stoma site is fully healed, after 2–3 weeks, bathing and swimming are allowed (NHS QIS 2007).
- Balloon devices should be deflated and re-inflated weekly to ensure that the correct amount of fluid remains in the balloon; however, this is dependent upon the make of the tube.

- When and how to change a balloon device – a replacement tube should be kept with the child (e.g. at school).
- Methods of unblocking tubes
  - Use a 50 mL syringe to attempt to gently flush (push/pull to instill) the tube using warm water or soda water (at least 10 mL)
  - Gently squeeze the tube between fingers and along its length (i.e. milking the tube)
  - If blockage persists draw back gently on syringe and attempt flush again
  - If still unable to unblock, consider changing tube, if PEG seek medical attention (sodium bicarbonate may be prescribed)
  - If there are problems with recurrent burst balloons or leaking valve ports a gastric aspirate should be taken and checked for yeasts, and if present, treated with fluconazole.
- The carer should observe the manufacturer's recommended life of button extension sets, as these vary considerably. They should also be aware of how to use a decompression tube, if applicable.

The aim of the CCN is to ensure that families are empowered to give the recommended nutritional support to their child, while maintaining as relaxed a home environment as possible. This is best achieved by ensuring a smooth transition from hospital to home and providing ongoing support from the appropriate members of the multidisciplinary team without overwhelming families with professional input. Respite care should, if possible, be offered, either by nursing staff or by carers trained to undertake this care.

DOS AND DON'TS

- Do always check that NG and gastrostomy tubes are correctly positioned before instilling anything into the tube.
- Do stop a NG feed immediately if the child experiences difficulty in breathing or develops cyanosis.
- Do aspirate and flush NG tubes 4-hourly to check position and maintain patency.
- Do secure a gastrostomy tube carefully to prevent peristalsis causing the tube to migrate into the wrong part of the intestine.
- Do secure the gastrostomy tube to prevent movement and granulation tissue forming.

- Do encourage the child who is not fed orally to use the mouth in play – blowing, kissing, touching the mouth and putting fingers into the mouth.
- Do take all measures to prevent bacterial contamination of feed.

- Do make an early referral to a speech and language therapist for children requiring long-term feeding.
- Do not *ever* use a NG or gastrostomy tube if there is any doubt that it is correctly placed in the stomach.

References

Anderton, A., 1995. Reducing bacterial contamination in enteral tube feeds. Br. J. Nurs. 4 (7), 368–376.

Anderton, A., Nivgough, C.E., 1991. Problems with the reuse of enteral feeding systems. A study of effectiveness of a range of cleaning and disinfection procedures. J. Hum. Nutr. Diet. 4, 25–32.

Booth, I.W., 1991. Enteral nutrition in childhood. Br. J. Hosp. Med. 46, 111–113.

Bowling, T., 2003. Nutritional support for adults and children: a handbook for hospital practice. Radcliffe Medical Press, Oxford.

Coldicutt, P., 1994. Children's options. Nurs. Times. 90 (13), 54–56.

Evans Morris, S., Dunn Klein, M., 1987. Pre-feeding skills. A comprehensive resource for feeding development. Therapy Skill Builders, San Antonio, pp. 320, 352.

Hambridge, K.M., Sokol, R.J., Krebs, N.F., 1995. Enteral and parenteral alimentation. In: Roy, A., Silverman, A., Alagille, D. (Eds.), Paediatric clinical gastroenterology, fourth ed. Mosby, St Louis, pp. 1030.

Hendry, P.J., Akyurekli, M.D., McIntyre, R., et al., 1986. Bronchopulmonary complications of nasogastric feeding tubes. Crit. Care Med. 14 (10), 892–894.

Holden, C.E., McDonald, A., Ward, M., et al., 1997. Psychological preparation for nasogastric feeding in children. Br. J. Nurs. 6 (7), 376–385.

Langley, P., 1994. From tube to table. Nurs. Times 90 (48), 43–46.

Lifshitz, F., Finch, N.M., Lifshitz, J.Z., 1991. Children's nutrition. Jones and Bartlett, Boston, pp. 518.

Lord, L.M., 1997. Enteral access devices. Nurs. Clin. North Am. 32 (4), 700.

Medical Devices Agency, 2004. Enteral feeding tubes (nasogastric). Medical Devices Section of the Medicines and Healthcare Products Regulatory Agency. Online. Available: www.medical-devices.gov.uk.

Merck, Tube manufacturer's guidelines. Merck Biomaterial, Alton, Hampshire.

Metheney, N., Reed, L., Wiersema, L., et al., 1993. Effectiveness of pH measurements in predicting tube placement: an update. Nurs. Res. 42 (6), 324–331.

Metheny, N., McSweeney, M., Wehrle, M.A., et al., 1990. Effectiveness of the auscultatory method in predicting feeding tube location. Nurs. Res. 39 (5), 14.

NHS QIS, 2007. Caring for children and young people in the community receiving enteral feeding. NHS QIS Scotland, Edinburgh September.

NPSA, 2005. National Patient Safety Agency Alert 09. Reducing the harm caused by nasal and orogastric feeding tubes in babies under the care of neonatal units. NPSA, London.

Nutritional Care, 2004. Best practice guidelines for confirmation of nasogastric tube placement safety. Birmingham Children's Hospital NHS Trust, Birmingham.

Patchell, C., Anderton, A., Holden, C., et al., 1998. Reducing bacterial contamination of enteral feeds. Arch. Dis. Child 78, 166–168.

Paul, L.A., Holden, C., Smith, A., et al., 1993. Tube feeding and you. Birmingham Children's Hospital NHS Trust, Birmingham.

Paul, L.A., Holden, C., Smith, A., et al., 1994. Gastrostomy feeding and you. Birmingham Children's Hospital NHS Trust, Birmingham.

Sidey, A., 1995. Enteral feeding in community settings. Paediatr. Nurs. 7 (6), 21–24.

Skipper, L., Cuffling, J., Pratelli, N., 2003. Enteral feeding infection control guidelines. Infection Control Nurses Association, London.

Taylor, S., McLaren, G., 1992. Nutritional support – a team approach. Wolfe Publishing, London, pp. 258, 273.

Further reading

Read All Booklets produced by the manufacturers of the devices.

Patchell, C.J., Anderton, A., MacDonald, A., et al., 1994. Bacterial contamination of enteral feeds. Arch. Dis. Child 70, 327–330.

Sidey, A., Torbet, S., 1995. Enteral feeding in community settings. Paediatr. Nurs. 7 (6), 21–23.

Chapter 41

Intravenous therapy

Nan D McIntosh

CHAPTER CONTENTS

Introduction 401
   Learning outcomes 401
   Factors to note 402

Intravenous infusions 402
   Equipment 402
   Method 402
   Observations and complications 403
   Dos and don'ts 404

Blood transfusions 404
   Factors to note 404
   Equipment 405
   Method 406
   Observations and complications 406
   Dos and don'ts 408

Platelet transfusion 408
   Factors to note 408
   Equipment 409
   Method 409
   Observations and complications 409
   Dos and don'ts 409

Parenteral nutrition 409
   Factors to note 409
   Equipment 410
   Method 410
   Observations and complications 410
   Dos and don'ts 412

INTRODUCTION

Intravenous infusions for fluid replacement and drug administration are commonplace in the paediatric ward, whereas blood transfusion, platelet administration and parenteral nutrition (PN) are seen more commonly in haematology, intensive care and neonatal units. The use of home PN has also increased to enable children with a variety of congenital and acquired gastrointestinal conditions to be cared for at home. Maintaining optimal function of intravenous infusions is of primary importance in children's nursing, as fluid overload and electrolyte imbalance are potentially life-threatening and the frequent re-siting of intravenous cannulae is stressful to the child and family (Fitzsimons 2001). Nurses must demonstrate and maintain their competency when administering any type of infusate to a child or young person (NMC 2008). This includes psychological care of the child/young person prior to and during the procedure (Morris 2006). Coping methods such as play and distraction therapy can reduce fear and anxiety (see Ch. 10).

LEARNING OUTCOMES

By the end of this section you should be able to:

- Understand the differences between a child's and an adult's body fluids distribution
- Recognise the need for intravenous fluid therapy
- Ensure the safe administration of intravenous fluid therapy

- Identify children who may require blood or blood products
- Safely administer blood and blood products
- Act appropriately should the child have a reaction to the treatment
- Understand the need for total parenteral nutrition
- Identify children who may require parenteral nutrition
- Safely administer parenteral nutrition.

FACTORS TO NOTE

- Body surface area differs in children and adults, with the infant and child having a proportionally greater body surface area than the adult. There is also a different distribution, e.g. the head constitutes 20% of the infant's body surface area compared with 7–9% of the adult's (Willock & Jewkes 2000).
- The proportion of body weight that consists of water is greater in the infant and child; 75–80% of the newborn's body weight is attributed to fluid compared with approximately 60–70% in adolescents. This reduces to between 50% and 60% in the adult, with females having slightly more body fluid.
- Body fluids are distributed between the intracellular and extracellular compartments. In adults, intracellular body fluid normally constitutes around two-thirds (67%) of total body fluid. The extracellular compartment constitutes the remaining third (33%). The extracellular fluid consists of plasma, lymph, interstitial fluid, bone water and connective tissue water. In infants and children, the majority of body fluid is found in the extracellular compartment; approximately one-half of this is exchanged daily to maintain homeostasis (Clancy & McVicar 2002).
- As a result of this distribution, dehydration will occur more quickly in the infant/child.
- Care should be taken when siting an intravenous cannula to be used for infusion of fluids to ensure that the child's dominant hand is not used.
- The intravenous site must never be covered. This ensures that the site can easily be observed at all times for extravasation. Routine removal of any bandaging for observation may result in the cannula being dislodged.

- A suitable size of intravenous cannula should be selected that not only reflects the size of the child's vascular access but also the intended use.
- Intravenous administration sets may or may not have an 'in-line' burette. It is preferential to use a set with an 'in-line' burette for both neonates and toddlers, as this will minimise the amount of fluid that the child receives should there be free flow of fluid (Dougherty 2002).

As there are numerous types of infusion pump available, the nurse must be educated and competent in the use of the device and have regular updates when new pumps are introduced into the workplace (NPSA 2004).

INTRAVENOUS INFUSIONS

The delivery of intravenous fluids is common within acute paediatric settings. Normally used to maintain hydrational status, intravenous infusions can also be used to administer drugs (Dougherty 2002, RCN 2007). Selection of the intravenous cannula site is important (see Ch. 33); sites should be chosen that present the best calibre vein and that can also be suitably immobilised. Once the intravenous cannula is inserted and secured, the intravenous infusion can be commenced.

EQUIPMENT

- Intravenous fluid for administration
- Intravenous administration set
- In-line burette (if required)
- Air inlet (if required)
- Intravenous infusion pump
- Splint to immobilise limb
- Surgical tape and/or bandage to secure cannula and prevent intravenous line trailing
- Non-sterile gloves and aprons should be worn.

METHOD

1. Identify the child/young person, verify the prescription and explain the need for the infusion and the procedure to the child and parent/carer (obtain verbal/written consent, dependent upon local guidance).
2. Ensure that hands are clean and dry.

3. Intravenous fluid should be checked by two members of the registered nursing staff (or as per local policy) against the medical prescription chart.

4. The expiry date and the batch number on the bag should be recorded on an intravenous infusion recording sheet or as per local policy.

5. Priming of the intravenous administration set is an aseptic procedure and care must be taken to avoid touching the spike or contaminating the system.

6. Remove the intravenous administration set from the sterile packaging.

7. Remove the in-line burette (if required) from the sterile packaging.

8. Insert the intravenous spike of the administration set into the exit line on the sterile burette ensuring that no key parts are touched (Rowley & Laird 2006).

9. Close all roller clamps attached to the burette and administration set.

10. Insert the spike of the burette into the appropriate port of the intravenous fluid bag. *Note:* If the intravenous fluid is in a bottle, the spike should be inserted into the appropriate place in the rubber stopper and an air inlet inserted. Clean the rubber stopper with 70% isopropyl alcohol (e.g. Mediwipes) and allow to dry prior to insertion of the spike and air inlet.

11. Fill the burette (if used) with around 20–30 mL of fluid by opening the roller clamp; then close the clamp.

12. Half fill the in-line bubble of the administration set with fluid by gently squeezing the bubble to expel air into the burette.

13. Open the clamp and allow fluid to flow into the administration set, thus expelling the remaining air. Once fluid has reached the end of the administration set, close the clamps and ensure that all air has been expelled.

14. Place the administration set into the intravenous infusion pump as per manufacturer's instructions.

15. Check patency of the child's intravenous cannula.

16. Attach the administration set to the child's intravenous cannula and secure with surgical tape.

Note: Non-sterile tape should not be placed directly over the insertion site (see Ch. 33).

17. Immobilise the child's limb if necessary with a splint, ensuring that the intravenous cannulation site can be easily observed.

18. Set the rate of infusion, as prescribed, on the infusion pump. Open all clamps and commence the infusion. Record time of commencement on appropriate chart.

OBSERVATIONS AND COMPLICATIONS

- Check the intravenous cannula insertion site, venous pressure (read from some computerised infusion pumps), volume infused, rate at which the fluid is infused and type of infusate hourly.

- Observe the intravenous cannula insertion site for signs of redness and swelling. The area approximately 2.5 cm (1 inch) above and below the insertion site should be easily observed.

- If the child complains of pain or there are signs of intravenous infiltration, stop the infusion immediately and report to medical staff. Infiltration can be graded, indicating the degree of possible damage to tissues (Table 41.1).

- Record the volume infused and the rate on a fluid balance chart.

- A running total of fluid infused should be maintained. This provides an accurate hourly fluid intake.

Table 41.1	Grading for intravenous infiltration
GRADE	**MANIFESTATIONS**
I	Painful intravenous site. No signs of swelling or redness
II	Painful site. Slight swelling, inflammation. Good pulse and capillary refill below infiltration site. No blanching evident
III	Painful site. Marked swelling with blanching and skin cool to touch. Good pulse below infiltration site with brisk capillary refill
IV	Very painful site. Marked swelling with blanching of skin. Skin cool to touch, pulses absent below infiltration with slow capillary refill (>4 s). Skin breakdown or necrosis may be present; however, this may be delayed

Infiltration may not traverse through all stages. Infiltration at Grade IV is possible on first detection. IV extravasation monitoring audit available online at: www.extravasation.org.uk

DOS AND DON'TS

- Do check the site on an hourly basis.
- Do stop the infusion if the child complains of pain. Inform the medical staff/nurse practitioner (Table 41.1).
- Do stop the infusion if there are any signs of extravasation.
- Do refer to local extravasation policy.
- Do not obscure the intravenous cannula insertion site.
- Do not bandage fully the limb on which a cannula is sited.
- Do not put the bandage on too tightly or obscure site.

BLOOD TRANSFUSIONS

Transfusion of blood or blood products is performed in children for a variety of reasons, including anaemia, acute haemorrhage, haematological disease, following surgery and in other acute and chronic conditions.

Advances in both surgery and medicine have been made possible partly through the availability of blood and blood products (McClelland 2001). The Serious Hazards of Transfusion reporting scheme (SHOT) is a confidential, anonymous reporting system for transfusion errors and severe transfusion reactions. The report emphasises the vital role of correct checking of component and patient details at every step in the transfusion process. It deals with the main practical aspects of blood and blood components (fresh frozen plasma, platelets, cryoprecipitate) with particular emphasis on a safe approach to the confirmation of component and patient identity. The aim is to ensure that the *right blood* is given to the *right patient* at the *right time*, every time (SHOT, RCN 2005). The recommendations are in keeping with the 'Guidelines for the Administration of Blood and Blood Components and the Management of Transfused Patients', drawn up by the Blood Transfusion Task Force (2005).

FACTORS TO NOTE

- Erythrocytes (red blood cells) are formed in the red bone marrow from haemocytoblasts. As the red blood cell matures it loses its nucleus and caves in on both sides, giving the characteristic biconcave disc shape.
- The usual life span of a red blood cell is 120 days. Once the cells grow old, their membranes become fragile and rupture, the contents being phagocytosed by the macrophages in the spleen, liver and bone marrow.
- The balance of production and destruction is equal under normal homeostasis.
- The main function of red blood cells is to transport oxygen, bound to haemoglobin, to all cells of the body. Other functions include the transport of waste carbon dioxide and the maintenance of blood pH.
- Fetal haemoglobin has a greater affinity for oxygen than adult haemoglobin, which is suitable for the fetal environment. Towards the later stages of pregnancy, the fetus begins to develop adult haemoglobin. The neonatal haemoglobin level is higher than that of children.
- Whole blood transfusion will replenish the volume, red blood cells and oxygen-carrying capacity of the blood. Packed red blood cells, referred to as packed cells, consist of blood in which some 80% of plasma has been removed. A packed cell transfusion aims at replenishing red blood cell mass and thus the oxygen-carrying capacity of the blood; however, a packed cell transfusion will not replenish volume (BCSH 2004, BTS 2007).
- Whole blood transfusion is normally reserved for exchange transfusion for rhesus incompatibility, severe haemorrhage with depletion of coagulation factors and situations where more appropriate blood products are not readily available (UK Blood Transfusion and Tissue Transplantation Services 2003).
- Washed red cells have had the plasma proteins, leucocytes and platelets removed by rinsing with a special solution; this decreases the chance of transfusion reaction. This type of prepared blood may be used in children who have frequent blood transfusions (BTS 2007).
- Following bone marrow transplant, children require to have blood products irradiated.
- Blood should be stored at 4°C; therefore it must be refrigerated in a specialised blood refrigerator. Blood can be stored for up to 36 days, after which it will have to be discarded (BCSH 2004).

- The blood transfusion should be commenced within 30 min following the arrival of blood from the blood bank (McClelland 2001, BTS 2007, Montgomery & Kumar 2008).
- There are no clear guidelines for the use of blood warmers and the decision is the responsibility of the consultant on each individual patient. This decision may be influenced by the temperature of the patient receiving the transfusion (i.e. hypothermic), the amount of blood being transfused, the duration of the transfusion, or patients with an antibody in their plasma which causes haemolysis when the temperature lowers (e.g. cryoglobulinaemia). A blood warmer actively warms the transfusion during administration by using tubing coils in a water bath. This may be performed during exchange transfusions or to prevent air embolism (Smith 2001, RCN 2005).
- Blood should be transfused over 4 hours Transfusions exceeding this time may become contaminated with bacteria. If the volume of blood cannot be transfused within 4 hours, it should be divided into smaller volumes (paedipacks) and stored accordingly in the blood bank until required (BCSH 2004, RCN 2005, BTS 2007).
- Blood is obtained from people who are between the ages of 18 and 65 years. Frequency of donations is normally two to three times per year.
- Since 1985, all donor blood has been tested for human immunodeficiency virus (HIV 1 and 2 antibody). Testing for hepatitis (A, B and C), syphilis and *Treponema pallidum* antibody are routine (BTS 2007). Selective testing for specific agents may be considered when administering blood to susceptible recipients, e.g. the testing for cytomegalovirus in immunosuppressed children. All donated blood has serologic tests performed to determine blood group (A, B, AB and O) as well as rhesus factor (Rh D +ve or −ve) (BTS 2007).
- Children with blood group AB can be transfused with blood groups AB, A, B and O. Children with blood group A can be transfused with groups A and O, and those with blood group B can be transfused with groups B and O. Those children with blood group O can only be transfused with blood group O (Table 41.2). However, the blood that a child is transfused with must be rhesus compatible, i.e. −ve must

Table 41.2	Blood product compatability		
PATIENT'S ABO GROUP	RED CELLS	PLATELETS	PLASMA
O	O	O, A, B	O, A, B, AB
A	A, O	A	A, AB
B	B, O	B, A	B, AB
AB	AB, A, B, O	A, B	AB, A

have −ve, but +ve can have +ve or −ve. Blood group O is regarded as the universal donor whereas blood group AB is the universal recipient (BTS 2007).

- Religious and cultural beliefs of the child and family must be taken into account when considering a blood transfusion. Families who are Jehovah's Witnesses may not agree to blood transfusions and substitutes may have to be considered. In cases where volume expansion is necessary, colloidal fluids may be as effective; however, if blood is a necessity, a court order may have to be obtained if the family does not give consent.

EQUIPMENT

Requirements are as for intravenous infusion. The following extra items are required:

- Blood or blood component administration set (this must be appropriate for the pump if one is being used), pack of blood or blood component
- Blood bank issue slip (supplied with the first unit of the batch sent from the blood bank. This includes details of each pack in the batch to be transfused); this should be readily available throughout the transfusion, located with the fluid administration chart at the child's bedside
- Blood components/products prescription
- Child's case notes, to enable checking of each unit administered
- 0.9% saline to prime the giving set
- In-line burette (if required)
- Infusion pump (e.g. Ivac pump).

Leucodepletion

Since 1999 all blood components have been leucodepleted ($<5 \times 10^6$/unit) at point of manufacture. This move was prompted by theoretical concerns about variant Creutzfeldt–Jakob disease (vCJD) transmission. Following this move, the use of bedside leucodepletion filters has become redundant.

Blood must be transfused through a blood giving set with an integral mesh filter (170–200 μm pore size). Platelets, fresh frozen plasma and cryoprecipitate must be administered through a normal blood administration set or through a platelet/cryoprecipitate giving set. Plasma protein solutions (4.5% albumin or 20% albumin) do not require to be infused through a giving set with a filter. A standard infusion set as used for crystalloids or synthetic colloids is suitable.

Filters

Each giving set designed for the administration of blood or blood components contains an integral 170–200 μm pore size mesh filter to remove macroaggregate or particulate matter. For the vast majority of transfusions, no additional filter is required.

Microaggregate filters

There are several filters available designed to hold back particles down to 20–40 μm in size (e.g. Pall Ultipore). There are few clinical indications, if any, for the use of these filters and their use for routine transfusions is unnecessary and expensive.

METHOD

1. Explain the procedure to the child and parent/carer and ensure that consent has been obtained. (This may be verbal or written depending on local policy.)
2. Wash and dry your hands.
3. Assemble the equipment and prime the administration set with 0.9% saline (see above). Check the blood for administration against the medical prescription, haematology/blood bank information, case records and with the child and/or parent/carer. The child's name, date of birth, hospital identification number, blood group, rhesus factor status, blood bag number and expiry date should be checked using the identification label attached to the bag of blood, the haematology/blood bank information slip, the child's hospital notes and the child's identification band. This check

should be done independently by two appropriately trained health professionals (Montgomery & Kumar 2008). Remember the final check must take place at the child's bedside (with the child) by the same two members of staff (BCSH 2004).

4. If the child is known to have any special transfusion needs (e.g. irradiated components), the prescription form must state this and pack labelling should be checked to ensure that these requirements have been met.
5. Check the bag of blood for abnormal colour, gas bubbles, clumping or any extraneous material. This may give an indication of bacterial contamination (Practice Guide 2006).
6. Attach the blood bag and prime the administration set with blood (if the child is not to receive the saline within the system, as may be the case if the child is fluid restricted) and attach to the child's cannula. Secure the child's limb as necessary (see above).
7. Monitor and record the transfusion as per intravenous infusions.
8. Once the transfusion is complete, flush the administration set with 0.9% saline and proceed as per medical instruction.

OBSERVATIONS AND COMPLICATIONS

- *Prior* to commencing the transfusion *of each unit*, record the child's temperature, respiratory rate, pulse and blood pressure on the appropriate chart (baseline recording). These observations must be recorded 15 min after commencement of each transfusion (United Kingdom Blood Services 2007) as per local policy. Additional recordings are at the discretion of each area but are essential if the child is unstable or if they appear to be experiencing an adverse reaction.
- The child is observed during the transfusion of blood and blood components to detect any adverse event as early as possible, in order that potentially life-saving action may be taken. Adverse reactions may be seen with all blood components and monitoring is therefore required even for patients receiving only fresh frozen plasma (FFP), platelets or cryoprecipitate. Severe reactions most commonly present during the first 15 min of a transfusion and the patient should be observed

Table 41.3   Reactions to blood transfusions

REACTION	MANIFESTATIONS	MANAGEMENT
Haemolytic reaction (Cause: incompatible blood. Rare)	Chills, fever, shaking, pain at i.v. site and along venous tract, breathlessness, abnormal bleeding, haematuria, progress to shock and renal failure	Stop transfusion Inform medical staff Retain sample of donor blood Obtain sample of child's blood Medical treatment to reverse shock
Febrile reactions (Cause: leucocyte, platelet or plasma protein antibodies)	Fever or chills	Stop transfusion Inform medical staff Administer prescribed antipyretic
Allergic reactions (Cause: allergens in donor's blood)	Urticaric rash, wheeze, breathlessness, laryngeal oedema	Stop transfusion Inform medical staff Epinephrine/steroid therapy may be used to counteract reaction Prophylactic antihistamines may be used in children who have a known reaction
Circulatory overload (Cause: rapid infusion)	Chest pain, cyanosis, noisy respirations, dyspnea, distended neck veins	Stop transfusion Inform medical staff Place child in upright position Use diuretics to diminish fluid overload in children who can pass urine

most closely during this period. These reactions can be categorised as haemolytic reactions, febrile reactions, allergic reactions and circulatory overload (Table 41.3). If a reaction occurs, stop the transfusion and inform medical staff immediately.

- Prior to commencing the transfusion, briefly explain the procedure to the patient/carer and advise them to notify staff immediately if they become aware of any changes/reaction that they may have, no matter how trivial they think it may be (such as shivering, flushing, urticarial rash, pain or shortness of breath).
- Wherever possible, transfusions should be given in areas where the patient can be readily observed by the clinical staff and during daytime hours.
- When the transfusion is commenced, record the relevant information on the appropriate charts.
- Adjust the flow-rate to achieve transfusion over the prescribed time period.
- Throughout the transfusion, observe the patient for any sign or symptom of incompatibility or adverse reaction, e.g. flushing, urticaria, vomiting, diarrhoea, fever, itching, headache, haemoglobinuria, rigor, severe backache, collapse or circulatory failure. Should any of

these be observed, the transfusion must be stopped immediately and the doctor informed. Keep the i.v. line open with a slow infusion of 0.9% saline.

- The transfusion of a single pack of red cells should be complete within 4–5 hours of removal from the blood fridge. Platelets and FFP are generally infused over 30–60 min. FFP must be infused within 4 hours once thawed.
- Any suspected transfusion reaction or incompatibility should be investigated and the blood bank informed. The blood pack and any empty packs should be returned to the blood bank (if requested by blood bank staff) in an appropriate, sealed polythene bag. Further investigation may be required.

Discontinuation

- Record the volume of blood transfused on the fluid balance chart (or 24-hours chart).
- Repeat the baseline observations 15 min after each infusion.
- In the event of blood transfusion being followed by other intravenous fluids, a change of giving set is required. It is not necessary to give a 0.9% saline 'flush' on completion of transfusion.

- When all units to be transfused have been administered, file the blood bank issue slip in the case sheet.

Disposal

If observation of the child at completion of the transfusion reveals no evidence of an adverse reaction, the bags may be placed in the standard 'clinical waste' bags (orange) for disposal. The giving set should be disposed of in an appropriate sharps container.

DOS AND DON'TS

- Do reassure child/young person/parents regarding the testing of blood and blood products.
- Do check with the child/young person/parents whether the child has had a previous reaction to blood or blood products. Report promptly to medical staff to ensure that appropriate safety measures/treatments are put in place.
- Do ensure that the blood is thoroughly checked by two registered members of staff prior to administration according to local and national policy (BTS 2007).
- Do stop the transfusion if there is any indication of a reaction.
- Do keep emergency equipment at hand in case of a severe haemolytic or anaphylactic reaction.
- Do report any errors/reactions to your local transfusion committee who will in turn inform SHOT.
- Do not, in the case of reaction, restart a transfusion until the child's condition has been fully medically evaluated.
- Do not administer any other medication intravenously using the same cannula during the transfusion.
- Do not give intravenous dextrose immediately before or after transfusion, as haemolysis and clotting may occur within the administration set (BTS 2007).

PLATELET TRANSFUSION

Platelets can be administered both prophylactically and therapeutically to children with thrombocytopenia, leukaemia or those undergoing chemotherapy. These children are at risk of bleeding, which can be fatal in some instances.

FACTORS TO NOTE

- Platelets are formed from cells within the bone marrow. They are disc-shaped cells and there are between 50 000 and 400 000 per cubic millimetre of blood (Tortora & Grabowski 2003).
- The normal life span of platelets is approximately 5–7 days; the life span of transfused platelets is 4 days (BCSH 2004, BTS 2007).
- Platelets arrest bleeding through platelet plug formation, wherein the platelets adhere to the damaged blood vessel. This adhesion changes the characteristics of the platelets by activating a series of reactions within them. This reaction forms a platelet plug which prevents blood loss in small vessels. Although initially loose, the plug eventually becomes tight by being reinforced with fibrin threads during coagulation (Tortora & Grabowski 2003).
- Ideally, platelets are matched according to their ABO and rhesus factors; however, in emergency situations, compatible (or even incompatible) platelet concentrates can be used (BTS 2007).
- Platelet transfusion may not increase platelet count in children with idiopathic thrombocytopenic purpura, disseminated intravascular coagulation or antibody reactions, because such conditions destroy platelets. However, platelet transfusion is of use in the treatment of severe haemorrhage in such children.
- Platelets are stored in the blood bank at 22°C and must *never* be refrigerated. Platelets are issued as single donations of matched platelets in a single pack obtained from one donor by apheresis or pools of four random donors. The total volume is stated on the pack. Ideally, this product should be infused over not more than 60 min. Packs which have been refrigerated inadvertently *must not be used* but should be returned to the blood bank.
- Platelets must be transfused immediately on arrival to the ward/theatre. Specific areas have facilities to enable packs to be constantly agitated for periods prior to transfusion, but this is not necessary during the transfusion period.
- Platelets will usually be group O or group A. As there will be a small amount of contaminating red cells, the appropriate Rhesus D group will be issued to avoid Rhesus D sensitisation in female children.

EQUIPMENT

- Platelets for infusion
- Platelet administration set containing an integral 170–200 μm pore size mesh filter to remove macroaggregate or particulate matter
- Appropriate infusion pump (if used)
- Apron and gloves.

METHOD

1. Explain the procedure to the child and parent/carer and ensure that consent has been obtained. (This may be verbal or written depending on local policy.)
2. Wash and dry your hands.
3. Check the platelets for infusion using the same criteria as those for blood (see above).
4. Prime the administration set (see above).
5. Place the administration set into the pump as per the manufacturer's instructions.
6. Attach the administration set to the child's intravenous cannula and secure.
7. Administer the platelets as instructed by the medical staff. Platelets are normally administered rapidly in 20–40 min (BTS 2007).
8. Once administration is complete, disconnect the platelet administration set and discard it according to hospital policy. Record the volume of platelets infused on the appropriate chart.

OBSERVATIONS AND COMPLICATIONS

- As the platelets are administered relatively rapidly, it is important that the child is constantly observed to monitor any adverse reactions and for the infusion being completed.
- Observe the child for signs of fever, chills or rash, as reaction to platelets can occur. Reactions to platelets are normally treated with antihistamine drug therapy. Report any reactions to the medical staff and stop the infusion until the child has been evaluated.

DOS AND DON'TS

- Do ensure that the platelets are agitated until they are to be transfused. This prevents them from clumping.

- Do administer the platelets rapidly.
- Do not administer platelets using a pump that is not designed for platelet infusion; refer to manufacturer's instructions (MHRA 2005).

PARENTERAL NUTRITION

The development of total parenteral nutrition (PN) has enabled children with a variety of conditions to survive (ASPEN 2002). Parenteral feeding is considered when a child cannot tolerate or absorb adequate nutrition orally or enterally. Parenteral nutrition is administered intravenously and refers to a nutrient solution which comprises dextrose, amino acids, fat, electrolytes, vitamins, micronutrients and water. TPN has associated risks and should only be considered when other feeding methods have failed (ASPEN 2002).

FACTORS TO NOTE

- PN is used in various settings and for various conditions such as short bowel syndrome, intestinal obstruction, persistent severe diarrhea, extensive burns and children receiving chemotherapy (RCN 2007).
- PN should ideally be administered through a central venous catheter, e.g. a Hickman line, or a peripheral cannula. The route of administration will be determined by the length of time that the child is to receive parenteral nutrition and the concentration of dextrose that is to be used. A concentration of dextrose and amino acids of 20–30% may cause vein sclerosis or burns if extravasation occurs; hence for this concentration a central venous catheter is used. For dextrose concentrations below 10% a peripheral cannula can be used (BMA & RPS 2003).
- Parenteral nutrition can be administered continuously throughout the day, as is often the case in the acutely ill, or can be administered overnight. Overnight administration would be considered for the child who is to receive long-term parenteral nutrition as it allows for more freedom of movement during the day.
- Parenteral nutrition is prepared on a daily basis and stored in a temperature-controlled refrigerator. If the child is acutely ill, electrolytes are altered in accordance with the child's own

biochemistry. Children who are to receive their nutrition for a longer period of time and who are stabilised may not require daily alterations to their nutrition.

- Dextrose is primarily used as a source of calories; amino acids are a source of nitrogen for protein synthesis. Electrolytes, minerals, trace elements and vitamins are added to meet the child's known nutritional requirements. Fat emulsions provide a major source of calories as well as preventing essential fatty acid deficiency states (RCN 2007).
- Fat solution, e.g. intralipid, is administered separately, as mixing it with dextrose solution may cause denaturing of the fat solution. However, the same cannula/central line can be used for administration. Fat and dextrose solution are infused into the same central line using a three-way tap or a Y extension.
- The dextrose constituent of the PN renders the child more prone to infection. An aseptic technique must therefore be used when changing bags of solution, and handling or changing intravenous lines (RCN 2007).
- Bags of nutrition should be stored in the refrigerator and removed around 30–60 min prior to the commencement of administration. This allows the solution to warm to room temperature (RCN 2007). Once opened, it should be infused or discarded within 24 h (RCN 2007).

EQUIPMENT

- Dextrose solution with additives
- Fat emulsion solution
- Amino acid solution, e.g. Vamin
- Intravenous administration set
- Intravenous infusion pump, e.g. Ivac pump
- Sterile drapes or dressing pack
- Sterile latex-free gloves
- Apron
- 2% chlorhexidine and 70% isopropyl alcohol
- Three-way tap or Y extension (if required).

METHOD

1. Explain the procedure to the child and parent/carer.
2. Wash and dry your hands.
3. Open all equipment and place on a sterile drape.

4. Two registered nurses (or as per local policy) should check the parenteral nutrition solution against the medical prescription. Check the solution for clarity, turbidity and particles. Check the expiry date.
5. Wearing sterile gloves, prime the intravenous administration set as described for intravenous infusions (see above); however, care should be taken to maintain asepsis.
6. Clean the child's central line/cannula injection site with alcohol solution 2.5 cm (1 inch) from the tip. If the child has an existing administration set attached, clean 2.5 cm (1 inch) on either side of the join. Allow the alcohol to dry.
7. Attach the administration set and thread the line through the infusion pump.
8. Commence the infusion.
9. Monitor and record the infusion as per intravenous infusions (see above).

OBSERVATIONS AND COMPLICATIONS

- Monitor fluid and electrolyte balance closely.
- Protect the bag of dextrose solution from sunlight, if necessary. Some additives degrade in sunlight; hence the solution bag may have to be covered, e.g. with a bag made out of paper or dark plastic. Coloured infusion sets can also be used. Guidance should be sought from the pharmacy department.
- Monitor and record the child's temperature 4-hourly. Pyrexia (temperature >38.5°C) may indicate sepsis and blood cultures should be obtained (Dougherty 2002).
- Monitor and record blood glucose 4-hourly. The frequency of monitoring can be gradually reduced in accordance with the child's condition, but the test should be performed at least daily. Urine may also be tested for glucose as per local policy.
- Monitor weight regularly (ASPEN 2002).
- Observe for any signs of oedema.
- Change the intravenous infusion set every 24 h (or as per local policy).
- To prevent oral dryness, perform oral hygiene frequently.
- If a central line is used, change the dressing in accordance with local policy.

- Sepsis, abnormalities in liver function, hyperglycaemia and hypocalcaemia are some complications of this therapy, therefore the child must be regularly monitored (ASPEN 2002, RCN 2007).

COMMUNITY PERSPECTIVE

There are many issues surrounding these procedures when undertaken in the home; however, providing these are addressed, with safety being paramount, home intravenous therapy may be implemented. The responsibility for instigating such treatment must be given due consideration and, should the Children Community Nurse (CCN) feel insufficiently experienced or trained, accountability in practice must be considered (NMC 2008). Specialist team input may be required, for example for the administration of TPN and immunoglobulin infusions (RCN 2007).

There will be situations where the CCN administers the infusion and others where the carers undertake the role (Mighten 2007). The suitability of the home environment should be assessed before any suggestion is made to the family. Not every environment will be suitable and the presence of boisterous siblings and pets, for example, must be taken into account. Even in the most motivated families, a moment's inattention to a toddler intent on grabbing an intravenous line could be disastrous. These issues need to be discussed with the family before any decision is made. It may be possible to recruit the help of a neighbour or friend in arranging a 'special outing' for the sibling(s) to coincide with a crucial period in the treatment. There are advantages for some families in that the child is likely to be more relaxed in the home environment and able to maintain a more normal lifestyle. The responsibility of undertaking this type of treatment, however, may be too overwhelming for some families, even with skilled teaching input and support from the CCN. This must be assessed, ensuring that carers are not left with feelings of guilt should they decide not to participate in this area of care. Other families may welcome the opportunity to be involved.

The carers will need an intensive teaching programme and issues such as cross-infection should be discussed. The CCN must feel confident in the ability of the carers to cope safely with the procedures. It is important that carers have access to a telephone. Support for paying telephone bills may be available with advice from social services.

General principles

It is necessary to ascertain whether clinical responsibility rests with the hospital paediatrician or with the GP.

The CCN will be responsible for ensuring that carers are fully informed about the therapy to be given, including side-effects and possible complications. They will need to be competent in the use of any pumps or syringe drivers which may be required and be able to recognise signs of infection, either local or systemic.

Where an intravenous pump is to be used, this should be capable of running on its own batteries for some hours, in case of power failure.

Anaphylaxis kits should be provided and carers given the guidelines and information concerning dosages and usage.

Whenever possible, home intravenous therapy should be checked by two people; this will include dose, drug, dilution and expiry date, and always with the prescription sheet which will be written in line with local policy (see Ch. 42). Carers must know who to contact at any time during the treatment and, if the CCN is unavailable, be given a link to the ward. Consideration should be given as to which intravenous system will be simplest for the families to use. This may not be the cheapest, and the CCN may need to convince the budget holder of the importance of this.

Commercial sharps boxes must be provided for safe disposal of ampoules, needles and syringes and disposed of as local policy dictates. This may entail making an arrangement with the council refuse department.

Specific considerations

Blood and blood products are only likely to be given in the community to enable a terminally ill child to remain at home. Should a child have had previous severe reactions then transfusion should not take place in the community (RCN 2001, Dimond 2006). The GP must be aware that the procedure is taking place and ensure that they or a member of the paediatric medical team is immediately contactable if necessary.

The CCN will need to remain in the home for the duration of the transfusion and for 30 min afterwards, monitoring vital signs throughout. Kits for dealing with any spillage should be available (RCN 2005).

Home parenteral nutrition

Close links need to be developed between hospital and community-based staff, specialist pharmacists, dietitians and specialist commercial homecare companies. A home PN information document containing procedures and troubleshooting guidelines should be provided.

It should always be remembered that parents are shouldering a tremendous responsibility and, however competent they become, will need ongoing support.

DOS AND DON'TS

- Do ensure that asepsis is maintained and manipulation of the line is kept to a minimum.
- Do ensure that the intravenous administration infusion set is changed every 24 hours.
- Do ensure, where necessary, that the bag of solution is protected from sunlight.
- Do ensure that parents are involved in care.
- Do not change intravenous lines without using aseptic technique.
- Do not use the same lumen of a central line or peripheral cannula for other drug or fluid administration while PN is in progress.

References

ASPEN American Society for Parenteral and Enteral Nutrition, 2002. Guidelines for the use of parenteral and enteral nutrition in adult and pediatric patients. J. Parenter. Enteral Nutr. 26, 1SA–138SA.

Blood Transfusion Task Force, 2005. Guidelines for the administration of blood and blood components and the management of transfused patients. BCSH, London.

BTS Blood Transfusion Service, 2007. Transfusion medicine handbook, fourth ed. The Blood Transfusion Service of the United Kingdom. HMSO, London. Online. Available: www.transfusionguidelines. org.uk.

BMA, RPS, 2003. British National Formulary for Children. BMA, RPS, London.

BCSH British Committee for Standards in Haematology, 2004. Blood Transfusion Task Force. Transfusion guidelines for neonates and older children. Br. J. Haematol. 124 (4), 433–453.

Clancy, J., McVicar, A., 2002. Physiology and anatomy: a homeostatic approach, second ed. Arnold, London.

Dimond, B., 2006. Intravenous therapy. Duty of care and liability. Br. J. Nurs. 15 (7), 392–393.

Dougherty, L., 2002. Delivery of intravenous therapy. Nurs. Stand. 16 (16), 45–52.

Fitzsimons, R., 2001. Intravenous cannulation. Paediatr. Nurs. 13 (3), 21–23.

McClelland, D.B.L., 2001. Handbook of transfusion medicine, third ed. TSO, London.

MHRA Medicines and Healthcare Products Regulatory Agency, 2005. Medical device alert MDA 2005/1 and device bulletin 2005/1. Reporting adverse incidents and disseminating Medical Device Alerts MHRA, London.

Mighten, J., 2007. Home intravenous therapy training for carers of children and young people. Br. J. Nurs. 16 (5), 272–276.

Montgomery, H., Kumar, J., 2008. Safe administration of blood and blood products. In: Kelsey, J., McEwing, G. (Eds.), Clinical skills in child health. Churchill Livingstone, Elsevier, London.

Morris, R., 2006. Intravenous drug administration: A skill for student nurses? Paediatr. Nurs. 18 (3), 35–38.

NPSA, 2004. Standardising and centralising infusion devices – a project to develop safety solutions for NHS trusts. NPSA, London.

NMC, 2008. The Code. Standards of Conduct, performance and ethics for nurses and midwives. NMC, London.

Practice Guide, 2006. Blood transfusion practice. Paediatr. Nurs. 18 (10), 18.

RCN Royal College of Nursing, 2001. Administering intravenous therapy to children in the community setting: guidance for nursing staff, third ed. Royal College of Nursing, London.

RCN Royal College of Nursing, 2005. Guidance for improving transfusion practice. RCN, London.

RCN Royal College of Nursing, 2007. Standards for infusion therapy. RCN, London.

Rowley, S., Laird, H., 2006. Aseptic non-touch technique. In: Trigg, E., Mohammed, T.A. (Eds.), Practices in children's nursing guidelines

for hospital and community.
Churchill Livingstone, Elsevier,
London.

SHOT Serious Hazards of
Transfusion Reporting Scheme,
Online. Available: www.shotuk.
org.

Smith, C.E., 2001. Principles of fluid
warming in trauma. In:
Smith, C.E., Rosenberg, A.D.,
Grande, C.M. (Eds.), Massive

transfusion and control of
haemorrhage in the trauma
patient, Seminars in Anaesthesia,
Peri-operative Medicine and Pain
20 51–59.

Tortora, G.J., Grabowski, S.R., 2003.
Principles of anatomy and
physiology, tenth ed. Harper
Collins, New York.

UK Blood Transfusion and
Tissue Transplantation

Services, 2003. Guidelines.
Online. Available: www.
transfusionguidelines.org.ok.

United Kingdom Blood Services,
2007. Handbook of Transfusion
Medicine, fourth ed. TSO,
London.

Willock, J., Jewkes, F., 2000. Making
sense of fluid balance in children.
Paediatr. Nurs. 12 (7), 37–42.

Further reading

British Committee for Standards in
Haematology (BCSH) guidelines,
Online. Available: www.
bcshguidelines.com.

Hughes, D.A., Milligan, A.,
Mehta, A., 2007. Home
therapy for lysosomal storage
disorders. Br. J. Nurs. 16 (22),
1384–1389.

Kassner, N.E., 2005. Blood
transfusion therapy. In:
Tomlonson, N.E., Kline, N.E.

(Eds.), Pediatric oncology
nursing. Springer, Berlin.

Kelsey, J., Blexham, N., 2008.
Peripheral intravenous
therapy. In: Kelsey, J.,
McEwing, G. (Eds.), Clinical
skills in child health practice.
Churchill Livingstone, Elsevier,
London.

Scottish Intercollegiate Guidelines
Network (SIGN), Guideline on
perioperative transfusion.

Online. Available: www.sign.ac.
uk/guidelines.

SHOT Guidelines – Annual Report
(Serious Hazards of Transfusion).
Available within each Hospital/
Trust.

SNBTS Scottish National Blood
Transfusion Service,
Compendium of Product
Information. Online. Available:
www.learnbloodtransfusion.
org.uk.

SECTION **6**

Medicines management

SECTION CONTENTS

42. The safe management of medicines for children   417

43. Oxygen therapy   446

44. Pain management   454

Chapter 42

The safe management of medicines for children

Louise Ford, Christina Maddox, Emma Moore, Rachel Sales

CHAPTER CONTENTS

Introduction   418
   Learning outcomes   418
   Rationale   418
   Factors to note   418
   Guidelines for administering medicines
   to children   419

Oral medication   423
   Equipment   424
   Technique   424

Nasogastric, orogastric or gastrostomy
medication   424
   Guidelines and precautions   424

Intravenous medication   425
   Equipment   425
   Method   426

Intramuscular medication   426
   Site   427
   Potential complications   428
   Equipment   428
   Technique   428

Subcutaneous medication   428
   Site   429
   Potential complications   429
   Equipment   429
   Technique   429

Intraosseous administration   430
   Equipment   430
   Method   430

Epidural infusions   430

Intrathecal medication   430

Chemotherapy   430

Rectal medication   431
   Potential complications   431
   Equipment   431
   Site   431
   Technique   431

Topical medication   431
   Equipment   432
   Technique   432

Transcutaneous medication   432
   Equipment   432
   Technique   432

Intra–aural/otic medication   432
   Equipment   432
   Technique   432

Intraocular/optic medication   433
   Equipment   433
   Technique   433

Anaphylaxis   434
   Causes   434
   Treatment of severe anaphylaxis   434
   Equipment and treatment   434

Inhaled therapy devices   436
   Guidelines   436
   Inhalers   438
   Spacers for babies and young children   438
   Nebulisers   439
   Potential complications   440
   Factors to note   440
   Dos and don'ts   441

INTRODUCTION

The Crown Report provides a comprehensive review of all aspects of drug administration that includes prescribing, supplying and administering medicines, and clearly states that: 'No health professional should undertake any aspect of patient care for which they are not trained and which is beyond their professional competence' (DoH 1999, p 23). Therefore, for students undertaking programmes to become registered children's nurses, recognition of personal limits, knowledge, understanding and skills are an essential part of the learning process. This is also endorsed within the Nursing and Midwifery Council (NMC) Standards for Medicine Management (NMC 2008a).

LEARNING OUTCOMES

After reading this section you should be able to:

● Understand the importance of administering medicines safely
● Understand the need to communicate effectively with the child and family
● Understand the importance of preparing children when administering medicines
● Understand the routes for the administration of medicines
● Understand the identification of suitable techniques for administration via each route.

RATIONALE

The administration of medicines to infants, children and teenagers requires a complex set of skills that must be grounded in a sound understanding of child development, not only in terms of biophysiological changes but also changes that occur from a psychological perspective (Watt 2003a). Knowledge and skills that are essential for children's nurses include understanding the relevant underpinning theory to support care, being numerically competent and being an effective communicator (Nicol & Thompson 2000, 2001, NMC 2008a). For this to be realised, registered nurses must have a sound knowledge base regarding the administration of medicines, that draws upon the currently available literature and use this to inform everyday practice.

FACTORS TO NOTE

The main pieces of legislation that influence the administration of medicines within the UK: the Medicines Act (1968) and the Misuse of Drugs Act (1971) and the EU Regulation of Paediatric Medicine (2006), which came into effect in January 2007. Within the European Union there are approximately 75 million children between the ages of 0 and 16 years, which represents approximately one-fifth of the total population (European Commission 2002). Choonara (2000, 2008) acknowledges that children have the right to receive medicines that are not only safe but effective for use specifically with this client group. Saint-Raymond and Seigneuret (2005) and Choonara and Bonati (2007) highlight the fact that European legislation encourages the pharmaceutical industry to provide an evidence base for the use of medications for children (Choonara & Bonati 2007). The EU legislation 'Better medicines for children' should also provide sufficient incentive for pharmaceutical companies to develop medicines for children (Wong et al 2006).

The majority of the world's children do not live in the UK or the USA where legislation supports and encourages the improvement of drug interventions; therefore the world's most vulnerable children are arguably still at risk. According to Choonara (2008), the majority of the world's children do not live where they have easy access to child appropriate medicines; within the UK in 2002, it was estimated that 200 million prescriptions for children and adolescents were issued (Costello et al 2004). In spite of these statistics, approximately 50–90% of all medicines administered to children have never been evaluated for use with children (Schaad 2001, European Commission 2002). This has had the effect of children becoming 'therapeutic orphans', which has led to the death of some children (Sutcliffe 2003). As a consequence, the European Commission proposed regulation of orphan medicinal products and this was adopted in December 1999 (European Commission 2002).

Within the UK, marketing authorisation is required from the Medicines Control Agency before medicines can be marketed and promoted (Wong et al 2006); however, it is common practice to prescribe unlicenced medicines (UL), also known as off label medicines (OL), to children; it is not illegal for a doctor to prescribe a medicine with different indicators or to children of different ages (McLay et al 2006, Stephenson 2000, 2001). Prescribing medicines that are off label is necessary when there is no suitable alternative (Watt 2003a). However, this practice of using 'off label medicines' is being associated with increased adverse reactions and has also been known to have fatal consequences particularly in neonatal care (Choonara & Conroy 2002). Of all admissions of children to hospital, at least one-third of the child population and 90% of infants in neonatal intensive care units, receive UL or OL drugs (Conroy et al 2000, Stephenson 2001); in primary care approximately 11–33% of prescriptions for children are UL or OL (McIntyre et al 2000). *Medicines for Children* (RCPCH 2003) is a relatively new formulary that provides practitioners with consensus views on correct dosages for children of all ages and is an important point of reference for all those involved in prescribing medicines to children. Please also note that the British National Formulary for children is an important reference point to use.

With reference to the administration of medicines, there are two key principles of common law, the first of which is the person's right to self-determination. Griffith et al (2003) cite Lord Goff in Airdale NHS Trust *v* Bland [1993] and maintain that self-determination requires healthcare professionals to respect the wishes of patients and carers. The second principle involves the practitioner's responsibility when administering medicines in any environment. A medicine that does have a product licence would be deemed to be unlicensed if, for example, tablets are crushed or capsules are opened, in which case the practitioner must be able to justify the reasons why this was done and may find themselves personally liable if harm comes to those receiving the medicine (Griffith et al 2003).

What is a medicine?

A medicinal product may be defined as any substance or combination of substances presented for treating or preventing disease in human beings or animals (Article 1.2 EC Directive 65/65 cited by the Crown Report, DoH 1999, p 79).

Within the Medicines Act (1968, section 130), there are three legal categories in which medicines can be grouped: according to potency, potential adverse effects and the need for the supply of some medicines to be professionally supervised (Crown Report, DoH 1999).

- *POM: prescription only medicines* – This group of medicines is sold or supplied with the signed authorisation of an 'appropriate practitioner'; this may be a doctor, dentist or, in some instances, a nurse prescriber. These medicines must be supplied by or under the supervision of a pharmacist.
- *P: pharmacy medicines* – These medicines must be supplied or sold by or under the supervision of a pharmacist on registered premises.
- *GSL: general sales list medicines* – These can be supplied and purchased directly by members of the public at 'any lockable business premises'.

GUIDELINES FOR ADMINISTERING MEDICINES TO CHILDREN

The National Service Framework for Children (DoH 2003) clearly states that the administration of medicines to children must be based on the best available evidence to underpin practice. The NMC Standards for Medicine Management (NMC 2008a) clearly indicate that it is not a rule book to be adhered to, covering all potential situations that may be encountered in practice; instead it is a set of guiding principles that must be used in conjunction with local trust/hospital policy (DoH 2003), thereby attempting to reduce the potential for errors in the administration of medicines (Watt 2003b). Standard 18 of the NMC (2008a) Standards for Medicine Management clearly states: *Students must never administer/supply medicinal products without direct supervision.*

The Standards for Medicine Management (NMC 2008a) must be used in conjunction with local trust/hospital policies on how to administer and who can administer medicines, as policies and protocols will vary to meet local needs. The NMC (2008a) requires that the registered nurse or midwife be able to administer medicines in a way that is technically safe and that they should also be able to contribute to any decisions regarding the prescription in a clinically competent and professional manner. Nurses are accountable for the drugs that they administer; therefore a prerequisite must be knowledge about drug actions, side-effects and dosages of any drugs that are administered to the child (Standard 8 of the Standards for Medicine Management, NMC 2008a). Kaushal et al (2001) suggest that Adverse Drug Events (ADEs) in children may be more common than had been originally thought; Ghaleb et al (2005) suggest that this is because what constitutes 'administering children's medications' is difficult to define.

Watt (2003b) identified the five 'Cs' as important principles to ensure the safe administration of medicines to all children:

- Correct child
- Correct medicine
- Correct dose
- Correct time
- Correct route.

To administer medication safely, the nurse must ensure that:

- The *correct child* receives the medication. The identity of the child must be checked. Name bands are used. However, if a parent is available, confirmation of identity by them is a useful resource. If in doubt, ask, because you may encounter children with similar names, or children from multiple births and potentially the patient can be confused with another child if engaging in activities on the ward or play room.
- The *correct medicine* must be given to the child. Hand-written prescriptions must be clear and unambiguous; in addition the label on the medicine to be dispensed must have guidelines that are also clear and easy to follow. There are times when seeing a drug written on a prescription may be assumed to be one thing when, in fact, it is something else (e.g. ceftazidime, cefotaxime). The nurse must be clear and understand exactly what is to be dispensed; if there is any element of doubt, the doctor must rewrite the prescription in a clear and legible manner. It is also important that the expiry dates on all medicines are checked for each drug, every time they are given.
- The *correct dose* must be given to the child. It is important that nurses ensure that the child receives the correct dose of medication; if in doubt there are numerous formularies to refer to, including *Medicines for Children* (RCPCH 2003) and the latest British National Formulary for children. The NMC (2008b) position is clear in that nurses must check the dose to be given. This requires numeracy skills that are not dependent upon the use of a calculator; relying on a calculator and a formula is not sufficient. If there is any element of doubt, *stop – do not give the medicine*. Check with the doctor and pharmacist and read the appropriate drug

information. Where there is more than one checker, calculations need to be completed independently and you should not feel intimidated if you arrive at different answers; check again separately and then with a third person if necessary (Watt 2003b). It is possible to administer an overdose if you do not understand the difference between milligrams (mg) and micrograms (µg). It is important to request that prescriptions are written out in full and abbreviations are not used, as this helps to avoid such confusion.

- The *correct time*. It is important that the medicine is given at the correct time; in some instances therapeutic doses need to be maintained. The NMC guidelines (2008b) state that when administering medicines, the checking of the route of administration as well as the time that the medicine is given are important parts of the process. Therefore all medicines that are administered must be an integral part of caring for the child and family and considered within the context of the child's current condition and other treatments that the child may be receiving. If there is any doubt that a dose has already been given but there is no evidence to indicate that the medicine has been administered, do not repeat the dose, but check with the person concerned and inform the doctor and ward manager. All events and actions taken must be documented in the nursing records (Watt 2003b).
- The *correct route*. Ensuring that the medicine is administered by the correct route is fundamental to the NMC's principles, which clearly indicate that nurses must consider the method of administration and its appropriateness and that the instructions written by the doctor match the information written on the medicine label (Dimond 2003b). If there are discrepancies, the doctor and pharmacist need to be alerted to the situation and this action documented in the child's nursing care records.

Record-keeping

Good record-keeping should be regarded as an important part of the process of administering medicines (NMC 2007b; see also local trust/hospital policies). It is the duty of the nurse administering the medicine to ensure that a record is made of the dose administered, the time given, the drug given and the administration route (Dimond 2003c). In the event of an error in medication administration being noted, it is important to follow trust policies for such an event; this usually includes ensuring the child is safe, informing the ward manager, doctor, parent and child. If appropriate, an incident form *must* be completed and the error documented in the patient's notes (Watt 2003b). Dimond (2003c) acknowledges that there is a danger that if a mistake is made by a nurse, they will not acknowledge that it has happened for fear of reprisals. In the event that an error in administration of a medicine occurs, the NMC's position is very clear in terms of advice to practitioners: What is important to recognise is that in the event that you do make an error in medicine administration, you must report it immediately to your line manager or employer (NMC 2008a). For individuals to admit when mistakes have been made, employers need to facilitate an open culture and one in which individuals are not fearful of reprisals. The NMC (2008b) is supportive of critical incident panels as a forum in which lessons can be learnt and improvements made to local practice, in light of such incidents (Dimond 2003c). As Dimond (2003c, p 761) highlights:

> The NMC takes great care to distinguish between those cases where the error was the result of reckless or incompetent practice or was concealed, and those that resulted from other causes, such as serious pressure of work, and where there was immediate, honest disclosure in the patient's interest.

Employers should therefore be encouraging a work culture in which it is considered to be normal working practice to challenge and question all members of the healthcare team, irrespective of who or what they do as a member of that team.

Storage of medicines

The manufacturers of medicines will usually indicate the type of storage conditions required, for example avoid sunlight or store at low temperatures, to ensure that drugs do not lose therapeutic effectiveness. There are legal obligations that each trust or care setting must adhere to as in cases where the manufacturer of a medicine is not known then the last person in the supply chain will

be deemed to be the manufacturer and can be held liable for any damages against the person (Griffith et al 2003). It is essential that all trusts/hospitals/care settings where medicines are administered keep accurate details of all supplies of medicines and ensure that they are securely stored (Griffith et al 2003).

The storage of all medicines is subject to legal requirements and statutory instruments (Dimond 2003a) and to local trust/hospital policies; therefore all practitioners working within a trust are responsible for familiarising themselves with those policies. These will include the following guiding principles, as adapted from Griffith et al (2003):

- Medicines should be stored and assembled in temperatures that remain below 25°C
- Medicines for taking orally (by mouth) should be stored in a locked trolley, cupboard or room
- All controlled drugs must be stored in a locked cabinet
- A locked refrigerator must be employed for the exclusive use of storing medicines and should have a thermometer to monitor the temperature on a daily basis.

Self-administration of medicines

The NHS Plan (DoH 2000) has, as a central theme, the importance of empowering patients to take an active role in their own care. The Audit Commission (2001) clearly indicates that patients are given the opportunity to learn about and take responsibility for their own medicines. Self-administration of medicines is not a new concept within the realms of adult care (DoH 2000), with many parts of the UK fully embracing this as everyday practice. However, self-administration in children's nursing is a less established practice. Wright et al (2002) maintain that the role of the nurse in terms of administering medicines to children is not that of a 'traditional role of administering'; adversely, it is now becoming a role that involves children and families managing their own medicines, with nurses focusing on education and facilitation of the child and family.

Nurse prescribing

To date, doctors, dentists and certain nurses are legally authorised to prescribe medicines. The Crown Report (DoH 1999) recommended the further development of the prescribing role and *The NHS Plan* (DoH 2000) highlighted that the prescribing of medicines and treatments is a key role for nurses. The Crown Report (DoH 1999) also identified that there needs to be training for the preparation of specific practitioners and needs to include Children's Nurses (Dimond 2003d, Hutchinson & Hall 2003, NMC 2006, Pontin & Jones 2007).

Gibson et al (2003) have been able to demonstrate how nurse prescribing can be seen as a means of improving care delivery to children and families, and the expansion of the role of the clinical nurse specialist (CNS) as a 'logical development' in the expanding role of nurses. While it is anticipated that nurses are the most likely group of healthcare professionals to develop prescribing skills, it is also important to note that other health professionals such as physiotherapists may be accommodated within the legislation in the future (Dimond 2003d).

Developmental issues for consideration

As students, you will be constantly reminded of the fact that children are not 'mini adults'. This is a complex phenomenon that includes social, cultural, ethnic, biological and physiological differences, which all impact on the ways in which children understand and make sense of their world and communicate with others. Therefore, gaining the child's trust and cooperation to effectively and safely administer medicines requires a sound understanding of the forces at play. There is an abundance of literature that explains the developmental progression of the infant through to adolescence, and this work has provided the basis for researchers to explore how children understand their bodies, health, illness and the experiences of being in hospital.

There is a growing body of evidence that explores children's knowledge and attitudes towards medication (Hämeen-Anttila et al 2006). Hämeen et al (2006) found that children's understanding of medicines and related topics increased and became more complex with chronological development; therefore when children are being given medications, it is important that they are offered an explanation/education that not only reflects chronological development but also takes into account cognitive development (Hämeen-Anttila et al 2006). Preparation of children for any

procedure is vital; this includes the giving of medicines and remembering to assess the child's understanding (Hämeen-Anttila et al 2006). By communicating effectively and getting to know the children and families that you are involved in caring for will begin to gain their trust, understanding and cooperation, not only when administering medicines but in all other aspects of care.

Routes of administration

The administration of medicines to children is frequently an aspect of nursing care that causes concern for the child, family and nurse. Medicines may vary in form and are given by a range of routes (see Table 42.1). The child's dignity, individuality and understanding need to be paramount when giving medicines (NMC 2008a, Standard 8), and whenever possible the family needs to be fully involved to reduce any trauma experienced by the child (Duff 2003). Additional consideration needs to be paid by the children's nurse to the individual child's cognitive development, communication and understanding throughout the whole procedure.

Principles of medicine administration

When administering any medicine to a child, certain key principles apply regardless of route. It is also important to note that in some hospitals/ trusts the local policy will require two people to check all medicines given.

For all routes, the following key aspects of technique/method apply:

- Full explanations need to be given to the child and family, prior to and during the procedure, which outline the ideal positioning, action to be taken and reason for the administration of the medication. It is also important that the nurse is honest about how the medication is to be given, including the possibility of pain, and any after-effects that may be experienced.
- Education of the child and family and the sharing of information are important roles which are the nurse's responsibility (NMC 2008b).
- Prior to any intervention, the nurse should undertake a thorough hand wash and wear gloves to reduce the possibility of cross-contamination and recurrent exposure to the medication.

Table 42.1   Medication administration routes

ROUTE	FORM
Gastric tube (via naso/oropharyngeal/direct)	Solutions, suspensions, syrups, elixirs, emulsions, oils
Inhaled (into the lung)	Compressed air nebulisers, metered dose inhalers, powder devices, sterile liquids
Injected:	
Subcutaneous (under the skin)	Dependent on route: aqueous solutions, suspensions, lipid (fat) solutions, dilutions
Intramuscular (into the muscle)	
Intravenous (into the vein)	
Intrathecal (into the cerebrospinal fluid)	
Intraosseous (into the bone)	
Arterially (into the artery)	
Intra-aural (into the ear)	Solutions, suspensions, drops
Intraocular (into the eye)	Solutions, suspensions, drops, ointments
Intravaginal (into the vagina)	Pessaries, liquids, solutions, ointments, creams, lotions
Nasally (into the nose)	Solutions, suspensions, drops, ointments, sprays
Orally (by mouth)	Liquid: solutions, suspensions, syrups, elixirs, emulsions, oils
	Solid: tablets, capsules, granules, lozenges, beads
Rectally (into the rectum)	Enemas, aqueous solutions, suspensions, oils, suppositories, ointments
Sublingual (beneath the tongue)	Capsules, beads, granules, tablets, drops
Topically (onto the skin)	Solutions, suspensions, ointments, sprays, creams, lotions, pastes, powders, shampoos, soaps, liquids

Adapted from Royal College of Paediatrics and Child Health 1999.

- The medication should be prepared according to the manufacturer's instructions and checked in accordance with the NMC Standards of Medicine Management (2008a) and individual NHS trust guidelines.
- All contaminated equipment should be disposed of immediately following the procedure.
- Following any intervention, the nurse should undertake a thorough hand wash to reduce the possibility of cross-contamination.
- The administration of medication, and site of injection where applicable, should be recorded in the child's health records (i.e. drug chart) (NMC 2007b).
- The child must be monitored following medication administration to ensure recognition of any reaction to the medication and prompt treatment to deal with this.

ORAL MEDICATION

In children, the most common route for administration of medicines is the oral route, i.e. medication administered by mouth. Most medications come in a choice of tablet or suspension form, and there are frequently a number of different strengths and flavours. If suspensions are unavailable, tablets can be crushed and mixed with sterile water, using a tablet crusher; however, advice should be sought from the pharmacist about whether such methods are suitable and which diluents are appropriate.

Some suspensions have a high sugar content, or the medication itself can cause damage to gums and teeth if used over a prolonged period (e.g. phenytoin); rinsing the mouth with water after administration and good oral hygiene are essential. Some tablets cannot be crushed or dissolved, for example those with enteric coating, or slow-release tablets. Care should be taken if dividing tablets to ensure as accurate a dose as possible. Medicines can be administered by spoon, syringe or cup; however, when using a syringe care must be taken not to force the syringe into the mouth or between the teeth, as trauma can result and the action may have the potential to trigger an oral aversion in the child. Oral syringes are available with connectors that cannot be fitted to intravenous equipment, thus making the risk of administering oral drugs through the intravenous route less likely.

EQUIPMENT

- Medication
- Medicine pots or cups, with measured volumes
- Oral syringes: various sizes
- Medicine spoons, again with measured graduations
- Tablet crusher
- Tablet divider
- Water (sterile water is required for babies)
- Formulary
- Prescription/medicine chart.

TECHNIQUE

When administering oral medications, solutions should be shaken before use and measured into an appropriate container at eye level and on a solid flat surface, or drawn up into a syringe to ensure accurate medication volume measurement. Advice should be sought from the pharmacist when tablets need to be cut or crushed. Following the administration of the medication, the child needs to be observed closely for any signs of aspiration or choking.

Young infants

The young infant is likely to have a strong attachment to a parent and may become anxious with a 'stranger'. The nurse's role is to encourage parental involvement, provide positive reinforcement and promote sensory soothing measures (i.e. cuddling and stroking the infant) throughout the procedure (Watt 2003b).

- Ask the parent to hold the infant firmly on their lap in a semi-reclining position
- Encourage the infant to open their mouth, and place the syringe onto their tongue
- Gently introduce the suspension into the infant's mouth
- Depressing the infant's tongue slightly with the syringe or gently stroking their cheek and under the chin will encourage the sucking and swallowing reflex and aid administration of the medication
- Record the medication administration in the child's health records (i.e. drug chart) (NMC 2007b, 2008a).

Toddlers

As a toddler, the child is considered to be developing autonomy and striving for independence (Watt 2003b). Characteristically, the toddler will need clear instructions and a firm direct approach. The toddler is likely to have a strong bond with their parents but may be interested in exploring new tastes and sensations; therefore, whenever possible, allow the child to participate and take the medication independently. Promote the full involvement of the parents and the use of positive reinforcement, encouragement and praise. Toddlers can be encouraged through play and fun; however, medications should not be disguised in a drink, such as a milk shake, as the full volume may not be taken and the child may feel betrayed if they discover the deception, and refuse to drink at all.

Older children

Older children need to be encouraged to participate fully in the administration of medicines. The sharing of information, communication and encouragement will encourage the child to cooperate fully and self-administer the oral medication. Children learn to swallow tablets at different ages, and this does require some coordination, but learning to swallow tablets is a skill worth encouraging, as tablets can be far easier to swallow and taste less bitter than suspensions. Swallowing tablets can also represent a welcome sign of growing up and learning new skills, especially important for children with chronic illness who may struggle to attain any independence.

NASOGASTRIC, OROGASTRIC OR GASTROSTOMY MEDICATION

Medication administration via the nasogastric, orogastric or gastrostomy route is directly into the stomach via a tube (see Ch. 40). For the child who has an indwelling tube placed directly into the stomach, medications may be prescribed via this route instead of orally. However, there are a number of precautions associated with this route.

GUIDELINES AND PRECAUTIONS

- Always check for correct placement of the tube.
- Always monitor the child for any sign of aspiration, distress or deterioration.

- Use an elixir or suspension preparation of the medication.
- Avoid the use of tablets whenever possible.
- If using tablets, crush to a fine powder and mix with sterile water.
- Never crush enteric-coated or sustained-release tablets.
- Avoid the use of fat/lipid-based medicines, as they tend to cling to the sides of the tube.
- Do not mix any medication with another solution, as interactions may occur (check with a pharmacist for compatibility).
- Administer medications at room temperature.
- Flush the tube with (sterile) water between medications and following use (utilise a flush volume appropriate to the size of the child and length/gauge of the tube) to avoid blockages and medication interactions.
- Record the medication administration in the child's health records (i.e. drug chart) (NMC 2007b, 2008a).

(See also Westhus 2004, Wyllie 2004, Beckstrand et al 2007, Clarke & Richardson 2007a,b.)

INTRAVENOUS MEDICATION

While there is a requirement that prior to registration a student nurse will have been involved in the monitoring and assessment of children receiving intravenous fluids (NMC 2007a), the administration of intravenous medication is a role that requires the completion and assessment competence after registration in line with local trust policy. Intravenous (i.v.) medication (administered directly into the vein) may be given by intermittent bolus injection, continuous or intermittent infusion, or via peripheral or central access devices (see Chs 34 and 41). The choice of technique will depend on the pharmacological characteristics of the medication (half-life, preferred plasma levels) and the lifestyle of the child (e.g. intermittent bolus injections may be preferable to continuous infusion in children who are at school).

Intravenous medication has the following benefits:

- It can sustain high plasma drug levels
- It can be used in an emergency when a child cannot swallow, and will have an immediate effect

- The drug will reach the 'target' rapidly when transported in the bloodstream
- The drug can be absorbed if gastrointestinal absorption is impossible
- It requires fewer needles than other forms of injection as it uses an *in situ* cannula, and is therefore less traumatic
- The intravenous route is the preferred route if the child is critically ill.

However, intravenous medication also carries with it the following potential complications:

- Anaphylaxis
- Once injected, reversal is almost impossible unless an antidote exists
- Contamination: microorganisms, foreign matter (e.g. latex from a rubber bung, drug precipitate)
- Extravasation (or 'tissuing', as the vein walls break down)
- Phlebitis (inflammation of the vein, causing localised pain)
- Air embolism
- Incompatibility if several infusions/bolus drugs are given at the same time
- Needlestick injury to child or nurse
- Fluid overload.

EQUIPMENT

The following should be available to the nurse administering intravenous medication:

- Clean surface: trolley, table top, etc.
- Medication
- Reconstitution solution if needed (see below)
- Sterile saline or heparinised saline for flush (see below)
- Needles
- Syringes
- Alcohol swabs
- Giving sets, connectors, bungs and lines: a large variety of types and sizes are available
- Gloves
- Infusion pump or syringe pump
- Medication chart
- 'Drug additive' or 'date and time' labels for line, syringe or burette.

Normally, intravenous medication will be given in an environment where emergency and resuscitation equipment is available. Because of the risk of anaphylaxis, adrenaline (epinephrine) should be available to nurses administering intravenous injections. Community nurses will usually carry packs of epinephrine, but must ensure that they are covered by local policy and appropriately trained to administer it in an emergency without a prescription or medical supervision.

METHOD

Reconstitution, dilution and length of infusion will all vary according to the drug being used. Nurses should refer to drug information sheets supplied with the medication as a first point of reference. These will often be the most up-to-date source of information, but recognised paediatric formularies (*Medicines for Children* (RCPCH 2003) and the British National Formulary for children should be used as further guidance. Some hospital pharmacies also supply their own drug information (e.g. with data about displacement volumes).

Displacement values/volume must be taken into account when reconstituting intravenous medications for children as failure to calculate the displacement value/volume can lead to an incorrect dose being given to the child NPSA (2007). The displacement value/volume is the volume occupied by the powder in a vial; for example the displacement value of a 250 mg vial of amoxicillin is 0.2 mL. If 4.8 mL of diluent is added to this vial, the resulting volume would be 5 mL; however, if 5 mL of diluent is added, the resulting volume would be 5.2 mL. Awareness of displacement values/volumes in children's nursing is important because children are often prescribed small doses which need to be part-drawn from a vial.

Administration

Many drugs require reconstitution. Some pharmacy departments offer a reconstitution service or centralised intravenous additives services (CIVAS) especially for cytotoxic or other potentially toxic drugs. In such a service, drugs are prepared under strict aseptic conditions, using lamina flow chambers. However, there will still be circumstances when drugs are reconstituted on the wards and in the community. This must be done in a clean environment, using a sterile technique and equipment. (See also Ch. 41.)

Method

The administration of intravenous medication is a role that should only be undertaken by a registered nurse and with appropriate trust/hospital training and assessment of skills.

● Medication may be added to a volume of fluid for infusion via bag or burette, or directly into the intravenous tubing or cannula through a bung near the entry site.
● If infusion lines are used, the amount of prime solution required should be considered when calculating the drug volume.

Doctors may sometimes administer medication directly into the vein through a hypodermic or 'butterfly' needle. This latter technique may only be used in an emergency or on induction of anaesthetic and can vary between hospitals and trusts.

Normal Saline (0.9%) (Le Duc 1997, Mok 2007) flush solutions can be used in the following circumstances:

● To check before intravenous administration whether the line is patent
● Between sequential injections or infusions, to ensure that incompatible drugs do not mix
● At the end of administration to ensure that no drug remains in the line, and to ensure that the vein remains patent.

Intravenous pumps should always be used to deliver infusions. There are many different types and makes of pump on the market. Nurses must ensure that they are familiar with each type of pump used in practice; evidence suggests that many drug errors occur because of staff's unfamiliarity with equipment (Quinn 2000, NPSA 2007).

INTRAMUSCULAR MEDICATION

Intramuscular (i.m.) injections (medication administered directly into the muscle) are rarely used routinely in children's care (Hemsworth 2000) other than in vaccine administration. Despite the fact that most medicines can be administered into the muscle, the i.m. route is now used only when other routes are not viable or do not allow effective absorption of the medication. Having an injection is not a pleasant thing for a child to experience and so every effort should be made to minimise the distress for the child – the use of distraction and the role of the family member should be discussed in order to achieve the best possible outcome for child and family.

SITE

Certain factors need to be considered when selecting an injection site, including:

- The size and age of the child; the site recommended may depend on the age/weight of the child
- The child's ability to maintain the required position safely
- The size and condition of the muscle; an accessible, well-developed, vascular muscle that will tolerate the volume of medication being administered should to be used
- The frequency or number of injections; a more developed muscle will preferentially be chosen for frequent use
- The type of medication being given and the manufacturer's instructions.

Four main sites are used for the administration of i.m. injections (Fig. 42.1):

1. *Deltoid muscle* (lateral aspect of the upper arm). This site is commonly used for small-volume i.m. injections (i.e. vaccinations) but caution must be exercised when using this site in children <5 years of age and is not recommended for repeated use or large volumes (Hemsworth 2000).

2. *Vastus lateralis* (lateral aspect of the thigh). This is a traditional site commonly used for i.m. injections, especially for children under 6 months of age. This is the preferred site for infant vaccinations (WHO 2002), as it has reduced risks of nerve or blood vessel damage and is easily accessible.

3. *Ventrogluteal site* (gluteus medius muscle). This is an appropriate choice for injection in children >7 months of age. It has reduced risks of nerve or blood vessel damage and is easily accessible in a variety of positions (Greenway 2004).

4. *Gluteus maximus muscle* (upper, outer quadrant of the buttock). This site is not recommended for use in children, mainly due to potential risks which include sciatic nerve damage or damage to the gluteal artery (due to the relatively small muscle mass in smaller children) and the risk of depositing the medication into fat rather than muscle due to the high level of fatty tissue found here. This muscle gains in volume once the child has begun walking and so may be suitable for large volume injections, such as immunoglobulin in older children (RCPCH 2003, RCPCH & RCN 2002).

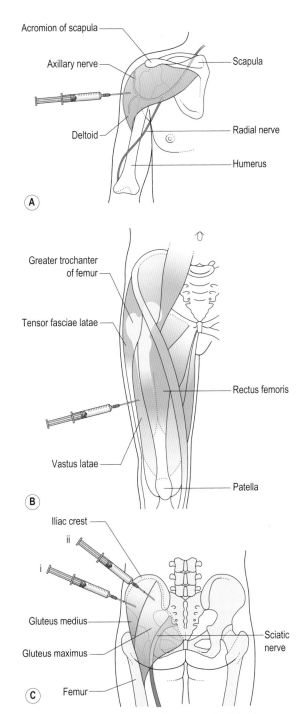

Figure 42.1 Common sites for intramuscular injections: (A) deltoid region; (B) lateral surface of the thigh; (Ci) gluteus maximus and (Cii) gluteus medius.

Volume

The exact volume that can be injected into each muscle is unclear and depends on the muscle development, medication used and viscosity of the solution (Hemsworth 2000).

POTENTIAL COMPLICATIONS

Attention needs to be paid to the possible complications of administration of a medication via the i.m. route. Potential complications (RCPCH 2003, RCPCH & RCN 2002, Hemsworth 2000) include:

- Nerve damage: ranges from foot drop to paralysis
- Muscle fibrosis and contractures: mainly reported following repeated use of the same site
- Necrosis and gangrene: rare but has occurred in neonates following large-volume injections
- Intramuscular haemorrhage: especially when i.m. injection is used for children with a clotting disorder
- Septic and sterile abscesses: secondary to large-volume injections
- Infection: relating to poor technique and multiple-use equipment
- Pain: necessitating the use of topical analgesics
- Allergic or anaphylactic reaction
- Needle phobia and mistrust: following poor technique and patient preparation (Duff 2003).

EQUIPMENT

- Dish or tray
- Medication and reconstitution solution (where appropriate)
- Prescription chart
- Needle: to 'draw up' the solution (remember to use a filter needle if accessing a snap-off glass vial)
- Syringe (size appropriate to the volume of solution)
- Needle: to 'give' the solution preferably 16 mm-long 25 gauge (Cook & Murtgh 2005).

TECHNIQUE

- Local anaesthetic (e.g. Ametop gel, EMLA cream, ethyl chloride spray or ice-packs) may block superficial pain but deep muscular pain, bruising, stiffness or 'soreness' may still occur.
- It is not necessary to swab clean skin (WHO 2004, DoH 2006).
- Distraction methods and the role of the parent/carer needs to have been discussed prior to the actual administration of the injection.
- The position of the child is essential in the safe, effective delivery of i.m. medication and may help the child to relax, thereby decreasing the pain and anxiety experienced.
- Once the medication is fully prepared, a new needle must be used to administer the solution.
- The skin at the injection site should be stretched, not bunched (DoH 2006). The needle should be inserted into the skin and muscle at a 90° angle. The needle should not be deep enough to touch bone but must penetrate deep into the muscle.
- Following insertion, there is no need to aspirate the syringe. The medication should be given as speedily as is pragmatic to reduce both the time of the injection and the child's discomfort (Ipp et al 2007).
- After administration of the medication the needle should be removed quickly while releasing the stretched skin (the Z technique) (see LPN 2005).
- Gentle pressure may be applied to the site using a sterile cotton wool ball or gauze pad but the site should not be rubbed as this may interfere with the drug absorption rate.
- The i.m. site needs to be reviewed regularly for signs of bruising or any other complication (Rodger & King 2000).
- Record the medication administration in the child's health records (i.e. drug chart) (NMC 2007b) and the site location in the child's care plan (NMC 2008a).

SUBCUTANEOUS MEDICATION

Subcutaneous (s.c.) injection or infusion medication is administered as a bolus directly below the dermis and epidermis layers of the skin and above the layer of muscle (Ansel et al 2002). Subcutaneous injections are a relatively convenient method of administering medication when other routes are not feasible (Cocoman & Barron 2008) and is a frequently used method used in caring for children, especially for the administration of anti-coagulants, analgesia, insulin and some anticancer drugs.

SITE

Certain factors need to be considered when selecting an injection site, including:

- The size and age of the child; the site recommended may depend on the age/weight of the child
- The frequency or number of injections; a more frequently used site may become fibrosed over time
- The type of medication given and manufacturer's instructions.

Common sites for the administration of s.c. injections are chosen for their deep fat layer and accessibility; these include the upper thigh, abdomen, upper arm and buttocks. Sites should be rotated, as a frequently used site may become fibrosed, which could reduce the absorption of the medication.

POTENTIAL COMPLICATIONS

Attention needs to be paid to the possible complications of administration of a medication via the s.c. route. Possible complications include:

- Tissue fibrosis: following multiple use of one site
- Infection: relating to poor technique and multiple-use equipment
- Pain: necessitating the use of topical analgesics
- Allergic or anaphylactic reaction
- Needle phobia and mistrust: following poor technique and patient preparation (Duff 2003)
- Medication errors: due to confusion between syringes measured in units (i.e. heparin, insulin) and those measured in millilitres (mL) (i.e. analgesia).

EQUIPMENT

- Dish or tray
- Medication and reconstitution solution (where appropriate)
- Prescription chart
- Needle – to 'draw up' the solution

- Syringe (size appropriate to the volume of solution)
- Needle – to 'give' the solution.

TECHNIQUE

- Local anaesthetic (e.g. Ametop gel, EMLA cream, ethyl chloride spray or ice-packs) may block superficial pain but bruising, stiffness or 'soreness' may still occur.
- It is not necessary to swab clean skin (WHO 2004, DoH 2006).
- Distraction methods and the role of the parent/carer needs to have been discussed prior to the actual administration of the injection.
- Once the medication is fully prepared, a new needle must be used to administer the solution. Many medications now come in prefilled syringes for ease of administration – in this case there would be no need to change the needle.
- The skin should be bunched not stretched in order to maximise the amount of adipose tissue available and minimise the risk of accidental intra-muscular administration. The needle should be inserted into the skin at an angle which ensures the tip of the needle remains in the subcutaneous layer.
- Following insertion, there is no need to aspirate the syringe. The injection should be administered as swiftly as the fluid and child allow in order to minimise injection time and child's discomfort (Ipp et al 2007).
- After administration of the medication the needle should be removed swiftly while releasing the bunched skin.
- Gentle pressure may be applied to the site using a sterile cotton wool ball or gauze pad, however the site should not be rubbed as this may affect the drug absorption rate.
- The s.c. site needs to be reviewed regularly for signs of bruising or any other complication.
- Record the medication administration in the child's health records (i.e. drug chart) (NMC 2007b) and record the site administration in the child's care plan (NMC 2008a).

Diabetes is the most common reasons for giving subcutaneous injections through the administration of insulin, the use of multiple injection sites is important to avoid lumps under the skin or infections occurring. It is important to note that absorption of drugs does vary depending on the site used with the quickest being the lower abdomen (Strauss et al 2002).

INTRAOSSEOUS ADMINISTRATION

Intraosseous (i.o.) administration (medication administered directly into the bone) is usually undertaken by medical staff; however, in some hospitals/trusts, nurses with EPLS training may also use i.o. methods in an emergency situation. This technique is used for quick vascular access, primarily in emergency situations, especially when veins are collapsing due to shock. The European Paediatric Life Support (EPLS 2005) guidelines recommend that this route be used if venous access cannot be established rapidly in infants or children who urgently require i.v. drugs or fluids. The i.o. needle is inserted aseptically into a long bone allowing fluids to be absorbed into the circulation via the vascular space within the bone.

EQUIPMENT

- Skin disinfectant
- Intraosseous 18G needle with trocar (at least 1.5 cm in length)
- Local anaesthetic
- 5 mL syringe
- 20 mL syringe
- Infusion fluid.

METHOD

When identifying the site for an i.o. needle, the anterior aspects of the upper tibial or lower femoral plate sites are preferred. Fractured bones must be avoided as should the tibia if the femur is fractured on the same side (EPLS 2005). The skin is cleaned and a local anaesthetic used. The needle is inserted at 90° to the skin and advanced until a 'give' is felt as the needle penetrates the cortex of the bone. The correct position of the needle is confirmed by aspirating blood using a 5 mL syringe. When confirmed, the needle is secured in place with sterile gauze and strapping. Intraosseous infusions should only be used in emergency situations and, to prevent infection, should be replaced as soon as a normal vein can be cannulated.

EPIDURAL INFUSIONS

Continuous epidural infusions, along with other forms of spinal nerve block, are becoming more commonly used in children, as they provide effective major pain relief without the side-effects of systemic opiates (see Ch. 44). The catheter is usually sited preoperatively in theatre under anaesthetic, by the anaesthetist or surgeon. Epidural infusions should be supervised by nursing and medical staff experienced and knowledgeable in their use. They should be used in conjunction with regular pain assessment. Epidurals may use a local anaesthetic agent (e.g. bupivacaine hydrochloride) and/or opiates for analgesia. If opiates are used, the patient should be observed closely for signs of respiratory depression. Other side-effects of opiate epidural analgesia include nausea and vomiting, or excessive sedation; therefore naloxone should always be available. If analgesia is insufficient, a technical cause such as local leakage or catheter disconnection should be sought before automatically increasing the infusion. Nurses should also observe for urinary retention as a result of local anaesthetic or opiates.

Common side-effects of epidurals in older patients, such as hypotension and lower limb temporary inability to move lower limbs, appear to be less common in children, but nurses must nonetheless remain alert for such signs (Clarke 2003, Ellis et al 2007).

INTRATHECAL MEDICATION

The intrathecal route of administration allows medications that cannot pass through the blood–brain barrier (a semi-permeable membrane that acts as a natural filter for substances from the blood to the brain) to enter cerebrospinal fluid via an implantable port or lumbar puncture. This method is commonly used within cancer treatments, pain management and severe spasticity/mobility problems.

CHEMOTHERAPY

Chemotherapy is the name given to a group of cytotoxic (cyto = cell; toxic = poison) drugs that are used mainly in the treatment of cancer. There are many different types of chemotherapy which fall naturally into a number of classes, each with characteristic cytotoxic activity, site of action and toxicity. Nevertheless, they all have the same role of destroying cancerous cells by damaging them so that they cannot divide and grow. However, they also affect normal non-cancerous cells, thereby producing side-effects. The handling of cytotoxic drugs has been acknowledged as an occupational hazard (HSE 2003); therefore hospital and trust policy surrounding chemotherapy is essential, as these drugs can be given by many different routes including oral and subcutaneous.

RECTAL MEDICATION

The rectal route (medication inserted into the rectum) is used when drugs cannot be absorbed orally, when the child is nil-by-mouth or when a local effect is required (see Ch. 12). Diarrhoea or impacted faeces are contraindications to the use of this route. In some countries, the rectal route is commonplace (e.g. France). However, in the UK there is a reluctance to administer via this route, perhaps owing to child protection concerns and cultural or sexual taboos. Because of these concerns, nurses must exercise great sensitivity in using this route, especially with older children and adolescents who may be totally unaware that this technique exists. Consent should be sought from the child and family, especially if the suppository is to be inserted in the recovery room or while the child is sedated; and a chaperone, preferably the parent, should be present (Rogers & Irwin 2003).

POTENTIAL COMPLICATIONS

Attention needs to be paid to the possible complications of administration of a medication via the rectal route. These include:

- Pain and discomfort
- Allergic or anaphylactic reaction
- Mistrust – following poor technique and patient preparation.

EQUIPMENT

- Medication chart
- Gloves

- Dish or tray containing:
  - Suppository
  - Lubricating gel
  - Swab or tissue.

SITE

The child should be on their side, with legs curled up in a fetal position. With babies, it is possible to lift the legs and flex the knees, as for changing a nappy.

TECHNIQUE

- Prior to any intervention the nurse should undertake a thorough hand wash to reduce the possibility of cross-contamination and put on a pair of clinical gloves.
- The suppository should be lubricated with a water-soluble gel (i.e. aqueous gel).
- The suppository should be gently inserted into the anus, just beyond the anal sphincter (Addison 2000).
- It may be necessary to hold the buttocks together for several minutes to prevent the immediate expulsion of the suppository.
- Record the medication administration in the child's health records (i.e. drug chart) (NMC 2007b, 2008a).
- Product literature will either recommend suppositories are inserted apex-first or make no recommendations at all; product details and hospital/trust policy must be checked when deciding which way a suppository should be inserted (Moppett 2000). According to Moppett (2000) there are no significant differences in expulsion rates when suppositories are inserted either blunt end or apex first; however, there is currently very little evidence to support this (Higgins 2007).

TOPICAL MEDICATION

Topical medication (medication applied directly to the skin), for example a cream, ointment or topical solution, may be prescribed for a variety of reasons, including:

- Treatment of eczema, dermatitis or *Candida*
- Local anaesthesia

- Severe excoriation
- Skin trauma (i.e. following a scald or burn).

The absorption of the medication through the skin may vary with age; medications administered topically may be absorbed systemically in neonates and infants (due to reduced skin density and maturity) when a localised response was intended (Prosser et al 2000). In order to prevent skin sensitisation and allergic reactions due to possible local inflammatory responses (Demoly & Bousquet 2001), gloves should be worn when administering any form of topical medication. Topical medications frequently have a variety of strengths and preparations; the children's nurse needs to be vigilant when checking the strength, dosage and preparation prescribed.

EQUIPMENT

- Medication
- Gloves
- Dressings/bandages as required.

TECHNIQUE

- Topical medication should always be single patient use to avoid cross-contamination and the administration of an incorrect dosage.
- Prepare the child and family.
- It is important that the person administering the medication wears gloves to reduce the potential of absorbing the medication through the skin of the hands.
- Administer the medication to the area stated in the prescription as per product instructions.
- Avoid contamination of the surrounding skin.
- Record the medication administration in the child's health records (i.e. drug chart) (NMC 2007b, 2008a) (see Ch. 11).

TRANSCUTANEOUS MEDICATION

The use of patches is increasing within both children's pain management and oncology. Transcutaneous absorption via patches or topical administration is greater in children than in adults (Prosser et al 2000). Although the use of skin patches can be considered, it must be borne in mind that absorption within neonates is altered and topical substances can damage the skin and internal organs (Bryan et al 2001).

EQUIPMENT

- Medication
- Gloves.

TECHNIQUE

- Prepare the child and family.
- Administer the medication to the area stated in the prescription as per product instructions.
- Record the medication administration in the child's health records (i.e. drug chart) (NMC 2007b, 2008a).

INTRA-AURAL/OTIC MEDICATION

Intra-aural/otic medication (medication inserted directly into the ear canal) is not a painful procedure; however, it can cause uncomfortable or unpleasant sensations for children. As with the administration of medication via any other route, it is paramount that the child and family are fully prepared and informed prior to the procedure. A potential problem associated with this route is the need to have the full cooperation of the child or to utilise gentle restraint to attain an optimum head position in order to insert the medication. As with the administration of all medications and procedures, the hands must be washed and dried thoroughly before and after the procedure.

EQUIPMENT

- Medication (frequently single-use ampoules and/or with a dropper attached)
- Syringe or dropper
- Swab or tissue.

TECHNIQUE

Medications for the ear often have a short shelf-life once opened, so expiry dates should be checked carefully. To help reduce the unpleasant/uncomfortable sensations associated with this administration route, remove medications stored in the refrigerator a few minutes before use to allow the medication to warm up to room temperature before instillation. If in doubt, check with the pharmacist or the manufacturer's recommendations.

- Lay the child on their back (supine) and turn their head to the appropriate side.
- Wash and dry hands thoroughly.
- For children <3 years of age, gently pull the pinna downwards and straight back in order to straighten the external auditory canal.
- For children >3 years of age, gently pull the pinna upward and back in order to straighten the auditory canal.
- Instil the drops, as prescribed, into the ear, without touching the dropper.
- After administration, encourage the child to remain still for a few minutes to allow the drops to be absorbed.
- Gentle massage of the area immediately anterior (in front of) the ear may help the droplets to descend and aid in relaxing the child.
- A swab or tissue should be used to absorb any exudate or leakage and to reduce skin contamination or irritation.
- Wash and dry hands thoroughly.
- The use of distraction techniques such as watching a DVD or the television are useful to alleviate boredom and to encourage the child to keep still.
- Record the medication administration in the child's health records (i.e. drug chart) (NMC 2007b, 2008a).

INTRAOCULAR/OPTIC MEDICATION

Intraocular/optic medication (medication administered directly onto the eye) may cause a significant level of discomfort, visual blurring and irritation to the child. As with the administration of medication via any other route, it is paramount that the child and family are fully prepared and informed prior to the procedure. A potential problem associated with this route is the need to have the full cooperation of the child or to utilise gentle restraint to attain an optimum head position in order to insert the medication. Administration of eye drops can be particularly difficult in young children and toddlers, who may struggle and close their eyes protectively. Play, patience and asking the parent to hold the child firmly on their lap, will help.

EQUIPMENT

- Medication (frequently single-use ampoules and/or with a dropper attached)
- Syringe or dropper
- Swab or tissue.

TECHNIQUE

Medications for the eye often have a short shelf-life once opened, so expiry dates should be checked carefully. To help reduce the unpleasant/uncomfortable sensations associated with this administration route, remove medications stored in the refrigerator a few minutes before use to allow the medication to warm up to room temperature before instillation. If in doubt, check with the pharmacist or the manufacturer's recommendations. Medicines for the eye need to be used exclusively for the left or right eye and not shared between patients; and as with the administration of all medications and procedures, the hands must be washed and dried thoroughly before and after the procedure.

- Lay the child flat on their back (supine) or sitting with head extended and ask them to look upwards, towards the ceiling; infants may need to be cuddled in a blanket.
- Use one hand to pull down the lower eyelid; rest the other hand on the child's forehead, so that it moves with the child and is therefore less likely to cause an injury if the child moves suddenly (Marsden & Shaw 2003).
- Drops: instil the prescribed number of drops, not directly onto the eyeball, but to the lower, inner corner of each eye.
- Ointment: squeeze the ointment along the inside of the lower lid.
- Do not touch the eye with the bottle, tube or your fingers, as the eye can easily become contaminated or damaged.
- Encourage the child to close their eyes, not squeeze together, and roll them around to disseminate the medication.
- A swab or tissue should be used to absorb any exudate or leakage and to reduce skin contamination or irritation.
- Record the medication administration in the child's health records (i.e. drug chart) (NMC 2007b, 2008a).

ANAPHYLAXIS

Anaphylaxis seems to be increasingly common and is almost certainly associated with an increase in the prevalence of allergic disease over the last few decades (Resuscitation Council UK 2008). Anaphylaxis can result from exposure to an agent or substance to which the body has previously been exposed or in which there has been no previous exposure (Jamieson et al 2002).

CAUSES

Anaphylactic reactions vary in severity and may follow exposure to a variety of agents, the most common of which are:

- Foods (e.g. peanut, tree nuts or other foods)
- Insect stings
- Medications (and contrast media)
- Latex.

Incidence

The speed at which an anaphylactic reaction may occur appears to depend on the hypersensitivity of the child to the agent encountered. Anaphylactic reactions vary in severity and can be rapid, slow or biphasic. A severe reaction will often occur immediately and recent studies showed that fatalities are unlikely after 6 h (Gupta et al 2007).

Recognition of anaphylactic reactions

The signs and symptoms of anaphylaxis vary in severity according to the hypersensitivity of the child to the agent encountered. Common signs and symptoms are shown in Box 42.1. To confirm a diagnosis of anaphylaxis the following should be present:

- Acute onset of illness
- Life threatening airway and/or breathing and/ or circulation problems
- Skin and/or mucosal changes.

TREATMENT OF SEVERE ANAPHYLAXIS

- Rapid treatment is important in life-threatening situations (Fig. 42.2)
- The child must be assessed using the ABCDE approach (Airway, Breathing, Circulation, Disability and Exposure)

BOX 42.1 Common signs and symptoms of anaphylactic reactions

- Angio-oedema
- Urticaria
- Dyspnoea
- Hypotension
- Skin colour change – pale or flushed
- Cardiovascular collapse
- Rhinitis
- Conjunctivitis
- Abdominal pain
- Vomiting
- Diarrhoea
- Sense of impending doom.

Adapted from Resuscitation Council UK 2008.

- Call for help (dial the emergency services (999) in the community or call the resuscitation team (2222) in a hospital setting)
- Position the child: if the child has an airway or breathing difficulty, sit the child up; if the child has a circulation problem you may wish to lie the child down with legs elevated
- Administer epinephrine using the child's pre-loaded epinephrine injection device into the outer aspect of the thigh – this can be injected through the child's clothing
- Remove the allergen wherever possible
- Monitor the child and transfer to specialist care ensuring they are aware of the treatment given so far
- Oxygen should be provided if available.

EQUIPMENT AND TREATMENT

- Equipment that should be in place includes oxygen, suction, etc.
- Rapid treatment is needed when an anaphylactic reaction occurs (Fig. 42.2)
- A full history and examination of the child should be undertaken
- The child's health records should be examined for any past sensitivity or reactions
- Any medications that the patient has received should be disclosed to the healthcare team
- Assess and monitor the child's condition and any physical symptoms, especially:
  - Airway
  - Breathing

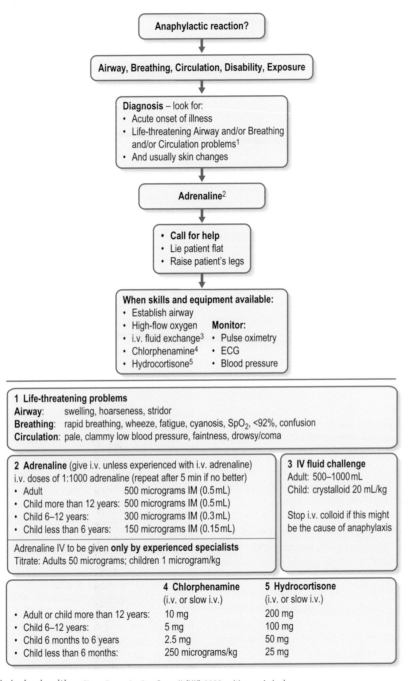

Figure 42.2 Anaphylaxis algorithm *(from Resuscitation Council (UK) 2008, with permission).*

– Pulse rate
– Blood pressure
– Skin colour
– Temperature
– Check for MedicAlert bracelet or necklace.

● If a severe reaction occurs, 'Call for Help' and ring for immediate medical assistance (either from the resuscitation team, in the hospital environment, or from the emergency services (999), in the community environment).

Table 42.2	Recommended i.m. epinephrine dosages in the treatment of a child with anaphylaxis
AGE GROUP	**EPINEPHRINE I.M. DOSAGE**
>12 years	500 micrograms i.m. (0.5 mL 1:1000 solution) 300 micrograms (0.3 mL) if child is small or prepubertal)
6–12 years	300 micrograms i.m. (0.3 mL 1:1000 solution)
>6 months to 6 years	150 micrograms i.m. (0.15 mL 1:1000 solution)
<6 months	150 micrograms i.m. (0.15 mL 1:1000 solution)

From Resuscitation Council (UK) 2008, p 22, with permission. Micrograms, μg; milliliters, mL.

Epinephrine

Epinephrine is regarded to be the most important medication for the treatment of severe anaphylactic reactions in both children and adults (Resuscitation Council UK 2008). The intramuscular route is effective in most cases, however where specialist facilities exist, this may be given via the intravenous route (see Table 42.2 for recommended dosages).

As the likelihood of a child experiencing an anaphylactic reaction continues to be a relatively rare occurrence, the majority of healthcare practitioners may not be familiar with the management and treatment of anaphylaxis. Therefore, pre-filled, dose-specific injection devices, such as the EpiPen, junior EpiPen or AnaPen, are recommended for use.

Unlike most other medications, the use of epinephrine for the treatment of anaphylaxis does not routinely require a medication prescription; however, the event should be documented in the child's records and local trust policy and guidance should detail the qualified (registered) children's nurses' responsibilities regarding the administration of medications in an emergency and outline any specific training requirements.

INHALED THERAPY DEVICES

Inhalation therapy is the most effective way to administer preventative and symptom-relieving drugs as used in the treatment of lung conditions such as asthma and cystic fibrosis (NICE 2000,

2002, 2005, O'Connor 2001, Madge 2002). Through inhalation, the drug will reach the lungs directly, requiring a lower dose and minimising any systemic side-effects (Watt 2003a). There are a variety of inhaled drugs, the pharmacology of which will not be discussed here. The nurse should refer to one of the formularies for drug and inhaler device clarification, prior to prescribing or using them.

GUIDELINES

Prescribing an inhaler suited to the child's cognitive and psychomotor ability is important. It is suggested that all children use an inhaler with a spacer device, because using the pressurised metered dose inhaler (pMDI) alone is complicated, requires high-level coordination and is least efficient (NICE 2000, 2002, 2005, Child et al 2002, Lissauer & Clayden 2002, SIGN 2004). Effective inhalation therapy and good symptom control are dependent upon adequate preparation of the child and parent. The spacer device will improve efficacy, increase the amount of drug reaching the lungs and reduce the amount of medication remaining in the throat (Jordan & White 2001, Child et al 2002). The NICE (2000, 2002, 2005) guidelines state that a pMDI with spacer device should be prescribed in the first instance. Only when the child has a high non-compliance rate when using the inhaler plus spacer device should other types of inhaler, such as dry powder (DPI) or breath-actuated inhalers, be considered. Although less cumbersome, both the DPI and breath-actuated inhaler require a significant inspiratory breath, which precludes their effectiveness during an exacerbation of symptoms (Child et al 2002, Roberts 2002). O'Callaghan and Barry (2000) maintain that there is no evidence to suggest that changing from a pMDI with spacer to DPI or breath-actuated inhaler will improve compliance (Peters et al 2002) and that they are not suitable for children under age 6 years; they also argue that as the inhaler plus spacer is mainly used on waking and going to bed, the size of the spacer should not be problematic as the device can remain at home. Furthermore, a study on infants and children under age 5 years by Castro-Rodriguez and Rodrigo (2004) has demonstrated that delivery of salbutamol via valved spacer is more effective in reducing the number of hospital admissions and clinical severity of symptoms than using a nebuliser during acute exacerbations.

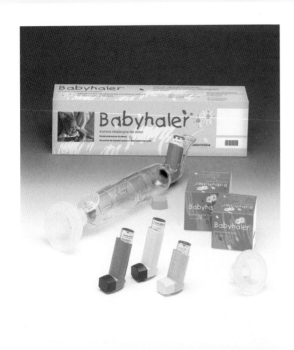

Figure 42.3 Babyhaler and volumatic plastic spacer devices *(courtesy of Glaxo Wellcome, UK).*

Nurses need to be aware of and teach children and families that plastic spacer devices such as the Volumatic and Babyhaler (Fig. 42.3) produce a positive charge that will attract the drug particles to the spacer walls, thus reducing the amount of drug inhaled. The best way to minimise this effect is to wash the spacer once a week in detergent and allow to air dry. This will leave a detergent coating on the spacer and reduce the electrostatic charge (Le Souif 1999, NICE 2000). An alternative to the plastic spacer is the Nebuchamber, a spacer made from stainless steel that is anti-static.

There are a number of different inhalers with different operating methods. It is important that nurses learn the correct technique for each type of inhaler, when used alone or with a spacer device. Teaching the child and family good inhaler technique and reviewing this regularly improves treatment adherence and symptom control and reduces the incidence of acute episodes (Francis 2001, O'Connor 2001, Roberts 2002).

In the case of asthma, a treatment plan should detail what medication is to be inhaled, the dosage, frequency, type of inhaler, how to monitor symptoms and what to do in the event of symptom exacerbation. Self-management plans have been developed for school-age children with the emphasis on improved symptom control and using peak flow measurement (Harrop 2002, Roberts 2002, Milnes & Callery 2003). The peak flow meter is a diagnostic and assessment tool that measures the peak expiratory flow rate.

Assessment should include observation of respiratory rate and effort (see Ch. 6). Skin colour and general well-being should be noted. Signs of increasing effort may include intercostal recession or using accessory muscles to aid breathing. The child may seek a position with the chest upright and head forward to increase lung expansion. Peak flow measurement (see below) is a useful test of lung function. Oxygen saturation measurement may give an early indication of any hypoxia. X-rays and other more detailed lung function tests can be performed. The history of the illness should be noted, especially as classic signs of chronic respiratory distress – chronic night-time coughing and shortness of breath after exercise (Caldwell 1998) – are still often ignored by parents and GPs.

Peak flow measurement

The peak expiratory flow rate (PEFR) is the fastest rate at which air can be expelled from the lungs and is measured in litres per minute (L/min). Regular PEFR measurement assists with good symptom control, gives early indication of disease exacerbation and can assist in identifying allergens (Singel & Lira 2001, Kennedy 2007). In order to monitor PEFR, a 'normal' peak flow value is calculated using the child's height. This is plotted on a nomogram, which details height on one axis and predicted peak flow on the other axis of the graph (Godfrey et al 1970, Lissauer & Clayden 2002). The child will also have a personal baseline rate, which is best measured when the child is in optimum health. The PEFR should be measured before inhalation and again 15 min after inhalation (Lissauer & Clayden 2002). Several types of peak flow meter are available for different age groups and the nurse must ensure the one used is suitable for the child as children will vary in their ability to understand according to their age and stage of development (Sleath et al 2003, Hämeen-Anttila et al 2006). To ensure understanding the nurse should clarify this by asking the child and/or parent(s) to repeat what is expected of them.

Measuring peak flow

The child should be taught the following steps:

1. Move the measurement bar on the meter to zero
2. Ask the child to stand up
3. Hold the meter horizontally
4. Open mouth, and slowly inhale as large a breath as possible
5. Put mouthpiece in the mouth, ensuring tongue is clear and seal with the lips
6. Blow out: a short, hard and fast breath
7. Relax and note reading
8. Repeat steps 1–7 three times
9. Record the best reading.

The reading should be compared with the child's own baseline measurement and the normal values for a child of their height, as detailed. Changes in PEFR will indicate an increase or decrease in the child's state of health.

Older children who are being taught self-management of their asthma may benefit from peak flow guidelines (Milnes & Callery 2003); these set levels above and below which certain medication should be taken or increased. While it is quite normal for morning readings to dip, variation above 15% may be significant.

INHALERS

Equipment

Tables 42.3 and 42.4 summarise the different features of common devices. As can be seen from these tables, children should be assessed individually to determine which device would be most suitable (Fig. 42.3).

Aerosol inhalers used to contain chlorofluorocarbons (CFCs), gases which contribute to the depletion of the ozone layer. As from 2003, all inhalers must be CFC-free (Lissauer & Clayden 2002). Hydrofluoroalkanes replaced CFCs but there may be some adjustment in switching from the older inhalers to the new CFC-free inhalers; they may look, feel, smell and taste different, but patients can be assured that they are equally effective (Shapiro et al 2000).

Method

The following common principles apply to all devices:

- Drugs should be checked and administered according to local policy and NMC guidelines (NMC 2006, 2008a)
- Always check expiry date of drug canister and inhaler
- Always remove the protective mouthpiece before use
- Ensure spacer device, if used, is clean, dry and assembled
- Record the medication administration in the child's health records (i.e. drug chart) (NMC 2007b, 2008a)

SPACERS FOR BABIES AND YOUNG CHILDREN

A large-volume spacer (such as Volumatic) should not be used with babies as the amount of drug absorption will be reduced. Instead, the smaller-volume, purpose-made Babyhaler has been shown

---

Table 42.3   Summary of features of dry powder inhalers (positive attributes in bold)

DEVICE FEATURES	CAPSULE INHALERS	DISKHALERS	MULTIDOSE DRY POWDER INHALERS
Preloading required	Yes	Yes	**No**
Multiple doses available	No	**Yes 8/4 doses**	**Yes 50, 100, 200 doses**
Indicator of doses taken/remaining	N/A	**Yes**	**Yes (last 20 only)**
Inspiratory flow rate (1/min)	60	60	30 (60 = optimum)
Lactose carrier	Yes	Yes	Varies with manufacturer

None of these devices is suitable for children under 5 years of age.
All the devices have the following attributes: Discreet and portable; do not contain CFCs; do not need shaking before use; do not require hand–lung coordination; no time lapse between actuations required.
Adapted from Warner & Gregson (1995).

Table 42.4   Summary of features of aerosol inhalers (positive attributes in bold)

DEVICE FEATURES	METERED-DOSE INHALER (MDI)	LARGE SPACER AND MDI	BREATH-ACTUATED MDI	SPINHALER
Discreet and portable	**Yes**	No	**Yes**	**Yes**
Require hand–lung synchronisation	Yes	**No**	**No**	Yes
Time lapse between actuations	Yes (30 s)	Yes (30 s)	Yes (60 s)	Yes (60 s)
Oropharyngeal impaction leading to inhibition of inhalation	Yes	**No**	Yes	Yes
Minimum age for use	7 years	**Infant**	7 years	No studies
Inspiratory flow rate (1/min)	30	22 (tidal volume breathing)	28–30	30
Medications available	All	Product specific	6	3

In addition, these devices have the following characteristics: no preloading required; multiple doses available; number of doses remaining/taken indicated; require shaking before use.
Adapted from Warner & Gregson (1995).

to increase drug deposition in the lungs and uses special valves that require minimum inspiratory volume to release drug particles, thus allowing the spacer to be used at any angle (Glaxo Wellcome; see Fig. 42.3). Contrary to popular belief, keeping the baby quiet, preferably sleeping, during inhalation gives the highest possible drug deposition (Iles et al 1999, O'Callaghan & Barry 2000, Esposito-Festen et al 2006).

Method

1. The medication should be checked against the prescription as per policy for administration of medications.
2. Remove the mouthpiece cover from the metered dose inhaler.
3. Shake the inhaler.
4. Insert the inhaler into the inhaler holder of the Babyhaler.
5. Place the facemask gently and securely over the baby's nose and mouth; try to keep the baby calm.
6. Hold the Babyhaler at an angle that is comfortable for the baby and the person administering.
7. Press down on the canister once to release a puff of medication into the Babyhaler.
8. Keep the Babyhaler facemask over the nose and mouth until the baby has taken at least 5–10 breaths.
9. Repeat steps 2–7 if necessary and check with the pharmacist if there is any doubt.

10. Remember to wipe the face of the baby after administration of inhaler.
11. Record the medication administration in the child's health records (i.e. drug chart) (NMC 2007b, 2008a).

NEBULISERS

Nebulisers can be used at home, in hospital during acute episodes, or to treat respiratory infections with inhaled antibiotics (e.g. cystic fibrosis). Depending on the child's ability, using a mouthpiece rather than a mask gives higher lung deposition, as much of the drug is lost through the mask vents (O'Callaghan & Barry 2000). Nebulisers do have the advantage that oxygen can be administered simultaneously, which is important if the child is hypoxic. The use of an inhaler plus spacer device is as effective at treating acute asthma exacerbation as the nebuliser (O'Callaghan & Barry 2000, Cates et al 2003, Castro-Rodriguez & Rodrigo 2004) and nurses should check the local trust protocol for treatment of acute asthma exacerbation in children.

Equipment

- Nebuliser unit or oxygen point
- Nebuliser pot and mask or mouthpiece.

Different sizes are available to suit all ages. O'Callaghan and Barry (2000) found that a mouthpiece gives higher lung deposition of nebulised drug. Some nebuliser types are better for specific drugs than others. If the child is ventilated, special connectors are available to connect the nebuliser to the ventilator tubing. The gas can be administered via a compressor, or via a bottled or piped gas supply. Oxygen should be used in acute asthma, as the child is likely to be hypoxic.

Method

- The medication should be checked against the prescription as per policy for administration of medications.
- To ensure adequate droplet formation, the nebuliser solution should be diluted to volume as recommended by the nebuliser manufacturer, for example 2.5 mL for Medic Aid nebulisers (MedicAid 1995). Even though some medications come in prepacked nebules, they may need further dilution if the volume is too small, for example when a small baby receives only a small proportion of the nebule, as a small volume of the fluid always remains in the pot (O'Callaghan & Barry 2000). The oxygen or airflow should reach 6–8 L/min to create a small particle vapour (Booker 2007).
- Booker (2007) observes that wherever possible, a mouthpiece should be used for nebulised ipratropium bromide to avoid contact of the mist with the eyes, as there is evidence that this can lead to acute glaucoma (Shah et al 1992).
- The child should be sitting comfortably, either in bed, on a chair, or on a parent's or nurse's lap.
- Tap the nebuliser during nebulisation to ensure that large droplets are shaken down.
- Observe the child's condition during and after using the nebuliser.
- After the nebuliser has finished, dry tubing using driven gas (use oxygen or air to run through the tubing to help dry), and wash and air dry nebuliser pot and mask. Store for that patient only.
- Record the medication administration in the child's health records (i.e. drug chart) (NMC 2007b, 2008a).

POTENTIAL COMPLICATIONS

The number of medications that may be given by inhaler precludes a comprehensive list of side-effects being given here. A thorough knowledge of pharmacology is, however, necessary to understand and identify these side-effects. Jordan and White (2001) and Roberts (2002) offer a good description of drugs used in asthma and their potential side-effects. It must be remembered that complications may occur, due both to the side-effects of the therapy and the natural history of the respiratory condition. Rinsing the mouth after the use of an inhaler may help to lessen any potential systemic side-effects (Hannemann 1999).

FACTORS TO NOTE

- Children with asthma should carry their relievers at all times.
- Regular and repeated teaching and follow-up checks of inhaler technique should improve compliance.
- Familiarise yourself with features of different devices in order to advise on the most suitable.
- Encourage mouthwashing/gargling in patients who use inhalers, especially if inhaled steroids are prescribed (Caldwell 1998, Roberts 2002).
- Ensure effective interprofessional liaison with all healthcare professionals involved in the child's care (Campbell 2002).

COMMUNITY PERSPECTIVE

The role of the community children's nurse (CCN) may range from supporting parents giving oral medication to administering complex drug regimens.

If it is necessary for the CCN to carry drugs, these should be transported in a sturdy container or cool box. If drugs have to be left in the car between visits, care must be taken to leave them unobtrusively in a securely locked car. Nurses must work within local guidelines in regard to the transport or carrying of controlled and cytotoxic drugs (RCN 2001). Drugs must be stored at the recommended temperatures. It may be necessary to supply the family with a drug refrigerator or freezer. A recommended resource is *Administering Intravenous Therapy to Children in the Community* (RCN 2001). As nurses are increasingly asked to undertake pioneering clinical work in the home, each practitioner must consider their own accountability.

All drugs must be administered according to local policy. Control of Substances Hazardous to Health (COSHH) Regulations (HSE 2002) apply in the home and the CCN is responsible for ensuring safe practice. This may include providing protective clothing for the administering nurse or parent and provision of spillage kits as appropriate.

The safety of the home environment for the preparation and administration of intravenous drugs will need to be assessed. Some homes may prove to be unsafe, either through inadequate standards of hygiene or lack of space, but this is the exception. The nurse will need to be able to create an aseptic field (see Ch. 34). Where parents are undertaking administration of drugs by injection, it is the responsibility of the CCN to ensure that appropriate training, supervision and written guidelines are in place. These must include information about side-effects and possible complications of therapy, including anaphylactic rescue.

Anaphylaxis kits containing adrenaline, chlorphenamine and hydrocortisone should be available to the nurse. These drugs should be prescribed and documented in the child's records by the hospital or GP. Wherever possible, two people should check intravenous drugs. The parent or an older child may be involved. However, preloaded syringes, prepared in a hospital pharmacy, are preferable.

When electrically powered syringe drivers or intravenous pumps are used, it is essential to ensure that they are capable of running on their own batteries, in case of power failure. Parents should know what they should do if the pump/driver fails to work, as it may be unrealistic to have spare pumps available. All equipment should be serviced regularly. When opioids are administered subcutaneously by syringe driver or intravenously via a pump, it may be necessary to have naloxone in the home as an antidote to respiratory depression. This is unlikely to occur as the majority of children on opioids are terminally ill and will have had their dosages increased gradually. Any clinical waste should be disposed of according to local policy.

Parents must know who to contact at any time should they have problems and the CCN must be aware of any potential problems that may occur with any of the devices in use, or the medication being administered.

DOS AND DON'TS

- Do be careful.
- Do allow sufficient time.
- Do ask for help if unsure of what you are being asked to do.
- Do your own calculations; if you disagree, say so.
- Do check with the doctor or pharmacist if unsure.
- Do check that the correct child receives the correct medication, in the correct dose, at the correct time, via the correct route.
- Do ensure that all medicines administered are recorded in the child's health records (i.e. drug chart) (NMC 2007b, 2008a).
- Do be familiar with equipment used in drug administration, e.g. pumps and nebulisers.
- Do emphasise that children with asthma should carry their relievers with them at all times.
- Do offer regular teaching sessions to check the use of inhalation devices.
- Do communicate with the school nurse regarding children's medications.
- Do encourage mouth washes in patients who have steroids via inhalers.
- Do not become rushed or distracted.
- Do not take 'short cuts' with checking procedures.

References

Addison, R., 2000. How to administer enemas and suppositories. Nurs. Times 10 (Suppl. 96), 3–4.

Ansel, H., Allen, L., Popovich, N., 2002. Pharmaceutical dosage forms and drug delivery systems, eighth ed. Lea and Febiger, Philadelphia.

Audit Commission, 2001. A spoonful of sugar: medicines management in the NHS hospitals. Audit Commission, London.

Beckstrand, J., Maarsha, L., Cirgin, E., et al., 2007. Predicting internal distance to the stomach for positioning nasogastric and orogastric feeding tubes in children. J. Adv. Nurs. 59 (3), 274–289.

Booker, R., 2007. Correct use of nebulizers. Nurs. Stand. 22 (8), 39–41.

Bryan, K.C., Cunningham, B.B., 2001. Topical anesthetics in children: agents and techniques that equally comfort patients, parents, and clinicians. Curr. Opin. Pediatr. 13, 324–330.

Caldwell, C., 1998. Management of acute asthma in children. Nurs. Stand. 12 (29), 49–54.

Campbell, A., 2002. Inter-professional collaboration and children with asthma. Paediatr. Nurs. 14 (10), 32–34.

Castro-Rodriguez, J., Rodrigo, G., 2004. Review: β agonist delivery by metered dose inhaler with a valved holding chamber (compared with a nebuliser) reduces admissions in preschool children and infants with acute asthma or wheezing. J. Pediatr. 145, 172–177.

Cates, C., Bara, A., Crilly, J., Rowe, B., 2003. Holding chambers versus nebulisers for beta-agonist treatment of acute asthma [systematic review]. Cochrane Airways Group, Cochrane Database 3.

Child, F., Davies, S., Clayton, S., et al., 2002. Inhaler devices for asthma: do we follow the guidelines? Arch. Dis. Child. 86 (3), 176–179.

Choonara, I., 2008. WHO wants safer medicines for children. Arch. Dis. Child. 93, 456–457.

Choonara, I., Bonati, M., 2007. European legislation to improve medicines for children. Paediatr. Perinat. Drug Ther. 8, 2–3.

Choonara, I., Conroy, S., 2002. Unlicensed and off-label drug use in children: implications for safety. Drug Saf. 25, 1–5.

Choonara, I., 2000. Clinical trials of medicines in children: US experience shows how to ensure that treatment of children is evidence based. Br. Med. J. 321 (7269), 1093–1094.

Clarke, S., Richardson, O., 2007a. A review of nasogastric tube management in children: Part 1: enteral feeding. Journal of Children's and Young People's Nursing 1 (2), 72–80.

Clarke, S., Richardson, O., 2007b. A review of nasogastric tube management in children: Part 2: position, placement, error and hydration. Journal of Children's and Young People's Nursing 1 (3), 119–128.

Clarke, S., 2003. Postoperative pain in children: a retrospective audit of continuous epidural analgesia in a paediatric orthopaedic ward. J. Orthop. Nurs. 7, 4–9.

Cocoman, A., Barron, C., 2008. Administering subcutaneous injections to children: what does the evidence say? Journal of Children's and Young People's Nursing 2 (2), 84–88.

Conroy, S., Choonara, I., Impicciatore, P., et al., 2000. Survey of unlicensed and off label drug use in paediatric wards in European countries. Br. Med. J. 320, 79–82.

Cook, I.F., Murtgh, J., 2005. Optimal technique for intramuscular injection of infants and toddlers: a randomised trial. Med. J. Aust. 183, 60–63.

Costello, I., Wong, I.C.K., Nunn, A.J., 2004. A literature review to identify interventions to improve the use of medicines in children. Child Care: Health Dev. 30 (6), 647–665.

Demoly, P., Bousquet, J., 2001. Epidemiology of drug allergy. Curr. Opin. Allergy Clin. Immunol. 1 (4), 305–310.

Department of Health, 2006. Immunisation against infectious disease. HMSO, London.

Department of Health, 1999. Review of prescribing, supply and administration of medicines. Final Report. TSO, London.

Department of Health, 2000. The NHS Plan. TSO, London.

Department of Health, 2003. Getting the right start: National Service Framework for children. Standard for hospital services. DoH, London.

Dimond, B., 2003a. The statutory framework for the control of medicines. Br. J. Nurs. 12 (7), 443–446.

Dimond, B., 2003b. Principles for the correct administration of medicines: 1. Br. J. Nurs. 12 (11), 682–685.

Dimond, B., 2003c. Principles for the correct administration of medicines: 2. Br. J. Nurs. 12 (12), 760–762.

Dimond, B., 2003d. The introduction of nurse prescribing 2. Final Crown Report. Br. J. Nurs. 12 (16), 980–983.

Duff, A.J.A., 2003. Incorporating psychological approaches into routine paediatric venepuncture. Arch. Dis. Child. 88, 931–937.

Ellis, J.A., Martelli, B., LaMontagne, C., et al., 2007. Evaluation of a continuous epidural analgesia program for postoperative pain in children. Pain Manag. Nurs. 8 (4), 146–155.

Esposito-Festen, J., Ijsselstijn, H., Hop, W., et al., 2006. Aerosol therapy by pressured metered-dose inhaler-spacer in sleeping young children: To do or not to do? Chest 130 (2), 487–492.

European Commission Enterprise Directorate-General, Better medicines for children. 2002. Proposed regulatory actions on paediatric medicinal products. European Commission, Brussels.

European Paediatric Life Support Group, 2005. Advanced paediatric life support: the practical approach, fourth ed. BMJ Publishing Group, London.

Francis, C., 2001. Setting up a school-based clinic to improve adolescent asthma. Community Nurse July/August, 19–22.

Ghaleb, M.A., Barber, N., Dean Franklin, B., et al., 2005. What constitutes a prescribing error in paediatrics? Qual. Saf. Health Care 14, 352–357.

Gibson, F., Khair, K., Pike, S., 2003. Nurse prescribing: children's nurses' views. Paediatr. Nurs. 15 (1), 20–25.

Godfrey, S., Kamburoff, P., Nairn, J., 1970. Spirometry, lung volumes and airway resistance in normal children aged 5 to 18 years. Br. J. Dis. Chest 64, 15–24.

Greenway, K., 2004. Using the ventrogluteal site for intramuscular injection. Nurs. Stand. 18 (25), 39–42.

Griffith, R., Griffiths, H., Jordan, S., 2003. Administration of medicines. Part 1: The law and nursing. Nurs. Stand. 18 (2), 47–54, 56.

Gupta, R., Sheikh, A., Strachan, D.P., et al., 2007. Time trends in allergic disorders in the UK. Thorax 62 (1), 91–96.

Hämeen-Anttila, K., Juvonen, M., Ahonen, R., et al., 2006. How well can children understand medicine related topics? Patient Educ. Couns. 60, 171–178.

Hannemann, L., 1999. What is new in asthma: new drug powder inhalers. J. Pediatr. Health Care 13, 159–165.

Harrop, M., 2002. Self-management plans in childhood asthma. Nurs. Stand. 17 (10), 38–42.

Health and Safety Commission, 1999. Control of substances hazardous to health regulations. Approved code of practice. TSO, London.

Health and Safety Executive, 2002. Control of substances hazardous to health regulations. TSO, London.

Health and Safety Executive, 2003. Safe handling of cytotoxic drugs: HSE Information Sheet MISC615. TSO, London.

Hemsworth, S., 2000. Intramuscular injection technique. Paediatr. Nurs. 12 (9), 17–20.

Higgins, D., 2007. Bowel care. Part 6: administration of a suppository. Nurs. Times 103 (47), 26–27.

Hutchinson, F., Hall, C., 2003. Nurse prescribing: issues for neonatal nurses. J. Neonatal Nurs. 9 (6), 203–206.

Iles, R., Lister, P., Edmunds, A., 1999. Crying significantly reduces absorption of aerolised drugs in infants. Arch. Dis. Child 81 (2), 163–165.

Ipp, M., Taddio, A., Sam, J., 2007. Vaccine-related pain: randomised controlled trial of two injection techniques. Arch. Dis. Child. 92, 1105–1108.

Jamieson, E.M., McCall, J.M., Blythe, R., 2002. Clinical nursing practices, fourth ed. Churchill Livingstone, Edinburgh.

Jordan, S., White, J., 2001. Bronchodilators: implications for nursing practice. Nurs. Stand. 15 (27), 45–55.

Kaushal, R., Bates, D.W., Clapp, M., et al., 2001. Medication errors and adverse events in pediatric inpatients. JAMA 285, 2114–2120.

Kennedy, M., 2007. Peak Flow Monitors Improve Asthma Control in Children. Am. J. Nurs. 107 (7), 22.

Le Duc, K., 1997. Efficacy of normal saline solution vs heparin solution for maintaining patency of peripheral intravenous catheters in children. J. Emerg. Nurs. 23 (4), 306–309.

Le Souif, P., 1999. Asthma in children. Medicine 27 (9), 54–58.

Lissauer, T., Clayden, G., 2002. Illustrated textbook of paediatrics, second ed. Mosby, London.

LPN, 2005. Z' is the key to I.M. injections. LPN 1 (6), 11–12.

Madge, S., 2002. Cystic fibrosis. Prof. Nurse 17 (6), 343–344.

Marsden, J., Shaw, M., 2003. Correct administration of topical eye treatment. Nurs. Stand. 17 (30), 42–44.

McIntyre, J., Conroy, S., Avery, A., et al., 2000. Unlicensed and off label drug use in general practice. Arch. Dis. Child. 83, 498–501.

McLay, J.S., Tanaka, M., Ekins-Daukes, P.J., Helms, P.J., 2006. A prospective questionnaire assessment of attitudes and experiences of off label prescribing among hospital based paediatricians. Arch. Dis. Child. 91, 584–587.

MedicAid, 1995. Information pack on nebulisers. Medic Aid, Pagham, Sussex.

Milnes, L., Callery, P., 2003. The adaptation of written self-management plans for children with asthma. J. Adv. Nurs. 41 (5), 444–453.

Mok, E., Kwong, T.K.Y., Fai Chan, M., 2007. A randomized controlled trial for maintaining peripheral intravenous lock in children. Int. J. Nurs. Pract. 13, 33–45.

Moppett, S., 2000. Which way is up for a suppository? Nurs. Times, NTPLUS 96 (19), 12–13.

NICE, 2000. Guidance on the use of inhaler systems (devices) in children under the age of 5 years with chronic asthma. Technology

Appraisal Guidance No. 10. National Institute for Clinical Excellence, London.

NICE, (reviewed 2005) 2002. Inhaler devices for routine treatment of chronic asthma in older children (aged 5–15 years). Technology Appraisal Guidance No. 38. National Institute for Clinical Excellence, London.

Nicol, M., Thompson, B., 2000. Causes of medication errors. Nurs. Prog. 8, 9–11.

Nicol, M., Thompson, B., 2001. Causes of medication errors. Part II. Nurs. Prog. 10, 17–19.

Nursing and Midwifery Council, 2006. Standards for the proficiency for nurse and midwife prescribers. NMC, London.

Nursing and Midwifery Council, 2007a. Essential Skills Clusters (ESCs) for Pre-registration Nursing Programmes NMC Circular 07/2007. NMC, London.

Nursing and Midwifery Council, 2007b. Record Keeping Advice Sheet. NMC, London.

Nursing and Midwifery Council, 2008a. Standards for Medicine Management. NMC, London.

Nursing and Midwifery Council, 2008b. The Code. Standards of Conduct, performance and ethics for nurses and midwives of professional conduct. NMC, London.

National Patient Safety Agency, 2007. Safety in doses: medication safety incidents in the NHS. The fourth report from the patient safety observatory. NPSA, London.

O'Callaghan, C., Barry, P., 2000. How to choose delivery devices for asthma. Arch. Dis. Child. 82 (3), 185–187.

O'Connor, B., 2001. Inhaler devices: compliance with steroid therapy. Nurs. Stand. 15 (48), 40–42.

Peters, J., Stevenson, M., Beverley, C., et al., 2002. The clinical effectiveness and cost effectiveness of inhaler devices used in the routine management of chronic asthma in older children: a systematic review and economic evaluation. Health Technol. Assess. 6 (5).

Pontin, D., Jones, S., 2007. Children's nurses and nurse prescribing: a case study identifying issues for developing training programmes in the UK.

Prosser, S., Worster, B., MacGregor, J., et al., 2000. Applied pharmacology. An introduction to pathophysiology and drug management for nurses and health care professionals. Mosby, London.

Quinn, C., 2000. Infusion devices: risks, functions and management. Nurs. Stand. 14 (26), 35–41.

Resuscitation Council UK, 2008. Emergency Treatment of Anaphylactic Reactions Guidelines for Health Providers. Resuscitation Council (UK), London. Online. Available: www.resus.org.uk.

Roberts, J., 2002. The management of poorly controlled asthma. Nurs. Stand. 16 (21), 45–53.

Rodger, M.A., King, L., 2000. Drawing up and administering intramuscular injections: a review of the literature. J. Adv. Nurs. 31 (3), 574–582.

Rogers, J., Irwin, K., 2003. Digital rectal examination. Guidance for nurses working with children and young people. Royal College of Nursing, London.

Royal College of Nursing, 2001. Administering intravenous therapy to children in the community. RCN, London.

Royal College of Paediatrics and Child Health, 2003. Medicines for children, second ed. RCPCH, London.

Royal College of Paediatrics and Child Health and Royal College of Nursing, 2002. Position statement on injection technique. RCPCH and RCN, London.

Saint-Raymond, A., Seigneuret, N., 2005. Medicines for children: time for Europe to act. Paediatric Perinatal Drug Therapy 6, 142–146.

Schaad, U.B., 2001. Drug therapy in children: still more art than science. Curr. Opin. Infect. Dis. 14 (3), 301–302.

Scottish Intercollegiate Guidelines Network, 2004. The British Thoracic Society. British guideline on the management of asthma. Quick reference guide. Royal College of Physicians, Edinburgh.

Shah, P., Dhurjon, L., Metcalfe, T., et al., 1992. Acute angle closure glaucoma associated with nebulised ipratropium bromide and salbutamol. Br. Med. J. 304 (6818), 40–41.

Shapiro, G., Bronsky, E., Murray, A., et al., 2000. Clinical comparability of Ventolin formulated with hydrofluoroalkanes or conventional chlorofluorocarbon propellants in children with asthma. Arch. Pediatr. Adolesc. Med. 154 (12), 1219–1225.

Singel, L., Lira, R., 2001. Yes, you can!': nurses create a template for teaching school-aged children to live with asthma. Am. J. Nurs. 101 (8), 24a–24c.

Sleath, B., Bush, P.J., Pradel, F.G., 2003. Communicating with children about medicines: a pharmacist's perspective. Am. J. Health Syst. Pharm. 60 (6), 604–607.

Stephenson, T., 2000. Implications of the Crown Report and nurse prescribing. Arch. Dis. Child. 83 (3), 199–202.

Stephenson, T., 2001. Medicines for children – the last century and the next. Arch. Dis. Child. 85 (3), 177–179.

Strauss, K., 2002. A pan-European epidemiologic study of insulin injection technique in patients with diabetes. Pract. Diab. Int. 19 (3), 71–76.

Sutcliffe, A.G., 2003. Testing new pharmaceutical products in children: a positive step, but ethical concerns remain. Br. Med. J. 326 (7380), 64–65.

Warner, J.O., Gregson, R.K., 1995. Asthma inhalers: developments or distractions? Matern. Child Health December, 383.

Watt, S., 2003a. Safe administration of medicines to children: part 2. Paediatr. Nurs. 15 (5), 40–44.

Watt, S., 2003b. Safe administration of medicines to children: part 1. Paediatr. Nurs. 15 (4), 40–43.

Westhus, N., 2004. Methods to Test Feeding Tube Placement in Children. MCN 29 (5), 282–291.

Wong, I.C.K., Basra, N., Yeung, V.W., Cope, J., 2006. Supply problems of unlicensed and off-label medicines after discharge. Arch. Dis. Child. 01, 686–688.

WHO, 2002. WHO task force on routine infant vaccination and child survival. WHO, Geneva.

WHO, 2004. Immunization in practice: a guide for health workers. World Health Organization. Online available from: www.who.int.

Wright, A., Falconer, J., Newman, C., 2002. Self-administration and reuse of medicines. Paediatr. Nurs. 14 (6), 14–17.

Wyllie, R., 2004. Changing the tube: a pediatrician's guide. Curr. Opin. Pediatr. 16, 542–544.

Further reading

Department of Health, 2000b. Pharmacy in the future – implementing the NHS plan. TSO, London.

Duff, A.J.A., 2003. Incorporating psychological approaches into routine paediatric venepuncture. Arch. Dis. Child. 88, 931–937.

Hunter, J., 2008. Intramuscular injection techniques. Nurs. Stand. 22 (24), 35–40.

Chapter 43

Oxygen therapy

Rebecca Clarke

CHAPTER CONTENTS

Introduction 446
    Learning outcomes 446
    Rationale 447
    Factors to note 447
    Guidelines 448

Delivery of oxygen therapy 448
    Equipment for headbox and body/trunk box delivery 448
    Equipment for nasal cannula delivery 449
    Equipment for oxygen mask delivery 449
    Method for headbox delivery 449
    Method for nasal cannula delivery 450
    Method for oxygen mask delivery 450
    Observations and complications 450
    Risks of oxygen therapy 451
    Dos and don'ts 452

INTRODUCTION

Adequate oxygenation is vital to prevent tissue damage. Prolonged hypoxia (a decreased availability of oxygen to the tissues) can result in cell death if allowed to persist, which ultimately leads to brain damage and multiorgan failure; 100% oxygen is therefore the first drug given in an emergency/resuscitation situation (Resuscitation Council UK 2005). Oxygen requirements can vary between individuals but are more significant in children as they have a lower pulmonary reserve and a higher metabolic rate than adults and can therefore decompensate more quickly if supplementary oxygen is not provided (Advanced Life Support Group 2005). Administering oxygen to children can be difficult, as they do not tolerate oxygen masks well, but nasal cannula and headboxes are often effective. Accuracy of the amount delivered can also be problematic as will be discussed later in this chapter. Oxygen can also be administered via an incubator but is not without problems (see Ch. 15).

LEARNING OUTCOMES

By the end of this section you should be able to:

- Assess the most appropriate delivery device for each child according to age, size, development and condition
- Assess whether or not the oxygen delivery system requires humidification
- Prepare the equipment necessary to deliver oxygen (humidified where necessary) via headbox, nasal cannula and oxygen mask

- State possible complications of oxygen administration.

RATIONALE

Administration of oxygen is a life-saving intervention commonly used in children's nursing and an important skill for a children's nurse to acquire.

FACTORS TO NOTE

Oxygen should be regarded as a drug and planned delivery of oxygen therapy should always be prescribed by a doctor (BMA 2006, Chandler 2001) As with any drug there can be adverse effects. Therefore, in any patient, oxygen should be delivered at the lowest concentration possible and for the shortest time possible (Chandler 2001, Wong et al 2002). Administration of oxygen to children is usually undertaken using one of three methods: via headbox, nasal cannula or oxygen mask. How much oxygen is delivered to the child is expressed as the fractional inspired oxygen concentration (FiO_2) – literally, the percentage concentration of oxygen the child is breathing in.

Headbox or body/trunk box

This method of oxygen delivery is normally most suitable for infants and small children. The advantages of these types of device are that they give effective oxygen delivery, it is possible to reliably monitor the FiO_2 and they are totally non-invasive. Disadvantages are that carbon dioxide re-breathing will occur at low oxygen flow rates, <4 L/min (Frey & Shann 2003), removal of the box quickly dilutes the oxygen delivered and a cold gas supply will quickly cool an infant. It is also desirable to humidify when prolonged oxygen therapy is required (Chandler 2001, Frey & Shann 2003, Pilkington 2004). Normally, inspired gas is warmed and humidified in the nasopharynx and reaches the upper trachea with a relative humidity of about 90% and a temperature of 32–36°C; it has reached a temperature of 37°C by the time it reaches the alveoli (Hazinski 1998). Mucociliary transport is impaired when relative humidity falls below 75% at 37°C (Pilkington 2004).

Nasal cannula

Nasal cannulae are available in different sizes, suitable for neonates through to adults. Advantages of nasal cannula are that they are reasonably well tolerated by children (particularly in comparison with an oxygen mask) and carbon dioxide re-breathing does not occur (Chandler 2001). Humidification is not necessary as the gas is entering via the nasal passages where it is warmed and moistened in the normal way (Frey & Shann 2003). Disadvantages are that nasal cannula are only suitable for use with a low flow of oxygen, i.e. maximum 2 L/min in neonates. Higher flows (>4 L/min) may be uncomfortable and dry the nasal mucosa (McGloin 2008). It is usually only possible to achieve an oxygen concentration of approximately 40–60% (EPLS 2006). In addition, a child who mouth breathes will dilute the FiO_2 with air and oxygen concentrations are very dependent upon the infant or child's breathing pattern.

One major hazard to be aware of is the risk of strangulation that nasal cannula can present if the child is not closely observed. This risk can be reduced by taking the tubing behind the child's head and not underneath their chin as is common in adult practice.

Oxygen masks

They are available in two sizes; paediatric and adult. Advantages are that oxygen masks without a reservoir bag can deliver concentrations of up to 60% and with a reservoir up to 95% or higher (EPLS 2006). Humidification can also be provided. Disadvantages are that the mask needs to be well fitting which can be problematic if a baby or child is in-between sizes of mask. Additionally, they can become hot and uncomfortable leading to non-compliance.

Healthy children

Healthy children should have an arterial oxygen saturation level of 95–98% (Balfour-Lyn et al 2005). However, some children with chronic lung disease or who have cyanotic heart conditions may have an oxygen saturation level well below this, even when otherwise healthy. It is therefore essential for nurses to be aware of the child's 'norm' and parents are a vital source of such information.

Neonates

Administration of continuous oxygen therapy to neonates must be monitored very carefully. High inspired oxygen concentrations have been clearly linked to the development of retinopathy of prematurity and prolonged exposure to high oxygen tensions may also cause pulmonary oxygen toxicity and permanent lung damage, e.g. bronchopulmonary dysplasia (BMA 2006, Kotecha & Allen 2002). However, very little is known about how much oxygen is safe to give and the target range of oxygen saturations in neonates is controversial (Tin & Gupta 2007). Recent studies have suggested that saturations of 92–94% in infants, particularly during the pre-term period, may be ideal (Askie et al 2003, Anon 2000).

Sick children

Children with respiratory problems may benefit from being nursed upright, well supported with pillows. An infant may benefit from being placed in a baby chair for periods of up to 4 h or longer if absolutely necessary. Any child should have a change of position 4-hourly if possible, to relieve pressure areas. If the child is too ill to sit up, consider tilting up the head of the bed or cot.

Recent studies have demonstrated that a child with chronic lung disease can and should have oxygen saturations maintained around 92–94% to provide a buffer zone against desaturation during sleeping and feeding. These targets also aim to reduce complications from pulmonary artery hypertension and promote growth (Kotecha & Allen 2002). However, in a small number of children with chronic lung disease, e.g. some children with cystic fibrosis, the dependence of respiratory drive on CO_2 and bicarbonate concentration is lost. In these children, inflammatory changes in the lungs result in increased alveolar CO_2 tension, which ultimately leads to a gross saturation of the chemoreceptors, making them dysfunctional. Administering high concentrations of oxygen to these children can cause carbon dioxide narcosis leading to unconsciousness (Chandler 2001). The BMA (2005) states that any patient with a chronic chest condition should not be administered more than 28% concentration of oxygen alongside repeated blood gas measurements.

GUIDELINES

Careful explanation to parents and child (if age and cognitive development allow) about the need for oxygen therapy will help to maximise cooperation.

Careful explanation of all the equipment involved is important to minimise anxiety by reducing fear of the unknown. Parents can be taught how to perform oral care to help maintain a moist, clean mouth if oxygen therapy is causing drying of the mucosa (see Ch. 9).

DELIVERY OF OXYGEN THERAPY

EQUIPMENT FOR HEADBOX AND BODY/ TRUNK BOX DELIVERY

- Oxygen supply (even if supply is piped, consider the need for a spare portable cylinder in case of emergencies, e.g. loss or failure of supply)
- Humidifier apparatus: preferably a warmed, water bath humidifier such as the Aquapak system; some humidifiers have temperature controls to enable the water to be heated to different temperatures (Fig. 43.1)

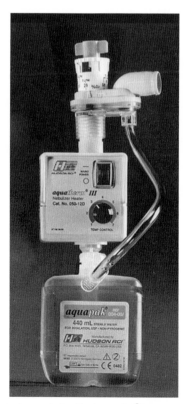

Figure 43.1 Aquapak (by Hudson RCI ®) humidification system with heater attached *(with permission of Teleflex Medical Europe Ltd).*

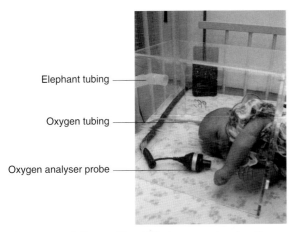

Elephant tubing

Oxygen tubing

Oxygen analyser probe

Figure 43.2 Delivery of humidified oxygen via a headbox (viewed from above).

- Apparatus to connect humidifier, water and oxygen together (usually supplied as a complete, sterile unit for once-only use, e.g. Aquapak system)
- Sterile water for humidification; tap water must not be used as it increases the risk of contamination with *Legionella bacteria*
- Elephant tubing
- Oxygen analyser
- Headbox of a size sufficient to enclose the baby's head while sitting over the baby's neck (Fig. 43.2)
- Oxygen saturation monitor and probe.

EQUIPMENT FOR NASAL CANNULA DELIVERY

- Oxygen supply
- Nasal cannula
- Oxygen saturation monitor and probe
- Tape for fastening the cannula in place
- Low-flow oxygen meter if required.

EQUIPMENT FOR OXYGEN MASK DELIVERY

- Oxygen supply
- Appropriate size oxygen mask
- Equipment to provide humidification (as per headbox delivery)
- Elephant tubing
- Oxygen saturation monitor and probe.

METHOD FOR HEADBOX DELIVERY

1. Explain the procedure to the parents to reduce fear of the unknown and aid compliance with the therapy.
2. If using a portable oxygen supply, ensure that the cylinder is full or nearly full. Determine how many hours' supply will be provided by the cylinder.
3. Set up the humidification system according to the manufacturer's instructions.
4. Test the alarm and set upper and lower alarm limits on the oxygen analyser. Calibrate the analyser to air and to 100% oxygen to ensure accuracy of monitoring.
5. Position the baby on their back or side in the cot and attach the oxygen saturation monitor probe. Turn on the saturation monitor. Set the upper and lower limit alarms for oxygen saturation and pulse rate (according to medical staff instructions) and record the child's oxygen saturation and pulse rate.
6. Place the headbox carefully on top of the baby's head, preferably with the shoulders outside. Sometimes the shoulders have to go inside the box as well, particularly in a smaller infant. Ensure that the box does not exert undue pressure anywhere on the baby's body. Do not block the gap around the infant's shoulders as this will cause carbon dioxide retention within the headbox.
7. Position the elephant tubing so that it delivers the oxygen through the purpose-built, larger hole and is behind the head or to one side of the baby's face.
8. Put the probe of the oxygen analyser into the headbox via the purpose-built (smaller) hole. Position the probe so that it is at the opposite side of the box to the point at which the oxygen is being delivered, near to the baby's face.
9. From the prescription sheet, determine the percentage oxygen to be delivered and turn on the oxygen to flow at 4.5 L/min minimum. The dial on the humidifier equipment will tell you how many litres of oxygen are needed for specific concentrations of oxygen.
10. Read the oxygen analyser and regulate the flow of oxygen until the prescribed percentage of oxygen is attained.

11. Monitor the effect on the baby's saturation level and record frequently (every 1–4 h depending on the child's condition). Report to medical staff if the prescribed percentage of oxygen does not maintain the baby's saturations at a level predetermined by the doctor. Report to medical staff if the saturations are decreasing despite prescribed oxygen flow.

12. Monitor the baby's respiratory rate and effort.

13. Monitor the amount of oxygen remaining in a portable oxygen cylinder at least hourly. Ensure that a replacement cylinder is available before the one in use empties.

14. Monitor the level of water in the humidifier bottle.

METHOD FOR NASAL CANNULA DELIVERY

1, 2. Follow steps 1 and 2 of headbox delivery.

3. Ensure that the child's nose is cleaned of any dried mucus. Take the nasal cannula and place it over the child's head. Position it so that the prongs slant towards the child's face and each of the two prongs sits in a nostril (Fig. 43.3).

4. Tighten the cannula to fit closely by sliding up the movable sheath at the back of the tubing.

5. If necessary, fasten the cannula in place by taping the tubes onto the child's cheeks. Ensure that the child is not allergic to the tape. If the skin is particularly delicate or sore, consider using a protective barrier such as a piece of extra-thin hydrocolloid sheet (e.g. Granuflex).

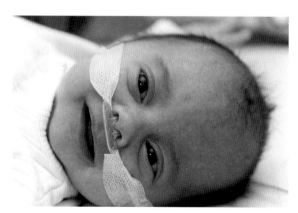

Figure 43.3 Delivery of oxygen via nasal cannula: nasal prongs *in situ*.

6. Attach the oxygen saturation monitor probe. Turn on the saturation monitor. Set the upper and lower limit alarms for oxygen saturation and pulse rate (according to medical staff instructions) and record the child's oxygen saturation and pulse rate.

7. Attach the end of the nasal cannula tubing to the oxygen supply.

8. From the prescription sheet, determine the oxygen flow rate to be delivered and turn on the oxygen accordingly.

9, 10. Follow steps 11 and 12 of headbox delivery.

METHOD FOR OXYGEN MASK DELIVERY

1–3. Follow steps 1–3 of headbox delivery.

4. Select appropriate sized oxygen mask and attach one end of the elephant tubing to the face mask and the other end to the humidification system.

5. From the prescription sheet, determine the percentage oxygen to be delivered and turn on the oxygen flow. The dial on the humidifier equipment will tell you how many litres of oxygen are needed for specific concentrations of oxygen.

6. Place the oxygen mask over the child's nose and mouth ensuring as good a fit as possible (Fig 43.4)

7. Attach the oxygen saturation monitor probe. Turn on the saturation monitor. Set the upper and lower limit alarms for oxygen saturation and pulse rate (according to medical staff instructions) and record the child's oxygen saturation and pulse rate

8–10. Follow steps 11–13 of headbox delivery.

OBSERVATIONS AND COMPLICATIONS

A child requiring oxygen therapy should always be monitored carefully. Oxygen saturations should be monitored continuously while oxygen is being delivered, using a pulse oximeter. Pulse oximetry will detect hypoxia long before clinical signs become apparent (Bilan et al 2006). The child's oxygen saturation level, respiratory rate and effort and percentage/flow rate of oxygen delivered should be monitored and recorded regularly, between 1- and 4-hourly depending on the stability of the child's condition. If using headbox oxygen,

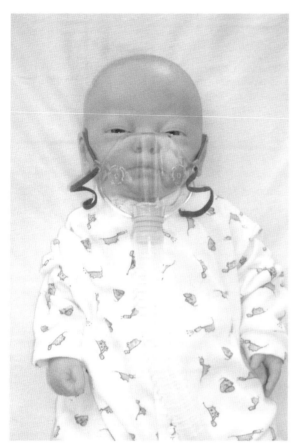

Figure 43.4 Delivery of humidified oxygen via oxygen mask.

for accuracy it is important to read the concentration of oxygen from the analyser which should be placed near the baby's mouth and not from the delivery system. Report any decrease in saturations and increase in respiratory rate and/or effort. If using a portable supply, check the cylinder regularly to ensure that sufficient oxygen remains in it.

Remember to change the humidifier water bottle when it is empty or in accordance with the manufacturer's instructions to prevent infection as humidifiers have been linked with Gram-negative bacilli and viruses associated with the respiratory system (Pilkington 2004).

Ensure that the infant or child's nostrils remain free from dried mucus; they may need gentle cleansing with warm water. Remember that some infants will not tolerate being removed from the headbox for washing, feeding, etc. They may require a source of oxygen close to their face during the time that they are removed from the headbox.

RISKS OF OXYGEN THERAPY

- There is a risk of eye damage associated with PO_2 above 15 kPa.
- There is a risk of lung damage associated with prolonged, continuous administration of high-pressure oxygen therapy.
- There is a risk of respiratory depression in children who have chronic obstructive respiratory disease.
- Whenever oxygen therapy is administered, remember that there is an increased risk of fire as oxygen is highly flammable.

COMMUNITY PERSPECTIVE

Prior to discharge
- Ensure that the parents are aware of all the constraints and problems that caring for a baby/child on long-term oxygen therapy can pose and consent to take on this role.
- Initiate a teaching programme for parents. This will need to cover:
  - Recognising normal and abnormal respiratory patterns in their child, including signs of desaturation
  - Knowing what action to take in the event of problems occurring
  - Training in resuscitation
  - Familiarisation with the use of the oxygen delivery system (e.g. oxygen cylinders, oxygen concentrator, liquid oxygen)
  - Knowing what action to take should there be problems with the equipment. They will also need the telephone number of the oxygen supplier and an engineer in case of emergencies
  - Training in order to gain competence in caring for their baby/child with nasal prongs in situ and being able to change the prongs when necessary
  - Familiarisation with the use of an apnoea monitor if one is in use
  - Information on the need to inform their insurance companies and the local fire station that they will be storing oxygen at home, and may carry cylinders in their car
  - Ensuring that they recognise the need for no smoking and are prepared to enforce this
  - Having the contact numbers of the CCN and the children's ward readily available.

■ A home visit by the CCN or special care baby unit (SCBU) liaison nurse will need to be arranged to check the suitability of the home and discuss the positioning and storage of the oxygen delivery system.

■ The parents will need to have a telephone and arrangements should be made to install one if necessary.

■ The medical practitioner responsible for prescribing the oxygen delivery system may vary locally between hospital and community.

■ Each child should have an individual management plan with information relating to clinical signs and symptoms. It should include:
  ■ Oxygen prescription
  ■ Amount of oxygen required (L/min)
  ■ Sliding scale of parameters or variables with indication of when to seek advice
  ■ Mode of delivery (e.g. face mask, nasal cannula)
  ■ Delivery system required
  ■ Equipment to be used (e.g. humidifier, pulse oximeter, apnoea monitor).

■ Discharge planning is essential, as is the transfer of information to all relevant professionals between hospital and community.

Equipment required

■ Apnoea monitor and possibly baby alarm
■ Nebuliser/nebuhaler if necessary
■ Portable oxygen cylinder
■ Low-flow head compatible with the cylinder and a carrying bag
■ Spare nasal prongs and tape
■ Humidifying device if necessary
■ Prescribed drugs including saline nasal drops as required

■ Equipment to measure oxygen saturation and heart rate if the child needs monitoring overnight.

The family will need to be in touch with a social worker in order to provide assistance with claiming any benefits to which they may be entitled. They may also require help to fill in the forms. Initially the family will need frequent home visits from the healthcare professionals involved in their baby/child's care, as they often feel very isolated at home. Ongoing support is also essential to enable the parents to cope with the oxygen-dependent baby or child. As they become more proficient and the child more stable, the CCN can advise the parents on future management to enable them to be more mobile.

DOS AND DON'TS

● Do ensure that the oxygen is prescribed.
● Do remember to check whether or not humidity is required.
● Do check whether the child has any chronic lung disease which could affect the normal functioning of the respiratory centre and therefore the child's response to oxygen therapy.
● Do monitor the duration and concentration of oxygen therapy at all times.
● Do secure portable O_2 when travelling and have sign in car advising compressed gases on board (O_2 company will supply stickers)
● Do not administer high concentrations of oxygen over prolonged periods without discussion with senior medical staff (particularly to the neonate or premature infant).
● Do not administer more than 4 L/min of oxygen via a nasal cannula, or more than 2 L/min in neonates and infants <6 months.

References

Advanced Life Support Group, 2005. Advanced paediatric life support – the practical approach, fourth ed. BMJ Publishing, London.

Anon, 2000. Supplemental therapeutic oxygen for prethreshold retinopathy of prematurity (STOP-ROP) a randomized controlled trial. Pediatrics 105, 295–310.

Askie, L.M., Henderson-Smart, D.J., Irwig, L., et al., 2003. Oxygen saturation targets and outcomes in extremely premature infants. N. Engl. J. Med. 349, 959–967.

Balfour-Lyn, I., Primhak, R., Shaw, B., 2005. Home oxygen for children: who, how and when? Thorax 60, 76–81.

Bilan, N., Abdinia, B., Mahallei, M., 2006. Validity of pulse oximetry of earlobe, toe and finger in the detection of pediatric hypoxemia. Med. J. Tabriz University of Medical Sciences 28 (3), 10.

British Medical Association, 2005. The neonatal and paediatric pharmacists group BNF for children. BMA, London.

British Medical Association, 2006.
British National Formulary for
children. British Medical Journal
Publishing Group, London.
Online. Available: www.bnfc.org.

Chandler, T., 2001. Oxygen
administration. Paediatr. Nurs.
13 (8), 37–43.

Frey, B., Shann, F., 2003. Oxygen
administration in infants. Arch.
Dis. Child 88 (2), F84–F88.

Hazinski, M.F., 1998. Manual of
pediatric critical care. Mosby,
St Louis.

Kotecha, S., Allen, J., 2002. Oxygen
therapy for infants with chronic

lung disease. Arch. Dis. Child.
87 (1), F11–F14.

McGloin, S., 2008. Administration of
oxygen therapy. Nurs. Stand.
22 (21), 46–48.

Pilkington, F., 2004. Humidification
for oxygen therapy for
nonventilated patients. Br. J. Nurs.
13 (2), 111–115.

Resuscitation Council (UK), 2005.
Paediatric advanced life support.
Resuscitation Guidelines.
Resuscitation Council (UK),
London. Online: www.resus.org.
uk/pages/pals.htm.

Resuscitation Council UK, 2006.
European paediatric life support,
second ed. Resuscitation Council
UK, London. Online. Available:
www.resus.org.uk July 2008.

Tin, W., Gupta, S., 2007. Optimum
oxygen therapy in preterm babies.
Arch. Dis. Child. Fetal Neonatal
Edition 92, F143–F147.

Wong, D.L., Hockenberry, M.,
Wilson, D., et al., 2002. Whaley
and Wong's nursing care of
infants and children, seventh ed.
Mosby Year Book, St Louis.

Chapter 44

Pain management

Rebecca Reaney, Catherine Trower

CHAPTER CONTENTS

Introduction   454
   Learning outcomes   454
   Rationale   455

Assessment of pain   455
   Guidelines   455
   Factors to note   456
   Conducting a pain assessment   457

Management of pain   459

Non-drug methods of pain management   459

Drug methods of pain control   459
   Routes of analgesia administration   459
   Analgesia   460
   Evaluation   462
   Sedation   463

Management of chronic pain   464
   Summary of pain assessment
   complications   465
   Dos and don'ts   465

INTRODUCTION

Pain is one of the most common experiences a child will have as a result of injury, illness or medical procedures. Pain is associated with anxiety, fear, stress and distress for the child and their family. The subjectivity and multidimensional experience of pain makes it inherently difficult to assess, particularly in children, who often lack the verbal or cognitive ability to express their feelings of pain (Gaffney et al 2003). However, pain assessment is essential, not only to detect pain but to evaluate the effectiveness of our pain management interventions if we are to provide optimal pain control (Howard 2003; Finley et al 2005).

LEARNING OUTCOMES

By the end of this section you should be able to:

- Be aware of the myths surrounding pain in children
- Recognise how your own feelings and beliefs may affect your assessment of pain in children
- Have developed an awareness of the different types of assessment tools and the factors affecting their application
- Understand the importance of routine pain assessment and documentation, involving the parent and, more importantly, the child, where possible
- Be aware of the commonly used analgesic drugs and the different routes of administration
- Understand the importance of administering balanced analgesia

- Have an insight into the assessment and treatment of chronic and recurrent pain in children
- Understand the need for sedation and have an insight into the principles of good sedation practice.

RATIONALE

The treatment and alleviation of pain is a basic human right that exists regardless of age (Schechter et al 2003). The consequences of untreated pain include a delay in mobilisation, psychological trauma, an increase in the risk of infections, slower recovery and a delay in discharge from hospital. The undertreatment of pain in children is evident in the literature (Wilson & Doyle 1996, Nikanne et al 1999, Van Hulle 2005, Stinson & McGrath 2007); however, over the past two decades, there has been growth in the quantity and quality of paediatric pain research evidence. This evidence has advanced our understanding of the physiology and management of pain in children. In 1993, in a publication entitled *Children First: A Study of Hospital Services*, the Audit Commission (1993) identified pain relief as an indicator for measuring quality of care for children in hospital. More recently, the *National Service Framework for Children* has outlined standards for managing pain in hospital (DoH 2003). Assessment of a child's pain is problematic but it is essential if we are to provide effective management and therefore it must be an integral part of our nursing care.

ASSESSMENT OF PAIN

GUIDELINES

The purpose of pain assessment is to provide as complete a picture as possible of a child's pain (Box 44.1).

BOX 44.1 Purpose of pain assessment

- Detect pain
- Assign a meaningful value for pain
- Evaluate effectiveness of treatment
- Enable re-assessment
- Aid decisions for treatment modification
- Aid decisions for treatment discontinuation
- Prevent unrelieved pain.

Good pain assessment contributes to the prevention and/or early recognition of pain as well as the effective assessment of pain (Finley et al 2005).

The family has an important role to play in ensuring that a child's pain is managed effectively (Liossi 2002). Where the situation permits, this involves determining a child's past pain experiences and whether these were good or bad. Children may use a variety of words to describe pain and these should be identified prior to potentially painful experiences (RCN 1999). A description of the child's behaviour, which would normally indicate the presence of pain should be sought from the parents. The family may already employ certain coping strategies; these, along with analgesics used at home, should be discussed. Parents can also be helpful in identifying the pain assessment scale that may be appropriate for their child. Parents can be a particularly valuable resource with children with complex needs. A variety of pain assessment tools are available to help guide the professional to assess the pain in this group of children (RCN 2001, Voepel-Lewis et al 2002). These children may be unable to articulate or express their pain verbally or behaviourally. Carter et al (2002) found that parents used various strategies to identify their child's pain based on their in-depth knowledge of their child. The identification of this skill is also supported by findings from a study by Stallard et al (2001).

Pain is difficult to measure accurately and reliably in children. There are several pain scales available for paediatric use; however, development of verbal skills and cognitive ability show wide variation in children and this must be taken into account. Sociocultural and environmental factors must also be noted. In addition to selecting the appropriate scale for an individual child, the nurse must consider several issues:

- The period of time that is available to teach the child how to use the assessment scale
- Whether the child is able to grasp the function of the scale, enabling the nurse to achieve an accurate assessment
- Whether the child is comfortable with using the scale; it is important that the nurse obtains the child's commitment to working with it
- If the child has a choice of pain scales, the nurse must abide by the choice and preference of the child.

It is vital that the nurse receives appropriate levels of education, training and preparation in the use of pain assessment tools and proficiency in using them (Treadwell et al 2002; Malviya et al 2006). The nurse's assessment of children's pain is subject to a range of individual bias, social, and contextual influences This is particularly important to note when caring for children who are too sick to use self-reporting scales, neonates/infants and children with special needs. Professionals need to be flexible and willing to develop more positive attitudes and beliefs regarding the attributes of children's pain (Salantera et al 1999). Pain assessment should be part of a holistic approach to the child. The nurse should be able to take the information provided by the child and interpret it with skill. For example, a report of pain described in a particular manner may indicate a full bladder and urinary retention rather than wound pain. This should be treated in a different way and it is important, therefore, that the information given is channelled correctly.

It is also vital that children who can comprehend the pain scale and self-report are made aware that if they are in pain the treatment of that pain is patient friendly. A self-report is the only truly direct measure of pain and is often considered to be the 'gold standard' of measurement. Pain assessment is the most accurate when children can describe their pain in an appropriate manner and relevant language for their age and development (Broome & Huth 2003). However, for certain patients this will not be possible.

FACTORS TO NOTE

Sick children

A very sick child may be too ill to comprehend instructions regarding the use of a pain scale. A child in an intensive care setting, who is perhaps ventilated, sedated or paralysed, will be unable to use a self-reporting scale that would normally be used for their age and development. With these patients, physiological and behavioural factors should be considered jointly to enable the nurse to judge whether the child is distressed by pain. The child may also become distressed by the requirement for suction, position change or oral hygiene and this should be taken into consideration. As the nurse develops a relationship with the patient, they will be able to differentiate between distress and pain and the pain scale will be an aid to this nursing skill.

Culture

It is accepted that culture can influence an individual's perception and response to pain (Bates 1987). However, over the years, most of the studies looking at culture have been in relation to adults (Bernstein & Pachter 2003). Recommendations have been made which suggest we should recognise the importance of cultural factors which affect the assessment of pain in children (RCN 1999). It is important that, while being aware of cultural differences in pain expression, we should try to avoid stereotyping (Bernstein & Pachter 2003).

Neonates

Neonates cannot communicate by verbal report, so they are dependent on caregivers to recognise that they are in pain. Physiological and behavioural signs must be observed and interpreted as an indication of pain being present. A variety of scales have been made available for neonates, taking into consideration physiological and behavioural factors such as facial expression, crying, body position, body movement, colour, oxygen saturation (SaO_2), respiratory rate, blood pressure and heart rate (Hodgkinson et al 1994, Krechel & Bildner 1995, Ghai et al 2008). However, it should be noted that these observations can be affected by a variety of factors as well as pain, such as ventilatory support, drugs and the neonate's clinical condition. The scales that take this into consideration may be more accurate (Sparshott 1996).

Infants/toddlers

Similar problems occur with infants and toddlers regarding the use of pain scales. Again the nurse should be able to pick up pain cues from the infant/toddler by observing physiological and behavioural signs and then act appropriately. Toddlers may clutch at the site of the surgery. They may also display the characteristic signs of frustration and unhappiness that they cannot communicate verbally.

Children (pre–school to 7 years)

Studies have shown that many 3 year olds can identify the presence and absence of pain and can report a pain intensity (Harbeck & Peterson 1992, Romsing et al 1996). It is recommended that the choice of pain intensity scores for this age group should be limited to around four choices. They can usually verbalise in appropriate language, to the nurse or their parents, a description of 'their hurting'. It is important to remember that younger children may choose extremes of measurement and some may even confuse the scales with measurements of happiness. Some children in this age group may experience behavioural disturbances due to the trauma of hospital admission. Regression to earlier stages in development, such as loss of speech, clinging to parents or a return to bed wetting, may be noticed. Aggression may be a form of identifying pain. Children may be in pain but unable or reluctant to indicate that it is present. Their behaviour becomes aggressive as a response to this pain. It is important that nursing staff can recognise this and educate parents of this response.

Older children (7 years to adolescence)

Older children of a normal developmental level can usually self-report their pain and understand the use of visual analogue scales. Although adolescents are developing quickly physically, emotional development can be at a different rate. It should be remembered that they will be anxious and frightened about hospitalisation. They may be aware of peer group pressure and may not admit to pain because of fear of ridicule or comparison with another child. Fear of treatment may also be a problem. The nurse should ensure that adolescent patients have complete privacy and quiet to report any pain and that they are aware of the 'patient-friendly' treatments.

CONDUCTING A PAIN ASSESSMENT

History taking

It is vital that the nurse, on admitting a child to the ward or unit, takes a pain history from the parents or guardian. The nurse should record the child's reaction to pain, the usual method for reporting pain (if developmentally able) and what happens in response to pain at home. This information should be incorporated into the nursing care plan. The appropriate scale should be selected at this time, if possible taking into account:

- Age
- Mechanical interventions that may be necessary
- Special needs
- Clinical condition
- Type of pain, i.e. acute, chronic or recurrent.

Documentation of pain assessments should occur and guidelines recommend that they be recorded on the routine observation chart (Royal College of Surgeons and the College of Anaesthetists 1990). This is important because there is evidence to suggest that accurate documentation increases the assessment of pain, administration of analgesia and improved pain management (Savedra et al 1993, Goddard & Pickup 1996, Treadwell et al 2002). For postoperative pain, for example, a pain scale should be used to assess a child's pain with the routine postoperative observations, decreasing in frequency as the observations decrease but more regularly if a child is complaining of pain or analgesia has been administered.

Pain assessment scales usually incorporate one or more of the following:

- Behavioural assessment
- Physiological assessment
- Self-report techniques.

Behavioural assessment

Behaviour is one of the first indicators that alerts caregivers to the presence of pain (Reaney 2007). It involves looking at how a child behaves in response to pain. Types of distress behaviour, e.g. facial expression, cry and body movements, have been associated with pain. However, difficulties include differentiating this behaviour from behaviour that results from anxiety or hunger (Gaffney et al 2003).

Several coding systems have been developed for infants; however, intense crying with high motor activity could indicate pain, while equally an infant that is withdrawn and quiet could also be in pain, highlighting the difficulties.

It must be remembered that behaviour can be affected by many things including drugs, splints, ventilation and prematurity.

Behavioural pain assessment has some advantages in that it is non-invasive, does not put any demands on the child and does not depend on their cognitive ability or language skills. Assessment of behavioural signs could indicate the presence of pain and help determine the effect the pain is having on the child or infant (Table 44.1).

Physiological assessment

Physiological signs vary greatly, particularly in premature infants (Stevens et al 1996).

Table 44.1 Behavioural pain assessment tools

SCALE	APPROPRIATE AGE RANGE	VALIDATED	RELIABLE	USEFULNESS	COMMENTS
FLACC	≥3 years	Yes	Yes	Simple, quick	Reliable for postoperative pain assessment
CHEOPS	≥1 month	Yes	Yes	Complicated	Wide age range
TPPPS	≥1 year	Yes	Yes	Simple, tracks effects of analgesia	Only validated in immediate postoperative period
Post-operative pain score	≥1 month	Yes	Yes	Complicated	Only validated in immediate postoperative period
COMFORT	≥1 month	Yes	Yes	Complicated	Uses physiological and behavioural indicators
NAPI	≥1 month	Yes	Yes	Good reliability	Adapted from CHEOPS
Paediatric objective pain score	≥2 months	Yes	Yes	Simple	Categories are similar
PPP	≥1 year	Yes	Yes	Links care from home to hospital	Pre-assessment of behaviours required

FLACC, Face, Legs, Activity, Cry, Consolability; CHEOPS, Children's Hospital of Eastern Ontario Pain Scale; TPPPS, Toddler–Preschooler Postoperative Pain Scale; NAPI, Nursing Assessment of Pain Intensity; PPP, Paediatric Pain Profile.

Different parameters have been examined, including:

- Pulse rate
- Respiratory rate
- Blood pressure
- Neurochemical and neurohormonal activity
- Palmar sweating
- SaO_2.

There is a debate surrounding the reliability of using physiological signs to determine the presence of pain (Carter 1994). There is in fact insufficient evidence to suggest that physiological signs are directly related to the pain experienced. Like behavioural responses, physiological responses can be affected by many things, resulting in problems of interpretation.

Self-report techniques

As pain is a subjective experience, self-reporting techniques are acknowledged as the most accurate indicators of pain (Broome & Huth 2003); however, they rely on children having the relevant language for their age and development and the ability to describe their pain in an appropriate manner. It must be remembered that a child's self-report of pain may be affected by contextual factors or concerns regarding the pain-relieving interventions that may be offered.

For many years there has been agreement that multidimensional assessment is essential. Stinson et al (2006) suggested that no individual behavioural, self-report or physiological measure is recommended for pain assessment across all children or all contexts. They suggested that healthcare professionals need to make informed choices about which tool to use to assess each individual child's individual pain (Table 44.2, Fig. 44.1). A well-established approach that takes these factors into account is QUESTT (Baker & Wong 1987):

- **Q**uestion the child; ideally prior to a painful episode. Obtain information on past pain experience. Identify specific words used for pain. Identify family's beliefs about pain.
- **U**se pain assessment scales; explain the pain assessment tool to the child. Allow choice of tool.
- **E**valuate behaviour and physiological signs; cry, facial expression, motor response, body posture, activity and appearance. Pulse, blood pressure, respirations, and oxygen saturation.
- **S**ecure the parents' involvement; encourage parental involvement; consider the stressful situation the family may be experiencing.
- **T**ake the cause of pain into account; have knowledge of the child's condition and type and amount of pain that may result.
- **T**ake action and evaluate results; give analgesia, provide distraction, evaluate actions.

Table 44.2   Self-report pain assessment tools

SCALE	APPROPRIATE AGE RANGE (YEARS)	VALIDATED	RELIABLE	USEFULNESS	COMMENTS
Faces	3–8	Yes	Yes	Simple, quick	Can be confused with happiness measure
Visual analogue	≥5	Yes	Yes	Quick, simple, versatile	Requires understanding of concept of proportionality
Numerical rating	≥5	Yes	Yes	Quick, simple	Child needs to be numerate
Poker-chip tool	≥4	Yes	Yes	Simple	Wide age-range
Colour	≥3	Yes	Yes	Exact site of pain described	Fun, engages interest

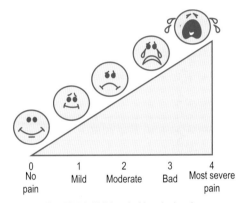

0
No
pain

1
Mild

2
Moderate

3
Bad

4
Most severe
pain

Figure 44.1 Sheffield Children's Hospital pain assessment tool. *(Adapted from Brown and Fisk 1992.)*

MANAGEMENT OF PAIN

Pain has both physical and psychological components and as a result, both physical and psychological methods of pain management can be employed.

NON-DRUG METHODS OF PAIN MANAGEMENT

Psychological interventions for pain include a wide variety of physiological, behavioural and cognitive techniques. These include guided imagery, where the child is encouraged to use positive thoughts and images, e.g. a favourite holiday destination, which has been shown to relieve pain (Duff 2003), and distraction, using interactive toys and games, e.g. pop-up books, music books, blowing bubbles. These techniques can all help to relax the child. Transcutaneous electrical nerve stimulation

(TENS) machines can relieve pain and be useful in reducing conventional analgesic requirements (Merkel et al 1999).

Massage, aromatherapy and reflexology have a role to play in pain management. For further information on these methods, see Chapter 5.

DRUG METHODS OF PAIN CONTROL

Broadly speaking, there are two types of analgesia: centrally acting and peripherally acting. These terms describe their specific sites of action in the nervous system: centrally acting drugs act on the opioid receptors in the brain and spinal cord; peripherally acting drugs inhibit the production of prostaglandins, which sensitise the nerve endings to pain. Analgesics are generally described as either opiates or non-opiates.

ROUTES OF ANALGESIA ADMINISTRATION

Oral

This tends to be the preferred route of analgesia administration in children because of their dislike of needles.

Rectal

This route is useful when children are experiencing nausea and vomiting or are nil by mouth.

Intravenous

Analgesia can be administered via this route as a bolus dose, a continuous infusion, patient-controlled analgesia (PCA) or nurse controlled analgesia (NCA) (see below). Paracetamol (Perfalgan) is also available for intravenous administration.

Intramuscular

This is the least preferred route of analgesia administration, often causing pain and anxiety.

Subcutaneous

The subcutaneous route, through a subcutaneous cannula, can be used as an alternative to intramuscular injections. Analgesia can be administered continuously or as a bolus dose when required.

Topical

The use of a topical local anaesthetic cream, e.g. EMLA or Ametop, or application of a medicated plaster for topical anaesthesia e.g. Rapydan can reduce the pain and discomfort a child may experience during intravenous cannulation or blood sampling.

Local/regional

For postoperative analgesia, blocks – including femoral nerve blocks, lumbar plexus blocks, penile blocks and ilio-inguinal blocks – are performed by the anaesthetist while a child is anaesthetised. Wound infiltration with local anaesthetics is also used for postoperative pain and for procedures in the A&E department. LAT (lidocaine, adrenalin and tetracaine) have been combined in a gel and can be applied as surface anaesthetic to lacerations of the skin. This can be used as an alternative to local anaesthetic wound infiltration prior to suturing of lacerations.

Inhalation

Entonox, for example, is a self-administered inhaled gas that will provide analgesia for procedural pain of short duration (see below).

Intrathecal

This is the instillation of drugs into the sub-arachnoid space to produce an analgesic effect.

Epidural

This is the instillation of drugs into the epidural space (extradural space). A caudal block is an epidural block using a sacral approach.

Transdermal

This is where an analgesic drug is absorbed through the skin, creating a systemic effect. Fentanyl patches are an example of transdermal analgesia.

Transmucosal

Drugs are rapidly absorbed across the mucous membranes. Examples of drugs used via this route are intranasal diamorphine, oral fentanyl (fentanyl lolly).

ANALGESIA

EMLA, Ametop and Rapydan

These are topical local anaesthetics that are used to reduce the pain experienced during blood tests and venous cannulation. When using either EMLA or Ametop, they need to be applied to the skin and then covered with an occlusive dressing. EMLA needs to be applied at least 60 min before the procedure and can be used for children over 1 year of age. Ametop works more quickly, needing to be applied 30–45 min prior to procedure. Ametop can be used with children and infants from 1 month of age upwards. Rapydan is a site-warming topical anaesthetic plaster which can be used in children from age 3 years. Rapydan needs to be applied 30 min prior to procedure.

Paracetamol

Although paracetamol is highly toxic in overdose, it is a safe and effective analgesic when administered in therapeutic doses (Hanson et al 1999). It has antipyretic properties but no demonstrable antiinflammatory activity.

Suboptimal doses of paracetamol have been shown not to provide analgesia postoperatively (Pickering et al 2002). The dose of paracetamol required for analgesia is greater than for an antipyretic effect (Anderson 2004) and the BNF for children 2008 gives clear guidance on appropriate analgesic dosages (BNFC 2008). The guidance includes appropriate loading and maintenance dosages, highlighting the dosages requirements recommended depending on the route of administration.

Ibuprofen and diclofenac

These are non-steroidal antiinflammatory drugs (NSAIDs). They produce an analgesic, antipyretic and antiinflammatory effect. Because of their mechanism of action NSAIDs have the potential to cause adverse effects. Extreme caution should be taken when administering NSAIDs to children who are asthmatic, children with coagulation defect and children with a history of peptic ulcer disease. Use with caution in children with severe eczema, multiple allergies and those with nasal polyps. NSAIDs should be avoided in liver failure. The use of combination therapy with NSAID and/ or paracetamol has been shown to more effectively manage pain.

Opioids

Morphine remains the most widely used and studied opioid in children and can be given by many routes of administration, e.g. oral, i.v., subcutaneous, epidural and rectal.

Some children, although not requiring opiates continually to control pain, may still require one or two doses of opiate during the postoperative period. Opioids are considered safe provided accepted dosing regimens are used and appropriate monitoring and staff education are in place.

Patient-controlled analgesia (PCA) is a method of intravenous analgesia administration, usually of an opioid such as morphine sulphate and is now widely used in children as young as age 5 years. The child controls their own analgesia by means of a hand-held button attached to a computerised pump. Patient selection will depend on the ability of the child to understand the concepts of PCA and the child's capacity to understand the need for pain relief and the mechanism for obtaining it (Gerick 2005). The pump is set up with a suitable dose of analgesia calculated on the child's body weight and age. The pump permits the child to self-administer a small pre-set amount of analgesia by pressing the handset. A maximum dose per hour and a lockout interval is programmed into the pump so that the child cannot overdose, thus ensuring safety. The child is then able to titrate

their own requirements of analgesia in an efficient and safe manner. Some studies have found that the administration of a background (continuous) infusion for the first night following surgery gives the child a better sleep pattern (Doyle et al 1993). The child also has the handset available for breakthrough pain but this continuous infusion seems to 'take the edge off' the pain and lets them sleep comfortably (Fisher 2000).

It is important that all children and parents are given a clear explanation regarding the use of PCA. This information can be given verbally and with the use of parent and child information leaflets (Figs 44.2, 44.3). It should always be stressed that for safety reasons, only the child presses the handset. Parents can encourage their child to press the button when they are sore and younger children need regular reinforcement of the idea to maintain optimal analgesia (Fisher 1999). Parents should never press the button for the child. If the child is unable to comprehend or physically press the handset, nurse-controlled analgesia should be considered. In many centres, PCA pumps have been used to allow the administration of a background infusion with intermittent boluses to be given by nursing staff, i.e. Nurse controlled analgesia (NCA). This allows a pre-set dose of analgesia to be administered safely, which is particularly useful prior to movement or procedural interventions.

Intravenous opioid infusions can be used to provide adequate analgesia with an acceptable level of side-effects. Side-effects include excessive sedation, respiratory depression, nausea, vomiting, pruritus and urinary retention. A child's vital signs should be monitored for complications and the child observed for side-effects. Regular pain assessments are necessary to determine if the morphine is having the desired effect.

Codeine phosphate and dihydrocodeine are oral opioids commonly administered for short-term treatment of moderate pain.

Entonox

Entonox is an analgesic gas composed of nitrous oxide and oxygen in equal proportions. It is an effective inhalation method of managing procedural pain of short duration. The gas is self-administered to the patient using a pressure regulator and demand valve, by using a mouthpiece under the supervision of an appropriately trained healthcare professional. The onset of analgesia is rapid, usually

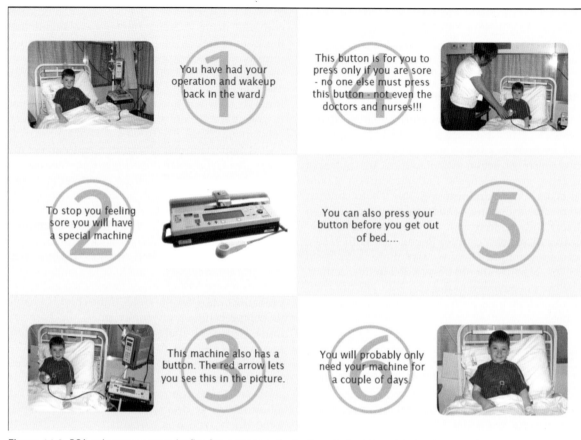

Figure 44.2 PCA pain management leaflet for younger patients. *(From the Royal Hospital for Sick Children in Glasgow, with permission.)*

within 2–3 min and the effects wear off quickly. It can be used alone or with analgesics and has few side-effects and contraindications (BOC 2007).

Entonox has been shown to be useful in several situations. It can be effective in the A&E department for many different procedures including fracture reduction (Gregory et al 1996) and chest drain removal (Bruce et al 2006). Supervision of a child self-administering Entonox can be carried out by a nurse who has received appropriate training. Nursing staff should be aware of the indications for use, the side-effects and contraindications, the administration equipment, the need to scavenge waste gases and the benefits of Entonox for managing procedural pain.

Balanced analgesia

Pain control and prevention can be enhanced by using a multimodal approach, using a combination of analgesics and non-drug methods, tailored to each child's individual needs (Morton 1993). A child using a morphine PCA pump, for example, will have their pain more effectively managed if an NSAID and/or paracetamol are administered. This will reduce the child's opiate requirements and therefore the potential for side-effects, while attacking the pain both centrally and peripherally. Also, the use of local and regional analgesia techniques can significantly reduce the amount of analgesia required postoperatively.

EVALUATION

Record-keeping is a fundamental part of nursing practice (NMC 2004, 2007). It is necessary to evaluate and document the efficacy of any pain-relieving interventions regularly. It is also important to observe that the child is not experiencing side-effects as a result of analgesia administration. It must be remembered that other factors can increase the pain experienced by a child, for example anxiety

What is PCA?

PCA is short for Patient Controlled Analgesia

- You will be able to administer your own pain relief medicine using a hand held button that is connected to a computerised pump

What does the system consist of?

- A syringe filled with a pain relief drug such as morphine this is fitted to the PCA pump
- An infusion line which is attached to the syringe then attached to a small plastic tube in the hand or arm or long line
- A button connected to the PCA pump which may be pressed by yourself when you feel uncomfortable or sore, this tells the pump to deliver a dose of the pain relief medicine

How does the system work?

- The Anaesthetist or the Pain Team will program the pump after discussion with your doctor. The Anaesthetist or pain team will work out a suitable dose for you which takes into account your weight
- The pump programme is not altered without discussion with the Pain Relief Team
- You cannot be overdosed with this medicine, as there is a safety device called a "Lockout" time. This is a period of time after you have received a dose of medicine when the machine will not deliver another dose - even if the button is pressed

- You may have a continuous infusion otherwise known as a background infusion of the pain relief medicine alongside the PCA

Observing you using PCA.

- The nurses on the ward will observe you closely when PCA is being used
- They will check the pump every hour to see how many times you use the pump to make sure that you are using it properly. The nurses will record a pain score on a chart every hour
- The nursing staff will encourage you to press the button and your carer should also encourage you to press the button if you are in discomfort. Nursing staff will contact the Pain Relief Service or Anaesthetist if you feel your pain is not fully controlled as they may need to adjust the amount of morphine which you are receiving
- If you are having regular mouth care carried out or anything that may cause discomfort, the nurses will ask you to press the button 10-15minutes beforehand, so you feel more comfortable during the procedure

You are the only person who should press the button, if you cannot do so or cannot understand the idea of PCA, you should have another form of pain relief.

It will not help you if someone else is pressing the button and may be harmful.

Figure 44.3 Information for adolescents about PCA. *(From the Royal Hospital for Sick Children in Glasgow, with permission.)*

and muscle tension, and this must be taken into account in planning pain-relieving interventions.

SEDATION

Invasive procedures such as lumbar punctures or bone marrow aspirations, the administration of intrathecal drugs or urinary catheterisation, etc. can be extremely distressing for children. It is often suggested that to reduce the distress or anxiety caused by these procedures, children should be sedated. Sedation is defined as 'a drug-induced depression of consciousness during which patients respond purposefully to verbal commands, either alone or accompanied by light tactile stimulation. No interventions are required to maintain a patent airway, and spontaneous ventilation is adequate' (SIGN 2004). Drugs with sedative properties usually do not provide analgesia and the choice of technique or drug should be determined by

considering if the procedure to be undertaken is painful or painless (SIGN 2004).

Studies indicate that few paediatric departments have protocols for the safe and effective sedation of children (Morton & Oomen 1998). The research suggests that available resources rather than scientific evidence influence practice. Non-pharmacological techniques are often not considered and the valuable resource of the play specialist not requested. All sedation techniques are considered to carry some sort of risk (Cote et al 2000). A Scottish guideline has therefore been developed to provide recommendations in the practice of sedation of children who are undergoing diagnostic and therapeutic procedures to minimise this risk (SIGN 2002). This guideline recommends the following principles of good sedation practice:

- A combination of non-pharmacological and pharmacological methods should be considered

- Some children may be unsuitable for sedation and may require general anaesthesia
- An individual approach should be taken for each child to minimise fear, anxiety, distress and pain
- Sedation should only be undertaken in an environment where the facilities, equipment and personnel to manage paediatric emergency situations are immediately available
- It is essential that informed consent be obtained prior to any procedures being undertaken with a clear explanation of the sedation technique proposed and possible adverse effects
- Monitoring should be commenced from the time of administration of the sedative agent until predetermined recovery criteria are met
- Discharge should not be initiated until all predetermined criteria are met.

The sedation of children should not be undertaken lightly. Cote et al (2000) found that children could suffer drug-related adverse outcomes after the administration of a variety of medicines and routes of administration. Every child undergoing sedation should receive an optimal standard of monitoring by experienced paediatric health professionals with facilities and equipment to manage paediatric emergency situations immediately available.

MANAGEMENT OF CHRONIC PAIN

Not all children experience pain continuously. Many children experience recurrent pains, the most common of which are abdominal pain, limb pain and headaches (Eccleston et al 2003).

Chronic or recurrent pain can be debilitating for both the child and family as it leads to a general reduction in activity, which in turn affects school attendance, participation in sports and leisure activities, resulting in loss of social contacts and isolation. The pain can result in lack of sleep, affecting concentration and schoolwork. All these factors eventually alter attitude and mood, creating a downward spiral of the child's confidence and self-esteem. Chronic pain assessment should follow the same decision-making processes from the nurse as the assessment of acute pain. Few validated pain assessment tools are available for the assessment of chronic pain in children, although it has been recognised that the paediatric chronic pain management centres in the UK have

developed local tools to aid the assessment process (Aitkenhead 2001).

History taking is vital and a thorough background report to the pain, including the following, should be undertaken:

- Pain details: When did the pain begin? Where is the pain? Is it present all the time? Can you get to sleep at night? Does the pain wake you up?
- Words to describe the pain (this is particularly helpful in the identification of neuropathic pain).
- How does the pain affect your life?
- What medications have helped or not helped (helpful in identifying non-opioid responsive pain).
- Is there anything else that helps the pain (non-pharmacological strategies)?
- Any trigger points?
- A drawing of the pain.

Whether or not an identifiable organic cause is found, children experiencing chronic or recurrent pain require specialised help and support to enable them to cope.

It has long been recognised that the management of chronic pain in adults benefits from a multidisciplinary approach, involving physiotherapy, psychological techniques and medication (Bonica 1953). This approach was first applied to the care of children experiencing chronic or recurrent pain in the late 1980s (Berde et al 1989), but many other paediatric centres are now developing this approach.

Whether a child is an in-patient or is being seen as an out-patient, it is important that the professionals work collaboratively through the use of an interdisciplinary model. This is where the child sees the professionals together in both the assessment and treatment process rather than being sent from professional to professional.

Due to the complex nature of chronic pain, a variety of treatments are often required which may include the following:

Physiotherapy

- General exercise programmes, stretching, relaxation and massage as part of an individual programme
- Advice regarding 'pacing' and graduated regaining of functional activities
- Transcutaneous electrical nerve stimulation and other methods such as ultrasound therapy may be used.

Psychology

- Hypnosis/guided imagery and relaxation to control anxiety and help reduce pain
- Cognitive-behavioural techniques to modify pain-related attitude and behaviour patterns
- Individual or family therapy.

Medicines

- Various types of analgesia
- Sedatives
- Antidepressants
- Anticonvulsants
- Regional or local nerve blocks.

Children experiencing chronic or recurrent pain and their families often present with a variety of medical, social and psychological difficulties. It is this variety of problems that creates a challenge for the professionals, demonstrating the need for a multidisciplinary approach.

SUMMARY OF PAIN ASSESSMENT COMPLICATIONS

- There may not be consistent behavioural and physiological changes in all infants and children experiencing pain.
- Many factors, including distress, can affect both behaviour and the physiological signs used to assess pain.
- It is difficult to distinguish between stress and pain, particularly in the infant or neonate.
- The ability to self-report depends on the cognitive ability and language skills of a child and may be affected by clinical condition, drugs or mechanical interventions.
- Children may report lower pain intensity than they are experiencing for fear of the consequences.
- A child's pain can be affected by previous pain experiences, cultural and social expectations and levels of anxiety.
- As nurses, our own experiences of pain and our preconceived ideas about how much an injury or certain type of surgery should hurt may affect our interpretation of a situation.

COMMUNITY PERSPECTIVE

Parents are likely to be more 'tuned in' to their child in pain than professionals. However, there will be times when parents lose their objectivity about this, especially during terminal care. Denying the level of pain may be a coping strategy for a parent but this takes away the rights of the child.

The role of the CCN is to be aware of the dynamics within the family and sensitively to lead the parents to a more objective assessment. For this to be possible, the family must have developed trust in the CCN and, when appropriate, other members of the team. Once their cooperation has been gained in titrating analgesia and they are able to recognise that the child is more settled and possibly able to participate in family life, a hurdle will have been surmounted, the child's pain will be better managed and the relationship between family and nurses strengthened.

Each individual case will need consideration as to whether the use of pain scales will be helpful. Although it may be appropriate to use them in an acute pain situation, for example the child with a fractured femur, it may be less so for the terminally ill child. Ongoing assessment of pain, however, is essential, whether this is undertaken using pain scales or as an ongoing assessment as part and parcel of family life. The preference of the child must be valued.

For the child with communication difficulties, the parents are almost without exception those who recognise when their child is in pain. The Pediatric Pain Profile is a validated and reliable behavioural pain assessment tool which is useful in linking care from home to hospital. It requires a thorough pre-assessment of pain behaviours but ensures specific pain behaviours are documented and the child's pain can then be more accurately assessed and treated in hospital. The role of the CCN here is to listen and learn from the parents and take action accordingly.

DOS AND DON'TS

- Do involve the parents and, more importantly, the child.
- Do take into account the child's age, clinical condition, type of pain, and any special needs or mechanical interventions.
- Do use a multidimensional pain assessment scale where possible.
- Do evaluate any pain-relief strategies.

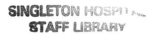

- Do consider the use of non-pharmacological pain-relieving strategies, either individually or in conjunction with pharmacological strategies.
- Do not let your own beliefs and values cloud your judgement when assessing pain.
- Do not let the common myths and misconceptions surrounding pain in children affect your assessment strategies.
- Do not be led to believe that:
  - Babies and infants do not feel pain
  - Children do not remember pain
  - Children who are playing or sleeping cannot be in pain
  - Children always tell the truth about their pain.

Remember that pain is a subjective experience, which is not solely dependent on the amount of tissue damage involved. It can be affected by many things which should be reflected in our assessment strategies and choice of assessment scales.

References

Aitkenhead, S., 2001. Managing chronic pain in children. Nurs. Times 97 (29), 34–35.

Anderson, B.J., 2004. Comparing the efficacy of NSAIDs and paracetamol in children. Paediatr. Anaesth. 14, 201–217.

Audit Commission, 1993. Children first: a study of hospital services. HMSO, London.

Baker, C., Wong, D., 1987. QUESTT: a process of pain assessment in children. Orthop. Nurs. 6 (1), 11–21.

Bates, M.S., 1987. Ethnicity and pain: a biocultural model. Soc. Sci. Med. 24 (1), 47–50.

Berde, C.B., Sethna, N.F., Maset, B., et al., 1989. Paediatric pain clinics: recommendations for their development. Paediatrician 16, 94–102.

Bernstein, B.A., Pachter, L.M., 2003. Cultural considerations in children's pain. In: Schechter, N.L., Berde, C.B., Yaster, M. (Eds.), Pain in infants, children and adolescents, second ed. Lippincott, Williams and Wilkins, Philadelphia.

Bonica, J.J., 1953. The management of pain. Lea and Febiger, Philadelphia.

BOC British Oxygen Company, 2007. Entonox controlled pain relief. Reference Guide 206690. BOC Medical, Manchester.

British National Formulary for children, 2008. Royal Pharmaceutical Society of Great Britain, London.

Broome, M.E., Huth, M.M., 2003. Nursing management of the child in pain. In: Schechter, N.L., Berde, C.B., Yester, M. (Eds.), Pain in infants, children and adolescents, second ed. Lippincott, Williams and Wilkins, Philadelphia.

Brown, T.C.K., Fisk, G.C., 1992. Anaesthesia for children. second ed. Blackwell Scientific, Oxford, p. 129.

Bruce, E., Franck, L., Howard, R.F., 2006. The efficacy of morphine and Entonox analgesia during chest drain removal in children. Pediatric Anesthesia 16, 302–308.

Carter, B., 1994. Child and infant pain. Chapman and Hall, London.

Carter, B., McArthur, E., Cunliffe, M., 2002. Dealing with uncertainty: parental assessment of pain in their children with profound special needs. J. Adv. Nurs. 38 (5), 449–457.

Cote, C.J., Karl, H.W., Notterman, D.A., et al., 2000. Adverse sedation events in pediatrics: analysis of medications used for sedation. Pediatrics 106, 633–644.

DoH Department of Health, 2003. Getting the right start. National Service Framework for children: standard for hospital services. DoH, London.

Doyle, E., Robinson, D., Morton, N.S., 1993. Comparison of patient controlled analgesia with and without a background infusion after lower abdominal surgery in children. Br. J. Anaesth. 71 (5), 670–673.

Duff, A.J.A., 2003. Incorporating psychological approaches into routine paediatric venepuncture. Arch. Dis. Child. 88, 931–937.

Eccleston, C., Malleson, P.N., Clinch, J., et al., 2003. Chronic pain in adolescents: evaluation of a programme of interdisciplinary cognitive behaviour therapy. Arch. Dis. Child. 88, 881–885.

Finley, G.A., Frank, L., Gruana, R., et al., 2005. Why children's pain matters. IASP, Seattle.

Fisher, S., 1999. Small relief. Nurs. Times 95 (23), 52–53.

Fisher, S., 2000. Postoperative pain management in paediatrics. Br. J. Perioper. Nurs. 10 (1), 80–84.

Gaffney, A., McGrath, P.J., Dick, B., 2003. Measuring pain in children: developmental and instrument issues. In: Schechter, N.L., Berde, C.B., Yaster, M. (Eds.), Pain in infants, children and adolescents. second ed. Lippincott, Williams and Wilkins, Philadelphia.

Gerick, S.M., 2005. Pain management in children: developmental considerations and mind-body therapies. South Med. J. 98, 295–302.

Ghai, B., Makkar, J.K., Wig, J., 2008. Postoperative pain assessment in preverbal children and children with cognitive impairment. Pediatr. Anaesth. 18, 462–477.

Gregory, P.R., Sullivan, J.A., 1996. Nitrous oxide compared with intravenous regional anaesthesia in paediatric forearm fracture manipulation. J. Paediatr. Orthop. 16 (2), 187–191.

Goddard, J.M., Pickup, S.E., 1996. Postoperative pain in children: combining audit and a nurse specialist to improve management. Anaesthesia 51, 588–590.

Hanson, T.G., O'Brien, K., Morton, N.S., et al., 1999. Plasma paracetamol concentrations and pharmacokinetics following rectal administration in neonates and young infants. Acta Anaesthesiol. Scand. 43 (8), 855–859.

Harbeck, C., Peterson, L., 1992. Elephants dancing in my head: a developmental approach to children's concepts of specific pains. Child Dev. 63 (1), 138–149.

Hodgkinson, K., Bear, M., Thorn, J., et al., 1994. Measuring pain in neonates: evaluating an instrument and developing a common language. Aust. J. Adv. Nurs. 12, 17–22.

Howard, R., 2003. Current status of pain management in children. J. Am. Med. Assoc. 290, 2464–2469.

Krechel, S.W., Bildner, J., 1995. CRIES: a new neonatal postoperative pain measurement score. Initial testing of validity and reliability. Paediatr. Anaesth. 5, 53–61.

Liossi, C., 2002. Procedure-related cancer pain in children. Radcliffe Medical Press, Abingdon.

Malviya, S., Voepel-Lewis, T., Burke, C., et al., 2006. The revised FLACC observational pain tool: Improved reliability and validity for pain assessment in children with cognitive impairment. Paediatr. Anaesth. 16, 258–265.

Merkel, S.I., Gustein, H.B., Malviya, S., 1999. Use of

transcutaneous electrical nerve stimulation in a young child with pain from open perineal lesions. J. Pain Symptom Manage. 18 (5), 376–381.

Morton, N.S., 1993. Development of a monitoring protocol for the safe use of opioids in children. Paediatr. Anaesth. 3, 179–184.

Morton, N.S., Oomen, G.J., 1998. Development of a selection and monitoring protocol for safe sedation of children. Paediatr. Anaesth. 8, 65–68.

Nikanne, E., Kokki, H., Tuovinen, K., 1999. Postoperative pain after adenoidectomy in children. Br. J. Anaesth. 82, 886–889.

NMC Nursing and Midwifery Council, 2004. Guidelines for records and record-keeping. NMC, London.

NMC Nursing and Midwifery Council, 2007. Record keeping and the law. NMC, London.

Pickering, A.E., Bridge, H.S., Nolan, J., et al., 2002. Double-blind, placebo controlled analgesic study of ibuprofen or rofecoxib in combination with paracetamol for tonsillectomy in children. Br. J. Anaesth. 88 (1), 72–77.

Reaney, R., 2007. Assessing pain in children. Anaesth. Intensive Care Med. 8.5, 180–183.

Romsing, J., Hertel, S., Moller-Sonnergaard, J., et al., 1996. Postoperative pain in children: comparison between ratings of children and nurses. J. Pain Symptom Manage. 11 (2), 42–46.

RCN Royal College of Nursing, Clinical practice guidelines. 1999. The recognition and assessment of acute pain in children: recommendations. RCN, London.

RCN Royal College of Nursing, Clinical practice guidelines. 2001. The recognition and assessment of acute pain in children: implementation guide. RCN, London.

Royal College of Surgeons and the College of Anaesthetists, Commission on the provision of surgical services. 1990. Report of the working party on pain after surgery. Royal College of Surgeons, London.

Salantera, S., Lauri, S., Salmi, T., et al., 1999. Nurses' knowledge about pharmacological and non pharmacological pain management. J. Pain Sympton Manage. 18 (4), 289–299.

Savedra, M.C., Holzemer, W.L., Tesler, M.D., et al., 1993. Assessment of postoperation pain in children and adolescents using the adolescent pediatric pain tool. Nurs. Res. 42 (1), 5–9.

Schechter, N.L., Berde, C.B., Yaster, M., 2003. Pain in infants, children and adolescents, second ed. Lippincott, Williams and Wilkins, Philadelphia.

SIGN Scottish Intercollegiate Guidelines Network, 2002. Safe sedation of children undergoing diagnostic and therapeutic procedures. SIGN, Edinburgh.

SIGN Scottish Intercollegiate Guidelines Network, Safe sedation of children undergoing diagnostic and therapeutic procedures. 2004. Quick reference guide. SIGN, Edinburgh.

Sparshott, M., 1996. The development of a clinical distress scale for ventilated infants: identification of pain and distress based on validated behavioural scores. J. Neonatal Nurs. 2, 5–11.

Stallard, P., Williams, L., Lenton, S., et al., 2001. Pain in cognitively impaired, non-communicating children. Arch. Dis. Child. 85 (6), 460–462.

Stevens, B., Johnston, C., Petryshen, P., et al., 1996. Premature infant pain profile (PIPP): development and initial validation. Clin. J. Pain 12, 13–22.

Stinson, J.N., McGrath, P., 2007. No pain – all gain. Advocating for improved paediatric pain management. Paediatric Child Health 12 (2), 93–94.

Treadwell, M.J., Frank, L.S., Vichinsky, E., 2002. Using quality improvement strategies to enhance pediatric pain assessment. Int. J. Qual. Health Care 14 (1), 39–47.

Van Hulle, V.C., 2005. Nurses' knowledge attitudes and practices regarding children's pain. MCN Am. J. Matern Child Nurs. 30 (3), 177–183.

Voepel-Lewis, T., Merkel, S., Tait, A.R., et al., 2002. The reliability and validity of the face, legs, activity, cry, consolability observational tool as a measure of pain in children with cognitive impairment. Anaesth. Analg. 95 (5), 1224–1229.

Wilson, G.A.M., Doyle, E., 1996. Validation of three paediatric pain scores for use by parents. Anaesthesia 51, 1005–1007.

Further reading

Ambuel, B., Hamlett, K.W., Marx, C.M., et al., 1992. Assessing distress in pediatric intensive care environments. The COMFORT scale. J. Pediatr. Psychol. 17, 95–109.

Campo, J.V., Comer, D.M., Jansen-McWilliams, L., et al., 2002. Recurrent pain, emotional distress, and health service use in childhood. J. Pediatr. 141 (1), 76–83.

Currie, J.M., 2006. Management of chronic pain in children. Arch. Dis. Child. Educ. Pract. 91, 111–114.

Harrison, A., 1991. Assessing patients' pain: identifying reasons for error. J. Adv. Nurs. 16, 1018–1025.

Kashikar-Zuck, S., Goldschneider, K.R., Powers, S.W., et al., 2001. Depression and functional disability in chronic pediatric pain. Clin. J. Pain 17 (4), 341–349.

Lawrence, J., Alcock, D., McGrath, P., et al., 1993. The development of a tool to assess neonatal pain. Neonatal Netw. 12, 59–65.

McGrath, P.A., Seifert, C.E., Speechley, K.N., et al., 1996. A new analogue scale for assessing children's pain – an initial validation study. Pain 64, 435–443.

In: Morton, N.S. (Ed.), 1998. Acute paediatric pain management: a practical guide. W B Saunders, London.

Munro, F.J., Fisher, S., Dickson, U., et al., 2002. The addition of antiemetics to the morphine solution in patient controlled analgesia syringes used by children after an appendicectomy does not reduce the incidence of postoperative nausea and vomiting. Paediatr. Anaesth. 12 (7), 600–603.

Pickup, S., Pagdin, J., 2000. Procedural pain: Entonox can help. Paediatr. Nurs. 12 (10), 33–36.

Royal College of Paediatrics and Child Health, 2003. Medicines for children. RCPCH Publications, London.

Sethna, N.F., Verghese, S.T., Hannallah, R.S., et al., 2005. A randomized controlled trial to evaluate S-Caine patch for reducing pain associated with vascular access in children. Anesthesiology 102, 403–408.

Stinson, J.N., Kavanagh, T., Yamada, et al., 2006. Systematic review of the psychometric properties, interpretability and feasibility of self-report pain intensity measures for use in clinical trials in children and adolescents. Pain 125, 143–157.

Sury, M.R., Hatch, D.J., Deeley, T., et al., 1999. Development of a nurse-led sedation service for paediatric magnetic resonance imaging. Lancet 353, 1667–1671.

Tarbell, S.E., Cohen, I.T., Marsh, J.L., 1992. The toddler-pre-school postoperative pain scale: an observational scale for measuring postoperative pain in children aged 1–5. Preliminary report. Pain 50, 273–280.

Walters, A.S., Williamson, G.M., 1999. The role of activity restriction in the association between pain and depression: a study of pediatric patients with chronic pain. Child. Health Care 28 (1), 33–50.

Wattenmaker, I., Kasser, J.R., McGravey, A., 1990. Self-administered nitrous oxide for fracture reduction in an emergency room setting. J. Orthop. Trauma 4 (1), 35–38.

Index

Notes: Page numbers followed by f refers to figures; t refers tables and b refers boxes.

A

ABC approach, 187
  assessment, 68–69
ABCDE, anaphylaxis treatment, 434
Abdominal examination, 76
Above-elbow casts, 202, 203f
Above-knee casts, 203, 203f
Abrasions, hand hygiene, 46–47
Absence seizures, 260
Academic programmes,
    accountability, 7
Accidents
  cardiopulmonary resuscitation, 94
  central line removal, 160
Accountability, 6–8
  academic programmes, 7
  community nursing, 7–8
  National Service Framework, 7
  Nursing and Midwifery Council,
    6–7
  Nursing and Midwifery Council's
    Guide for Students, 6
Accu-Check Advantage blood glucose
    meter, 369, 370, 371f
Action for Sick Children, day-care
    surgery, 229
Active listening, communication, 25
Acute compartment syndrome, 306
Acute infections, neonatal seizures,
    258
Acutely sick children, positioning,
    217–218
Acute wounds, 354
Additional needs children,
    communication, 30

Adelaide Scale, 183
Adolescents
  hygiene, 112
  pain assessment, 457
  patient-controlled analgesia, 463f
  physical examination, 71
  seizures, 259
  stoma, 267
  traction, 303
Adrenaline, paediatric life support,
    101
Advanced Life Support Group, coma
    scales, 183, 185t
Advanced paediatric life support, 98
Advocacy, 8–10
  The NHS Plan, 8, 9
AeroChamber, tracheostomies, 297
Aerosol inhalers, 438, 439t
Age
  assessment, 70–71
  infants *see* Infant(s)
  pressure area care, 237
  see also Adolescents; Babies; Infant
    (s); Premature babies
Age-appropriate preoperative care, 231
Agenda for Change, 5
Air-borne transmission, 44
Air embolism, central lines, 160
Air enemas, radiography, 245–246
Airway distress, tracheostomies, 285
Airway maintenance, 98–100
  basic paediatric life support, 96–97
  endotracheal intubation, 99–100
  equipment, 98
  method, 98–100
  radiography, 244

Alcohol hand-rubs, 46–47, 332
Alginate wound dressings, 362t
Allergies
  aromatherapy, 60–61
  occupational health, 53
  weaning, 385
  see also Anaphylaxis
Ametop, 460
Amiodarone, 101
Amoebic dysentery, 348
Anaemia, wound healing, 357
Anaesthesia
  general, radiography, 244–245
  local *see* Local anaesthetics
  postoperative care, 223
Anaesthetic lubricants, urethral
    catheterisation, 311
Anaesthetics, topical *see* Topical
    anaesthetics
Analgesia, 459–464
  administration routes, 459–460
    see also specific routes
  balanced, 462
  chronic pain management,
    465
  evaluation, 462–463
  postoperative care, 225
  traction, 304
  see also specific analgesic drugs
Anaphylaxis, 434–436
  incidence, 434
  recognition, 434
  signs and symptoms, 434b
  treatment, 434, 435f
Angiography, 249
Antegrade continence stoma, 266

Antibiotics/antimicrobials, specimen collection, 345, 351
Anticonvulsant drugs
epilepsy, 259
rectal administration, 260–261, 262
Antipyretic drugs, 282
ANTT *see* Aseptic non-touch techniques (ANTT)
Appearance, communication, 25
Appointments, adolescents, 128
Aromatherapy, 60–61
Arteries, anatomy, 321
Artificial feeding, 380–384
casein dominant feeds, 381*t*
follow-on formula, 381, 381*t*
hand washing, 383
parental choice, 381
preparation of, 382
supplements, 381
whey dominant feeds, 381, 381*t*
see also Bottle-feeding
Aseptic fields, 332–333
Aseptic non-touch techniques (ANTT), 327–336, 330*f*, 333–334
aseptic fields, 332–333
audit cycle, 330
community nursing, 334
complications, 334–335
definition, 330
diagnosis-independence, 330–331
environmental/air contamination, 332
equipment, 333–334
gloves, 332
intravenous care, 330
observations, 334–335
risk assessment, 333–334
stages, 333–334, 333*f*, 334*b*
terminology, 330, 331*b*
venepuncture, 333
see also Hand washing
Aseptic techniques, 331
chest drain removal, 168
wound drain removal, 253
Assessment, 65–80
age-specific approaches, 70–71
community nursing, 78
complications, 78
ear care, 117
eye care, 116–117
growth information, 76–77
models, 68
nutrition information, 76–77
objective information *see* Physical examination
observation *see* Physical examination
physical examination *see* Physical examination

pressure area care, 235
radiography, 243
rationale, 68
subjective information (history), 69
treatment options, 77
wound care, 357–365, 359*f*
Ataxic children, 219
Athetoid children, 219
Atonic seizures, 260
Atopic eczema, 134–135
emollients, 134
lichenification, 135
pimecrolimus, 135
Staphylococcus aureus, 135
tacrolimus, 135
Atropine, 101
Auditing practice
aseptic non-touch techniques, 330
infection control, 53
Auscultation
cardiovascular examination, 73
physical examination, 72
Autolytic wound debridement, 358*t*
Automatic electrical defibrillators (AEDs), 101
Autonomy, adolescents, 28
AVPU scales, neurological examination, 74

B

Babies
body temperature maintenance, 171
breastfeeding support, 377, 377*f*
hygiene *see* Hygiene
stoma, 266–267
Baby baths, 108
contact and interaction, 108
equipment, 109
full-term infants, 107–108
methods, 109–110
top and tail wash, 108
Baby rooting, breastfeeding, 378, 378*f*
Baby toothbrushes, 115
Backache, lumbar puncture, 177–178
'Back to Sleep' campaign, 212
Bacterial infections, urethral catheterization, 314
Bag specimens, urine collection, 310, 349
Balanced analgesia, 462
Balanced traction, 300
Balloon changing, gastrostomy tubes, 394
Balloon water changing, gastrostomy tubes, 394–395
Baptism, 85–86
Barium contrast enemas, 245

Barium meals, 245
Barium studies, 245
Basic paediatric life support, 96–98
airway opening, 96–97
method, 96–97
pulse, 97, 97*f*
Bathing
babies *see* Baby baths
bed baths *see* Bed baths
bottle-feeding, 296
casts, 206–207
fragile skin, 137
psoriasis, 136
skin fragility, 137
wound care, 360–361
Bed baths
hygiene, 112–114
older children, 112
parental involvement, 112
Bedpans, casts, 206
Behavioural problems, radiography, 244
Below-elbow casts, 202, 202*f*
Below-knee casts, 202, 203*f*
Benzodiazepines, 259
Bereavement care, 81–93
community nursing, 91
complications, 90–92
coroner referrals, 84*b*
equipment needed, 87–88
expected deaths, 82–83
guidelines, 87–92
home deaths, 82
informed people, 90*t*
long-term care, 87
observations, 90
organ donation *see* Organ donation
organ retention, 83–84
other family members, 82–83
parents, 87
non-presence at death, 83–85
photographs, 88
postmortem *see* Postmortems
religious views, 85–87, 86*b*
Christian families, 85–86
Hindu families, 86
Jewish families, 86
Muslim families, 86
organ donation, 85
Sikh families, 86–87
under resuscitation, 83
staff, 87
Best practice guidelines, wound care, 361*b*
Bilirubin, 196
conjugated, 196
unconjugated, 196
Biofilms, 43

Biological wound debridement, 358t
Biopsy material, 352
Birth trauma, neonatal seizures, 258
Bisacodyl (Dulco-lax), 146
Bivona tracheostomy tubes, 288
Bladder irrigation, urethral
        catheterisation, 316–317
Blood
    clotting see Blood clotting
    glucose measurement see Blood
        glucose measurement
    samples see Blood samples
    spillages, 346
    storage, 404
    transfusions see Blood transfusions
Blood borne transmission, 44
Blood clotting, 355–356
    platelets, 408
Blood donation, 405
Blood flow, intravenous cannulation,
        324
Blood glucose measurement, 367–373
    Accu-Check Advantage blood
        glucose meter, 369, 370, 371f
    blood sample, 371, 372f
    complications, 372
    education, 370–373
    equipment, 370
    guidelines, 370
    method, 370–372
    observations, 372
    parenteral nutrition, 410
Blood pressure cuffs, 74, 74f
Blood pressure measurement
    cardiovascular examination, 73–74
    neurological assessment, 188
Blood samples
    blood glucose estimation, 371, 372f
    specimen collection, 350
Blood transfusions, 404–408
    blood storage, 404
    blood warmers, 405
    compatibility, 405, 405t
    complications, 406–408
    discontinuation, 407–408
    donation, 405
    equipment, 405–406
    explanations, 410
    filters, 406
    leucodepletion, 405–406
    microaggregate filters, 406
    observations, 406–408
    packed cell, 404
    reactions to, 407t
    religious objections, 405
    screening, 405
    temperature recording, 406
    time taken, 405

variant Creutzfeldt–Jakob disease,
        405–406
    washed red cells, 404
    whole blood, 404
Blood warmers, blood transfusions,
        405
Body fluid distribution, intravenous
        therapy, 402
Body mass index (BMI), 77
Body surface area, intravenous
        therapy, 402
Body temperature
    control see below
    daily fluctuation, 281
Body temperature control, 280–283
    babies, 171
    community nursing, 282
    complications, 282
    environmental interventions, 282
    hypothalamus, 280
    observations, 282
    pharmacological intervention, 282
    pre-term infant, 171
Body temperature taking/recording,
        281
    blood transfusions, 406
    neurological assessment, 188
    parenteral nutrition, 410
    phototherapy, 197
    physical examination, 75–76
Body/trunk box, oxygen therapy, 447,
        448–449
Body weight
    intravenous therapy, 402
    pressure area care, 235
Bolus drug administration, central
        lines, 155–156
Bolus feeds, enteral feeding,
        396–397
Bone scans, nuclear medicine, 247
Bottle changing, chest drainage,
        168
Bottle-feeding, 382–384
    baby position, 383
    complications, 384
    observations, 384
    tracheostomies, 296
Bowel care, 139–151
    evidence-based care, 143
    growth/development issues,
        142–143
    nursing practice, 145
    psychosocial issues, 143
    rationale, 142
    terminology, 142
Bowel movements, 141, 143–144
    changes in, 144
    children, 144
    daily frequency, 142

developmental delay, 144
    infants, 143
    see also Constipation; Diarrhoea
Braden Q Scale, pressure area care,
        237
Bradycardia, suctioning, 278
Brain stem herniation, lumbar
        puncture, 177
Breakage, central lines, 160–161
Breastfeeding, 375–380
    advantages, 375b
    baby position, 377, 377f
    baby rooting, 378, 378f
    baby support, 377, 377f
    complications/difficulties,
        378–379
    elimination, 380
    emotional bonding, 378
    frequency, 376
    good infant attachment, 378, 378f
    help with, 380
    HIV-positive mothers, 380
    length of, 376
    lying, 376f
    malnourished mother, 380
    mother's comfort, 376, 378
    observations, 378
    premature cessation, 375b
    sitting, 376f
    stress, 378
Breast milk, 375–376
    expression of, 379–380
    pasteurization, 380
    storage, 380
Breast milk jaundice, 196
Breathing
    play, 126
    problems, positioning, 218
British Medical Association (BMA),
        parental responsibilities, 12
Broomstick casts, 203, 204f
Broviac line, 153
Bubbles, play, 125
Buccal administration, 261
Burns frame, 301

C

Candida albicans infection (thrush), 133
Cardiac arrest
    cardiopulmonary resuscitation,
        94–95
    definition, 96
Cardiac pacemakers, magnetic
        resonance imaging, 246
Cardiopulmonary arrest
    respiratory infections, 95
    sepsis, 95

Cardiopulmonary resuscitation (CPR), 94–103
 accidents, 94
 adults *vs.*, 95
 cardiac arrest, 94–95
 chest compression, 95
 ventricular fibrillation, 96
 ventricular tachycardia, 96
 see also Paediatric life support
Cardiovascular examination, 73–74
 auscultation, 73
 blood pressure recording, 73–74
 inspection, 73
 normal blood pressure, 74*t*
 normal heart rates, 73, 73*t*
 palpation (pulse), 73, 73*t*
Cardiovascular system, chest drainage, 167
Care coordination, community children's nursing, 35–36
Care Coordination UK (CCNUK), 35
Carers
 cast application, 202
 community care nursing, 36
 moving and handling, 212–213
Caring for Children in the Health Service, day-care surgery, 229
Carrier oils, 60–61
Car seats, tracheostomies, 297
Casein dominant feeds, 381*t*
Casts, 200–210
 application, 204–206
 casting materials, 201–202
  see also specific materials
 clothing, 207
 community nursing, 208
 complications, 205–206
 drinking, 207
 eating, 207
 family, effects on, 202
 hygiene, 206–207
 mobility, 207
 multidisciplinary team, 203–204
 positioning, 207
 rationale, 200
 removal, 207–209
 safety, 207
 skin care, 206–207
 sleeping, 207
 types, 202–203
  see also specific types
Cast saws, 208
Catheter(s)
 blockages, 316
 care, 314–315
 material, 313
 misplacement, 160
 suctioning, 275

tracheostomy suction, 289
 urine specimens, 349
Centralised intravenous additives service, 426
Central lines, 152–162, 248
 accidental removal, 160
 air embolism, 160
 bolus drug administration, 155–156
 breakage, 160–161
 catheter misplacement, 160
 central venous line exit care, 158–159
 community nursing, 161
 complications, 159–161, 160*t*
  see also specific complications
 connecting/changing infusion set, 156
 dressings, 158, 159–161
 drug administration, 155
 heparinisation, 155
 implanted ports *see* Implanted ports
 infections, 159
 Luer lock changing, 155
 non-tunnelled long line, 154
 occlusions, 160
 parenteral nutrition, 409
 peripherally inserted central catheters, 154
 septicaemia, 159, 350
 superior vena cava syndrome, 160
 tunnelled, 153, 153*f*
 types, 153*t*
  see also specific types
 uses, 152–153
 venous tunnelled, 153
Central nervous system (CNS), positioning, 218
Central venous lines (CVL)
 exit care, 158–159
 radiographic guidance, 248
Cerebrospinal fluid (CSF)
 lumbar puncture, 178
 specimen collection, 352
Cerumen (ear wax), 117
Chain of infection, infection control, 43–44
Chaperones, urethral catheterisation, 314
Chemotherapy, 430–431
 infection risk factors, 45*t*
CHEOPS (Childrens Hospital of Eastern Ontario Pain Scale), 458*t*
Chest, anatomy, 164
Chest compression, cardiopulmonary resuscitation, 95
Chest drainage, 163–169
 bottle changing, 168
 cardiovascular system care, 167

chest drain, 165
 clamping, 168–169
 complications, 166
 drain removal, 168
 equipment care, 167–168
 method, 166
 'milking,' 168
 observation, 166
 pathophysiology, 164
 respiratory system care, 166–167
 systems, 165, 165*f*
 underwater seal system, 165*f*
Child abuse, 16
Child Accident Prevention Trust (CAPT), 109
Child Adolescent Mental Health (CAMH), 68, 69
Child Growth Foundation, 76–77
Children
 bed baths, 112
 bowel movements, 144
 hygiene, 112–118
 neurological assessment, 186–187
 oral medication, 424
 seizures, 258
 stoma, 267
Children (Scotland) Act (1995), 10
The Children Act England and Wales (1989)
 consent, 10
 moving and handling, 213
 restraint guidelines, 29
Children First: A Study of Hospital Services
 pain management, 455
 preoperative care, 230–231
Chinese herbalists, 58
Chlamydia infection
 eye swabs, 346
 vaginal swabs, 350
Christianity, bereavement care, 85–86
Chronic conditions, positioning, 218
Chronic pain management, 464–466
Chronic wounds, 354
Circulation
 casts, 205
 problems, traction, 306
Circulatory overload, blood transfusions, 407*t*
Clamping, chest drainage, 168–169
Clean-catch techniques, urine collection, 310, 349
Clean contaminated wounds, 252
Cleaning
 curtains, 341
 infection control, 51–52
 mop heads, 341
 solutions, central line care, 155, 158
Clean wounds, 252

Clinical audits, pressure area care, 238
Clinical effectiveness, pressure area care, 238
Clinical governance, 12–15, 18
  Information Focus, 12–13
  Leadership, 12–13
  National Service Framework, 13
  Patient Focus, 12–13
  pressure area care, 238
  Quality Improvement, 12–13
  Staff Focus, 12–13
Clinical waste, isolation nursing, 340
Closed appliances, stoma, 269*f*
Closed questions, 23
Clostridium difficile, 338
Clothes/clothing
  babies, 173
  casts, 207
  magnetic resonance imaging, 247
  preoperative care, 232
Coal tar preparations, psoriasis, 136
Coconut oils, skin care, 132
Codeine phosphate, 461
Collection pads, urine collection, 310
Colostomy, stoma, 265
Colour-coding, waste disposal, 50*t*
Coma scales, neurological assessment, 183
Comforters, preoperative care, 231
COMFORT, pain assessment, 458*t*
Commando crawling, casts, 207
Common Assessment Framework, 36
Communication, 22–31
  additional need children, 30
  adverse factors, 29
  breakdown of, 29–30
  casts/casting, 200
  child's ability, 25–28
  community children's nursing, 35
  creative, 28
  Essential Care Clusters, 22
  hygiene, 105
  isolation nursing, 341
  lumbar puncture procedure, 176
  non-verbal *see* Non-verbal communication
  parents, 23
  play, 28, 28*t*
  puberty, 28
  question types, 23–24, 24*b*
  radiography, 243
  risk management, 14
  stage 1 (sensory motor child (birth to 2 years)), 26–27, 26*t*
  stage 2 (pre-operational child (2-7 years)), 26*t*, 27
  stage 3 (concrete operational child (7-11 years)), 26*t*, 27

stage 4 (formal operational child (11-18)), 26*t*, 27–28
  verbal *see* Verbal communication
Community children's nursing (CCN), 32–40
  accountability, 7–8
  aseptic non-touch techniques, 334
  assessment, 78
  bereavement care, 91
  care coordination, 35–36
  casts, 208
  central lines, 161
  challenges, 36–37
  communication, 35
  constipation, 148
  continuing care, 35–36
  disabilities, 32–33
  enteral feeding, 398
  family partnership, 35
  future work, 38–39
  gastrostomy tubes, 399
  hospital–home transition, 34
  hygiene, 118
  interpersonal skills, 34
  intravenous cannulation, 325
  isolation, 8
  medication administration, 440
  nasogastric tubes, 398–399
  neurological assessment, 193
  oxygen therapy, 451
  pain management, 465
  parental care, 34
  parenteral nutrition, 412
  play, 121–122
  positioning, 219
  postoperative care, 226
  premature babies, 32
  preoperative care, 232
  pressure area care, 238
  seizures, 262
  service delivery models, 33
  skin care, 137
  specimen collection, 352
  stoma, 272
  suctioning, 278
  support, 37–38
  temperature control, 282
  tracheostomies, 297
  traction, 306
  workload evaluation, 38
  wound care, 364
  wound drain removal, 255
Competence, consent, 11
Complementary therapies, 58*b*, 57–64
  benefits, 58, 58*b*
  consent, 59–60
  definition, 57
  disadvantages, 58

  environment, 62
  prevalence, 57–58
  provision, 59
  risk reduction, 59
  see also specific types
Complex partial seizures, 260
Compressions, basic paediatric life support, 97
Computed tomography (CT), 241, 246
Conduction, heat loss, 171
Confidantes, protection (of children), 16
Congenital abnormalities
  infection risk factors, 45*t*
  tracheostomies, 284
  see also specific diseases/disorders
Conjugated bilirubin, 196
Connecting/changing infusion set, central lines, 156
Consciousness, decreased, 186*b*
Conscious sedation, lumbar puncture, 177
Consent, 10–11
  Children (Scotland) Act (1995), 10
  The Children Act England and Wales (1989), 10
  competence, 11
  complementary therapies, 59–60
  definition, 11
  hygiene, 105
  lumbar puncture, 176–177
  parental responsibilities, 12
  postmortems, 84
  rectal administration, 431
  specimen collection, 345
  therapeutic massage, 61
  Victoria Gillick case, 10
Constipation, 144–147
  causes, 144–145
    see also specific causes
  community nurses, 148
  definition, 142
  dietary fibre, 142–143
  management, 145–146
    medications, 146–147
    see also specific medications
  pain, 142
  potty training, 143
  school problems, 143
  traction, 305
Contact transmission, 44
Contamination
  specimen collection, 345
  wounds, 252
Continuing care, community children's nursing, 35–36
Continuous enteral feeding, 396–397
Contrast agents
  computed tomography, 246
  magnetic resonance imaging, 247

Convection, heat loss, 172
Convulsions *see* Seizures
Cooling measures, febrile convulsions, 262
Cornea, organ donation, 85*t*
Coroner referrals, bereavement care, 84*b*
Cots, incubators, transition from, 173
Counting, play, 126
CPR *see* Cardiopulmonary resuscitation (CPR)
Cradle cap/seborrhoeic dermatitis, 132–133
Cramps
  casts, 207
  stoma, 271
Cranial nerves, function assessment, 75
Creative communication, 28
Cross-infection prevention, 331
Cuffed tracheostomy tubes, 288
Cultural issues
  hygiene, 106–107
  pain assessment, 456
  skin care, 132
Curtains, cleaning, 341
Cuts, hand hygiene, 46–47
Cyanosis
  phototherapy, 197
  tracheostomies, 285
Cylinder casts, 203, 203*f*
Cytotoxic drugs, wound healing, 357

D

Day-care surgery, preoperative care, 229–230
Deaths, expected, 82–83
Decannulation, tracheostomies, 297
Decerebrate posturing, 191, 191*f*
Decontamination, isolation nursing, 341
Decorticate posturing, 191, 191*f*
Defecation *see* Bowel movements; Constipation; Diarrhoea
Defibrillation, paediatric life support, 101–102
Dehydration assessment
  diarrhoea, 148, 148*t*
  postoperative care, 225
Deltoid muscle, medicine administration, 427, 427*f*
Dental care, hygiene, 114–115
Developmental issues
  bowel care, 142–143
  bowel movements, 144
  community care nursing, 36
  enteral feeding, 398
  hygiene, 106–107
  isolation nursing, 338–342

medications, 422
pressure area care, 237
traction, 302–303
Dextrose, parenteral nutrition, 410
Diabetes mellitus
  subcutaneous medication, 429–430
  wound healing, 356
Diagnosis-independence, aseptic non-touch techniques, 330–331
Diarrhoea, 147–149
  definition, 142
  dehydration assessment, 148, 148*t*
  management, 147
  specimen collection, 348
Diclofenac, 461
Dietary fibre, constipation, 142–143, 145
Diet, constipation, 144, 145
^{99m}Tc Diethylenetriamine-pentaacetic acid (DTPA), nuclear medicine, 247–248
Dieticians
  enteral feeding, 389
  traction, 304
Digital rectal examination (DRE), 142
Dignity, hygiene, 106
Dihydrocodeine, 461
^{99m}Tc Dimercaptosuccinic acid (DMSA), nuclear medicine, 247–248
Dioctyl (docusate sodium), 146
Dipsticks, urine testing, 348
Dirty wounds, 252
Disabilities
  community children's nursing, 32–33
  preoperative care, 230
  radiography, 243
Disability discrimination Act, 213
Discharge from hospital
  postoperative care, 226–227
  stoma care, 271–272
Discomfort, traction, 305
Discontinuation, blood transfusions, 407
Disinfectants, 51–52
  see also specific disinfectants
Disposable gloves, 48
Disposable nappies, urine collection, 349
Distraction techniques, 126*t*
  intramuscular medication, 428
  play, 125, 126*t*
  preoperative care, 230
  subcutaneous medication, 429
  see also Play
Documentation
  hygiene, 106
  isolation nursing, 341
Docusate sodium (Dioctyl), 146

Doses, medications, 420
Drainable stoma appliances, 268*f*
Drainable urostomy appliances, 270*f*
Drains
  non-suction, 253
  suction, 253
Dressings
  central lines, 158, 159–161
  chest drain care, 167
  implanted ports, 159
Drinking
  casts, 207
  hip spica casts, 207
  traction, 305
Drop attacks, 260
Droplet transmission, 44
Drug-induced constipation, 144
Drug precipitates, central line occlusion, 160
Drugs *see* Medication(s)
Dry powder inhalers (DPI), 436, 438*t*
Dry skin, care, 132
Dulco-lax (Bisacodyl), 146
Dunlop traction, 301, 302*f*

E

Ear care, 117–118
Early warning systems, neurological assessment, 183
Ear swabs, 347
Ear wax (cerumen), 117
Eating
  casts, 207
  hip spica casts, 207
  traction, 305
  utensils, infection control, 51
  see also Nutrition
Eczema, atopic *see* Atopic eczema
Eczema herpeticum, 133
  herpes simplex virus, 133
Education
  blood glucose estimation, 370–373
  medications, 422
  pressure area care, 237
Electric pump, breast milk expression, 379, 379*f*
Electrolytes, parenteral nutrition, 410
Electron microscopy, vesicular fluid, 351
Elimination
  breastfeeding, 380
  traction, 305
Emergencies
  lumbar puncture, 175
  preoperative care, 229
  traction, 300

Emergency flow chart, tracheostomies, 287f
Emergency trolley, paediatric life support, 98, 99b
EMLA cream, 460
  venepuncture, 322
Emollients
  atopic eczema, 134
  fragile skin, 137
  psoriasis, 136
Emotional bonding, breastfeeding, 378
Encopresis, 142
Endotracheal intubation, 99–100
Endotracheal suction, 275, 277–278
Enemas, 147
Enteral feeding, 388–400
  bolus feeds, 396–397
  community nursing, 398
  complications, 397–399
  continuous feeds, 396–397
  developmental delay, 398
  dieticians, 389
  gastroenteritis, 398
  guidelines, 392
  infection prevention, 391
  nasogastric tubes see Nasogastric tubes
  need for, 388–392
  nutritional care specialists, 389
  observations, 397
  postoperative care, 225
  rationale, 388
  research-based practice, 390–392
  speech therapists, 389
  syringe size, 391–392
  tube blockages, 398
  vomiting, 398
Enterobius vermicularis (threadworm/ pinworm), 348
Enterococcus faecalis, 348
Entonox, 461–462
Environment
  aseptic non-touch techniques, 332
  cleaning, 341
  community care nursing, 36
  complementary therapies, 62
  infection transmission, 44
  temperature control, 282
Enzymic wound debridement, 358t
Epidermolysis bullosa (EB), 136–137
Epidural routes, 430
  analgesics, 460
Epiglottitis, suctioning, 276
Epilepsy, 259–260
  anticonvulsant drugs, 259
  see also Seizures
Epinephrine, 434, 436, 436t

Equipment
  cleaning methods, 52
    moving and handling, 215
  decontamination, 52
  isolation nursing, 339
Erythrocytes see Red blood cells (erythrocytes)
Essence of Care, 234–235
Essential Care Clusters, communication, 22
Essential oils, 60
Essential Steps to Safe Clean Care: Reducing healthcare-associated infection, 42
EU Regulation of Paediatric Medicine, 418
Evaporation, heat loss, 172
Every Child Matters, 4
  community care nursing, 36
  protection (of children), 16
Evidence-based bowel care, 143
Evidence-based practice (EPIC), infection control, 42
Exercise, 215
  constipation, 146
Exhaustion, tracheostomies, 285
Expected deaths, bereavement care, 82–83
Explanations
  blood glucose estimation, 372
  blood transfusions, 410
  cast removal, 208
  medications, 422
  neurological assessment, 188
  radiography, 242
  suctioning, 276
  wound dressing, 364
Eye care, 115–116
Eye drops, 433
Eye protection, phototherapy, 198
Eye swabs, 346
  Chlamydia infection, 346

F

Facial expression
  communication, 25
  pain assessment, 459t
Facial protection, 49
Faecal specimens
  amoebic dysentery, 348
  collection, 348
  Enterobius vermicularis (threadworm/pinworm), 348
Family, 10
  casts, effects of, 202
  community children's nursing, 35, 36

hygiene, 105
isolation nursing, 338–342
postoperative care, 226
risk management, 14–15
tracheostomies, 286
traction, effects of, 300
Fasciotomy, casts, 205
Fasting, preoperative care, 231
Febrile convulsions, 258, 281
  cooling measures, 262
Febrile reactions, blood transfusions, 407t
Feeding, 374–387
  enteral see Enteral feeding
  nutritional status assessment, 375
  parenteral nutrition see Parenteral nutrition (PN)
  written guidance, 374
  see also Artificial feeding; Bottle-feeding; Breastfeeding; Nutrition
Fenestrated tracheostomy tubes, 288
Fetal haemoglobin, 404
Fever, 281
  convulsions see Febrile convulsions
  prostaglandins, 281
  see also Body temperature control
Fibreglass, casts, 201
Fibrin clots, central line occlusion, 160
Fibroblasts, wound healing, 356
Film wound dressings, 362t
Filters, blood transfusions, 406
Fingernails, 134
First-stage foods, weaning, 384
Fits see Seizures
Fixed traction, 300
FLACC (Face, Legs, Activity, Cry, Consolability), 458t
Floppy children, 218–219
Fluid intake
  constipation, 144, 145
  phototherapy, 197
Fluid requirements, 381t
  postoperative care, 224, 225
Fluid therapy, paediatric life support, 100–101
Foam packs, 252
  removal, 255
Foam sponges, teeth cleaning, 115
Foam wound dressings, 362t
Focus, communication, 24
Focused rigidity casting (FRC), 201
Follow-on formula, 381, 381t
Food-borne transmission, 44
Footwear, 49
Foreign bodies
  ear care, 117–118
  tracheostomies, 284

Foreign travel, stoma supplies, 271
Fractures *see* Casts
Fragile skin
  bathing, 137
  emollients, 137
  epidermolysis bullosa, 136–137
Full-term infants, baby baths,
    107–108
Fungal specimen collection, 351

G

Gallows traction, 300, 301*f*
Gaseous exchange, positioning,
    217–218
Gastric washing, 351–352
Gastroenteritis
  enteral feeding, 398
  stoma, 271
Gastrostomy button, 389, 390*f*
Gastrostomy tubes, 389
  accidental removal, 395
  balloon changing, 394
  balloon water changing, 394–395
  community nursing, 399
  feeding via, 395–400
  gastrostomy button, 389, 390*f*
  granulation tissue, 395
  guidelines, 424–425
  infection, 395
  leakage, 395
  medication, 424–425
  passing of, 394
  patency maintenance, 390
  percutaneous endoscopic tube,
    389–390, 390*f*
  precautions, 424–425
Gaze, communication, 25
General anaesthetics, radiography,
    244–245
Generalised seizures, 259
General sales list medicines, 419
Genitourinary examination, 76
Gestational age, infection risk
    factors, 45*t*
Getting Ahead of the Curve, 41–42
Glasgow Coma Scale (GCS), 183
Gloves, 332
  aseptic non-touch techniques,
    332
  hand washing, 331–332
  isolation nursing, 340
Glucose
  blood *see* Blood glucose
    measurement
  paediatric life support, 101
Gluteus maximus muscle, medicine
    administration, 427, 427*f*

Gluteus medius muscle (ventrogluteal
    site), medicine administration,
    427, 427*f*
Good infant attachment,
    breastfeeding, 378, 378*f*
Good Practice Implementation Guide, 11
Gowns, 49
Grading, intravenous cannulation,
    403*t*
Grand mal seizures, 259–260
Granulation tissue, gastrostomy
    tubes, 395
Grimace score, 186, 186*t*, 190, 191*f*
Groshong catheter, 153
Growth information, assessment,
    76–77
Guided imagery, 61–62, 126–127
Guidelines
  enteral feeding, 392
  hygiene, 107
  moving and handling, 213

H

Haemoglobin, fetal, 404
Haemolytic reaction, blood
    transfusions, 407*t*
Haemorrhages, postoperative care,
    223–224
Haemothorax, 164
Hair care, 114
  casts, 206–207
Hair samples, 351
Halo traction, 301
Halter neck traction, 301, 303*f*
Hamilton–Russell traction, 301, 303*f*
Hand hygiene, 46–48, 47*t*
  alcohol gel hand rubs, 46–47
  cuts/abrasions, 46–47
  infection risk factors, 47–48
  isolation nursing, 339
  methods, 47, 47*f*
  requirements, 47
  tracheostomy care, 287
  see also Hand washing
Handling *see* Moving and handling
Hand pump, breast milk expression,
    379, 379*f*
Hand washing, 331–332
  alcohol hand-rubs, 332
  artificial feeding, 383
  central line care, 154
  cross-infection prevention, 106, 331
  gloves, 331–332
  isolation nursing, 339
  medication administration, 422
  nasogastric tubes, 392
  soap and water, 332

specimen collection, 345
toddler feeding, 385
Headache, lumbar puncture,
    177–178
Headbox, oxygen therapy, 447,
    448–450
Head lice, 114
Headtilt/chin lift, 96, 96*f*
Head trauma, seizures, 258
Headwear, 49
*The Healthcare Act 2006: Code of Practice
    for the Prevention and Control of
    Healthcare-associated Infections*,
    infection control, 42
Healthcare-associated infections
    (HCAI), 329
  control *see* Infection control
  mortality, 42–43
Health promotion, 107
Health Protection Agency (HPA), 42, 53
Healthy infants, positioning, 212
Heart
  anatomy, 164
  organ donation, 85*t*
Heart and lung, donation, 85*t*
Heart valves, donation, 85*t*
Heat loss, 171
Heparinization
  central lines, 155
  implanted port, 155, 157–158
Hepatitis, donated blood screening,
    405
Herpes simplex virus (HSV), eczema
    herpeticum, 133
Hickman line, 153
High-dependency unit (HDU), 223
High-efficiency particulate air filters
    (HEPA), 338
Hindu families, 86
Hip spica casts, 203, 204*f*
  eating/drinking problems, 207
History-taking
  assessment, 69
  chronic pain assessment, 464
  pain assessment, 457
HIV infection
  breastfeeding, 380
  donated blood screening, 405
Hoists, moving and handling, 214
Home deaths, 82
Homeopathy, 62
Home, play, 121–122
Hoop traction, 301
Hospital–home transition, 34
Hospital service recommendations,
    National Service Framework, 5
Human Rights Act (1998), 213
Humidifier apparatus, oxygen
    therapy, 448, 448*f*, 449, 451

Hydration
  postoperative care, 224–225
  pressure area care, 236
Hydrocolloid dressings, 362t
  nasogastric tubes, 392, 392f
Hydrofibre wound dressings,
    362t
Hydrogel wound dressings, 362t
Hygiene, 104–119
  adolescents, 112
  babies, 107–109
    baby baths see Baby baths
    mouthing objects, 108
    nail care, 111
    nappy area care, 110–111
    umbilical cord care, 111
  bed baths, 112–114
  casts, 206–207
  communication, 105
  community nursing, 118
  consent, 105
  cultural needs, 106–107
  dental care, 114–115
  developmental needs, 106–107
  dignity, 106
  documentation, 106
  ear care, 117–118
  eye care, 115–116
  family inclusion, 105
  guidelines, 107
  hair care, 114
  health promotion, 107
  independence, 105
  isolation nursing, 338
  observation, 107
  older children, 112–118
  oral care, 114–115
  patient participation, 105
  play, 107
  privacy, 106
  rationales, 104–105
  risk assessment, 105–106
  safe practice, 105, 106
  toddlers/pre-schoolers, 111–112
  toileting, 114
  see also Infection control
Hyperbilirubinaemia (jaundice),
    195
  urobilinogen, 196
Hypertension, suctioning, 278
Hypnotherapy, 62
Hypochlorite disinfectants, 52
  blood fluid spillages, 346
Hypoglycaemia, 369
  neonates, 369
Hypotension, suctioning, 278
Hypothalamus, temperature control,
    280
Hypoxia, suctioning, 278

I

Ibuprofen, 461
  temperature control, 282
Ileal conduit, 266
Ileostomy, 265
Imagination, play, 126
Immediate recovery period, 223–224
Immunisations, employment
    recommendations, 53
Immunosuppressed patients
  infection control, 51
  wound healing, 357
  see also HIV infection
Immunosuppressive therapies,
    occupational health, 53
Impetigo, 133
  Staphylococcus aureus, 133
Implanted ports, 153–154, 154f
  accessing, 156–157
  dressing, 159
  heparinization, 155, 157–158
Incontinence, pressure area care, 236
Incubator care, 170–174
  complications, 173
  cot, transition to, 173
  methods, 172
  neutral thermal environment,
    170, 172t
Independence, hygiene, 105
Infant(s)
  bowel movements, 143
  pain assessment, 456
Infant Feeding Survey, 375
Infant-led breastfeeding, 376
Infected linen, waste disposal, 50
Infection(s)
  central lines, 159
  control see Infection control
  gastrostomy tubes, 395
  hosts, 44
  isolation nursing, 341
  lumbar puncture, 178
  risk factors, 45t
  seizures, 258
  tracheostomies, 284
  transmission, 44
    air-borne, 44
    blood borne, 44
    contact, 44
    droplet, 44
    food-borne, 44
    vector-borne, 44
  see also specific infections
Infection control, 41–56
  auditing practice, 53
  chain of infection, 43–44
  cleaning, 51–52
  cross-infection prevention, 106

disinfectants, 51–52
eating utensils, 51
enteral feeding, 391
equipment decontamination, 52
evidence-based practice, 42
hand hygiene see Hand hygiene
microorganisms, 43
occupational health, 53
protective clothing see Personal
    protective equipment (PPE)
source, 43–44
standard precautions, 45–46
sterilization, 51
surveillance, 53
transmission-based controls, 46
waste disposal see Waste disposal
see also Aseptic non-touch
    techniques (ANTT); Hygiene;
    Isolation nursing
Infectious diarrhoea, 147
Infectious specimen collection, 345
Inflammatory phase, wound healing,
    355–356
Information Focus, clinical
    governance, 12–13
Information gathering, 23
Informed consent see Consent
Informed people, bereavement
    care, 90t
Inhalation, analgesics, 460
Inhalers, 436–441
  complications, 440
  dry powder inhalers, 436, 438t
  guidelines, 436–438
  spacers, 437f, 438–439
  see also specific types
Insects, ear care, 117–118
Inspection
  abdominal examination, 76
  cardiovascular examination, 73
  physical examination, 71
  skin examination, 75
Intensive care unit (ICU)
  neurological assessment, 193
  postoperative care, 223
  tracheostomies, 286
Interactive websites, adolescents, 128
Intercostal recession, 285f
  tracheostomies, 285
Intermittent urethral catheterisation,
    312
Interpersonal skills, community
    children's nursing, 34
Interventional radiography, 241,
    248–249
Intra-aural/otic medications,
    432–433
Intracranial pressure, raised see Raised
    intracranial pressure

Intramuscular medication, 426–428
  analgesics, 460
  complications, 428
  distraction techniques, 428
  sites, 427–428
    see also specific sites
Intraocular/optic medications, 433
Intraosseous medication, 430
  paediatric life support, 100
Intrathecal medication, 430
  analgesics, 460
  lumbar puncture, 176–178
Intravenous cannulation, 323–325
  aseptic non-touch techniques, 330
  care of, 325
  community nursing, 325
  complications, 324–325
  grading, 403*t*
  limb immobilization, 324, 324*f*,
    325
  observations, 324–325
  pain, 403
  scalp vein, 323, 324, 324*f*
  taping, 324, 324*f*, 325
  see also Venepuncture
Intravenous therapy, 401–414, 425–426
  analgesics, 459–460
  blood transfusions *see* Blood
    transfusions
  body fluid distribution, 402
  body surface area, 402
  body weight, 402
  centralised intravenous additives
    service, 426
  complications, 403, 425
  equipment, 402
  observations, 403
  parenteral nutrition *see* Parenteral
    nutrition (PN)
  platelet transfusion *see* Platelet
    transfusion
  see also Central lines; Intravenous
    cannulation
Irrigation
  tracheostomy care, 287
  wound care, 360
Irritability, neurological assessment,
  188
Irritation, skin care, 132
Islam, bereavement care, 86
Isolation nursing, 337–343
  clinical waste, 340
  communication, 341
  community nursing, 8
  decontamination, 341
  developmental considerations,
    338–342
  documentation, 341
  environmental cleaning, 341

equipment, 339
family, 338–342
general principles, 338–339
gloves, 340
hand hygiene, 339
high-efficiency particulate air filters,
  338
hygiene, 338
infection control, 46
infection risks, 341
linen/laundry, 340–341
personal protective equipment, 339,
  340, 341
planning of care, 341
privacy, 338
prophylactic antibiotics, 339
protective isolation, 337
sharps, 340
single-occupancy rooms, 338
specimen collection, 340
stress, 341
toys, 338
written information, 341
see also Infection control

J

Japanese frame, 301
Jaundice *see* Hyperbilirubinaemia
  (jaundice)
Jaw thrust, 96
Jewish families, bereavement
  care, 86
Joint problems, traction, 306
Just for the Day, 230

K

Keratolytic agents, psoriasis, 136
Kernicterus, phototherapy, 195
Ketones, urine testing, 309
Kidney donation, 85*t*
Kidney transplants, ^{99m}Tc
  diethylenetriamine-pentaacetic
  acid imaging, 248
Klebsiella, 338

L

Labelling
  chest drain care, 167
  specimen collection, 345
Lactose intolerance, neonatal stoma,
  266
Lactulose, 146

Laming report, protection (of
  children), 16–17, 17*b*
Language specialists *see* Speech and
  language therapists
Laryngospasm, suctioning, 278
Larynx, cardiopulmonary
  resuscitation, 95
Lateral decubitus position, lumbar
  puncture, 179
Leadership, clinical governance,
  12–13
Leakage, gastrostomy tubes, 395
Learning from Bristol, 4
Legislation, 6
  medications, 418–419
  moving and handling, 213
Leucocyte esterase, urine testing,
  310
Leucodepletion, blood transfusions,
  405–406
Lichenification, atopic eczema, 135
Lifestyle, constipation, 144
Life support, paediatric *see* Paediatric
  life support
Limb immobilization, intravenous
  cannulation, 324, 324*f*, 325
Limb movement, neurological
  assessment, 192
Line kinking, central line occlusion,
  160
Linen/laundry, isolation nursing,
  340–341
Liquid paraffin, 146
Liver donation, 85*t*
Local anaesthetics
  lumbar puncture, 177
  subcutaneous medication, 429
Local routes, analgesics, 460
Lone working, community care
  nursing, 36–37
Long-term bereavement care, 87
Lorazepam, 261
Low birth weight, infection risk
  factors, 45*t*
Low friction sheets, moving and
  handling, 214
Luer lock changing, central lines,
  155
Lumbar puncture, 175–181
  adverse reactions, 177–178
  cerebrospinal fluid collection, 352
  complications, 177–178
  contraindications, 180*b*
  emergency settings, 175
  equipment, 178–179
  intrathecal drug administration,
    176–178
  manual handling risks, 178
  nurses role, 178

pain, 177
positioning, 178, 179f
post-lumbar puncture activity,
179–180
preparation, 176–177
procedure, 179–180
rationale, 176
risks, 177–178
Lungs
anatomy, 164
drainage, positioning, 217, 217t
Lying
breastfeeding, 376
communication problems, 29

M

Macrophages, wound healing, 356
Maggots, wound debridement, 358t
Magnetic resonance imaging (MRI),
241, 246–247
sedation, 244
Malnourished mother, breastfeeding,
380
Managers, community care nursing, 37
Manual defibrillators, 101
Manual handling *see* Moving and
handling
Manual Handling Operations
Regulations, 213
Maturative phase, wound healing, 356
Mechanical wound debridement, 358t
Medication(s), 415–445
definition, 419
developmental issues, 422
education, 422
explanations, 422
legislation, 418–419
neurological assessment, 188–192
nurse prescribing, 421–422
paediatric life support, 100–101
pressure area care, 236
rationale, 418
storage, 421
temperature control, 282
wound healing, 356–357
Medication administration
central lines, 155
community nursing, 440
correct child, 420
correct medicine, 420
dose, 420
guidelines, 419–423
hand washing, 422
principles, 422–423
record-keeping, 420–421
routes of, 420, 422, 423t
see also specific routes

self-administration, 421
timings, 420
Medicine Councils Agency, 418–419
Medicines Act (1968), 418, 419
Mental Capacity Act (2005), 9
competence in consent, 11
Mental health, 7
assessment, 68–69
Messy play, 125
Metabolic disorders
constipation, 144
neonatal seizures, 258
seizures, 258
Methaemoglobinaemia, 322
Methicillin-resistant *Staphylococcus
aureus* (MRSA), 41–42, 338
Microaggregate filters, blood
transfusions, 406
Microatelectasis, suctioning, 278
Microorganisms, 337, 338
infection control, 43
Micturating cystograms, 245
Midazolam, 261
Midstream urine collection,
310, 349
'Milking,' chest drainage, 168
Minerals, parenteral nutrition, 410
Misuse of Drugs Act (1971), 418
Mitrofanoff stoma, 266
urine collection, 349–350
Mobility
casts, 207
pressure area care, 236
Modernising Nursing Careers, 5
Moist heat sterilization, 52
Monocytes, wound healing,
355–356
Mop heads, cleaning, 341
Morphine, 461
Mother's comfort, breastfeeding,
376, 378
Motor responses, neurological
assessment, 191
Mouthing objects, baby hygiene, 108
Movicol®, 146
Moving and handling, 212–215
carer protection, 212–213
controversial techniques, 212–213
equipment cleaning, 215
guidelines/legislation, 213
hoists, 214
low friction sheets, 214
lumbar puncture, 178
musculoskeletal injuries, 212
patient sling, 214
PATslide, 214
risk assessments, 213
training, 215
transfer boards, 214

Mucus overproduction, suctioning,
275
Multidisciplinary teams, 33
casts, 203–204
traction, 303–304
Muscles, casts, 205–206
Muscular problems, traction, 306
Musculoskeletal injuries, moving
and handling, 212
Muslims, bereavement care, 86
Mycobacterium tuberculosis
gastric washings, 351–352
wound swabs, 348
Myoclonic seizures, 260

N

Nail care, 111
Nail samples, 351
NAPI (Nursing assessment of Pain
Intensity), 458t
Nappy area care, 110–111
casts, 206
Nappy rash, 110–111, 133
Candida albicans infection (thrush),
133
Nasal cannula, oxygen therapy, 447,
449, 450, 450f
Nasal flaring, tracheostomies, 285
Nasogastric medication, 424–425
Nasogastric tubes, 389–390
community nursing, 398–399
feeding via, 395–400
guidelines, 424–425
hand washing, 392
hydrocolloid dressings,
392, 392f
length, 393f
misplacement, 397
passing of, 392–395
patency maintenance, 390
precautions, 424–425
Nasopharyngeal suction, 275, 276, 277,
277f
National association for the Welfare
of Children in Hospital
(NAWCH), 230
National Institute for Clinical
Excellence (NICE)
Asthma Guidelines, 71
ultrasound placement of central
lines, 248
National Patient Safety Agency, 14
National Service Framework (NSF), 4
accountability, 7
clinical governance, 13
hospital service recommendations, 5
medications, 419

National Service Framework (NSF)
(*Continued*)
pain management, 455
radiography, 242
National Society for the Prevention of
Cruelty to Children (NSPCC), 16
Nebulisers, 439–440
tracheostomies, 297
Needle play, 124–125
Neonates
hypoglycaemia, 369
neurological assessment, 186
oxygenation, 447–448
pain assessment, 456
postoperative care, 223
pressure area care, 235
seizures, 258
stoma, 266–267
see also Premature babies
Nerves
casts, 206
traction, 306
Neurological assessment, 74–75,
182–194
children, 186–187
coma scales, 183
community nursing, 193
complications, 193
early warning systems, 183
equipment, 187
guidelines, 187
initial observations, 187–188
neonates, 186
pain application, 183–186
palpation, 74
rapid assessment, 183
rationale, 182–183
special sense examination, 75
Neurological impairment
cardiopulmonary resuscitation, 95
positioning, 219
Neurovascular assessment, traction,
305
Neutral thermal environment,
incubator care, 170, 172t
Neutrophils, wound healing, 355–356
The NHS Plan
advocacy, 8, 9
medicine self-administration, 421
90–90 traction, 301, 302f
Nitrate tests, urine testing, 309
Non-adherent wound dressings, 362t
Non-steroidal anti-inflammatory
drugs (NSAIDs), 461
Non-suction drains, 253
Non-tunnelled long central lines, 154
Non-verbal communication, 24–25, 27
Normal blood pressure, 74t
Normal heart rates, 73, 73t

Nose swabs, 347
Nosocomial infections *see* Infection
control
Notification of Death certificates, 90
NSPCC, 16
Nuclear medicine, 247–248
bone scans, 247
^{99m}Tc diethylenetriamine-
pentaacetic acid, 247–248
^{99m}Tc dimercaptosuccinic acid,
247–248
Numerical rating, pain assessment,
459t
Nurse-led sedation programmes,
radiography, 244
Nurse prescribing, 421–422
Nurses, risk management, 15
Nursing and Midwifery Council
accountability, 6–7
venepuncture guidelines, 321
*Nursing and Midwifery Council's Guide
for Students*, 6
Nursing care, traction, 305
Nursing practice, bowel care, 145
Nutrients, parenteral nutrition, 410
Nutrition
infection risk factors, 45t
parenteral nutrition *see* Parenteral
nutrition (PN)
phenylketonuria, 380
pressure area care, 236
wound healing, 356
see also Eating
Nutritional care specialists, enteral
feeding, 389
Nutritional status assessment, 375
Nutrition information, 76–77

O

Observations
hygiene, 107
postoperative care, 224
traction, 305–307
Occlusions, central lines, 160
Occupational health
immunosuppressive therapies, 53
infection control, 53
Occupational therapists, traction,
303
Oedematous stoma, 271
Off label medicines, 418–419
Olive oils, skin care, 132
Open questions, 23
Open wards, traction, 302–303
Opioids, 461
patient-controlled analgesia, 461

Opisthotonos, neurological
assessment, 191, 192f
Oral hygiene, 114–115
medications, 423
Oral medication, 423–424
analgesics, 459
older children, 424
toddlers, 424
young infants, 424
Organ donation, 84–85, 85t
religious objections, 85
Organs, retention of, 83–84
Orientation, communication, 25
Orogastric medication, 424–425
Oropharyngeal airways, 99
Oropharyngeal suction, 275, 276, 277,
277f
Osteomyelitis, traction, 306–307
Outer the counter (OTC) remedies, 58
Overheating, sudden infant death
syndrome, 281
Oxygen masks, 447, 449, 450, 451f
Oxygen saturation
physical examination, 72–73
suctioning, 276
Oxygen supply
endotracheal suction, 277–278
neonates, 447–448
normal levels, 447
postoperative care, 223, 224
sick children, 448
Oxygen therapy, 446–453
body/trunk box, 447, 448–449
community nursing, 451
complications, 450–451
guidelines, 448
headbox, 447, 448–450
humidifier apparatus, 448, 448f,
449, 451
nasal cannula, 447, 449, 450, 450f
observations, 450–451
oxygen masks, 447, 449, 450, 451f
positioning, 449
rationale, 447
risks, 451–452
tracheostomies, 297

P

Packed cell blood transfusions, 404
Packs, 252
Pads, urine collection, 349
Paediatric Early Warning System
(PEWS), 68
assessment, 68
lumbar puncture, 180
neurological observation, 183
Paediatric Glasgow Coma Scale
(PGCS), 183, 184t, 185t

Paediatric life support
    advanced, 98
    airway maintenance *see* Airway
        maintenance
    basic *see* Basic paediatric life support
    defibrillation, 101–102
    drug therapy, 100–101
    emergency trolley, 98, 99*b*
    fluid therapy, 100–101
    intraosseous access, 100
    vascular access, 100
    venous access, 100
Paediatric Objective Pain Score, 458*t*
Pain
    assessment *see below*
    constipation, 142, 144
    intravenous cannulation, 324, 403
    lumbar puncture, 177
    neurological assessment, 183–186
    postoperative care, 225
    skin care, 132
    specimen collection, 345
    traction, 305
    untreated, 455
Pain assessment, 455–458
    behavioural assessment, 457, 458*t*
    children (pre-school to 7),
        456–457
    complications, 465
    culture, 456
    guidelines, 455–456, 455*b*
    history taking, 457
    infants/toddlers, 456
    neonates, 456
    older children (7 to adolescence),
        457
    parental role, 455
    physiological assessment, 457–458
    self-report techniques, 458,
        459*f*, 459*t*
    sick children, 456
    see also specific tests
Pain management, 454–468
    chronic pain, 464–466
    community nursing, 465
    drugs *see* Analgesia
    non-drug methods, 459
    parental role, 455
    rationales, 455
    see also Analgesia
Pallor, tracheostomies, 285
Palpation, 70
    abdominal examination, 76
    cardiovascular examination, 73, 73*t*
    physical examination, 71–72
    skin examination, 75
Pancreas donation, 85*t*
Paracetamol, 460–461
    temperature control, 282

Paraldehyde, rectal administration, 261
Parent(s)
    bereavement care, 83–85, 87
    communication, 23
Parental roles/responsibilities, 10
    artificial feeding, 381
    bed baths, 112
    British Medical Association, 12
    community children's nursing,
        34, 36
    consent, 12
    lumbar puncture, 176
    pain assessment, 455
    pain management, 455
    postoperative care, 224, 225
    preoperative care, 231
    rectal drug administration, 263
    seizures, 260–261, 263
    traction, 304
Parenteral nutrition (PN), 409–412
    blood glucose monitoring, 410
    central lines, 409
    community nursing, 412
    complications, 410–412
    dextrose, 410
    nutrients, 410
    observations, 410–412
    postoperative care, 225
    preparation and storage, 409, 410
    sepsis, 411
    temperature monitoring, 410
Partial seizures, 260
Passive movements, floppy children,
    218
Pasteurization, breast milk, 380
Patient-controlled analgesia (PCA),
    459–460, 462*f*
    adolescents, 463*f*
    opioids, 461
    postoperative care, 225
Patient Focus, clinical governance,
    12–13
Patient sling, moving and handling,
    214
PATslide, moving and handling, 214
Peak flow expiratory rate (PFER),
    437–438
Peer pressure, non-compliance, 28
Pelvic traction, 301
Percussion, 71–72
Percutaneous endoscopic tube (PEG),
    389–390, 390*f*
Periosteal skin soreness, stoma, 271
Peripherally inserted central catheters,
    154
Pernasal swabs, 347
Personal protective equipment (PPE),
    48–49, 48*f*
    facial protection, 49

footwear, 49
gloves, 48, 332
headwear, 49
isolation nursing, 339, 340, 341
plastic aprons, 49
protective gowns, 49
Perthes disease, slings and springs
    traction, 301
Petit mal seizures, 260
PEWS *see* Paediatric Early Warning
    System (PEWS)
Pharmacy medicines, 419
Phenylketonuria, nutrition, 380
Phlebotomy technicians, 322
Photographs
    bereavement care, 88
    preparation play, 123
Phototherapy, 195–199
    complications, 197–198
    equipment, 196
    method, 197–198, 197*f*
pH, urine testing, 309
Physical examination, 69–70, 71–76
    abdominal examination, 76
    adolescents, 71
    auscultation, 72
    body mass index, 77
    cardiovascular system
        see Cardiovascular examination
    genitourinary examination, 76
    inspection, 71
    neurology *see* Neurological
        assessment
    oxygen saturation, 72–73
    palpation, 70, 71–72
    percussion, 71–72
    preparation, 68–71
    pre-schoolers, 70–71
    pulse oximetry, 72–73
    reflexes, 70
    respiratory examination, 71
    respiratory rates, 70, 70*t*
    school-age child, 71
    separation anxieties, 70
    skin examination, 75–76
    STAMP (Screening Tool for the
        Assessment of Malnutrition in
        Paediatrics), 77
    stranger anxieties, 70
    temperature taking/recording,
        75–76
    weighing, 77
Physiological pain assessment,
    457–458
Physiological problems, constipation,
    144
Physiotherapy/physiotherapists
    casts, 204
    chronic pain management, 464

Physiotherapy/physiotherapists
(*Continued*)
  suctioning, 276
  traction, 303
Pimecrolimus, atopic eczema, 135
Pinworm, 348
Plain X-rays, 245
Planned surgery, preoperative care, 229
Plaster of Paris, 201
Plastic aprons, 49
Platelets
  blood clotting, 408
  formation, 408
  functions, 408
  life span, 408
  storage, 408
Platelet transfusion, 408–409
  complications, 409
  observations, 409
Play, 120–130
  adolescents, 127–128
    appointments, 128
    choices, 127
    interactive websites, 128
    privacy, 128
    resources, 128
    routine, 128
  assessment, 69–70
  benefits, 129*f*
  breathing, 126
  bubbles, 125
  communication, 28, 28*t*
  community nurse, 121–122
  counting, 126
  distraction therapy, 125, 126*t*
  fear alleviation example, 124*b*
  future work, 129
  at home, 121–122
  hygiene, 107
  imagination, 126
  messy play, 125
  needle play, 124–125
  positioning, 212, 218
  praise and rewards, 128
  pre-admission programmes,
    124–126
  preparation, 122–127
  programmes, 120–121
  puppets, 122, 126
  radiography, 242
  relaxation tapes, 126
  shouting, 126
  siblings, 128
  squeezing, 126
  sticky bubbles, 126
  therapeutic play, 122
  traction, 303–304
  types, 122
    see also specific types of play

Pleural cavity, anatomy, 164
Pleural effusion/empyema, 164–165
PN *see* Parenteral nutrition (PN)
Pneumothorax, 164
  chest drains, 168
  suctioning, 278
Poker-chip pain assessment, 459*t*
Policy context, 4–5
Polyurethane-based materials, casts,
  201
Port-a-Cath *see* Implanted ports
Ports, implanted *see* Implanted ports
Positioning, 211–221
  acutely sick children, 217–218
  anaphylaxis treatment, 434
  bottle-feeding, 383
  breastfeeding, 377, 377*f*
  casts, 207
  central nervous system, 218
  chronic conditions, 218
  community nursing, 219
  complications, 219–220
  healthy infants, 212
  lumbar puncture, 178, 179*f*
  neurological assessment, 188
  neurological impairment, 219
  observations, 219–220
  oxygen therapy, 449
  play, 212, 218
  pre-term babies, 215–217, 216*f*
  radiography, 243
  rationale, 211–212
  respiratory system, 212, 217–218
  skin problems, 218
  traction, 305
  wound dressing, 364
Postal services, specimen collection,
  346
Post-lumbar puncture activity,
  179–180
Postmortems, 83–84
  consent, 84
  religious views, 84*b*
Postoperative care, 222–227
  community nursing, 226
  discharge planning, 226–227
  family, 226
  hydration, 224–225
  immediate recovery period, 223–224
  pain, 225
  rationale, 222
  return to ward, 224–226
  stoma, 270
Post-Operative Pain Score, 458*t*
Potty training, constipation, 143
PPP (Paediatric Pain Profile), 458*t*
Praise
  play, 128
  radiography, 244

Pre-admission programmes
  play, 124–126
  preoperative care, 229
Pregnancy
  occupational health, 53
  radiography, 241
Premature babies
  body temperature maintenance,
    171
  community children's nursing, 32
  nutritional concerns, 380
  positioning, 215–217, 216*f*
  skin care, 136
Premedication, preoperative care, 232
Preoperative care, 228–233
  age-appropriate preparation, 231
  community nursing, 232
  day-care surgery, 229–230
  disabilities, 230
  emergency surgery, 229
  fasting, 231
  parents, 231
  planned surgery, 229
  preparation, 231
  rationale, 228–229
  setting standards, 230–231
  toys/comforters, 231
Pre-schoolers
  hygiene, 111–112
  physical examination, 70–71
Prescription only medicines (POMs),
  419
Pressure area care, 234–239
  assessment tools, 235
  body weight, 235
  clinical governance, 238
  community nursing, 238
  continence problems, 236
  developmental considerations,
    237
  education, 237
  hydration, 236
  medication, 236
  mobility, 236
  nutrition, 236
  pressure sores, 236–237
  prevention, 237
  rationale, 234–235
  risk factors, 235–236
  risks due to, 238
  skin integrity, 236
  wound management, 237–238
  see also Pressure sores
Pressured metered dose inhaler
  (PMDI), 436
Pressure-relieving mattresses, 237
Pressure sores
  casts, 206
  pressure area care, 236–237

Primary intention, wound healing, 252, 355
Privacy
  adolescents, 128
  hygiene, 106
  isolation nursing, 338
  radiography, 243
  stoma care, 267
  traction, 302–303
Professional framework, 6
Prolapse, stoma, 271
Proliferative phase, wound healing, 356
Prone positioning, pre-term babies, 216, 216f, 217f
Prophylactic antibiotics, isolation nursing, 339
Prostaglandins, fever, 281
Protection (of children), 16–17, 18, 18b
  child abuse, 16
  confidantes, 16
  Every Child Matters, 16
  Laming report, 16–17, 17b
  NSPCC, 16
  referrals, 18f
  Victoria Climbié inquiry, 16
Protection, radiography, 243
Protective clothing *see* Personal protective equipment (PPE)
Protective gowns, 49
Protective isolation, 337
Protein(s)
  deficiency, wound healing, 356
  pressure area care, 236
  urine testing, 309
Provision and Use of Working Equipment Regulations, 215
Proximity, communication, 25
Psoriasis, 135–136
  bathing, 136
  coal tar preparations, 136
  emollients, 136
  keratolytic agents, 136
Psychological preparation, preoperative care, 229
Psychology, chronic pain management, 465
Psychosocial issues, bowel care, 143
Puberty, communication, 28
Public Health (Infectious Disease) Regulations, 41–42
Pulse, 73, 73t
  basic paediatric life support, 97, 97f
Pulse oximetry, physical examination, 72–73
Pulse rate, neurological assessment, 188

Pupillary response, neurological assessment, 189, 189f, 190f
Puppets, play, 122, 126
Purse-string sutures, chest drains, 168

Q

Quality Improvement, clinical governance, 12–13
Question types, communication, 23–24, 24b
QUESTT, self-reporting pain assessment, 458–459

R

Radiation
  doses, 241
  heat loss, 172
Radiography, 240–250
  air enemas, 245–246
  barium studies, 245
  disabilities, 243
  general anaesthetics, 244–245
  general environment, 242
  interventional, 241, 248–249
  investigation, 245–249
  micturating cystograms, 245
  plain X-rays, 245
  positioning, 243
  praise and reward, 244
  preparations, 242–243
  privacy, 243
  protection, 243
  rationale, 241
  sedation, 244–245
Radiotherapy, wound healing, 357
Raised intracranial pressure
  positioning, 218
  radiography, 244
Rapid assessment, neurological assessment, 183
Rapydan, 460
Reagent strips, urine testing, 310
Record Keeping Guidance for Nurses and Midwives, 106
Records
  infection control surveillance, 53
  medication administration, 420–421
  neurological assessment, 188, 192
Recovery units, postoperative care, 223
Rectal discharges, stoma, 271
Rectal medications, 431
  analgesics, 459
  anticonvulsant drugs, 260–261, 262

consent, 431
  paraldehyde, seizures, 261
  parental care, 263
Rectal temperature recording, 75–76
Red blood cells (erythrocytes)
  formation, 404
  functions, 404
  life span, 404
  normal life history, 196, 196f
Referrals, protection (of children), 18f
Reflexes, physical examination, 70
Reflexology, 61
Reflex zone therapy, 61
Relaxation tapes, 126
Religious views
  blood transfusions, 405
  postmortems, 84b
  see also Bereavement care
Removal, accidental, central lines, 160
Renal biopsy, radiographic guidance, 249
Requests, radiography, 241
Research-based practice, enteral feeding, 390–392
Respiratory infections, cardiopulmonary arrest, 95
Respiratory rates
  neurological assessment, 188
  physical examination, 70, 70t
  tracheostomies, 285
Respiratory system
  chest drainage care, 166–167
  examination, 71
  positioning, 212, 217–218
Restraints, 9
  Children Act (1989), 29
Resuscitation equipment, 165
Resuscitation, suctioning, 275–279
Resuscitation trolley, 287
Retention of organs, 83–84
Retraction, stoma, 271
Rewards, radiography, 244
Ribbon gauze pack removal, 254–255
Risk assessments
  aseptic non-touch techniques, 333–334
  cleaning methods, 52
  hygiene, 105–106
  moving and handling, 213
  specimen collection, 345
Risk factors, infections, 45t
Risk management, 12–15
  communication difficulties, 14
  community care nursing, 37
  family-centred care, 14–15
  National Patient Safety Agency, 14
  for nurses, 15
  pressure area care, 238
  written instructions, 15
Room temperature, incubators, 172

Routine, adolescents, 128
Royal College of Nursing, community care nursing, 38
Royal Liverpool Children's Inquiry (2001), organ retention, 83

S

Safe Management of Healthcare Waste, 49
Safe practice, hygiene, 105, 106
Safety, casts, 207
Safety equipment, tracheostomies, 286
Saving Lives: A delivery programme to reduce healthcare-associated infections including MRCA, 42
Scalp vein cannulation, 323, 324, 324*f*
Scaphoid casts, 202, 203*f*
School problems, constipation, 143
Scottish Surveillance of Healthcare-associated Infection Programme (SSHAIP), 53
Screening, blood transfusions, 405
Secondary intention, wound healing, 252, 355
Secondary socialization, 3–4
Sedation, 463–464
    conscious, lumbar puncture, 177
    magnetic resonance imaging, 244
    radiography, 244–245
Seizures, 257–264
    absences (petit mal), 260
    adolescents, 259
    atonic (drop attacks), 260
    children, 258
    community nursing, 262
    complex partial, 260
    complications, 262–263
    generalised seizures, 259
    guidelines, 260–261
    myoclonic, 260
    neonates, 258
    observations, 262–263
    parental care, 260–261, 263
    partial, 260
    rationale, 257–258
    rectal paraldehyde administration, 261
    simple partial, 260
    tonic-clonic (grand mal), 259–260
    see also specific types
Self-administration, 421
Self-feeding, toddlers, 386
Self-reporting pain assessment, 458, 459*f*, 459*t*
Semi-rigid casts, 202
Senna, 146
Separation anxieties, 70

Sepsis
    cardiopulmonary arrest, 95
    parenteral nutrition, 411
    suctioning, 278
Septicaemia, central lines, 159, 350
Serious Hazards of Transfusion (SHOT) reporting scheme, 404
Service delivery models, community children's nursing, 33
Setting standards, preoperative care, 230–231
Sharps
    isolation nursing, 340
    waste disposal, 50
Sheffield tracheostomy tubes, 289, 289*f*
Shiley tracheostomy tubes, 288, 288*f*
Shivering, 171, 280
Shouting, play, 126
Showering, wound care, 360–361
Siblings, play, 128
Side finger pressure, neurological observation, 184, 185*f*
Side-lying positioning, 218
    pre-term babies, 217, 217*f*
Sikh families, bereavement care, 86–87
Silence, communication, 24
Silicone Medical Adhesive Remover (SMAR), 136
Silver wound dressings, 362*t*
Simple leg traction, 300
Simple partial seizures, 260
Single-occupancy rooms, 338
Single-use items, 52
Site cleaning, tracheostomies, 291
Sitting, breastfeeding, 376
Skeletal traction, 300–301
Skin care, 131–138
    casts, 206–207
    coconut oils, 132
    community nursing, 137
    cultural issues, 132
    dry skin, 132
    equipment, 132
    olive oils, 132
    pain/irritation, 132
    pre-term infant, 136
    rationale, 132
    skin fragility, 136–138
    traction, 305
    see also specific diseases/disorders
Skin damage, pressure area care, 237
Skin examination, 75–76
Skin fragility
    bathing, 137
    care, 136–138
    general care, 137

Skin granulation, tracheostomies, 291, 291*f*
Skin integrity, pressure area care, 236
Skin problems, positioning, 218
Skin samples, 351
Skin traction, 300
    application, 304–305
    equipment, 304
Sleeping, casts, 207
Slings and springs traction, 301
Soap and water, hand washing, 332
Societal change, 3
Sodium bicarbonate, 101
Sodium dichloroisocyanurate (NaDCC), blood fluid spillages, 346
Softening agents, 146
Soiling, 142
Source isolation, 337
Spacers, inhalers, 437*f*, 438–439
Specific gravity, urine testing, 309
Specimen collection, 344–353
    antibiotic level measurement, 351
    biopsy material, 352
    blood samples, 350
    cerebrospinal fluid, 352
    community nursing, 352
    consent, 345
    contamination, 345
    ear swabs, 347
    equipment, 346
    eye swabs, 346
    faeces, 348
    fungal samples, 351
    gastric washing, 351–352
    hair samples, 351
    hand washing, 345
    infectious specimens, 345
    isolation nursing, 340
    labelling, 345
    nail samples, 351
    nose swabs, 347
    pain, 345
    pernasal swabs, 347
    postal services, 346
    pre-antimicrobial therapy, 345
    risk assessments, 345
    skin samples, 351
    sputum, 347
    throat swabs, 347
    transport medium, 346
    urine *see* Urine collection
    vaginal swabs, 350
    vesicular fluid, 351
    viral haemorrhagic fevers, 346
    wound swabs, 347–348
Speech and language therapists
    enteral feeding, 389
    tracheostomies, 296–297

Spina bifida, bowel care, 144
Spleen, blood cell breakdown, 196
Sputum specimens, 347
Squeezing, play, 126
Staff Focus, clinical governance, 12–13
STAMP (Screening Tool for the Assessment of Malnutrition in Paediatrics), 77
Standards for Medication Management, 419–420
Standing hoists, 214
Staphylococcus aureus
  atopic eczema, 135
  impetigo, 133
  nose swabs, 347
Status epilepticus, 259
Sterile techniques, 331
Sterilization, 51
Sternal recession, 285*f*
  tracheostomies, 285
Steroids, wound healing, 357
Stertor, tracheostomies, 285
Stethoscopes, 72
Sticky bubbles, play, 126
Stockinettes, casts, 204
Stoma, 265–273
  adolescents, 267
  antegrade continence stoma, 266
  babies, 266–267
  bag changing, 267–271
  children, 267
  closed appliances, 269*f*
  colostomy, 265
  community nursing, 272
  complications, 270–271
  on discharge, 271–272
  drainable appliances, 268*f*
  drainable urostomy appliances, 270*f*
  ileostomy, 265
  Mitrofanoff, 266
  neonates, 266–267
  observations, 270–271
  postoperative care, 270
  pouch design, 268, 268*f*, 269*f*, 270*f*
  rationale, 266
  urinary diversion, 265, 270*f*
Stoma caps, 267, 267*f*
Storage, breast milk, 380
Stranger anxieties, physical examination, 70
Stress
  breastfeeding, 378
  cast application, 202
  isolation nursing, 341
Stridor, tracheostomies, 285
Subcutaneous medication, 428–430

analgesics, 460
complications, 429
diabetes mellitus, 429–430
distraction techniques, 429
local anaesthetics, 429
sites, 429
Subjective information, assessment, 69
Subjective, objective, assessment plan (SOAP) model, 68
  assessment, 68
Suction drains, 253
Suctioning, 274–279
  catheters, 275
  community nursing, 278
  complications, 278–279
  endotracheal suction, 275, 277–278
  equipment, 275
  indications, 276
  mucus overproduction, 275
  nasopharyngeal suction, 275, 276, 277, 277*f*
  observations, 278
  oropharyngeal suction, 275, 276, 277, 277*f*
  postoperative care, 224
  preparation, 276
  rationale, 274–275
  resuscitation, 275–279
  technique, 276–278
  tracheostomy suction, 275, 276, 278
Sudden infant death syndrome (SIDS), 281
Superior vena cava syndrome, 160
Supervision, community care nursing, 38
Supine positions, 216, 216*f*
Supplements, artificial feeding, 381
Support, community children's nursing, 37–38
Supportive comments, 24
Suppositories, 147
Suprapubic aspiration, urine collection, 310, 317–318
Suprapubic urethral catheterisation, 313
Surface bleeding, stoma, 271
Surgery
  infection risk factors, 45*t*
  wound debridement, 358*t*
Surveillance, infection control, 53
Suspensions, 423
Sutures, wound drain removal, 254
Swelling, casts, 206
Syphilis, donated blood screening, 405
Syringe size, enteral feeding, 391–392

T

Tablets, 423
Tachycardia
  suctioning, 278
  tracheostomies, 285
Tacrolimus, atopic eczema, 135
Tag questions, 23
Tangible rewards, communication, 24
Tapeworms, faecal specimens, 348
Taping, intravenous cannulation, 324, 324*f*, 325
Tempadot, 75–76
Therapeutic massage, 61
Therapeutic play, 122
Thomas splint traction, 300, 301*f*
Threadworm, 348
Throat swabs, 347
Thrush *see Candida albicans* infection (thrush)
Tightness problems, casts, 206
TIME framework, 357–358
Time taken, blood transfusions, 405
Timings, medication administration, 420
TIVAD *see* Implanted ports
Toddlers
  feeding, 385–386
    complications, 386
    hand washing, 385
    observations, 386
    self-feeding, 386
  hygiene, 111–112
  oral medication, 424
  pain assessment, 456
Toileting, hygiene, 114
Toilet training, 111
Tonic-clonic seizures, 259–260
Top and tail wash, 108
Topical anaesthetics
  day-care surgery, 230
  venepuncture, 321, 322
Topical medications, 431–432
  analgesics, 460
Total parenteral nutrition (TPN), neonatal stoma, 266
Touch, communication, 25
Toxicity, aromatherapy, 60
Toys
  isolation nursing, 338
  preoperative care, 231
TPPPS (Toddler-Preschooler Postoperative Pain Scale), 458*t*
Trace elements, parenteral nutrition, 410
Tracheal dilators, tracheostomy care, 287

Tracheostomies, 284–298
AeroChamber, 297
bottle-feeding, 296
car seats, 297
community nursing, 297
day-to-day life, 296–297
decannulation, 297
definition, 284, 285f
emergency flow chart, 287f
family support, 286
family training, 286
indications, 284–285
nebulisers, 297
observations, 296
oxygen therapy, 297
rationale, 286
safety equipment, 286
site cleaning, 291
speech and language therapists, 296–297
suction *see below*
tube changing, 292–297, 293f, 294f, 295f, 296f
tube selection, 287–289
tube tape changing, 292
Tracheostomy suction, 275, 276, 278, 286, 289–290
catheters, 289
method, 290
observations, 290
trauma safeguards, 290
Traction, 299–307
circulatory system problems, 306
community nursing, 306
complications, 305–307
developmental issues, 302–303
eating and drinking, 305
elimination, 305
equipment, 300–301
family, effects on, 300
joint problems, 306
multidisciplinary team, 303–304
muscular problems, 306
nerves, 306
nursing care, 305
observations, 305–307
osteomyelitis, 306–307
pain/discomfort, 305
parental participation, 304
positioning, 305
rationale, 299
skin care, 305
types, 300–301
see also specific types
Training, 5–6
moving and handling, 215
Transcutaneous bilirubin monitors, 196
Transcutaneous medications, 432

Transcutaneous nerve stimulation (TENS), 465
Transdermal routes, analgesics, 460
Transfer boards, 214
Transmission-based infection control, 46
Transmucosal routes, analgesics, 460
Transport medium, specimen collection, 346
Trauma
tracheostomies, 284
tracheostomy suction, 290
traction, 300
Tunnelled central lines, 153, 153f
Tympanic temperature recording, 75–76

U

UK Infant Feeding Survey, 384
Ultrasound, 246
central venous access, 248
Umbilical cord care, 111
Umbilical cord stump, infection risk factors, 45t
Unconjugated bilirubin, 196
Understanding, communication, 24
Underwater seal system, chest drainage, 165f
Ureterostomy, 266
Urethral catheterisation, 311–314
anaesthetic lubricants, 311
bladder irrigation, 316–317
blockages, 316
catheter care, 314–315
catheter material, 313
chaperones, 314
complications, 314
equipment, 313
intermittent, 312
observations, 314
removal, 316
size selection, 312t
suprapubic, 313
Urinary diversion, stoma, 265, 270f
Urinary tract infections (UTIs), 76
traction, 305
urinary diversions, 271
Urine collection, 310, 348–350
bag specimens, 310, 349
catheter specimens, 349
clean-catch techniques, 310, 349
collection pads, 310
disposable nappies, 349
midstream collection, 310, 349
Mitrofanoff stoma, 349–350
pads, 349
suprapubic aspiration, 310, 317–318

Urine, daily output, 309
Urine testing, 310–311
complications, 311
dipsticks, 348
ketones, 309
leucocyte esterase, 310
nitrate tests, 309
observations, 311
pH, 309
protein, 309
reagent strips, 310
specific gravity, 309
urobilinogen, 309
Urobilinogen, 196
urine testing, 309

V

Vaccinations, employment recommendations, 53
Vaginal swabs
Chlamydia infection, 350
specimen collection, 350
Vancomycin-resistant enterococcus (VRE), 338
Variant Creutzfeldt–Jakob disease, 405–406
Vascular access, paediatric life support, 100
Vascuport *see* Implanted ports
Vasoconstriction, 280
Vastus lateralis, medicine administration, 427, 427f
Vector-borne transmission, 44
Vegan diets, 385
Vegetarian diets, 385
Veins
anatomy, 321
size, 321
Venepuncture, 322–323
aseptic non-touch techniques, 333
equipment, 322
method, 322–323
rationale, 321
sites, 321f, 322
topical anaesthetics, 321, 322
Venous access, paediatric life support, 100
Venous tunnelled central lines, 153
Ventricular fibrillation (VF), 96
Ventricular tachycardia (VT), 96
Ventrogluteal site (gluteus medius muscle), medicine administration, 427, 427f
Verbal communication, 23–24
neurological assessment, 190
Vernix caseosa, 107

Vesicostomy, 266
Vesicular fluid, specimen collection, 351
Victoria Climbié inquiry, 16
Victoria Gillick case, 10
Viral haemorrhagic fevers, specimen collection, 346
Visual analogue scale (VAS), 459t
Visualization, 61–62
Vital sign monitoring, postoperative care, 223
Vitamin C
  pressure area care, 236
  urinary diversions, 267
Vitamin C deficiency, wound healing, 356
Vitamin E, pressure area care, 236
Vitamin supplements, 381–382
Volkmann's ischaemic contracture, traction, 306
Vomiting, enteral feeding, 398

W

Walking hoists, 214
Ward-based teaching, traction, 304
Washed red cell transfusions, 404
Waste disposal, 49–51
  colour-coding, 50t
  infected linen, 50
  sharps, 50
Waterhouse Report (2000), 4
Water temperature, baths, 109, 111–112
Weaning, 384–385
  allergies, 385
  first-stage foods, 384
  UK Infant Feeding Survey, 384
Weighing, physical examination, 77

Whey dominant feeds, artificial feeding, 381, 381t
Whole blood transfusions, 404
Wick packs, 252
Winning Ways: working together to reduce healthcare-associated infections in England, 42b, 41–42
Workload evaluation, community children's nursing, 38
Wound(s)
  acute, 354
  chronic, 354
  clean, 252
  clean contaminated, 252
  contaminated, 252
  definition, 354
  dirty, 252
  healing *see* Wound healing
  infection, 206
  specimen collection, 347–348
  types, 252
Wound care, 354–366
  aims, 355b
  assessment, 357–365, 359f
  bathing/showering, 360–361
  best practice guidelines, 361b
  cleansing (debridement), 358t, 359–360, 364
  community nursing, 361
  dressings *see below*
  guidelines, 358–361
  irrigation, 360
  pressure area care, 237–238
Wound drain(s)
  shortening, 254
  types of, 252–253
Wound drain removal, 251–256
  aseptic techniques, 253
  community nursing, 255

methods, 253–254
  rationale, 251
Wound dressings, 361, 362t
  methods, 364
  requirements, 357–358, 357b
  TIME framework, 357–358
Wound healing, 252, 354–357
  affecting factors, 356–357
  diseases/disorders, 356–357
  immunosuppressed patients, 357
  inflammatory phase, 355–356
  maturative phase, 356
  medication, 356–357
  nutrition, 356
  primary intention, 252, 355
  proliferative phase, 356
  secondary intention, 252, 355
Wrappings, babies, 173
Written information, 29
  day-care surgery, 230
  feeding, 374
  isolation nursing, 341
  risk management, 15

X

X-rays *see* Radiography

Y

Young infants, oral medication, 424

Z

Zinc deficiency, wound healing, 356
Zinc, pressure area care, 236